NURSING THEORIES

THE BASE FOR PROFESSIONAL NURSING PRACTICE

SIXTH EDITION

Julia B. George, RN, PhD

Department of Nursing

California State University, Fullerton

Fullerton, CA

Pearson

Boston   Columbus   Indianapolis   New York   San Francisco   Upper Saddle River
Amsterdam   Cape Town   Dubai   London   Madrid   Milan   Munich   Paris   Montreal   Toronto
Delhi   Mexico City   Sao Paulo   Sydney   Hong Kong   Seoul   Singapore   Taipei   Tokyo

Library of Congress Cataloging-in-Publication Data

Nursing theories: the base for professional nursing practice / [edited by] Julia B. George.—6th ed.
    p. cm.
  Includes bibliographical references and index.
  ISBN-13: 978-0-13-513583-9 (alk. paper)
  ISBN-10: 0-13-513583-4 (alk. paper)
  1. Nursing—Philosophy. I. George, Julia B.
  [DNLM: 1. Nursing Theory. 2. Models, Nursing. WY 86 N9755 2010]
  RT84.5.N89 2010
  610.7301—dc22

                                           2010000641

Publisher: Julie Levin Alexander
Publisher's Assistant: Regina Bruno
Editor-in-Chief: Maura Connor
Executive Acquisitions Editor: Pamela Fuller
Editorial Assistant: Lisa Pierce
Managing Production Editor: Patrick Walsh
Senior Production Project Manager: Cathy O'Connell
Production Editor: Smitha Pillai S4 Carlisle
Publishing Services

Manufacturing Manager: Ilene Sanford
Creative Director: Jayne Conte
Cover Design: Bruce Kenselaar
Marketing Specialist: Michael Sirinides
Marketing Assistant: Crystal Gonzalez
Media Project Manager: Rachel Collett
Composition: S4 Carlisle Publishing Services
Printer/Binder: STP/RRD/Harrisonburg
Cover Printer: STP/RRD/Harrisonburg

Notice: Care has been taken to confirm the accuracy of information presented in this book. The authors, editors, and the publisher, however, cannot accept any responsibility for errors or omissions or for consequences from application of the information in this book and make no warranty, express or implied, with respect to its contents.

The authors and publisher have exerted every effort to ensure that drug selections and dosages set forth in this text are in accord with current recommendations and practice at time of publication. However, in view of ongoing research, changes in government regulations, and the constant flow of information relating to drug therapy and drug reactions, the reader is urged to check the package inserts of all drugs for any change in indications of dosage and for added warnings and precautions. This is particularly important when the recommended agent is a new and/or infrequently employed drug.

Pearson® is a registered trademark of Pearson plc

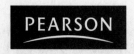

www.pearsonhighered.com

10 9 8 7 6 5 4 3 2
ISBN-10:   0-13-513583-4
ISBN-13: 978-0-13-513583-9

Dedication

Dedicated to all the theorists, meta-theorists, and students of theory who have made this book possible.

THANK YOU

Thanks go to our colleagues from schools of nursing across the world, who generously gave their time to help create this book. These professionals helped us plan and shape our book by contributing their collective experience and expertise as nurses and teachers, and we made many improvements based on their efforts.

Contributors

Jan V. R. Belcher, RN, PhD, NEA, PMHCNS-BC
Associate Professor
College of Nursing and Health
Wright State University
Dayton, Ohio

Susan Stanwyck Bowman, PhD, RN
Professor Emeritus, Nursing
Humboldt State University
Arcata, California

Noreen Cavan Frisch, PhD, RN
Director and Professor
School of Nursing
University of Victoria
Canada, Victoria BC

Peggy Coldwell Foster, RN, cEFM
Perinatal Clinical Nurse Specialist
Kettering Medical Center
Dayton, Ohio

Julia Gallagher Galbreath, RN, MS
Director of Nursing
Department of Nursing
Edison Community College
Piqua, Ohio

Maryanne Garon RN, DNSc
Associate Professor
Department of Nursing
California State University, Fullerton
Fullerton, California

Julia B. George, RN, PhD
Professor Emeritus, Nursing
California State University, Fullerton
Fullerton, California

Bobbe Ann Gray, PhD, RNC-OB
Associate Professor and Director
Doctor of Nursing Practice Program
Wright State University—Miami Valley
College of Nursing and Health
Dayton, Ohio

Janet S. Hickman, RN, EdD
Interim Dean, Graduate Studies a
Extended Education
Professor of Nursing
West Chester University
West Chester, Pennsylvania

Brenda P. Johnson, RN, PhD
Professor
Department of Nursing
Southeast Missouri State University
Cape Girardeau, Missouri

Jane H. Kelley, RN, PhD
Professor
RN-BSN outreach campus
Indiana Wesleyan University
Louisville, Kentucky

Marie L. Lobo, PhD, RN, FAAN
Professor
University of New Mexico
College of Nursing
Albuquerque, New Mexico

Reviewers

Nagia S. Ali, PhD, RN
Professor
Ball State University, School
of Nursing
Muncie, Indiana

Jo Azzarello, PhD, RN
Associate Professor
University of Oklahoma, College
of Nursing
Oklahoma City, Oklahoma

Martha C. Baker, PhD, RN,
CNE, APRN-BC
Director of BSN Program
St. John's College of Nursing—Southwest
Baptist University
Bolivar, Missouri

Mary Baumberger-Henry, RN, DNSc
Associate Professor
Widener University, School of Nursing
Chester, Pennsylvania

Esther Levine-Brill, PhD,
APRN-BC, ANP
Professor, Chairperson
Long Island University, School of Nursing
Brooklyn, New York

Mirella Vasquez Brooks, PhD, APRN,
FNP-BC
Assistant Professor
University of Hawaii
Honolulu, Hawaii

Lynn H. Buckalew, MSN, RN
Instructor
Mississippi College
Clinton, Mississippi

Lenny Chiang-Hanisko, PhD, RN
Assistant Professor, Chair
Kent State University, College of Nursing
Kent, Ohio

Thomas W. Connelly, Jr., PhD, RN
Assistant Professor
University of Massachusetts
Boston, Massachusetts

Alice E. Conway, PhD, CRNP, APRN-BC
Professor
Edinboro University of Pennsylvania
Edinboro, Pennsylvania

Mary Ann Dailey, DNSc, RN
Assistant Professor and
Chairperson
Kutztown University
Kutztown, Pennsylvania

Catherine Dearman, RN, PhD
Professor and Department Chair
University of South Alabama,
College of Nursing
Mobile, Alabama

Elizabeth Diener, RN, PhD, CPNP
Assistant Professor
D'Youville College
Buffalo, New York

Margie Eckroth-Bucher, DNSc,
APRN-BC
Associate Professor
Bloomsburg University
Bloomsburg, Pennsylvania

Sharon K. Falkenstern, PhD, CRNP
Assistant Professor
The Pennsylvania State University
University Park, Pennsylvania

Pauline M. Green, PhD, RN, CNE
Professor
Howard University
Washington, D.C.

Gladys L. Husted, RN, PhD, CNE
Distinguished Professor Emeritus
Duquesne University
Pittsburgh, Pennsylvania

Vicky P. Kent, PhD, RN, CNE
Clinical Associate Professor
Towson University
Towson, Maryland

Joyce M. Knestrick, PhD, CRNP
Instructor
Frontier School of Midwifery
and Family Nursing
Hyden, Kentucky

Kathleen Masters, DNS, RN
Associate Director for Undergraduate
Programs
University of Southern Mississippi, School
of Nursing
Hattiesburg, Mississippi

Marilyn Meder, RN, PhD, CFCN
Assistant Professor
Kutztown University
Kutztown, Pennsylvania

Elizabeth Pross, PhD, RN
Director
Christine E Lynn College of
Nursing—Florida Atlantic University
Port St. Lucie, Florida

Sheryl J. Samuelson PhD, RN
Associate Professor
Millikin University, School of Nursing
Decatur, Illinois

Bonnie L. Saucier, PhD, RN
Dean of Nursing
Linfield College
McMinnville, Oregon

Phyllis Skorga, PhD, RN, CCM
Professor
Arkansas State University
Jonesboro, Arkansas

Kathleen L. Skrabut, EdD, RN, CRRN
Professor and Graduate Program
Coordinator
Salem State School of Nursing
Salem, Massachusetts

Darlene Sredl, PhD, RN
Assistant Professor
University of Missouri—St. Louis
St. Louis, Missouri

Judith M. Stanley, RN, DHSc
Assistant Professor
D'Youville College
Buffalo, New York

Anne Stiles, PhD, RN
Professor, Associate Dean
Texas Woman's University College
of Nursing
Denton, Texas

Donna Scott Tilley, RN, PhD, CNE
Associate Professor
Texas Christian University
Fort Worth, Texas

Marilyn L. Weitzel, RN, CNL, PhD
Assistant Professor
Cleveland State University
Cleveland, Ohio

PREFACE

It has been over three decades since the idea for a text on nursing theories germinated among a group of faculty at Wright State University, Dayton, Ohio. The germinating seed was a recognized need for the various extant concepts, models, and theories specific to nursing to be gathered in one volume with application to nursing practice to help individuals, both students and practitioners, make optimum use of theory in practice. Who could have foreseen how that seed would grow and flower? Who could have foreseen how nursing theories would grow and flower? Literature and research about nursing theories can now be found literally around the world, a world that seems to have shrunk with the multitude of technological changes. Technology has not only made a huge impact on the delivery of nursing care but has also facilitated access to knowledge about nursing theory. Technology has enhanced our ability to search for, locate, and even possibly download immediately the relevant literature. Online searches support the international use of, and publications about, nursing theory.

The first edition of *Nursing Theories: The Base for Professional Nursing Practice* focused on 12 theories. This sixth edition includes information on 29 theories. With the multitude of theoretical works being published, it was a major challenge to choose what works to include in this text. The choices were made with the assistance of a number of nursing faculty who responded to a survey conducted by Pearson Health Science about what they believed should be included in such a textbook. Respondents were asked to rate 44 nursing theories as "critical, must be included," "nice to have, but not critical," "do not include," and "no opinion, makes no difference," as well as given the opportunity to suggest additional theories for inclusion. No additional nursing theories were suggested. Criteria for selecting theories for inclusion were all theories receiving 80% or greater on "critical, must be included" plus "nice to have, but not critical" were included as full chapters; those receiving 50% to 79% on "critical" and "nice to have" were included in summary chapters, and those receiving less than 50% in "critical" and "nice to have" were not included. This resulted in the incorporation of nine theories not previously included: those of Joyce Travelbee, Kathy Barnard, Nola Pender, Patricia Benner, Ramona Mercer, Merle H. Mishel, Juliet Corbin and Anselm Strauss, Kathy Kolcaba, and Afaf Meleis.

Expansion to 29 theories forced us to examine how to present the material. After much consideration, it was decided to include both full and summary chapters. Full chapters continue to follow the format of previous editions, with a biography of the theorist(s), a summary of the theory, discussion of the theory and four concepts of nursing's metaparadigm, application of the theory to nursing practice (previously primarily within the nursing process, in this edition expanded to application as appropriate to the theory), and a critique and discussion of the strengths and limitations of the theory and thought questions about the theory. Each summary chapter includes more than one theory with a brief biography of each theorist, an overview of each theory, and highlights of research- and practice-based publications about each theory. Both types of chapters will have references and possibly a bibliography. Where there is a significant body of literature, whether research, practice, or theoretical in nature, about the work discussed in the chapter, an annotated bibliography of selected publications may be provided. Most bibliographies do not reflect the complete work of the theorist(s) but may reflect either more current or most relevant works.

It is important to recognize that this text serves as a secondary source in relation to the statements and purposes of the theorists who are discussed. It is intended as a tool for thoughtful and considered application of theoretical works in nursing to the practice of nursing. The intent is not to provide a comprehensive view or critique of each of the included works but to provide information to stimulate the reader's thought processes about the characteristics of a theory and about a particular work. The terms *theory, model, conceptual framework,* and *conceptual model* are not used consistently in the nursing literature. We have sought to reflect the language of the theorist(s). Thus, the work being presented in a given chapter may be strongly supported in the responses to the critique questions and still not be labeled as a theory.

Some of the theorists, as appropriate to their times, used *she* to refer to the nurse, *he* to refer to the recipient of care, and *man* to refer to human beings in general. In some chapters, it would have been awkward to change the theorist's use of such words. In some situations, we have indicated that the use is that of the original author. In like manner, we have tried to reflect the original author's use of the terms *patient* and *client*.

ACKNOWLEDGMENTS

A very special thank you is due to those who responded to the survey and helped shape the content of this edition. It would not have been the same without you!

Thanks and appreciation also go to the many staff members at Pearson Education Health Science who have participated in the development of this sixth edition. The process has been a long and arduous one, impacted by changes in society and the economy, as well as changes in staff and contributors. Perhaps the greatest thrill for all of us is seeing the process come to completion.

Suggestions and comments from users of this text are both requested and welcomed.

Julia B. George

CONTENTS

CHAPTER 1

An Introduction to Nursing Theory

Janet S. Hickman

The purpose of this chapter is to provide the learner with the tools necessary to understand the nursing theories presented in this book. These tools include learning the language and definitions of theoretical thinking, acquiring a perspective of the historical development of nursing theories, and learning methods to analyze and evaluate nursing theories. Understanding nursing theory is the prerequisite to choosing and using a theory to guide one's nursing practice.

Nursing theories have developed from the choices and assumptions about the nature of what a particular theorist believes about nursing, what the basis of nursing knowledge is, and what nurses do or how they practice in the real world. Each theory carries with it a worldview, a way of seeing nursing and human events that highlights certain aspects of reality and possibly shades or ignores aspects in other areas (Ray, 1998). Each theorist was influenced by her or his own values, the historical context of the discipline of nursing, and a knowledge base rooted in the world of nursing science.

A FEW WORDS ABOUT NURSING SCIENCE . . .

What nursing science is, and what it is not, is a topic of significant debate in the current nursing literature. This is especially true now in the early years of a new century, after nearly two decades of cost containment, nursing shortages, staffing reductions, and managed care. Despite (or in spite of) a health care delivery situation in the United States that is unfriendly for both nurses and clients, thinking about nursing science has achieved some areas of consensus on an international level. In 1997, *Nursing Science Quarterly* presented an international dialogue on the question: "What is nursing science?" (Barrett et al., 1997). In the following responses, note the patterns of agreement of thinking from the different respondents.

Dr. John Daly—Australia:

> Nursing science is an identifiable, discrete body of knowledge comprising paradigms, frameworks, and theories. . . . This structure is vested in nursing's totality and simultaneity paradigms. These competing paradigms posit

mutually exclusive perspectives on the human-universe inter-relationship, health, and the central phenomenon of nursing. . . . Nursing science is in development; it will continue to evolve. . . . (p. 10)

Dr. Gail J. Mitchell—Canada:

Nursing science represents clusters of precisely selected beliefs and values that are crafted into distinct theoretical structures. Theoretical structures exist for the purpose of giving direction and meaning to practice and research activities. . . . Nursing theories can be learned through committed study, but to understand a theory's contribution to humankind, it must be experienced as a way of being with others. It is within the nurse-person process or the researcher-participant process, that theory can be judged as meaningful, or not . . . (p. 10)

Dr. Brian Millar—Great Britain:

. . . nursing science is that body of knowledge developed from questions raised by nurses and investigated by them, concerning the relationship of the human-health-environment. (p. 11)

Dr. Renzo Zanotti—Italy:

. . . The goal of nursing science is to test new interpretations and to explore different explanations, under general laws, about phenomena referring to caring, well-being, and autonomy of persons as harmonious entities. . . . (p. 11)

Dr. Teruko Takahashi—Japan:

Nursing science is a unique human science which focuses on phenomena related to human health. . . . Unlike natural sciences such as medicine, nursing science focuses on the quality of life for each person. Therefore, nursing science does not investigate health phenomena based on causality. Health as lived experience is investigated from the point of view of healthcare consumers. . . . (p. 11)

Dr. Elizabeth Ann Manhart Barrett—United States of America:

Nursing science is the substantive, abstract knowledge describing nursing's unique phenomenon of concern, the integral nature of unitary human beings and their environments. The creation of this knowledge occurs through synthesis as well as qualitative and quantitative modes of inquiry. . . . Nursing science-based practice is the imaginative and creative use of nursing knowledge to promote the health and well-being of all people. . . . (p. 12)

Dr. William K. Cody—United States of America:

The discipline of nursing requires knowledge and methods other than nursing science, *but nursing science is the essence of nursing as a scholarly discipline;* without it, there would be no *nursing,* only care. . . . As a *science,* nursing's *richness* is manifest in the availability of cutting-edge philosophies and theories to provide guidance for practice, . . . and a growing body of literature describing nursing theory-based practice . . . (pp. 12–13).

ANOTHER VIEW

Meleis (2007) speaks specifically of nursing as a human science that focuses on human beings as wholes and has at its core an understanding of experiences as lived by its members. She states that, from a human science view, the art and science of nursing are inseparable. Nursing as a human science is concerned with the experiences of human beings with health and illness and requires both quantitative and qualitative research methodologies.

THE LANGUAGE OF THEORETICAL THINKING

The previous section of this chapter presented current thinking about the definition of nursing science from international experts. Clearly it has been a long journey from Nightingale's *Notes on Nursing* (1859/1992) to the state of nursing science in the early 21st century! This chapter will provide you with the tools to examine the theories that were developed by nurses during this more than 140-year period. As you proceed through this textbook, the commentary in the previous section will take on new and different meanings. You are about to begin a new journey that will take you into the realm of theoretical thinking in nursing as it evolved in the context of nursing history. This journey will provide you with an appreciation of the implications of nursing theory for professional nursing practice, nursing science, and nursing research.

Concepts

The first unit to consider in the language of theoretical thinking is the *concept*. A concept is an idea, thought, or notion conceived in the mind. Concepts may be empirical or abstract, depending on their ability to be observed in the real world. Concepts are said to *empirical* when they can be observed or experienced through the senses. A stethoscope is an example of an empirical concept; it can be seen and touched. *Abstract* concepts are those that are not observable, such as caring, hope, and infinity. All concepts become abstractions in the absence of the object. For example, once you have become familiar with a stethoscope, you are able to see the concept of a stethoscope in your mind, without having one physically present. Abstractions such as caring, hope, or infinity are more difficult to picture, as one has never had the opportunity to observe these concepts in reality.

To understand the presentations of nursing theories in this book, it will be of critical importance to look at the definitions of the concepts provided. Some of the theories will use concepts with which you are familiar, but they may be used in unfamiliar ways; others will introduce new concepts, some with new or unfamiliar labels.

The term *metaparadigm* is defined as the core content of a discipline, stated in the most global or abstract of terms. Kim (1989) states that the functions of a metaparadigm are to summarize the intellectual and social missions of a discipline and to place a boundary on the subject matter of that discipline. Until the 1990s there was general agreement in the literature that the metaparadigm of the discipline of nursing consisted of four major concepts: person, health, environment, and nursing. Each of these four concepts was presented as an abstraction. Specific definitions of each of the four concepts differed depending on the author. For the purposes of this text, the following general definitions will be used. *Person* may represent an individual, a family, a community, or all of humankind. In this context, person is the focus of nursing practice. *Health* represents a state of well-being as defined by the person or mutually decided on by the person and the nurse. *Environment* represents the person's physical surroundings, the community, or the universe and all it contains. *Nursing* is the practice of the science and art of the discipline.

Some of the current literature suggests that a four-concept metaparadigm for the discipline of nursing is too restrictive. Meleis (2007) maintains that the domain of nursing knowledge encompasses seven concepts: nursing client, transitions, interaction, nursing process, environment, nursing therapeutics, and health. Parse (1995a) states that the major phenomena of concern to nursing include self-care, adaptation, interpersonal relations, goal attainment, caring, energy fields, human becoming, and others. To these, Cody (1996) adds the concerns of nursing's unique traditions of respect for human dignity and the uniqueness of each client—dimensions of the discipline that he believes find no expression in a metaparadigm limited to concepts and their definitions. Malinski (1995) suggests dropping the entire idea of a metaparadigm of nursing, as she considers it to be no longer warranted. She states that as nursing is now more diverse than homogeneous, any attempt to define the scope of the discipline will be so broad as to be meaningless.

Despite the scholarly controversies regarding metaparadigms and their current status (or lack of status) in nursing science, it is important to consider their impact on theory development in nursing. In analyzing the theories in this book, the reader will be able to identify the presence (or absence) of global or metaparadigm concepts upon which the different theories are based (or not based). For purposes of consistency, each chapter will discuss the theorists' definitions or viewpoints on the original four-concept metaparadigm of person, health, environment, and nursing as well as consider other concepts in each theory.

THEORIES

Concepts are the elements used to generate theories. Chinn and Kramer (2004) define a theory as "a creative and rigorous structuring of ideas that projects a tentative, purposeful, and systematic view of phenomena" (p. 58). They state that the word *creative* underscores the role of human imagination and vision in theory development but caution that the creative processes are also rigorous, systematic, and disciplined. In their view, theories are *tentative* and, as such, are open to revision as new evidence emerges. Their definition of theory requires that there be a purpose for the theory. Simply stated, a theory suggests a direction in how to view facts and events.

Theories cannot be equated with scientific laws, which predict the results of given experiments 100% of the time. Laws compose the basis of most of the natural sciences. As nursing is a human science, the rigor and objectivity of the laboratory-produced data are both inappropriate and impossible to replicate. The predictability of nursing theories becomes more reliable as the research base from which theories develop grows.

Meleis (2007) defines nursing theory as ". . . a conceptualization of some aspect of nursing reality communicated for the purpose of describing phenomena, explaining relationships between phenomena, predicting consequences, or prescribing nursing care" (p. 37). This definition includes the importance of communicating nursing theory and the purpose of prescribing nursing care.

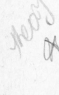
Theories are composed of concepts (and their definitions) and propositions that explain the relationships between the concepts. For example, Nightingale *proposed* a beneficial relationship between fresh air and health. Theories are based on stated assumptions that are presented as givens. Theoretical assumptions may be taken as "truth" because they cannot be empirically tested, such as in a value statement or ethic. Theories may be presented as models that provide a diagram or map of the theory's content.

Barnum (1998) states that a complete nursing theory is one that contains context, content, and process. Context is the environment in which the nursing act takes place.

Content is the subject of the theory. Process is the method by which the nurse acts in using the theory. The nurse acts on, with, or through the content elements of the theory.

Smith and Liehr (2003) suggest picturing a ladder of abstraction consisting of three rungs. In this model, the highest rung represents the philosophical, the middle rung represents the theoretical, and the lowest rung represents the empirical. The philosophical level "represents [the] beliefs and assumptions that are accepted as true and fundamental to a theory" (p. 1). The theoretical rung is abstract and consists of the symbols, ideas, and concepts that form the theory. The third rung, the empirical, is concrete and represents what can be observed by the senses.

While some texts differentiate between "theories," "conceptual models," and "conceptual frameworks" of nursing, the majority of authors believe that this is an artificial distinction. Meleis (2007) goes so far as to say, "The attempt to differentiate between them has frequently taken on the dimension of splitting hairs and has only added to the confusion" (p. 151). For the purposes of this text, the existing nursing conceptualizations presented *are* theories.

LEVELS OF THEORY

The level of a theory refers to the scope or range of phenomena to which the theory applies. The level of abstraction of the concepts in the theory is closely tied to its scope. Chinn and Kramer (2004) state that theory may be characterized as *micro, macro, midrange, atomistic,* or *wholistic* (p. 94). Micro and atomistic suggest relatively narrow-range phenomena, while macro and wholistic imply that the theory covers a broad scope. Midrange (or middle range) theories deal with a portion of nursing's total concern but not with the totality of the discipline. Chinn and Kramer provide the example of pain alleviation as a midrange theory and the explanation of the physiology of the phenomena known as pain as a possible micro theory. Both of these deal with a portion of the person. Macro theories deal with persons as a whole. These labels are arbitrary and may differ in different disciplines.

Grand theory is a term used in the literature to mean theory that covers broad areas of concern within a discipline. In the same vein, a *school of thought* has been defined by Parse (1997b) as "a theoretical point of view held by a community of scholars" (p. 74). It is a tradition, including specific assumptions and principles, a specified focus of inquiry, and congruent approaches to research and practice. *Metatheory* is a term used to label theory about the theoretical process and theory development.

Merton (1968) describes *middle range theories* as those "that lie between the minor but necessary working hypotheses that evolve in abundance during day-to-day research and the all-inclusive systematic efforts to develop unified theory that will explain all the observed uniformities of social behavior, social organization and social change" (p. 39). Descriptions of middle range theory in the nursing literature reflect congruency with Merton. Nurse authors have described middle range theory as follows:

- Narrower in scope than grand theories (Fawcett, 2005a; Suppe, 1996)
- Composed of a limited number of concepts and propositions that are written at a level that is concrete and specific (Fawcett, 2005a; McKenna, 1997)
- Concerned with less abstract, more specific phenomena (Fawcett, 2005a; Meleis, 2007)
- More applicable to practice (Fawcett, 2005a; Liehr & Smith, 1999)

Im (2005) describes a "ready-to-wear" level of theory. *Ready-to-wear* refers to easy applicability to research and practice. She describes situation-specific theory as one type of ready-to-wear theory. *Situation-specific theories* are defined as those that focus on specific nursing phenomena, reflect clinical practice, and are limited to specific populations or specific fields of practice (Im & Meleis, 1999a). Situation-specific theories are also labeled as *microtheories* or *practice theories*. Im (2005) goes on to caution that situation-specific theories are not intended to be universal theories that can be applied to any time or setting but are rather intended to be more clinically specific, reflect a particular context, and include blueprints for nursing action(s). An example of a situation-specific theory is that proposed by Im and Meleis (1999b), which was aimed only at the specific population of menopausal low-income Korean immigrant women in the United States.

Im (2005) states that situation-specific theories may or may not be testable. Theories that are developed on the philosophical bases of hermeneutics, phenomenology, or critical theory do not have testable hypotheses. These theories, rather, aim at understanding and explaining the lived experience of human beings experiencing a phenomenon.

Another way of looking at levels of theory is to look at what it is that the theory does. For Dickoff and James (1968), theory develops on four levels: factor-isolating, factor-relating, situation-relating, and situation-producing. Level 1, factor-isolating, is descriptive in nature. It involves naming or classifying facts/events. Level 2, factor-relating, requires correlating or associating factors in such a way that they meaningfully depict a larger situation. Level 3, situation-relating, explains and predicts how situations are related. Level 4, situation-producing, requires sufficient knowledge about how and why situations are related, so that when using the theory as a guide, valued situations can be produced. When using this method, one speaks of the relative power of the theory, with Level 4 being the most powerful, as it controls (or does more than describe, explain, or predict).

Fawcett (2005a) uses similar labels when describing middle range theory. She states that middle range theories describe what a phenomena is, explain why it occurs, or predict how it occurs. Middle range *descriptive* theories are the most basic type of theory, may include only one concept, and describe or classify a phenomenon. Middle range *explanatory* theories specify relations between two or more concepts, while middle range *predictive* theories predict precise relationships between concepts or the effects of one or more concepts on one or more other concepts (p. 19).

WORLDVIEWS

A worldview is one's philosophical frame of reference in looking at one's world. The worldview of the philosophy of science is that of logical empiricism. This worldview requires that all truths must be confirmed by sensory experiences. Logical empiricism requires objectivity and is relatively value free. Objectivity requires study of the smallest parts of phenomena with use of the scientific method. In this worldview, the whole is equal to the sum of its parts. In the literature, this worldview is also called the *received view*. It is from this view of nursing science that the nursing process was created.

One of the worldviews, which opposes logical empiricism, is that of the human science or the *perceived view*. A human science worldview focuses on human beings as wholes and their lived experiences within a given context.

Parse (1987) posits two worldviews of nursing related to the received and the perceived views. Her description of the totality paradigm reflects the received view, while her description of the simultaneity paradigm reflects the perceived view. A basic difference in these paradigms is the perception of person. The totality paradigm looks at the bio-psycho-social-spiritual aspects of person, while the simultaneity paradigm views person as an irreducible whole in constant interrelationship with the universe. Theorists of the totality paradigm tend to define health as a state of well-being as measured against norms, while simultaneity paradigm theorists view health as something the client determines individually. Cody (1995) affirms Parse's position on paradigms. He states, "Basic assumptions that Parse made about the totality and simultaneity paradigms ten years ago hold true today. There really are only two sets of essential beliefs about human beings and health in nursing" (p. 146).

Fawcett (2003, p. 273) proposed changing the language of the metaparadigm of nursing. She suggests that the word *person* be changed to *human beings*, that *health* should refer to human processes of living and dying, and that *nursing* actions can be viewed as a process between participants in nursing and nurses. She further suggests that the linkages between human beings, environment, health, and nursing can be stated in a way that is more inclusive of both the totality and simultaneity paradigms. The discipline of nursing is concerned with the following:

1. Principles that govern human processes of living and dying
2. Patterning of human health experiences
3. Nursing actions or processes that are beneficial to human beings
4. Human processes of living and dying, recognizing that human beings are in continuous mutual process with their environments

CIRCULAR NATURE OF THEORY-RESEARCH-PRACTICE

It is important to understand that theory, research, and practice impact each other in circular ways. Middle range theories can be tested in clinical practice by nursing research. The research process may validate the theory, cause it to be modified, or invalidate it. When research validates a theory, it provides the *evidence* required for *evidence-based practice*. As more research is conducted about a specific theory, more evidence is provided to support practice. Practice is based on the theories of the discipline that are validated through research (see Figure 1-1). Research findings are published in the periodical literature and books, are presented at conferences, and are available through abstracts, such as Dissertation Abstracts International.

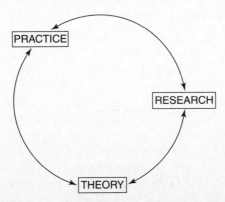

FIGURE 1-1 Circular nature of theory, research, and practice

Liehr and Smith (1999, p. 88) propose five approaches for middle range theory generation in the 21st century:

1. Induction through research and practice
2. Deduction from research and practice applications of grand nursing theories
3. Combination of existing nursing and non-nursing middle range theories
4. Derivation from theories of other disciplines that relate to nursing's disciplinary perspective
5. Derivation from practice guidelines and standards rooted in research

Research may be based on the received or perceived worldview. Received-view research is *quantitative*, where statistical data represent empirical facts and events. The methodology of the research is based on the scientific method. Perceived-view research is *qualitative* in nature, based on the thoughts, feelings, and beliefs of the research subjects. Numerous methodologies have been proposed to conduct qualitative research.

Polit and Beck (2004) state that *quantitative research* tends to emphasize deductive reasoning, the rules of logic, and the measurable attributes of human experience. They state that quantitative research methods *generally* focus on a small number of concepts, begin with hunches as to how the concepts are related, use formal instruments and structured processes to collect data (under conditions of control), emphasize objectivity in both data collection and analysis, and analyze numerical data using statistical procedures (pp. 15–16).

Qualitative research is described by Polit and Beck (2004) as emphasizing the dynamic, holistic, and individual aspects of the human experience and attempting to capture those aspects in their entirety, within the context of those experiencing them. They state that research using qualitative methods *generally* focuses on attempts to understand the entirety of some phenomenon rather than focusing on specific concepts; relies on the subject's interpretation of events rather than hunches of the researcher; collects data without formal, structured instruments; does not attempt to control the context of the research but rather attempts to capture it in its entirety; capitalizes on the subjectivity of the data as a means for understanding and interpreting human experiences; and analyzes narrative data in an organized but intuitive fashion (pp. 16–17).

Speziale and Carpenter (2007) caution that not all qualitative studies lead to theory development but that certain approaches used in qualitative research can lead to theory development. They state that in the instance of grounded theory, the method is dedicated to the discovery of theory.

According to Haase and Meyers (1988, p. 132), quantitative and qualitative approaches differ in the following ways:

1. Quantitative methods assume a singular reality, while qualitative methods assume multiple interrelated realities
2. Quantitative methods assume that objective reality is its appropriate domain, while qualitative methods assume that subjective experiences are also legitimate
3. Quantitative methods are reductionistic, whereas qualitative methods take an ecological view—that is, they attempt to gain a full understanding of the reality
4. Quantitative methods reveal the whole through its parts, whereas qualitative methods assume that the whole is greater than the sum of its parts
5. Quantitative methods assume that discrepancies are to be accounted for or eliminated, while qualitative methods recognize that discrepancies may be existentially real

Table 1-1 provides a comparison of quantitative and qualitative research methods.

TABLE 1-1   Comparison of Research Methods

Quantitative	Qualitative
Cause-and-effect relationships	Patterns of association
Context free	Context dependent
Data expressed in numerical values	Data expressed in narrative descriptions
Deductive processes	Inductive processes
Emphasis on concepts	Emphasis on the whole
Fixed design	Flexible design
Measurable	Interpretative
Mechanistic	Organismic
Objective	Subjectivity is desirable
One reality	Multiple subjective realities
Reduction, control, prediction	Discovery, description, and understanding
Report statistical analyses	Report rich narrative
Researcher is independent	Researcher interacts with subjects
Subjects	Participants

Modified from Streubert & Carpenter (1995, p. 12).

HISTORICAL PERSPECTIVE

The history of theory development and theoretical thinking in nursing began with the writings of Florence Nightingale and continues to the present. This section highlights significant events in this history.

Florence Nightingale

Nightingale's (1859/1992) *Notes on Nursing* presents the first nursing theory that focuses on the manipulation of the environment for the benefit of the patient. Although Nightingale did not present her work as a "nursing theory," it has directed nursing practice for over 150 years.

The Columbia School—The 1950s

In the 1950s the need to prepare nurses at the graduate level for administrative and faculty positions was recognized. Columbia University's Teachers College developed graduate education programs to meet these functional needs. The first theoretical conceptualizations of nursing science came from graduates of these programs. These nurse theorists include Peplau (1952/1988), Henderson (Harmer & Henderson, 1955), Hall (1959), and Abdellah (Abdellah, Beland, Martin, & Metheney, 1960).

    Theorists of this decade operated from a biomedical model that focused primarily on what nurses do, that is, their functional roles. They considered patient problems and needs to be the practice focus. Independent of the Columbia theorists, Johnson (at the University of California at Los Angeles) suggested that nursing knowledge is based on a theory of nursing diagnosis that is different from medical diagnosis (Meleis, 2007).

The Yale School—The 1960s

In the 1960s the focus of theoretical thinking in nursing moved from a problem/need and functional role focus to the relationship between the nurse and the patient. The Yale

School's theoretical position was influenced by the Columbia Teacher's College graduates who became faculty members there (Henderson, 1960, 1966; Orlando, 1961/1990; Wiedenbach, 1964, 1969).

Theorists of the Yale School view nursing as a process rather than an end in itself. Their theories look at how nurses do what they do and how the patient perceives his situation. Theorists of this school include Henderson, Orlando, and Wiedenbach. Independent of the Yale School, Levine (1967) presented her four conservation principles of nursing.

In 1967, Yale faculty Dickoff, James, and Wiedenbach (two philosophers and a nurse, respectively) presented a definition of nursing theory and goals for theory development in nursing. Their paper was published in *Nursing Research* a year later and has become a classic document in the history of theoretical thinking in nursing (Dickoff, James, & Wiedenbach, 1968).

Also in this decade, Joyce Travelbee presented her Human-to-Human Relationship Theory in her book *Interpersonal Aspects of Nursing* (1966, 1971). This theory extended the interpersonal relationship theories of Peplau and Orlando. Travelbee emphasized caring, empathy, sympathy, and the emotional aspects of nursing.

It is important to note that in 1965 the American Nurses Association published a position paper on nursing education. This document changed the landscape of nursing education forever by recommending two levels of education for nursing: the professional nurse educated at the baccalaureate level and the technical nurse educated at the associate degree level. It was during this decade that federal monies were made available for doctoral study for nurse educators. The resulting doctorally prepared individuals became the next wave of nurse theorists.

Table 1-2 lists the theorists of this decade and their publications.

The 1970s

The 1970s was the decade in which many nursing theories were first presented. Most of these theories have been revised since their original presentations. It is of note to mention that as of the mid-1970s, the National League for Nursing (NLN) required schools of nursing to select, develop, and implement a conceptual framework for the curricula as an accreditation standard. This requirement focused theoretical thinking on the application of theory to nursing education.

In 1978, the first edition of *Advances in Nursing Science* was published. This journal focuses on nursing science, including the construction, analysis, and application of

TABLE 1-2 Nursing Theories of the 1960s

Theorist	Year	Title
V. Henderson	1960	*Basic Principles of Nursing Care*
	1966	*The Nature of Nursing*
I. J. Orlando	1961	*The Dynamic Nurse-Patient Relationship: Function, Process, and Principles*
E. Wiedenbach	1964	*Clinical Nursing: A Helping Art*
	1969	*Meeting the Realities in Clinical Teaching*
L. E. Hall	1966	*Another View of Nursing Care and Quality*
J. Travelbee	1966	*Interpersonal Aspects of Nursing*
M. E. Levine	1967	*The Four Conservation Principles of Nursing*

TABLE 1-3   Nursing Theories of the 1970s

Theorist	Year	Title
M. Rogers	1970	*An Introduction to the Theoretical Basis of Nursing*
I. King	1971	*Toward a Theory for Nursing*
D. Orem	1971	*Nursing: Concepts of Practice*
J. Travelbee	1971	*Interpersonal Aspects of Nursing,* 2nd ed.
M. Levine	1973	*Introduction to Clinical Nursing*
B. Neuman	1974	*The Betty Neuman Health-Care Systems Model*
A. I. Meleis	1975	*Role Insufficiency and Role Supplementation: A Conceptual Framewor*
J. Paterson & L. T. Zderad	1976	*Humanistic Nursing*
Sr. C. Roy	1976	*Introduction to Nursing: An Adaptation Model*
K. E. Barnard	1978	*Nursing Child Assessment and Training*
M. Newman	1979	*Theory Development in Nursing*
J. Watson	1979	*Nursing: The Philosophy and Science of Caring*

theory (Chinn, 1978). *Advances in Nursing Science* quickly provided a forum for discussion and debate about theoretical thinking in nursing.

Table 1-3 lists the theoretical publications of this decade.

The 1980s

In the 1980s, many nursing theories were revised based on research findings that expanded them. In addition, the works of Johnson, Benner, Parse, Leininger, Meleis, Pender, Riehl-Sisca, and Erickson, Tomlin, and Swain were added to the body of theoretical thought in nursing. The theoretical publications of the 1980s are presented in Table 1-4.

The 1990s

In the 1990s, research studies to test and expand nursing theory were numerous. *Nursing Science Quarterly* (edited by Rosemarie Rizzo Parse and published by Chestnut House, 1988–1998, and Sage, 1999–present) is devoted exclusively to the presentation of theory-based research findings and theoretical topics.

Rogers published "Nursing: A Science of Unitary, Irreducible, Human Beings: Update 1990 (in *Visions of Rogers' Science-Based Nursing*, edited by Barrett), her final refinement of her theory. Barrett's text contains 24 additional chapters about Rogers's theory and its implications for practice, research, education, and the future.

In 1992, Parse changed the language of her theory from "man-living-health" to the theory of "human becoming." She explained that the reason for the change was that contemporary dictionary definitions of "man" tend to be gender based as opposed to meaning *humankind.* The assumptions and principles of the theory remained the same; only the language was new. In 1998, Parse published *The Human Becoming School of Thought—A Perspective for Nurses and Other Health Professionals.*

In 1993, Boykin and Schoenhofer published their theory of *Nursing as Caring.* They presented this theory as a grand theory, with caring as a moral imperative for nursing.

The 1990s were marked by the proliferation of middle range theories to guide nursing practice. The circle of theory-research-practice provides the base for evidence-based practice and best practices in clinical nursing. Another landmark or milestone of the

TABLE 1-4   Nursing Theories of the 1980s

Theorist	Year	Title
	NEW	
D. Johnson	1980	*The Behavioral System Model for Nursing*
J. Riehl-Sisca	1980, 1989	*The Riehl Interaction Model; The Riehl Interaction Model: An Update*
R. Parse	1981	*Man-Living-Health: A Theory for Nursing*
N. Pender	1982, 1987	*Health Promotion in Nursing Practice*
H. Erickson, E. Tomlin, & M. Swain	1983	*Modeling and Role Modeling*
J. Fizpatrick	1983	*Conceptual Models of Nursing* (with A. Whall)
P. Benner	1984	*From Novice to Expert: Excellence and Power in Clinical Practice*
	1989	*The Primacy of Caring: Stress and Coping in Health and Illness* (with J. Wrubel)
A. I. Meleis	1986	*Transitions: A Nursing Concern* (with N. Chick)
M. Mishel	1988	*Uncertainty in Illness Theory*
	REVISED/EVOLVING	
M. Leininger	1980	*Caring: A Central Focus of Nursing and Health Care Services*
	1981	*The Phenomenon of Caring: Importance, Research, Questions, and Theoretical Considerations*
	1985	*Transcultural Care Diversity and Universality*
	1988	*Leininger's Theory of Nursing: Culture Care, Diversity and Universality*
D. Orem	1980	*Nursing: Concepts of Practice*, 2nd ed.
	1985	*Nursing: Concepts of Practice*, 3rd ed.
M. Rogers	1980	*Nursing: A Science of Unitary Man*
	1983	*Science of Unitary Human Beings: A Paradigm for Nursing*
	1989	*Nursing: A Science of Unitary Human Beings*
C. Roy	1980	*The Roy Adaptation Model*
	1981	*Theory Construction in Nursing: An Adaptation Model* (with S. Roberts)
	1984	*Introduction to Nursing: An Adaptation Model*, 2nd ed.
	1989	*The Roy Adaptation Model*
I. King	1981	*A Theory for Nursing: Systems, Concepts, Process*
	1989	*King's General Systems Framework and Theory*
B. Neuman	1982	*The Neuman Systems Model*
	1989	*The Neuman Systems Model*, 2nd ed.
M. Newman	1983	*Newman's Health Theory*
	1986	*Health as Expanding Consciousness*
J. Watson	1985/1988	*Nursing: Human Science and Human Care*
	1989	*Watson's Philosophy and Theory of Human Caring in Nursing*
R. Parse	1987	*Nursing Science: Major Paradigms, Theories, Critiques*
	1989	*Man-Living-Health: A Theory of Nursing*
M. Levine	1989	*The Conservation Principles: Twenty Years Later*

1990s is the internationalization of the nursing theory movement, as evidenced by international conferences and theoretical publications.

Kolcaba published a concept analysis of comfort with her husband (Kolcaba & Kolcaba, 1991), diagrammed the aspects of comfort (1991), operationalized comfort as an outcome of care (1992), presented the middle-range theory of comfort (1994), and tested the theory in an intervention study (Kolcaba & Fox, 1999). Mercer's theory of maternal role attainment (1995) is a middle range theory based on her extensive research about mothers, fathers, infants, and parenting.

From the mid-1990s to the present, theorists have published both commentaries about and revisions of their theories. Selected publications are reflected in Table 1-5.

The Future

In the early part of the 21st century, nursing theory is characterized by diversity. After decades of struggling with questions about how and what theories could or should guide the discipline of nursing, diversity of theoretical thought is now both accepted and embraced. As the discipline of nursing focuses on humans, health and illness, interactions, caring, relationships, therapeutics, environmental factors, and ethics, pluralism and diversity are both warranted and appropriate. This pluralism has provided a fertile ground for the development of middle range theories that guide research and evidence-based practice.

In 1992, Meleis predicted that six characteristics of the discipline of nursing would direct theory development in the 21st century. These predictions, which follow, are still valid today:

1. The discipline of nursing is the human science underlying the discipline that "is predicated on understanding the meanings of daily lived experiences as they are perceived by the members or the participants of the science" (p. 112).
2. Increased emphasis on practice-orientation.
3. Nursing's mission is to develop theories to empower nurses, the discipline, and clients.
4. "Acceptance of the fact that women may have different strategies and approaches to knowledge development than men" (p. 113).
5. Nursing's attempt to "understand consumers' experiences for the purpose of empowering them to receive optimum care and to maintain optimum health" (p. 114).
6. "The effort to broaden nursing's perspective which includes efforts to understand the practice of nursing in third world countries" (p. 114).

Contemporary nursing literature supports the validity of these predictions. Writing almost a decade later, Liehr and Smith (1999) describe and analyze a decade of middle range theory products that establish the foundation for the new millennium. They state that the current context urges a focus on the human development potential of health and healing and supports a nursing knowledge base that synthesizes art and science as well as practice and research.

Research

Many contemporary authors state that qualitative and quantitative research are *equally* essential for the development of the discipline of nursing. Theories involved in this research may be single-domain theories that describe, explain, or predict a phenomenon within a specific descriptive and explanatory context, or they may be prescriptive. Prescriptive theories reflect guidelines for caregivers and for providing appropriate actions.

TABLE 1-5   Nursing Theory, 1990–2007

Theorist	Year	Title
	1990–1999	
M. H. Mishel	1990	*Reconceptualization of the Uncertainty in Illness Theory*
D. E. Orem	1991, 1995	*Nursing: Concepts of Practice*, 4th and 5th eds.
	1995	*Orem's Nursing Theory and Positive Mental Health* (with E. M. Vardiman)
	1997	*Views of Human Beings Specific to Nursing*
K. Kolcaba	1994	*A Theory of Holistic Comfort for Nursing*
A. I. Meleis	1994	*Facilitating Transitions: Redefinition of the Nursing Mission* (with P. A. Trangenstein)
M. A. Newman	1994	*Health as Expanding Consciousness*, 2nd ed.
	1997	*Evolution of the Theory of Health as Expanding Consciousness*
I. M. King	1995a	*A System's Framework for Nursing*
	1995b	*The Theory of Goal Attainment*
	1996	*The Theory of Goal Attainment in Research and Practice*
	1997a	*Reflections on the Past and a Vision for the Future*
	1997b	*King's Theory of Goal Attainment in Practice*
	1999	*A Theory of Goal Attainment: Philosophical and Ethical Implications*
M. E. Levine	1995	*The Rhetoric of Nursing Theory*
	1996	*The Conservation Principles: A Retrospective*
R. T. Mercer	1995	*Becoming a Mother*
B. Neuman	1995	*The Neuman Systems Model*, 3rd ed.
	1996	*The Neuman Systems Model in Research and Practice*
P. Benner	1996	*Expertise in Nursing Practice* (with C. Tanner & C. Chesla)
M. Leininger	1996	*Culture Care Theory, Research, and Practice*
J. Corbin	1992	*A Nursing Model for Chronic Illness Management Based Upon the Trajectory Framework* (with A. Strauss)
	1998	*The Corbin and Strauss Illness Trajectory Model*
R. R. Parse	1995a	*Building the Realm of Nursing Knowledge*
	1995b	*Illuminations: The Human Becoming Theory in Practice and Research*
	1996a	*Building Knowledge Through Qualitative Research: The Road Less Traveled*
	1996b	*The Human Becoming Theory: Challenges in Practice and Research*
	1997a	*The Human Becoming Theory: The Was, Is, and Will Be*
	1998	*The Human Becoming School of Thought*
	1999	*Hope: An International Human Becoming Perspective*
N. J. Pender	1996	*Health Promotion in Nursing Practice*, 3rd ed.
H. E. Peplau	1997	*Peplau's Theory of Interpersonal Relations*

Theorist	Year	Title
C. Roy	1997	*Future of the Roy Model: Challenge to Redefine Adaptation*
J. Watson	1997	*The Theory of Human Caring: Retrospective and Prospective*
	1999	*Postmodern Nursing and Beyond*
2000–2007		
A. Meleis and others	2000	*Experiencing Transitions*
A. Meleis	2007	*Theoretical Nursing: Development and Progress*
K. Kolcaba	2003	*Comfort Theory and Practice*
R. R. Parse	2003	*Community: A Human Becoming Perspective*
R. T. Mercer	2004	*Becoming a Mother Versus Maternal Role Attainment*
P. Benner	2005	*Using the Dreyfus Model of Skill Acquisition to Describe and Interpret Skill Acquisition and Clinical Judgment in Nursing Practice and Education*
M. M. Leininger	2006	*Culture Care Diversity and Universality* McFarland
N. Pender	2002, 2006	*Health Promotion in Nursing Practice,* 4th and 5th eds. (with C. L. Murdaugh & M. A. Parsons)

ANALYSIS AND EVALUATION OF THEORY

Smith (2003) states, "Evaluation is one of the most popular indoor sports of the organizations in which we live" (p. 190). She advocates that theories should be evaluated with the aspects of appreciation, recognition, and affirmation balanced with the identification of any theoretical weaknesses. She reminds us that nursing scholars who contribute to the development of nursing science are innovative pioneers who courageously offer their ideas for the advancement of the discipline. She cautions that the evaluator must be a responsible steward of the discipline with an obligation to care about the nature of evolution of nursing knowledge.

Review of the Literature on Theory Analysis and Evaluation

Parse (1997b, 2005) proposes a design for critical appraisal that is appropriate for all frameworks and theories and is comprised of structure and process. Structure criteria refer to the *historical evolution* of the theory, the *foundational elements* (assumptions and concepts), and *relational statements* (principles created from the concepts into human-universe-health process written at an abstract level). The process criteria include *correspondence* (semantic integrity and simplicity), *coherence* (syntax and aesthetics), and *pragmatics*. Syntax is recognized by the precision and logical flow with which ideas are presented. *Aesthetics* is recognized by the beauty of the presentation of theory, that is, the symmetry and harmony of the elements. *Pragmatics* refers to effectiveness and heuristic potential. *Effectiveness* is recognized by the way the theory is used as a guide to research and practice. *Heuristic potential* refers to the possibilities for inquiry.

Barnum (1998) proposes analytic criteria of content, process, context, and goals. Her evaluative criteria of internal criticism include clarity, consistency, adequacy, logical development, and level of theory development. Her criteria for external evaluation include reality convergence, utility, significance, discrimination, scope of theory, and complexity.

Smith (2003) proposes a structure for the evaluation of middle range theories that includes consideration of the theory's substantive foundations, structural integrity, and functional adequacy. Functional adequacy speaks specifically to application to practice, research, and generalizability.

Chinn and Kramer (2004) describe theory in terms of purpose, concepts, definitions, relationships, structure, and assumptions. They offer a pragmatic guide to critical reflection of theory. They suggest that one should consider the following five criteria: clarity, simplicity, generality, accessibility, and importance.

Fawcett (2005a) describes the *analysis* of conceptual models of nursing as the objective and systematic way of examining the origin, focus, and content of a theory *without* evaluating or making subjective value judgments about the theory. In her guidelines for *analysis*, the following areas are addressed: origins of the model, focus of the model, and content of the model. She provides questions to be answered for each of the areas. Fawcett states that *evaluation* of a nursing model is accomplished by comparing its content with the following criteria: significance, internal consistency, parsimony, testability, empirical adequacy, and pragmatic adequacy. As with the areas for analysis, Fawcett provides specific questions to be answered for each area of evaluation. The questions for testability and empirical adequacy differ for grand theories and middle range theories (Fawcett, 2005b).

Johnson and Webber (2005) propose a criterion-based critique model for nursing theories that contains the following elements:

Phase I—Intent of the Theory

> Criterion 1: The meaning is clear and understandable.
> Criterion 2: Boundaries are consistent with nursing practice.
> Criterion 3: Language is understandable and includes minimal jargon.

Phase II—Concepts and Propositions

> Criterion 4: Major concepts are identified and defined.
> Criterion 5: Concepts stimulate the formulation of propositions.
> Criterion 6: Variables and assumptions help understand and interpret propositions.

Phase III—Usefulness in Nursing Practice

> Criterion 7: Theoretical knowledge helps explain and predict phenomena.
> Criterion 8: Theoretical knowledge influences nursing practice. (p. 207)

Parker (2006) states that readers should look carefully at the theory, read the theory as presented by the theorist, and read what others have written about the theory. She cautions readers to study the whole theory, as the parts will not be fully meaningful and may lead to misunderstanding (p. 20).

Meleis (2007) suggests a model that defines theory evaluation as encompassing description, analysis, critique, testing, and support. This model also includes a unique aspect that she calls the "circle of contagiousness of a theory." This concept refers to the popularity of usage of the theory to guide nursing practice and research.

Guidelines for This Text

For the purposes of this text, theories will be critiqued using a synthesis of the analysis and evaluation frameworks of Barnum (1998), Chinn and Kramer (2004), Johnson and

Webber (2005), Fawcett (2005a, 2005b), and Meleis (2007). Critique, by definition, is the art of analyzing or evaluating a work of art or literature (*Webster's,* 1991). It is assumed that there are both objective and subjective elements to the process of critiquing.

Currently, case management and integrated health care systems focus on the bottom line, or the profit that can be realized from health care delivery. The system expects favorable outcomes to be delivered in increasingly shorter time frames in order to reduce costs. Advanced practice nurses are being utilized in many settings, and nurse practitioner programs have grown rapidly. While this situation has put the discipline of nursing solidly into all realms of care as a primary provider of service, this focus has diverted attention away from nursing knowledge and toward biomedical knowledge as the base for nursing practice (Fawcett, 1997).

In order to analyze and evaluate nursing theory in the 21st century, it seems appropriate to use the best elements of the traditional academic sense of critique. It is hoped that this synthesis of methods provides the best practices of academic critique while retaining the idea that nursing theory is the base for professional nursing practice.

QUESTIONS FOR CRITIQUE OF A NURSING THEORY

1. *What is the historical context of the theory?*   This first question requires the reader to look carefully at the assumptions upon which the theory is built. Are the assumptions based on a specific philosophy and/or another theory—from nursing or a related discipline? Does one need additional study or information to understand the assumptions? Where does this theory fit in the history of nursing theory? Can it be identified as belonging within the totality or simultaneity paradigm, or does it rest on a different metaparadigm entirely?

2. *What are the basic concepts and relationships presented by the theory?*   Are the concepts of the theory defined and used in a consistent fashion? Are the relationships presented logically and based upon the stated assumptions? Are the concepts and relationships clear and understandable to the reader?

3. *What major phenomena of concern to nursing are presented? These phenomena may include* **but are not limited to** *human beings, environment, health, interpersonal relations, caring, goal attainment, adaptation, and energy fields.*   Current literature in nursing theory suggests the presence of more than the "original" four metaparadigm concepts of man, health, environment, and nursing. A theory need not address all of the major phenomenon of concern to nursing, but for the purpose of critique it is important to identify those phenomena that *are* addressed by the theory.

4. *To whom does this theory apply? In what situations? In what ways?*   What is the scope of the theory? Does it apply to all recipients of nursing care in all possible situations? If not, to whom, and where will the theory have meaning? Does the theory describe, explain, or predict phenomena?

5. *By what method or methods can this theory be tested?*   Can the concepts and relationships of this theory be observed, measured, and tested using qualitative or quantitative methods? Has testing of this theory occurred? What findings have been presented in the literature?

6. *Does this theory direct nursing actions that lead to favorable outcomes?*   Does the research conducted about theory-directed practice demonstrate favorable client outcomes? With what frequency? In what situations?

7. *How contagious is this theory?*   Who is using this theory? In what context? Is this theory directing nursing practice, nursing education, and/or nursing administration?

Summary

Nursing science provides the basis for professional nursing practice. Nursing theories provide the critical thinking structures to direct the clinical decision-making process of professional nursing practice. The relationship between theory, research, and practice is circular in nature. As new knowledge and discoveries emerge in each of these realms, the cutting edge of the art and science of the discipline of nursing evolves.

Theory development began with Nightingale and was revived in the 1950s. Theory development has been described from the historical context as well as the current state-of-the-art of theory development at the start of the new millennium.

A framework for the critique of a theory has been presented and will be used throughout this text for the theories presented. Please refer to the individual chapters for these critiques.

PEARSON

EXPLORE **mynursingkit™**

MyNursingKit is your one stop for online chapter review materials and resources. Prepare for success with additional NCLEX®-style practice questions, interactive assignments and activities, web links, animations and videos, and more!

Register your access code from the front of your book at
www.mynursingkit.com.

References

Abdellah, F. G., Beland, I. L., Martin, A., & Matheney, R. V. (1960). *Patient-centered approaches to nursing.* New York: Macmillan. [out of print]

Barnard, K. E. (1978). *Nursing child assessment and training: Learning resource manual.* Seattle: University of Washington.

Barnum, B. J. S. (1998). *Nursing theory: Analysis, application, and evaluation* (5th ed.). Philadelphia: Lippincott.

Barrett, E. A. M. (1990). *Visions of Rogers' science based nursing.* New York: National League for Nursing.

Barrett, E. A. M., Cody, W. K., Daly, J., Millar, B., Mitchell, G. J., Takahasi, T., et al. (1997). What is nursing science? An international dialogue. *Nursing Science Quarterly, 10,* 8–13.

Benner, P. (1984). *From novice to expert: Excellence and power in clinical nursing practice.* Menlo Park, CA: Addison-Wesley.

Benner, P. (2005). Using the Dreyfus model of skill acquisition to describe and interpret skill acquisition and clinical judgment in nursing practice and education. *The Bulletin of Science, Technology and Society Special Issue: Human Expertise in the Age of the Computer, 24*(3), 188–199.

Benner, P., Tanner, C., & Chesla, C. (1996). *Expertise in nursing practice; Caring, clinical judgment, and ethics.* New York: Springer.

Benner, P., & Wrubel, J. (1989). *The primacy of caring: Stress and coping in health and illness.* Menlo Park, CA: Addison-Wesley.

Boykin, A., & Schoenhofer, S. (1993). *Nursing as caring: A model for transforming practice.* New York: National League for Nursing.

Chick, N., & Meleis, A. I. (1986). Transitions: A nursing concern. In P. L. Chinn (Ed.), *Nursing research methodology.* Boulder, CO: Aspen.

Chinn, P. L. (1978). A model for theory development in nursing. *Advances in Nursing Science, 1,* 1–11.

Chinn, P. L., & Kramer, M. K. (2004). *Integrated knowledge development in nursing* (6th ed.). St. Louis: Mosby.

Cody, W. K. (1995). About all those paradigms: Many in the universe, two in nursing. *Nursing Science Quarterly, 8,* 144–147.

Cody, W. K. (1996). Response: On the requirements of a metaparadigm: An invitation to dialogue. *Nursing Science Quarterly, 9,* 97–99.

Corbin, J. (1998). The Corbin and Strauss illness trajectory model. *Scholarly Inquiry for Nursing Practice, 12,* 33–41.

Corbin, J. M., & Strauss, A. (1992). A nursing model for chronic illness management based upon the trajectory framework. In P. Woog (Ed.), *The Chronic Illness Trajectory Framework: The Corbin and Strauss Nursing Model* (pp. 9–28). New York: Springer.

Dickoff, J., & James, P. (1968). A theory of theories: A position paper. *Nursing Research, 17,* 197–203.

Dickoff, J., James, P., & Wiedenbach, E. (1968). Theory in a practice discipline, part 1—Practice-oriented theory. *Nursing Research, 17,* 415–435.

Erickson, H. C., Tomlin, E. M., & Swain, M. A. P. (1983). *Modeling and role modeling.* Lexington, SC: Pine Press.

Fawcett, J. (1997). Conceptual models of nursing, nursing theories, and nursing practice: Focus on the future. In M. R. Alligood & A. Marriner-Tomey (Eds.), *Nursing theory: Utilization and application* (pp. 211–221). St. Louis: Mosby.

Fawcett, J. (2003). Critiquing contemporary nursing knowledge: A dialogue. *Nursing Science Quarterly, 16,* 273–276.

Fawcett, J. (2005a). *Contemporary nursing knowledge: Analysis and evaluation of nursing models and theories* (2nd ed.). Philadelphia: F. A. Davis.

Fawcett, J. (2005b). Criterion of evaluation of theory. *Nursing Science Quarterly, 18,* 131–135.

Fitzpatrick, J. J., & Whall, A. L. (1983). *Conceptual models of nursing: Analysis and application.* Bowie MD: Robert J. Brady. [out of print]

Haase, J. E., & Meyers, S. T. (1988). Reconciling paradigm assumptions of qualitative and quantitative research. *Western Journal of Nursing Research, 10,* 132.

Hall, L. E. (1959). Nursing . . . what is it? Published by the Virginia Nurses Association.

Hall, L. E. (1966). Another view of nursing care and quality. In K. M. Straub & K. S. Parker (Eds.), *Continuity in patient care: The role of nursing.* Washington, DC: Catholic University Press.

Harmer, B., & Henderson, V. (1955). *Textbook of the principles and practice of nursing* (5th ed.). New York: Macmillan.

Henderson, V. (1960). *Basic principles of nursing care.* Geneva: ICN.

Henderson, V. (1966). *The nature of nursing.* New York: Macmillan. [out of print]

Im, E. O. (2005). Development of situation-specific theories: An integrative approach. *Advances in Nursing Science, 28,* 137–151.

Im, E. O., & Meleis, A. I. (1999a). Situation-specific theories: Philosophical roots, properties, and approach. *Advances in Nursing Science, 22,* 11–24.

Im, E. O., & Meleis, A. I. (1999b). A situation-specific theory of Korean immigrant women's menopausal transition. *Image, 31,* 333–338.

Johnson, B. M., & Webber, P. B. (2005). *An introduction to theory and reasoning in nursing* (2nd ed.). Philadelphia: Lippincott Williams & Wilkins.

Johnson, D. E. (1980). The behavioral system model for nursing. In J. P. Riehl & C. Roy (Eds.), *Conceptual models for nursing practice* (2nd ed., pp. 207–216). New York: Appleton-Century-Crofts. [out of print]

Kim, H. S. (1989). Theoretical thinking in nursing: Problems and perspectives. *Advances in Nursing Science, 24,* 106–122.

King, I. M. (1971). *Toward a theory for nursing: General concepts of human behavior.* New York: Wiley.

King, I. M. (1981) *A theory for nursing: System, concepts, process.* New York: Wiley. (Reissued 1991, Albany, NY: Delmar)

King, I. M. (1989). King's general systems framework and theory. In J. Riehl-Sisca (Ed.), *Conceptual models for nursing practice* (3rd ed., pp. 149–158). Norwalk, CT: Appleton & Lange.

King, I. M. (1995a). A systems framework for nursing. In M. A. Frey & C. L. Sieloff (Eds.), *Advancing King's systems framework and theory of nursing* (pp. 14–22). Thousand Oaks, CA: Sage.

King, I. M. (1995b). The theory of goal attainment. In M. A. Frey & C. L. Sieloff (Eds.), *Advancing King's systems framework and theory of nursing* (pp. 23–32). Thousand Oaks, CA: Sage.

King, I. M. (1996). The theory of goal attainment in research and practice. *Nursing Science Quarterly, 9,* 61–66.

King, I. M. (1997a). Reflections on the past and a vision for the future. *Nursing Science Quarterly, 10,* 15–17.

King, I. M. (1997b). King's theory of goal attainment in practice. *Nursing Science Quarterly, 10,* 180–185.

King, I. M. (1999). A theory of goal attainment: Philosophical and ethical implications. *Nursing Science Quarterly, 12,* 292–296.

Kolcaba, K. (1991). A taxonomic structure for the concept of comfort. *Image: The Journal of Nursing Scholarship 23,* 237–240.

Kolcaba, K. (1992). Holistic comfort: Operationalizing the construct as a nurse-sensitive outcome. *Advances in Nursing Science, 15*, 1–10.

Kolcaba, K. (1994) A theory of holistic comfort for nursing. *Journal of Advanced Nursing, 19*, 1178–1184.

Kolcaba, K. (2003). *Comfort theory and practice: A vision for holistic health care and research.* New York: Springer.

Kolcaba, K., & Fox, C. (1999). The effects of guided imagery on comfort of women with early stage breast cancer undergoing radiation therapy. *Oncology Nursing Forum, 26*(1), 67–92.

Kolcaba, K., & Kolcaba, R. (1991) An analysis of the concept of comfort. *Journal of Advanced Nursing, 16*, 1301–1310.

Leininger, M. M. (1980). Caring: A central focus of nursing and health care services. *Nursing and Health Care, 1*, 135–143, 176.

Leininger, M. M. (1981). The phenomenon of caring: Importance, research questions, and theoretical considerations. In M. M. Leininger (Ed.), *Caring: An essential human need* (pp. 3–15). Thorofare, NJ: Slack. [out of print]

Leininger, M. M. (1985). Transcultural care diversity and universality: A theory of nursing. *Nursing and Health Care, 6*, 209–212.

Leininger, M. M. (1988). Leininger's theory of nursing: Culture care diversity and universality. *Nursing Science Quarterly, 1*, 152–169.

Leininger, M. M. (1996). Culture care theory, research and practice. *Nursing Science Quarterly, 9*, 71–78.

Leininger, M. M., & McFarland, M. R. (2006). *Culture care diversity and universality: A worldwide nursing theory.* Sudbury, MA: Jones & Bartlett.

Levine, M. E. (1967). The four conservation principles. *Nursing Forum, 6*, 45–59.

Levine, M. E. (1973). *Introduction to clinical nursing.* Philadelphia: F. A. Davis.

Levine, M. E. (1989). The conservation principles: Twenty years later. In J. Riehl-Sisca (Ed.), *Conceptual models for nursing practice* (3rd ed., pp. 325–337). Norwalk, CT: Appleton & Lange.

Levine, M. E. (1995). The rhetoric of nursing theory. *Image: The Journal of Nursing Scholarship, 27*, 11–14.

Levine, M. E. (1996). The conservation principles: A retrospective. *Nursing Science Quarterly, 9*(1), 38–41.

Liehr, P., & Smith, M. J. (1999). Middle range theory: Spinning research and practice to create knowledge for the new millennium. *Advances in Nursing Science, 21*(4), 81–91.

Malinski, V. M. (1995). Response: Notes on book review of *Analysis and evaluation of nursing theories. Nursing Science Quarterly, 8*, 58–59.

McKenna, H. (1997). *Nursing theories and models.* London: Routledge.

Meleis, A. I. (1975). Role inefficiency and role supplementation: A conceptual framework. *Nursing Research, 24*, 264–271.

Meleis, A. I. (1992). Directions for nursing theory development in the 21st century. *Nursing Science Quarterly 5*, 112–117.

Meleis, A. I. (2007). *Theoretical nursing: Development and progress* (4th ed.). Philadelphia: Lippincott Williams & Wilkins.

Meleis, A. I., Sawyer, L. M., Im, E., Messias, D. K. H., & Shumacher, K. (2000). Experiencing transitions: An emerging middle-range theory. *Advances in Nursing Science, 23*, 12–28.

Meleis, A. I., & Trangenstein, P. A. (1994). Facilitating transitions: Redefinition of the nursing mission. *Nursing Outlook, 42*, 255–259.

Mercer, R. T. (1995). *Becoming a mother: Research on maternal identity from Rubin to the present.* New York: Springer.

Mercer, R. T. (2004). Becoming a mother versus maternal role attainment. *Journal of Nursing Scholarship, 36*, 226–232.

Merton, R. K. (1968). *Social theory and social structure.* New York: Free Press.

Mishel, M. H. (1988). Uncertainty in illness. *Image: The Journal of Nursing Scholarship, 20*, 225–231.

Mishel, M. H. (1990). Reconceptualization of the uncertainty in illness theory. *Image: The Journal of Nursing Scholarship, 22*, 256–262.

Neuman, B. (1974). The Betty Neuman health care systems model: A total person approach to patient problems. In J. P. Riehl & C. Roy (Eds.), *Conceptual models of nursing practice* (pp. 99–114). New York: Appleton-Century Crofts. [out of print]

Neuman, B. (1982). *The Neuman Systems Model.* Norwalk, CT: Appleton & Lange. [out of print]

Neuman, B. (1989). *The Neuman Systems Model* (2nd ed.). Norwalk, CT: Appleton & Lange.

Neuman, B. (1995). *The Neuman Systems Model* (3rd ed.). Norwalk, CT: Appleton & Lange.

Neuman, B. (1996). The Neuman Systems Model in research and practice. *Nursing Science Quarterly, 9*, 67–70.

Newman, M. A. (1979). *Theory development in nursing.* Philadelphia: F. A. Davis.

Newman, M. A. (1983). Newman's health theory. In I. W. Clements & F. B. Roberts (Eds.), *Family health: A theoretical approach to nursing care* (pp. 161–175). New York: Wiley.

Newman, M. A. (1986). *Health as expanding consciousness.* St. Louis: Mosby.

Newman, M. A. (1994). *Health as expanding consciousness* (2nd ed.). New York: National League for Nursing.

Newman, M. A. (1997). Evolution of the theory of health as expanding consciousness. *Nursing Science Quarterly, 10,* 22–25.

Nightingale, F. (1992). *Notes on Nursing: What it is and what it is not* (Com. ed.). Philadelphia: Lippincott. (Original work published 1859)

Orem, D. E. (1971). *Nursing: Concepts of practice.* New York: McGraw-Hill. [out of print]

Orem, D. E. (1980). *Nursing: Concepts of practice* (2nd ed.). New York: McGraw-Hill. [out of print]

Orem, D. E. (1985). *Nursing: Concepts of practice* (3rd ed.). New York: McGraw-Hill.

Orem, D. E. (1991). *Nursing: Concepts of practice* (4th ed.). St. Louis: Mosby. [out of print]

Orem, D. E. (1995). *Nursing: Concepts of practice* (5th ed.). St. Louis: Mosby-Yearbook

Orem, D. E. (1997). Views of human beings specific to nursing. *Nursing Science Quarterly, 10,* 26–31.

Orem, D. E., & Vardiman, E. M. (1995). Orem's nursing theory and positive mental health: Practical considerations. *Nursing Science Quarterly, 8,* 165–173.

Orlando, I. J. (1961). *The dynamic nurse-patient relationship.* New York: G. P. Putman's Sons.

Orlando, I. J. (1990). *The dynamic nurse-patient relationship: Function, process, and principles.* New York: National League for Nursing. (Reprinted from 1961, G. P. Putman's Sons)

Parker, M. E. (2006). Studying nursing theory: Choosing, analyzing, evaluating. In M. E. Parker (Ed.), *Nursing theories and nursing practice* (2nd ed., pp. 14–22). Philadelphia: F. A. Davis.

Parse, R. R. (1981) *Man-living-health: A theory for nursing.* New York: Wiley.

Parse, R. R. (1987). *Nursing science: Major paradigms, theories, and critiques.* Philadelphia: Saunders.

Parse, R. R. (1989). Man-living-health: A theory of nursing. In J. P. Riehl-Sisca (Ed.), *Conceptual models for nursing practice* (3rd ed., pp. 253–257). Norwalk, CT: Appleton & Lange.

Parse, R. R. (1992). Human becoming: Parse's theory of nursing. *Nursing Science Quarterly, 5,* 35–42.

Parse, R. R. (1995a). Building the realm of nursing knowledge. *Nursing Science Quarterly, 8,* 51.

Parse, R. R. (1995b). *Illuminations: The human becoming theory in practice and research.* New York: National League for Nursing Press.

Parse, R. R. (1996a). Building knowledge through qualitative research: The road less traveled. *Nursing Science Quarterly, 9,* 10–16.

Parse, R. R. (1996b). The human becoming theory: Challenges in practice and research. *Nursing Science Quarterly, 9,* 55–60.

Parse, R. R. (1997a). The human becoming theory: The was, is, and will be. *Nursing Science Quarterly, 10,* 32–38.

Parse, R. R. (1997b). The language of nursing knowledge: Saying what we mean. In I. M. King & J. Fawcett (Eds.), *The language of nursing theory and metatheory* (pp. 73–77). Indianapolis: Center Nursing Press.

Parse, R. R. (1998). *The human becoming school of thought.* Thousand Oaks, CA: Sage.

Parse, R. R. (1999). *Hope: An international human becoming perspective.* New York: NLN Press.

Parse, R. R. (2003). *Community: A human becoming perspective.* Sudbury, MA: Jones & Bartlett.

Parse, R. R. (2005) Parse's criteria for evaluation of theory with a comparison of Fawcett's and Parse's approaches. *Nursing Science Quarterly, 18,* 135–137.

Paterson, J. G., & Zderad, L. T. (1976). *Humanistic nursing.* New York: Wiley. (Reissued 1988, New York: National League for Nursing)

Pender, N. (1982). *Health promotion in nursing practice.* New York: Appleton-Century-Crofts. [out of print]

Pender, N. J. (1987). *Health promotion in nursing practice* (2nd ed.). Stamford, CT: Appleton & Lange. [out of print]

Pender, N. J. (1996). *Health promotion in nursing practice* (3rd ed.). Stamford, CT: Appleton & Lange. [out of print]

Pender, N. J., Murdaugh, C. L., & Parsons, M. A. (2002). *Health promotion in nursing practice* (4th ed.). Upper Saddle River, NJ : Prentice Hall. [out of print]

Pender, N. J., Murdaugh, C. L., & Parsons, M. A. (2006). *Health promotion in nursing practice* (5th ed.). Upper Saddle River, NJ: Pearson Prentice Hall.

Peplau, H. E. (1988). *Interpersonal relations in nursing.* New York: Springer. (Original work published 1952, New York: G. P. Putnam's Sons)

Peplau, H. E. (1997). Peplau's theory of interpersonal relations. *Nursing Science Quarterly, 10*, 162–167.

Polit, D. F., & Beck, C. T. (2004). *Nursing research: Principles and methods* (6th ed.). Philadelphia: Lippincott Williams & Wilkins.

Ray, M. A. (1998). Complexity and nursing science. *Nursing Science Quarterly, 11*, 91–93.

Riehl, J. P. (1980). The Riehl interaction model. In J. P. Riehl & C. Roy (Eds.), *Conceptual models for nursing practice* (2nd ed., pp. 350–356). New York: Appleton-Century-Crofts.

Riehl-Sisca, J. P. (1989) The Riehl interaction model: An update. In J. P. Riehl-Sisca (Ed.), *Conceptual models for nursing practice* (3rd ed., pp. 383–402). New York: Appleton & Lange.

Rogers, M. E. (1970). *An introduction to the theoretical basis of nursing.* Philadelphia: F. A. Davis. [out of print]

Rogers, M. E. (1980). Nursing: A science of unitary man. In J. Riehl & C. Roy (Eds.), *Conceptual models for nursing practice* (2nd ed., pp. 329–337). New York: Appleton-Century- Crofts.

Rogers, M. E. (1983). Science of unitary human beings: A paradigm for nursing. In I. W. Clements & F. B. Roberts (Eds.), *Family health: A theoretical approach to nursing care* (pp. 221–228). New York: Wiley. [out of print]

Rogers, M. E. (1989). Nursing: A science of unitary human beings. In J. Riehl-Sisca (Ed.), *Conceptual models for nursing practice* (3rd ed., pp. 181–188). Norwalk, CT: Appleton & Lange.

Rogers, M. E. (1990). Nursing: A science of unitary, irreducible human beings. In E. A. M. Barrett (Ed.), *Visions of Rogers' science based nursing* (pp. 5–11). New York: National League for Nursing.

Roy, C. (1976). *Introduction to nursing: An adaptation model.* Englewood Cliffs, NJ: Prentice Hall. [out of print]

Roy, C. (1980). The Roy Adaptation Model. In J. P. Riehl & C. Roy (Eds.), *Conceptual models for nursing practice* (2nd ed., pp. 179–188). New York: Appleton-Century-Crofts. [out of print]

Roy, C. (1984). *Introduction to nursing: An adaptation model* (2nd ed.). Norwalk, CT: Appleton-Century-Crofts.

Roy, C. (1989). The Roy Adaptation Model. In J. Riehl-Sisca (Ed.), *Conceptual models for nursing practice* (3rd ed., pp. 105–114). Norwalk, CT: Appleton & Lange.

Roy, C. (1997). Future of the Roy Model: Challenge to redefine adaptation. *Nursing Science Quarterly, 10*, 42–48.

Roy, C., & Andrews, H. A. (1999). *The Roy Adaptation Model* (2nd ed.). Norwalk, CT: Appleton & Lange.

Roy, C., & Roberts, S. (1981). *Theory construction in nursing: An adaptation model.* Englewood Cliffs, NJ: Prentice Hall. [out of print]

Smith, M. C. (2003). Evaluation of middle range theories for the discipline of nursing. In M. J. Smith & P. R. Liehr (Eds.), *Middle range theory for nursing* (pp. 189–205). New York: Springer.

Smith, M. J., & Liehr, P. R. (Eds.). (2003). *Middle range theory for nursing.* New York: Springer.

Speziale, H. J. S., & Carpenter, D. R. (2007). *Qualitative research in nursing* (4th ed.). Philadelphia: Lippincott, Williams & Wilkins.

Streubert, H. J., & Carpenter, D. R. (1995). *Qualitative research in nursing.* Philadelphia: Lippincott.

Suppe, F. (1996). Middle range theory: Role in research and practice. In *Proceedings of the Sixth Rosemary Ellis Scholar's Retreat, nursing science implications for the 21st century.* Cleveland, OH: Frances Payne Bolton School of Nursing, Case Western Reserve University.

Travelbee, J. (1966). *Interpersonal aspects of nursing.* Philadelphia: F. A. Davis.

Travelbee, J. (1971). *Interpersonal aspects of nursing* (2nd ed.).Philadelphia: F. A. Davis.

Watson, J. (1979). *Nursing: The philosophy and science of caring.* Boston: Little, Brown. [out of print]

Watson, J. (1985). *Nursing: Human science and human care.* Norwalk, CT: Appleton-Century-Crofts. (Reissued 1988, New York: National League for Nursing)

Watson, J. (1989). Watson's philosophy and theory of human caring. In J. Riehl-Sisca (Ed.), *Conceptual models for nursing practice* (3rd ed., pp. 219–236). Norwalk, CT: Appleton & Lange.

Watson, J. (1997). The theory of human caring: Retrospective and prospective. *Nursing Science Quarterly, 10*, 49–51.

Watson, J. (1999). *Postmodern nursing and beyond.* Edinburgh, UK: Churchill Livingstone.

Webster's ninth new collegiate dictionary. (1991). Springfield, MA: Merriam.

Wiedenbach, E. (1964). *Clinical nursing—A helping art.* New York: Springer.

Wiedenbach, E. (1969). *Meeting the realities in clinical teaching.* New York: Springer.

CHAPTER 2

Nursing Theory and Clinical Practice

Julia B. George

A major characteristic of a profession is the identification and development of its own body of knowledge. The models and theories discussed in this book are representative of this characteristic for nursing. A body of knowledge in a practice discipline such as nursing is developed through research and through use in practice. Use of nursing theory in practice may involve application within the framework of the nursing process (also used in the American Nurses Association standards of practice) through the use of critical thinking, patterns and ways of knowing, and evidence-based practice knowledge. These topics will be briefly summarized. The reader is encouraged to read more in depth on each of these topics, beginning with the references cited in this chapter.

APPLICATION IN PRACTICE

The American Nurses Association identifies six standards of practice: assessment, diagnosis, outcomes identification, planning, implementation, and evaluation (2004). These standards of practice may also be identified as the *nursing process*. Assessment represents the collection and analysis of information, diagnosis is the identification of a problem, outcomes identification involves specifying what goal(s) is/are to be reached, planning encompasses the decisions about who is to do what in an effort to reach the identified goals, implementation is the carrying out of the planned activities, and evaluation is ongoing throughout the process as to the accuracy and success of the information and activities. While these standards or steps are described as discrete entities, in practice each is constantly ongoing as newly available data lead to the identification of new problems or modification of the previously identified one so that outcomes may be changed, which leads to the need to alter planning and implementation.

Scriven and Paul (2004) provide a complex definition of *critical thinking*: "the intellectually disciplined process of actively and skillfully conceptualizing, applying, analyzing, synthesizing, and/or evaluating information gathered from, or generated by, observation, experience, reflection, reasoning, or communication, as a guide to belief and action." More simply, Paul and Elder (2002) define critical thinking as "the disciplined art of ensuring that you use the best thinking you are capable of in any set of circumstances"(p.7). Kataoka-Yohira and Saylor (1994) identify five components for critical thinking in nursing: specific knowledge base, experience, competencies, attitudes, and standards. A study to define critical thinking in nursing resulted in a consensus statement that nurses who are critical thinkers exhibit "confidence, contextual perspective, creativity, flexibility, inquisitiveness, intellectual integrity, intuition, open-mindedness, perseverance, and reflection" (Rubenfeld & Scheffer, 1999, p. 5). The nursing process represents one form of critical thinking.

Various *patterns of knowing* are important to nursing. Four major patterns of knowing were first identified by Carper (1978/2004) and discussed further by Chinn and Kramer (2004, pp. 3–12). These two sources provide the basis for the following summary. Carper identified four patterns of knowing in nursing through a thorough review of the nursing literature. The first pattern of knowing is identified by Carper as *empirics*, or the science of nursing, based on observable, measurable information obtained through quantitative methods. Chinn and Kramer state the critical questions for empirical knowing are *what is this?* and *how does it work?* The second pattern of knowing is *aesthetics*, or the art of nursing, and involves the recognition of and reaction to the meaning of situations. The critical questions are *what does this mean?* and *how is this significant?* The third pattern of knowing is that of *personal knowledge*, seeking to know the self rather than about the self. The critical questions are *do I know what I do?* and *do I do what I know?* The fourth pattern of knowing is ethics, or the moral component. The critical questions are *is this right?* and *is this responsible?*

Patterns of knowing are similar to but should not be confused with *ways of knowing* described in the literature. Perry (1970) described how college students' conceptions of knowledge and their understanding of themselves as knowers evolved over the years of their college experience. He identified them as beginning with a position of basic dualism, an either/or view—right or wrong, black or white (no gray)—with learning as a passive process, accepting what comes from authorities. Next is multiplicity, with a move to understanding that the authority does not know everything and the student has a right to his or her own opinion. The third position is that of relative subordinate, in which analytical evaluation and the scientific method predominate. The fourth position is that of relativism, with recognition of the importance of context and change. Belenky, Clinchy, Goldberger, and Tarule (1986) were concerned that the subjects in Perry's study were all male and sought to investigate the applicability of Perry's positions to women, using a research methodology similar to Perry's. They found both similarities and differences in women's ways of knowing. The first way of knowing they describe is silence, in which the knower is seen but not heard, experiences disconnection, and views authority as all powerful. The second way of knowing is received knowing, in which listening to others is a way of knowing. The third way of knowing is subjective knowing, in which women begin to listen to their inner voice and identify a sense of self. Next is procedural knowing, which involves reason, objectivity, and knowing that is both separate from others and connected to others. Finally there is constructed knowing, in which women seek to integrate knowledge that they instinctively know is of personal importance with knowledge received from others. A major difference between the ways of knowing described by Perry and by Belenky et al. is that Perry's presented his ways of knowing as linear, and the women's ways of knowing are described as being context dependent—a constructed knower in most areas may be a silent knower when dealing with totally new information, for example.

Concerns about evidence-based nursing, which limits the evidence to that drawn only from randomized clinical trials, have been expressed by a number of leading thinkers in nursing, for example, Fawcett, Watson, Neuman, Walker, and Fitzpatrick (2001). While some definitions of evidence-based practice rely primarily upon quantitative or empirical evidence, Melnyk and Fineout-Overholt (2005) discuss components of evidence-based practice in nursing that are more compatible with Carper's ways of knowing in nursing. They identify evidence-based practice in nursing as a problem-solving approach that integrates evidence from research, evidence-based theories, opinion leaders or expert panels, one's own clinical experience, and information about the patient's preferences and values (pp. 6–7). Hasseler (2006) describes evidence-based nursing as based on scientific knowledge integrated into the individual's circumstances that provides both an instrument for decision making and the concept of lifelong learning with the multiple aims of providing successful and cost-effective nursing care, improving the quality of care, and optimizing nursing outcomes. Within this text, the type of evidence most appropriate for application of a theory will vary from theory to theory. For some, empirical evidence is entirely appropriate; for others, only qualitative evidence is appropriate. In considering each of the theories for use in practice, think about the relationship of each theory to the nursing process, critical thinking, patterns of knowing, and evidence-based nursing.

Using Nursing Theory in Clinical Practice

To assist the reader in comparing and contrasting them, this chapter provides a review of the models and theories discussed in this text. Following this review, each of these will be discussed in relation to nursing practice using the same case study. The resulting comparison should assist the readers in identifying those models and theories of greatest interest or utility for their own practice. Where applicable, the six-step nursing process format described earlier will be used in this comparison.

Florence Nightingale believed that the force for healing resides within the human being and that, if the environment is appropriately supportive, humans will seek to heal themselves. Her 13 canons indicate the areas of environment of concern to nursing. These are ventilation and warming, health of houses (pure air, pure water, efficient drainage, cleanliness, and light), petty management (today known as continuity of care), noise, variety, taking food, what food, bed and bedding, light, cleanliness of rooms and walls, personal cleanliness, chattering hopes and advices, and observation of the sick.

Hildegard E. Peplau focused on the interpersonal relationship between the nurse and the patient. The three phases of this relationship are orientation, working, and termination. The relationship is initiated by the patient's felt need and termination occurs when the need is met. Both the nurse and the patient grow as a result of their interaction.

Virginia Henderson first defined nursing as doing for others what they lack the strength, will, or knowledge to do for themselves and then identified 14 components of care. These components provide a guide to identifying areas in which a person may lack the strength, will, or knowledge to meet personal needs. They include breathing, eating and drinking, eliminating, moving, sleeping and resting, dressing and undressing appropriately, maintaining body temperature, keeping clean and protecting the skin, avoiding dangers and injury to others, communicating, worshiping, working, playing, and learning.

Dorothea E. Orem identified three theories of self-care, self-care deficit, and nursing systems. The ability of the person to meet daily requirements is known as self-care, and carrying out those activities is self-care agency. Parents serve as dependent care agents for their children. The ability to provide self-care is influenced by basic conditioning factors including but not limited to age, gender, and developmental state. Self-care needs are partially determined by the self-care requisites, which are categorized as universal (air, water, food, elimination, activity and rest, solitude and social interaction, hazard prevention, function within social groups), developmental, and health deviation (needs arising from injury or illness and from efforts to treat the injury or illness). The total demands created by the self-care requisites are identified as therapeutic self-care demand. When the therapeutic self-care demand exceeds self-care agency, a self-care deficit exists, and nursing is needed. Based on the needs, the nurse designs nursing systems that are wholly compensatory (the nurse provides all needed care), partly compensatory (the nurse and the patient provide care together), or supportive-educative (the nurse provides needed support and education for the patient to exercise self-care).

Dorothy E. Johnson stated that nursing's area of concern is the behavioral system that consists of seven subsystems. The subsystems are attachment or affiliative, dependency, ingestive, eliminative, sexual, aggressive, and achievement. The behaviors for each of the subsystems occur as a result of the drive, set, choices, and goal of the subsystem. The purpose of the behaviors is to reduce tensions and keep the behavioral system in balance.

Ida Jean Orlando described a disciplined nursing process. Her process is initiated by the patient's behavior. This behavior engenders a reaction in the nurse, described as an automatic perception, thought, or feeling. The nurse shares the reaction with the patient, identifying it as the nurse's perception, thought, or feeling, and seeking validation of the accuracy of the reaction. Once the nurse and the patient have agreed on the immediate need that led to the patient's behavior and to the action to be taken by the nurse to meet that need, the nurse carries out a deliberative action. Any action taken by the nurse for reasons other than meeting the patient's immediate need is an automatic action.

Lydia E. Hall believed that persons over the age of 16 who were past the acute stage of illness required a different focus for their care than during the acute stage. She described the circles of care, core, and cure. Activities in the care circle belong solely to nursing and involve bodily care and comfort. Activities in the core circle are shared with all members of the health care team and involve the person and therapeutic use of self. Hall believed the drive to recovery must come from within the person. Activities in the cure circle also are shared with other members of the health care team and may include the patient's family. The cure circle focuses on the disease and the medical care.

Faye G. Abdellah sought to change the focus of care from the disease to the patient and thus proposed patient-centered approaches to care. She identified 21 nursing problems, or areas vital to the growth and functioning of humans that require support from nurses when persons are for some reason limited in carrying out the activities needed to provide such growth. These areas are hygiene and comfort, activity (including exercise, rest, and sleep), safety, body mechanics, oxygen, nutrition, elimination, fluid and electrolyte balance, recognition of physiological responses to disease, regulatory mechanisms, sensory functions, emotions, interrelatedness of emotions and illness, communication, interpersonal relationships, spiritual goals, therapeutic environment, individuality, optimal goals, use of community resources, and role of society.

Ernestine Wiedenbach proposed a prescriptive theory that involves the nurse's central purpose, prescription to fulfill that purpose, and the realities that influence the ability to fulfill the central purpose (the nurse, the patient, the goal, the means, and the framework or environment). Nursing involves the identification of the patient's need for help, the ministration of help, and validation that the efforts made were indeed helpful. Her principles of helping indicate the nurse should look for patient behaviors that are not consistent with what is expected, should continue helping efforts in spite of encountering difficulties, and should recognize personal limitations and seek help from others as needed. Nursing actions may be reflex or spontaneous and based on sensations, conditioned or automatic and based on perceptions, impulsive and based on assumptions, or deliberate or responsible and based on realization, insight, design, and decision that involves discussion and joint planning with the patient.

Joyce Travelbee was concerned with the interpersonal process between the professional nurse and that nurse's client, whether an individual, family, or community. The functions of the nurse–client, or human-to-human, relationship are to prevent or cope with illness or suffering and to find meaning in illness or suffering. This relationship requires a disciplined, intellectual approach, with the nurse employing a therapeutic use of self. The five phases of the human-to-human relationship are encounter, identities, empathy, sympathy, and rapport.

Myra Estrin Levine described adaptation as the process by which conservation is achieved, with the purpose of conservation being integrity, or preservation of the whole of the person. Adaptation is based on past experiences of effective responses (historicity), the use of responses specific to the demands being made (specificity), and more than one level of response (redundancy). Adaptation seeks the best fit between the person and the environment. The principles of conservation deal with conservation of energy, structural integrity, personal integrity, and social integrity of the individual.

Imogene M. King presented both a systems-based conceptual framework of personal, interpersonal, and social systems and a theory of goal attainment. The concepts of the theory of goal attainment are interaction, perception, communication, transaction, self, role, stress, growth and development, time, and personal space. The nurse and the client usually meet as strangers. Each brings to this meeting perceptions and judgments about the situation and the other; each acts and then reacts to the other's action. The reactions lead to interaction, which, when effective, leads to transaction or movement toward mutually agreed-on goals. She emphasizes that both the nurse and the patient bring important knowledge and information to this goal-attainment process.

Martha E. Rogers identified the basic science of nursing as the Science of Unitary Human Beings. The human being is a whole, not a collection of parts. She presented the human being and the environment as energy fields that are integral with each other. The human being does not have an energy field but is an energy field. These fields can be identified by their pattern, described as a distinguishing characteristic that is perceived as a single wave. These patterns occur in a pandimensional world. Rogers's principles are resonancy, or continuous change to higher frequency; helicy, or unpredictable movement toward increasing diversity; and integrality, or the continuous mutual process of the human field and the environmental field.

Sister Callista Roy proposed the Roy Adaptation Model. The person or group responds to stimuli from the internal or external environment through control processes or coping mechanisms identified as the regulator and cognator (stabilizer and innovator for the group) subsystems. The regulator processes are essentially automatic, while the cognator processes involve perception, learning, judgment, and emotion. The results of the processing by these coping mechanisms are behaviors in one of four modes. These modes are the physiological–physical mode (oxygenation; nutrition; elimination; activity and rest; protection; senses; fluid, electrolyte, and acid–base balance; and endocrine function for individuals and resource adequacy for groups), self-concept–group identity mode, role function mode, and interdependence mode. These behaviors may be either adaptive (promoting the integrity of the human system) or ineffective (not promoting such integrity). The nurse assesses the behaviors in each of the modes and identifies those adaptive behaviors that need support and those ineffective behaviors that require intervention. For each of these behaviors, the nurse then seeks to identify the associated stimuli. The stimulus most directly associated with the behavior is the focal stimulus; all other stimuli that are verified as influencing the behavior are contextual stimuli. Any stimuli that may be influencing the behavior but that have not been verified as doing so are residual stimuli. Once the stimuli are identified, the nurse, in cooperation with the patient, plans and carries out interventions to alter stimuli and support adaptive behaviors. The effectiveness of the actions taken is evaluated.

Betty Neuman developed the Neuman Systems Model. Systems have three environments—the internal, the external, and the created environment. Each system, whether an individual or a group, has several structures. The basic structure or core is where the energy resources reside. This core is protected by lines of resistance that in turn are surrounded by the normal line of defense and finally the flexible line of defense. Each of the structures consists of the five variables of physiological, psychological, sociocultural, developmental, and spiritual characteristics. Each variable is influenced by intrapersonal, interpersonal, and extrapersonal factors. The system seeks a state of equilibrium that may be disrupted by stressors. Stressors, either existing or potential, first encounter the flexible line of defense. If the flexible line of defense cannot counteract the stressor, then the normal line of defense is activated. If the normal line of defense is breached, the stressor enters the system and leads to a reaction, associated with the lines of resistance. This reaction is what is usually termed *symptoms*. If the lines of resistance allow the stressor to reach the core, depletion of energy resources and death are threatened. In the Neuman Systems Model, there are three levels of prevention. Primary prevention occurs before a stressor enters the system and causes a reaction. Secondary prevention occurs in response to the symptoms, and tertiary prevention seeks to support maintenance of stability and to prevent future occurrences.

Kathryn E. Barnard's focus is on the circumstances that enhance the development of the young child. In her Child Health Assessment Interaction Model, the key components are the child, the caregiver, the environment, and the interactions between child and caregiver. Contributions made by the child include temperament and ability to regulate and by the caregiver physical health, mental health, coping, and level of education. The environment includes both animate and inanimate resources. In assessing interaction, the parent is assessed in relation to sensibility to cues, fostering emotional growth, and fostering cognitive growth. The infant is assessed in relation to clarity of cue given and responsiveness to parent.

Josephine E. Paterson and *Loretta T. Zderad* presented humanistic nursing. Humans are seen as becoming through choices, and health is a personal value of more-being and well-being. Humanistic nursing involves dialogue, community, and phenomenologic nursology. Dialogue occurs through meeting the other, relating with the other, being in presence together, and sharing through call and response. Community is the sense of "we." Phenomenologic nursology involves the nurse preparing to know another, having intuitive responses to another, learning about the other scientifically, synthesizing information about the other with information already known, and developing a truth that is both uniquely personal and generally applicable.

Madeleine M. Leininger provided a guide to the inclusion of culture as a vital aspect of nursing practice. Her Sunrise Model posits that important dimensions of culture and social structure are technology, religion, philosophy, kinship and other related social factors, cultural values and lifeways, politics, law, economics, and education within the context of language and environment. All of these influence care patterns and expressions that impact the health or well-being of individuals, families, groups, and institutions. The diverse health systems include the folk care systems and the professional care systems that are linked by nursing. To provide culture congruent care, nursing decisions and actions should seek to provide culture care preservation or maintenance, culture care accommodation or negotiation, or culture care repatterning or restructuring.

Margaret Newman described health as expanding consciousness. Important concepts are consciousness (the information capacity of the system), pattern (movement, diversity, and rhythm of the whole), pattern recognition (identification within the observer of the whole of another), and transformation (change). Health and disease are seen as reflections of the larger whole rather than as different entities. She proposed (with Sime and Corcoran-Perry) the unitary–transformative paradigm in which human beings are viewed as unitary phenomenon. These phenomenon are identified by pattern, and change is unpredictable, toward diversity, and transformative. Stages of disorganization, or choice points, lead to change, and health is the evolving pattern of the whole as the system moves to higher levels of consciousness. The nurse enters into process with a client and does not serve as a problem solver.

Jean Watson described nursing as human science and human care. Her clinical caritas processes include practicing loving-kindness and equanimity within a context of caring consciousness; being authentically present and enabling and sustaining the deep belief system and subjective life world of self and one-being-cared-for; cultivating one's own spiritual practice and transpersonal self, developing and sustaining helping-trusting in an authentic caring relationship; being present to and supportive of the expression of positive and negative feelings as a connection with the deeper spirit of self and the one-being-cared-for; creatively using self and all ways of knowing as a part of the caring process to engage in artistry of caring-healing practices; engaging in a genuine teaching-learning experience that attends to unity of being and meaning while attempting to stay within other's frame of reference; creating healing environments at all levels, physical as well as nonphysical, within a subtle environment of energy and consciousness, whereby the potentials of wholeness, beauty, comfort, dignity, and peace are enhanced; assisting with basic needs, with an intentional caring consciousness, to potentiate alignment of mind/body/spirit, wholeness, and unity of being in all aspects of care; tending to both embodied spirit and evolving spiritual emergence; opening and attending to spiritual-mysterious and existential dimensions of one's own life-death; and soul care for self and the one-being-cared-for. These caritas processes occur within a transpersonal caring relationship and a caring occasion and caring moment as the nurse and other come together and share with each other. The transpersonal caring relationship seeks to provide mental and spiritual growth for both participants while seeking to restore or improve the harmony and unity within the personhood of the other.

Rosemarie Rizzo Parse developed the theory of *Humanbecoming* within the simultaneity paradigm that views human beings as developing meaning through freedom to choose and as more than and different from a sum of parts. Her practice methodology has three dimensions, each with a related process. The first is illuminating meaning, or explicating, or making clear through talking about it, what was, is, and will be. The second is synchronizing rhythms, or dwelling with or being immersed with the process of connecting and separating within the rhythms of the exchange between the human and the universe. The third is mobilizing transcendence, or moving beyond or moving toward what is envisioned, the moment to what has not yet occurred. In the theory of Humanbecoming, the nurse is an interpersonal guide, with the responsibility for decision making (or making of choices) residing in the client. The nurse provides support but not counseling. However, the traditional role of teaching does fall within illuminating meaning, and serving as a change agent is congruent with mobilizing transcendence.

Helen C. Erickson, Evelyn M. Tomlin, and *Mary Ann P. Swain* presented the theory of Modeling and Role-Modeling. Both modeling and role-modeling involve an art and a science. Modeling requires the nurse to seek an understanding of the client's view of the world. The art of modeling involves the use of empathy in developing this understanding. The science of modeling involves the use of the nurse's knowledge in analyzing the information collected to create the model. Role-modeling seeks to facilitate health. The art of role-modeling lies in individualizing the facilitations, while the science lies in the use of the nurse's theoretical knowledge base to plan and implement care. The aims of intervention are to build trust, promote the client's positive orientation of self, promote the client's perception of being in control, promote the client's strengths, and set mutual health-directed goals. The client has self-care knowledge about what his needs are and self-care resources to help meet these needs and takes self-care action to use the resources to meet the needs. In addition, a major motivation for human behavior is the drive for affiliated individuation, or having a personal identity while being connected to others. The individual's ability to mobilize resources is identified as adaptive potential. Adaptive potential may be identified as adaptive equilibrium (a nonstress state in which resources are utilized appropriately), maladaptive equilibrium (a nonstress state in which resource utilization is placing one or more subsystems in jeopardy), arousal (a stress state in which the client is having difficulty mobilizing resources), or impoverishment (a stress state in which resources are diminished or depleted). Interventions differ according to the adaptive potential. Those in adaptive equilibrium can be encouraged to continue and may require only facilitation of their self-care actions. Those in maladaptive equilibrium present the challenge of seeing no reason to change since they are in equilibrium. Here motivation strategies to seek to change are needed. Those in arousal are best supported by actions that facilitate change and support individuation; these are likely to include teaching, guidance, direction, and other assistance. Those in impoverishment have strong affiliation needs, need their internal strengths promoted, and need to have resources provided.

Nola J. Pender developed the Health Promotion Model (revised) with the goal of achieving outcomes of health-promoting behavior. Areas identified to help understand personal choices made in relation to health-promoting behavior include perceived benefits of action, perceived barriers to action, perceived self-efficacy (or ability to carry out the action), activity-related affect, interpersonal influences, situation influences, commitment to a plan of action, and immediate competing demands and preferences.

Patricia Benner described expert nursing practice and identified five stages of skill acquisition as novice, advanced beginner, competent, proficient, and expert. She discusses a number of concepts in relation to these stages, including agency, assumptions, expectations and set, background meaning, caring, clinical forethought, clinical judgment, clinical knowledge, clinical reasoning, clinical transitions, common meanings, concern, coping, skill acquisition, domains of practice, embodied intelligence, embodied knowledge, emotions, ethical judgment, experience, graded qualitative distinctions, intuition, knowing the patient, maxims, paradigm cases and personal knowledge, reasoning-in-transition, social embeddedness, stress, temporality, thinking-in-action, and unplanned practices.

Juliet Corbin and *Anselm L. Strauss* developed the Chronic Illness Trajectory Framework, in which they describe the course of illness and the actions taken to shape that course. The phases of the framework are pretrajectory, trajectory onset, stable, unstable, acute, crisis, comeback, downward, and dying. A trajectory projection is one's personal vision of the illness, and a trajectory scheme is the plan of actions to shape the course of the illness, control associated symptoms, and handle disability. Important also are one's biography or life story and one's everyday life activities (similar to activities of daily living).

Anne Boykin and *Savina Schoenhofer* present nursing as caring in a grand theory that may be used in combination with other theories. Persons are caring by virtue of being human; are caring, moment to moment; are whole and complete in the moment; and are already complete while growing in completeness. Personhood is the process of living grounded in caring and is enhanced through nurturing relationships. Nursing as a discipline is a being, knowing, living, and valuing response to a social call. As a profession, nursing is based on a social call and uses a body of knowledge to respond to that call. The focus of nursing is nurturing persons living in caring and growing in caring. This nurturing occurs in the nursing situation, or the lived experience shared between the nurse and the nursed, in which personhood is enhanced. The call for nursing is not based on a need or a deficit and thus focuses on helping the other celebrate the fullness of being rather than seeking to fix something. Boykin and Schoenhofer encourage the use of storytelling to make evident the service of nursing.

Katharine Kolcaba developed a comfort theory in which she describes comfort, comfort care, comfort measures, and comfort needs as well as health-seeking behavior, institutional integrity, and intervening variables. She speaks of comfort as physical, psychospiritual, environmental, and sociocultural and describes technical comfort measures, coaching for comfort, and comfort food for the soul.

Ramona Mercer describes the process of becoming a mother in the four stages of commitment, attachment, and preparation; acquaintance, learning, and physical restoration; moving toward a new normal; and achievement of the maternal identity. The stages occur with the three nested living environments of family and friends, community, and society at large.

Afaf Meleis, in her theory of transitions, identifies four types of transitions: developmental, situational, health–illness, and organizational. Properties of the transition experience include awareness, engagement, change and difference, time span, critical points, and events. Personal conditions include meanings, cultural beliefs and attitudes, socioeconomic status, and preparation and knowledge. Community conditions include family support, information available, health care resources, and role models. Process indicators are feeling connected, interacting, location, and being situated and developing confidence and coping. Outcome indicators include mastery and fluid integrative processes.

Merle H. Mishel describes uncertainty in illness with the three major themes of antecedents of uncertainty, appraisal of uncertainty, and coping with uncertainty. Antecedents of uncertainty are the stimuli frame, including symptom pattern, event familiarity, and event congruence; cognitive capacity or informational processing ability; and structure providers, such as education, social support, and credible authorities. Appraisal of uncertainty includes both inference (use of past experience to evaluate an event) and illusion (creating beliefs from uncertainty with a positive outlook). Coping with uncertainty includes danger, opportunity, coping, and adaptation. The Reconceptualized Uncertainty in Illness Theory adds self-organization and probabilistic thinking and changes the goal from return to previous level of functioning to growth to a new value system.

Each of these models or theories will be applied to clinical practice with the following case study:

> May Allenski, an 84-year-old White female, had emergency femoral-popliteal bypass surgery two days ago. She has severe peripheral vascular disease, and a clot blocked 90% of the circulation to her right leg one week ago. The grafts were taken from her left leg, so there are long incisions in each leg. She lives in a small town about 75 miles from the medical center. The initial clotting occurred late on Friday night; she did not see a doctor until Monday. The first physician referred her to a vascular specialist, who then referred her to the medical center. Her 90-year-old husband drove her to the medical center on Tuesday. You anticipate she will be discharged to home on the fourth postoperative day, as is standard procedure. She is learning to transfer to and from bed and toilet to wheelchair.

Table 2-1 shows examples of application in clinical practice that are not complete but are intended to provide only a partial example for each. Study of these examples can provide ideas or suggestions for use in clinical practice. Readers are encouraged to develop further detail as appropriate to their practice.

TABLE 2-1   Application of Theories in Clinical Practice

Florence Nightingale's Environmental Focus
Assessment
Ventilation and warming: Room temperature controlled; uses an extra blanket because she is "always cold"
Health of houses (pure air, pure water, efficient drainage, cleanliness, and light), bed and bedding, cleanliness of rooms and walls: Hospital environment meets these satisfactorily
Petty management: There is a written plan of care for the nursing staff
Noise: 2-bed room is located near nurses' station: MA states she has trouble sleeping at night due to the noise
Variety: Able to move about the unit in wheelchair
Taking food: Can feed herself; states she is not very hungry
What food: On a low sodium diet
Light: Large window in the room provides natural lighting; well lit at night
Personal cleanliness: Able to bathe with assistance
Chattering hopes and advices: Only visitor is her husband
Observation of the sick: Vital signs are near her baseline data; wounds are healing normally

Diagnosis
Sleep pattern disturbance related to noisy environment

Outcomes
Adequate amount of sleep to support healing

Planning
Encourage night staff to hold all conversations quietly
Close door to room
Be certain lights are dimmed in room and that call light is within reach
Offer earplugs

Implementation
Planned activities were carried out—earplugs refused

Evaluation
On 4th postoperative day, reported "slept better last night"

Hildegard E. Peplau's Interpersonal Relationships
Assessment
Orientation: MA's expressed felt need is to go home

Diagnosis
Orientation: Relocation stress syndrome related to hospitalization

Outcomes
Working: To have access to needed care at home

Planning
Working: Home health nurse in hometown to provide support

Implementation
Working: Referral made to appropriate home health agency

Evaluation
Termination: MA discharged from medical center on 4th post op day (a Sunday). Monday is a holiday; home health agency personnel not available before Tuesday—outcome only partially met

(continued)

TABLE 2-1   **Continued**

Virginia Henderson's Definition and 14 Components
Assessment
Breathing: R 18; skin pink
Eating and drinking: States not very hungry; fluid intake 100 cc
Eliminating: Voiding without discomfort; no bowel movement since surgery, normally has at one daily
Moving: Able to move self about in bed; learning to transfer to wheelchair
Sleeping and resting: States not sleeping well due to noisy environment
Dressing and undressing appropriately: Dressed in hospital gown and own robe and slippers
Maintaining body temperature: T 98.9° F.*Keeping clean and protecting the skin:* Needs assistance with washing back and feet.
Avoiding dangers and injury to others: Learning safe transfer techniques; needs information on dressing changes
Communicating: Hears best when wearing glasses; expresses self clearly
Worshiping: No information available
Working: Has always cared for own home
Playing: Enjoys reading and watching tennis on television
Learning: Reads for information; avid TV news watcher

Diagnosis
Risk of constipation related to low fiber and fluid intake and to decrease in exercise

Outcomes
Restoration of normal bowel function

Planning
Have fluid and fiber intake adequate to restore normal bowel functioning within one week

Implementation
Identify favorite foods and fluids
Identify who will be fixing meals at home
Ascertain her knowledge about fluid and fiber intake (her college education was in home economics). Mutually develop a plan of tempting sources of fiber and fluids to increase her intake

Evaluation
By discharge had increased fluid intake to 250 cc daily; fiber intake remained limited.
State not hungry or interested in food.
Reassessment: Need to investigate if this disinterest is evidence of depression.

Dorothea E. Orem's Theories of Self-Care
Assessment
Universal self-care requisites:
Air—Breathing normally, lung sounds clear
Water—Fluid intake of 100cc qd
Food—States has no appetite, eating about ¼ of what is served on each meal tray
Elimination—Voiding adequately; no bowel movement since surgery
Activity and rest—Can position self in bed, learning to transfer to and from wheelchair
Solitude and social interaction—Only visitor is her husband. No family living in area. Interacts with roommate
Hazard prevention—bed rails are kept up, call bell within reach
Function within social groups—at home interacts with friends through their visits to her home; used to play bridge but she and husband are the only members of the group still living

Development self-care requisites: See function within social groups

Health deviation self-care requisites: Cannot walk due to surgical involvement of both legs; has fresh incision bilaterally, history of hypertension

Diagnosis
Self-care deficit in ability to continue to care for self and home independently

Outcomes
Safe and adequate care at home for self and husband

Planning
Identify changed areas of self-care needs.

Identify sources of meeting each of these needs.

Assist the family in making contact with these sources.

Implementation
Discuss with MA and her husband how they can handle meal preparation, housekeeping, and health deviation care needs.

Evaluation
After they return home, Mr. A will find a housekeeper who help with meals, housecleaning, laundry, and MA's dressing and hygiene needs.

Dorothy E. Johnson's Behavioral System

Assessment
Attachment or affiliative: Husband drove her to the medical center and has stayed in a nearby motel. He visits daily.

Dependency: MA hesitates to ask for needed help—states she is used to being able to care for herself and it is hard to have others do for her.

Ingestive: Likes her coffee hot and ice cream cold.

Eliminative: Usually has a bowel movement every morning after breakfast.

Sexual: Kisses her husband each time he leaves.

Aggressive: No data

Achievement: No data

Diagnosis
Discrepancy in dependency subsystem: has difficulty asking for needed help.

Outcomes
Able to seek help appropriately

Planning
MA will identify areas in which she needs help.

Ma will plan how to seek the needed help.

Implementation
Discuss with MA what she can do for herself, and what she needs help to do.

Discuss what would make her more comfortable in accepting help.

Plan with her how she can seek and accept help in a way that is comfortable for her.

Evaluation
By discharge, MA is calling the nurse for supervision in transferring from bed to chair and is clearly verbalizing exactly what she needs.

(continued)

TABLE 2-1 Continued

Ida Jean Orlando's Disciplined Nursing Process

Assessment

MA's behavior: Rubbing one hand with the other

Nurse's reaction: Perception—she is anxious or worried. Perception is shared—MA says, no, her joints hurt from arthritis and she has not had her medication for it.

Diagnosis

Immediate need: Relief from arthritis pain

Outcomes

Comfort

Planning

Within one hour after receiving pain medication, the joint pain will be alleviated.

Implementation

Deliberative action: MA and the nurse agree that the ordered NSAID would be appropriate; the nurse obtains the medication for MA

Evaluation

In one hour, MA reports her hands feel much better.

Lydia E. Hall's Care, Core, and Cure

Assessment

Care: Able to provide most of own hygiene, needs help bathing back and feet. Having little pain from surgical sites but needs pain relief for arthritis pain in hands and hips.

Core: Does not like being in hospital, wants to be at home. Will not discuss how she will be cared for at home.

Cure: Incisions are healing normally, pedal pulses present in both feet although diminished on the right.

Diagnosis

Relocation stress syndrome related to hospitalization

Outcomes

Have MA involved in solving the challenges associated with her care needs at home

Planning

Develop a plan of care to be used at home

Implementation

Identify with MA what she can do for herself.

Identify with MA what she will need help doing (for example, dressing changes, preparing meals, housekeeping chores).

Include MA in problem solving how these needs can be met—e.g., home health referral.

Evaluation

MA agreed to home health referral and indicated her husband will find someone to help with the housekeeping. Also, he can cook.

Faye G. Abdellah's Patient-Centered Approach to Care

Assessment

Hygiene and comfort: Can position self in bed; needs medication for arthritis pain; needs assistance washing back and feet.

Activity (including exercise, rest, and sleep): Cannot walk on own at present; states not sleeping well due to noise from nurses' station

Safety: Bed rails are up when in bed; call bell in reach

Body mechanics: Learning appropriate transfer techniques.

Oxygen: R 18, lung sounds clear, skin pink

Nutrition: Eating about ¼ of food served at each meal; fluid intake 100 cc in 24 hours

Elimination: Voiding adequately, urine clear and yellow; no bowel movement since surgery

Fluid and electrolyte balance: Lab values WNL

Recognition of physiological responses to disease: Reduced pedal pulse on right

Regulatory mechanisms: Lab values WNL

Sensory functions: Wears glasses, slightly hard of hearing, states often cannot tell if she has a good grip on an object or not

Emotions: Teary about this sudden change in her ability to be independent

Interrelatedness of emotions and illness: Recognizes her emotional responses to this illness

Communication: Communicates clearly

Interpersonal relationships: Husband visits daily

Spiritual goals: Not expressed

Therapeutic environment: Says would feel better at home

Individuality: Able to select desired foods—little other opportunity to express her individuality

Optimal goals: To function independently and care for her own home again

Use of community resources: Will need home health referral

Role of society: No apparent social contribution to current problems

Diagnosis
Risk for activity intolerance

Outcomes
Able to carry out activities of daily living independently

Planning
Will be able to transfer to and from wheelchair safely by discharge
Will gradually resume walking, first using a walker and then independently

Implementation
Physical therapy twice daily to teach about and prepare muscles for transfer activities Home health referral for physical therapy at home to assist in walking

Evaluation
Able to safely transfer by time of discharge. Home health referral made for physical therapy at home

Ernestine Wiedenbach's Prescriptive Theory of Nursing
Assessment
The nurse's central purpose is to educate her patients so they can care for themselves effectively. The nurse (the agent) assesses that MA (the recipient) will need to know how to assess healing of her incisions (the goal).

Diagnosis
Altered protection related to compromised circulation secondary to severe peripheral vascular disease

Outcomes
Cleanly healed surgical incisions

Planning
MA will describe the signs and symptoms of healing and of delayed healing.

Implementation
The means: teach MA about the signs and symptoms to be observed and actions to be taken to support healing or in response to delayed healing.

(continued)

TABLE 2-1 Continued

Ernestine Wiedenbach's Prescriptive Theory of Nursing

Evaluation

By discharge, the nurse had not been able to have this discussion with MA due to the time MA spent in physical therapy and the nurse's days off.

Joyce Travelbee's

Nurse SP seeks to establish a human-to-human relationship with MA through knowing herself and MA— meeting as strangers, moving to recognizing uniquenesses. SP, moving into empathy recognizes MA's lack of appetite is associated with her feelings about being away from home and concerns about every being able to take care of her home again. SP pats MA's hand when MA tears up talking about this (sympathy). From this, rapport grows and MA feels SP at least somewhat understands her situation.

Myra E. Levine's Adaptation and Principles of Conservation

Assessment

Conservation of energy: Vital signs and lab values WNL. MA naps in room after returning from physical therapy.

Conservation of structural integrity: Surgical wounds are seeping and are slightly reddened

Conservation of personal integrity: MA does not want to talk about herself

Conservation of social integrity: MA's husband brought her to the medical center and visits daily.

Diagnosis

Need to conserve structural integrity: ensure wound healing

Outcomes

Clean healing of surgical wounds.

Planning

Avoid infection of surgical wounds

Implementation

Keep wounds clean, expose to air at least four hours a day.

Position with legs elevated to encourage circulation

Evaluation

At discharge, wounds are seeping serous fluid, no indication of infection.

Imogene M. King's Theory of Goal Attainment

Assessment

Growth and development: "Senior citizen," accustomed to caring for self and home

View of self: Independently functioning, self-sufficient person

Perception of current health status: Ability to care for self and home now limited due to mobility difficulties

Communication patterns: Does not talk much about self and her emotions

Role: Wife, homemaker, mother, and grandmother

Sensory system: At times cannot tell if she has a grip on an object, wears glasses, slightly hard of hearing, very sensitive skin on shoulder where had shingles

Education: College graduate, taught in a one-room school before marriage. Reads and watches TV to keep current

Drug history: Has taken medication for high blood pressure for 40 years, also takes NSAIDs for arthritis.

Diet history: Has followed low-fat, low-sodium diet for 35 to 40 years.

Diagnosis

Altered role performance related to surgery

Outcomes
Adjustment to changes in role

Planning
Mutually establish goal for MA to be able to work with support services at home

Implementation
Help MA identify what would increase her comfort level with having help at home—how to let them know what she would like done and how she would like for it to be done without feeling she is being too demanding.

Evaluation
At time of discharge MA not able to make such identifications—included as a need in home health referral

Martha E. Rogers' Science of Unitary Human Beings

Pattern manifestation knowing indicates that the energy field patterns of the human and environmental fields point to a disruption due to environmental noise disturbing sleep. Voluntary mutual patterning indicates MA's preference is to go home but in the meantime she suggests closing the door to the room during the night hours and asks for pain medication at hs. After the first night, she indicates she slept a little bit better.

Sister Callista Roy's Adaptation Model

Assessment
Physiological-physical mode:
Oxygenation—R 18, skin pink, lung sounds clear
Nutrition—eating about ¼ of food served, fluid intake 100 cc
Elimination—voiding adequately, no bowel movement since surgery
Activity and rest—reports not sleeping well at night; learning to transfer to and from wheelchair
Protection—protective dressings on leg wounds
Senses—wears glasses, slightly hard of hearing
Fluid, electrolyte, and acid-base balance—Lab values WNL
Endocrine function—Lab values WNL
Self-concept-group identity mode: A senior citizen
Role function mode: Married, has cared for own home
Interdependence mode: Social contact with others occurs through visits to her home and via telephone. Primary relationship is with husband.
Focal stimulus: Noise at night
Contextual stimuli: Different bed, postoperative discomfort
Residual stimuli: Arthritis

Diagnosis
Sleep pattern disruption

Outcomes
Adequate rest to support healing

Planning
Will sleep seven to eight hours at night by time of discharge.

Implementation
Since she is stable postoperatively, move her to a room farther from the nurses' station.
Offer pain medication at hs.
Close door to room at hs.

(continued)

TABLE 2-1 Continued

Sister Callista Roy's Adaptation Model
Evaluation
On day of discharge, indicates she slept better last night— at least six hours, more like at home.

Betty Neuman's Systems Model
Assessment
Major stressor: Blood clot that led to secondary prevention of emergency surgery
Life-style patterns: Maintained own home with husband
Coping patterns: "Grin and bear it," do what is necessary
Perception of future: Hope to return to independence
Ability to help self: Will do what doctors say
Care from others: Husband will help and maybe daughter, who is a nurse, will be able to come help out for a few days
Physical factors: History of hypertension, severe peripheral vascular disease. Bilateral incisions on legs
Psycho-sociocultural factors: Lives with husband in own home
Development: Normal for age
Spiritual beliefs: No information
Resources: Adequate finances; on Medicare

Diagnosis
To regain system stability, need to heal surgical incisions, regain strength to walk again and regain independence

Outcomes
Regain independence

Planning
By two weeks after surgery, incisions will be healing without sign of infection.
By one month after surgery will be ambulatory.
By two months after surgery, will be independent except for housecleaning.

Implementation
Teach MA how to care for incisions and observations to make.
Make referral for home health physical therapy.

Evaluation
At time of discharge, signs of healing were appropriate.
Data not yet available for longer time frames.

Katharyn Barnard's Child Health Assessment Interaction Model
Not applicable; however, the concepts of cues and responses could be used to assess communication patterns

Josephine E. Paterson and Loretta T. Zderad's Humanistic Nursing
Assessment
Nurse preparing to know: The nurse has a B.S.N. and five-years experience on the vascular surgery unit.
Nurse knowing other intuitively: Nurse perceives MA as unhappy to be in the hospital and dealing with the stress as best she can.
Nursing knowing other scientifically: Notes history of hypertension, lab values within normal limits.

Diagnosis
Synthesizing information about the other with information already known, and developing a truth that is both uniquely personal and generally applicable: Normal reaction to emergency surgery

Outcomes
Be with MA and encourage and support her efforts to regain well-being and develop more-being
Consider educational needs of MA and her family members.

Madeleine M. Leininger's Theory of Culture Care Diversity and Universality
Assessment
In addition to the information she already has about MA, the nurse learns that MA's culture places emphasis on the importance of independence and taking care of one's self and one's family. She believes in seeking professional care when symptoms lie outside the range of her folk care system knowledge. She also believes that it is important to follow the directions of the professional care provider.

Diagnosis
Altered role performance related to surgery

Outcomes
Regain ability to perform role

Planning
Through culture congruent care, heal from surgery and walk again.

Implementation
Culture care preservation: Provide foods she likes prepared in the manner she prefers.
Culture care accommodation: Provide small frequent meals to tempt failing appetite
Culture care repatterning: If she is not able to walk, provide ramp for the front porch so she can enter and exit the house.

Evaluation
At time of discharge, appetite remained poor. Activities need to be ongoing.

Margaret Newman's Health as Expanding Consciousness
MA is at a choice point as she must function differently, at least temporarily. The nurse seeks to be present with her, providing support and information as called for by MA's pattern.

Jean Watson's Theory of Transpersonal Caring
Assessment
Caring interaction identifies functional deficits in relation to food and fluid intake, bowel elimination, mobility.

Diagnosis
Altered nutrition: Less than body requirements related to decreased appetite

Outcomes
Nutritional intake adequate to support healing and regaining function

Planning
By time of discharge, fluid intake will be at least 500 cc daily and nutrient intake will be at least 1200 calories.

Implementation
Explore with MA what foods and fluids are among her favorites. Provide them in frequent, small amounts.

Evaluation
By discharge, fluid intake 250 cc, nutrient intake 900 calories. Movement toward desired outcome but goal not reached.

(continued)

TABLE 2-1   Continued

Rosemarie Rizzo Parse's Theory of Human Becoming

The nurse seeks to be in true presence with MA—the nurse prepares to be open to MA and to focus on the moment at hand. In illuminating meaning, MA indicates this surgery is "the pits" because it limits her ability to continue in her accustomed life style; in synchronizing rhythms, MA is not willing (or not yet able) to discuss the changes she will be making in her lifestyle, and in mobilizing transcendence, MA is able to talk about what it might be like to prepare to go home.

Helen C. Erickson, Evelyn M. Tomlin, and Mary Ann P. Swain's Modeling and Role-Modeling

Assessment
MA is in a stress state due to the emergency surgery. She has not yet mobilized resources but is interested in doing so.

Diagnosis
MA is in a state of arousal.

Outcomes
MA's self-care actions will provide for appropriate use of resources and coping mechanisms.

Planning
MA will be facilitated in changing how she reaches her goals.
MA will be informed about techniques she can use to meet her self-care needs.

Implementation
As MA identifies her self-care needs, teaching and support will be provided to help her meet those needs.

Evaluation
Discharge 4 days postoperatively occurred before MA felt confident in her ability to meet her self-care needs. She could identify the needs but did not yet feel comfortable about the resources to meet them

Nola J. Pender's Health Promotion Model (revised)

Assessment
Personal: 84 year old, married white female, height 5'3", weight 105 #, able to care for self and home prior to surgery. Views herself as a capable person who has had relatively good health "considering my age," born and raised in the state, college education, husband's retirement income allows them to live comfortably
Perceived benefits: Being able to care for self and home again.
Perceived barriers: Not certain she has the physical strength in her hands and arms to use a wheelchair, and then a walker for physical therapy and to get around
Self-efficacy: "I can usually do whatever I set out to do, but I'm not so sure this time."
Interpersonal: husband hopes she'll get better and tries to encourage her
Situational: Options: can exercise to gain upper body strength or can just "sit there and grow mold"
Demand: primary desire is to be better
Environment: home is on one level which will be easier to navigate; but it is an older house and the doorways are barely wide enough for a wheelchair
Commitment: "I will do physical therapy both in the hospital and at home to get back on my feet."
Immediate demands and preferences:
Pain control and dressings make moving around difficult

Diagnosis
Immediately post surgery with health promotion need to heal incisions and regain strength to walk independently

Outcomes
Able to walk independently and care for self and home again

Planning

Encourage regular participation in Physical Therapy

Ensure referral to home health includes need for Physical Therapy

Implementation

Arrange care activities around PT schedule to avoid creating barriers to this therapy

Write home health referral to include PT

Evaluation

Five weeks post discharge, MA is able to get around at home via wheelchair; very limited use of the walker; unable to stand independently. During 5th post operative week is rehospitalized due to poor wound healing secondary to poor circulation.

Patricia Benner's Expert Nursing Practice

Assessment

Advanced Beginner

Surgical incisions have light drainage

Expert

Teary eyed when discussing the recent, abrupt changes in her life

Diagnosis

Advanced Beginner

Normal post surgical healing

Expert

Grieving loss of former independence

Anxious about the future

Outcomes

Advanced Beginner

Cleanly healed wounds

Expert

Regain as much independence as possible

Planning

Advanced Beginner

Follow care plan—elevate feet, change dressings

Expert

Provide opportunities for MS to talk about her concerns

Help MS explore how to deal with the areas of concern

Implementation

Advanced Beginner

Care plan followed

Expert

Sat with MA for a few quiet moments each day

Evaluation

Advanced Beginner

Wounds healing normally at discharge

Expert

MA's reluctance to talk about herself, and an early discharge, prevented any detailed discussion

(continued)

TABLE 2-1   Continued

Ramona Mercer's Becoming a Mother
Not applicable

Afaf Meleis' Theory of Transition
Assessment
Awareness: can explain events that led to surgery
Engagement: asking what she needs to do to care for the incisions
Change and difference: activity level changed from self care to dependence
Time span: Change to being ill has occurred over a relatively brief period of time; recovery is predicted to take weeks to months
Marker event: "My leg turned black"
Also assess personal, community and societal conditions

Diagnosis
Health-illness transition

Outcomes
Mastery of new skills needed to regain ability to care for self

Planning
Teach her incision care

Implementation
Demonstrate appropriate dressing change technique.
Discuss bathing procedures for cleanliness and to facilitate healing.
Provide home nursing referral for assistance with dressing changes after discharge home.

Evaluation
Wounds healing normally at discharge.
Home health referral made.

Merle Mishel's Uncertainty in Illness
Assessment
Antecedents of uncertainty: Totally new experience; never been in this hospital or had emergency surgery
Cognitive capacity: Alert and oriented; responds appropriately to new information
Structure: Education—needs information on wound care, exercise patterns; Social Support—husband is present; Credible authority—MA and husband respect health care providers and the information they offer
Appraisal of Uncertainty: very new experience with a high degree of uncertainty
Coping: Danger continues as do not yet know if circulation is adequately restored; seeking help on how to cope.
Self-organization: has dealt with chronic illness for decades; this is a new challenge to be incorporated into the rhythm of her life

Diagnosis
Increased uncertainty associated with sudden change in health status

Outcomes
Incorporate uncertainty into new life rhythm

Planning
Provide information and assistance needed to enhance ability to care for self

Implementation
Teach how to check circulation in her extremities to help her feel more informed about her healing process
Provide home health referral for dressing changes and help with ambulation

Evaluation
Assessment of circulation led to rehospitalization in a few weeks due to evidence of poor circulation

Juliet Corbin and Anselm L. Strauss's Chronic Illness Trajectory Framework

Assessment
Post surgery for circulatory impairment

40 year history of treatment for hypertension

Diagnosis
In crisis phase of the trajectory framework

Outcomes
Remove the threat to circulation

Move to comeback stage of the framework

Planning
Promote healing of wounds from surgery

Assist in regaining ability to provide care for self

Implementation
Keep feet elevated when sitting, change dressings as needed

Include physical therapy in helping MA learn bed to chair transfers

Evaluation
The immediate threat was removed by the surgery—continued evaluation needed.

MA able to transfer with minimal assistance

Anne Boykin and Savina Schoenhofer's Theory of Nursing as Caring
MA says she cannot sleep. The nurse offers a brief back rub to help her relax. After the back rub, the nurse straightens the linens and helps MA achieve a position of comfort in bed—on her side with a pillow at her back and another supporting her upper leg. The next morning MA reports having slept as well as she does at home and credits the caring response of the nurse, including the experience of human touch that occurred through the back rub, as making a major contribution to her ability to rest

Kathy Kolcaba's Comfort Theory

Assessment
Physical: pain from fresh incisions in both legs; arthritis in hands

Psychospiritual: "Will I ever be able to fix a meal in my kitchen again?"

Environment: "It is so noisy at night that I don't sleep well."

Sociocultural: lives with husband in own home with adequate finances

Diagnosis
Real or potential discomfort physically, psychospiritually, and environmentally

Outcomes
Pain relief for both incisional and arthritic pain

Long term goal—able to care for her home again

Able to sleep seven to eight hours each night

Planning
Give pain meds, including NSAIDs, in patterns she determines effective

Start limited physical activity—bed to wheelchair and wheelchair to toilet transfers

Provide quieter environment at night

(continued)

TABLE 2-1 Continued

Kathy Kolcaba's Comfort Theory

Implementation

NSAIDs given every six hours as she requested (unless she is sleeping)

Physical therapy to help MS learn transfer techniques

Change her room to one further away for the center of activity; at bedtime, dim the lights and pull her door closed after helping her settle into her desired sleeping position

Evaluation

MA indicates pain control is similar to what she had at home

Able to transfer to-from bed/wheelchair and toilet/wheelchair safely

Reports she is sleeping about six hours a night

PEARSON

EXPLORE mynursingkit™

MyNursingKit is your one stop for online chapter review materials and resources. Prepare for success with additional NCLEX®-style practice questions, interactive assignments and activities, web links, animations and videos, and more!

Register your access code from the front of your book at
www.mynursingkit.com.

References

American Nurses Association. (2004). *Nursing: Scope and standards of practice.* Washington, DC: Author.

Belenky, M. F., Clinchy, B. M., Goldberger, N. R., & Tarule, J. M. (1986). *Women's ways of knowing: The development of self, voice, and mind.* New York: Basic Books.

Carper, B. A. (2004). Fundamental patterns of knowing in nursing. In P. G. Reed, N. C. Shearer, & L. H. Nicoll (Eds.), *Perspectives on nursing theory* (pp. 221–228). Philadelphia: Lippincott Williams & Wilkins. (Reprinted from *Advances in Nursing Science, 1*[1], pp. 13–23)

Chinn, P. L., & Kramer, M. K. (2004). *Integrated knowledge development in nursing.* St. Louis: Mosby.

Fawcett, J., Watson, J., Neuman, B., Walker, P. H., & Fitzpatrick, J. J. (2004). On nursing theories and evidence. In P. G. Reed, N. C. Shearer, & L. H. Nicoll (Eds.), *Perspectives on nursing theory* (pp. 285–292). Philadelphia: Lippincott Williams & Wilkins. (Reprinted from *Journal of Nursing Scholarship, 33*[2], pp. 115–119)

Hasseler, M. (2006). Evidence based nursing practice and science. In H. S. Kim & I. Kollak (Eds.),

Nursing theories: Conceptual and philosophical foundations (pp. 215–235). New York: Springer.

Kataoka-Yahoro, M., & Saylor, C. (1994). A critical thinking model for nursing judgment. *Journal of Nursing Education, 33,* 351–356.

Melnyk, B. M., & Fineout-Overholt, E. (2005). *Evidence-based practice in nursing and healthcare: A guide to best practice.* Philadelphia: Lippincott Williams & Wilkins.

Paul, R. W., & Elder, L. (2002). *Critical thinking: Tools for taking charge of your professional and personal life.* Upper Saddle River, NJ: Prentice Hall.

Perry, W. G. (1970). *Forms of intellectual and ethical development in the college years.* New York: Holt, Rinehart & Winston.

Rubenfeld, M. G., & Scheffer, B. K. (1999). *Critical thinking in nursing: An interactive approach* (2nd ed.). Philadelphia: Lippincott.

Scriven, M., & Paul, R. (2004). *Defining critical thinking.* Retrieved April 15, 2007, from http://www.criticalthinking.org/aboutCT/definingCT.shtml

CHAPTER 3

Environmental Model
Florence Nightingale

Marie L. Lobo

Florence Nightingale was born in Florence, Italy, on May 12, 1820, during one of her parents' extensive trips abroad. As she grew up, her father provided her with a very broad education, which was unusual for Victorian women. According to her biographer, Sir Thomas Cook, Nightingale was a linguist; had a broad knowledge of science, mathematics, literature, and the arts; was well read in philosophy, history, politics, and economics; and as well was knowledgeable about the workings of government. She wanted to do more with her life than become the idle wife of an aristocrat. She had a strong belief in God, and for a time believed she had a religious calling.

Nightingale became a heroine in Great Britain as a result of her work in the Crimean War. Her description of the very poor sanitary conditions in the hospital wards at Scutari is overwhelming. She fought the bureaucracy for bandages, food, fresh bedding, and cleaning supplies for the invalid soldiers. At times she bought supplies with her own money. She demonstrated great concern for the well-being of the English soldier—well, injured, or sick—including assisting with the establishment of a laundry, a library, assistance with letter writing, a banking system so the soldiers could save their pay, and a hospital for the families who accompanied the soldiers to war. As well, she provided comfort to the critically ill and dying. Her managerial skills were often greater than those of many officers in the army. She spent the years after the Crimean War establishing schools of nursing and influencing public policy by lobbying her acquaintances about various of her concerns.

Nightingale was romanticized by Henry Wadsworth Longfellow in his poem "The Lady with the Lamp." Although this poem was meant to honor Nightingale, it may have done a great disservice to her because it ignored her superb management skills and ability to provide nursing care to both healthy and ill soldiers. Nightingale died on August 13, 1910, and she is honored each year in a commemorative service at St. Margaret's Church, East Wellow, Great Britain, where she is buried.

Nightingale is viewed as the mother of modern nursing. She synthesized information gathered in many of her life experiences to assist her in the development of modern nursing. Her place in history has been established. To understand how

Nightingale developed her conceptualization of nursing, it is helpful to review her roots. As noted, she was highly educated for a woman of the Victorian era. In seeking to use her knowledge, she was frustrated by prevailing social norms. Her desire to have a position that was useful to society was incompatible with nineteenth-century upper-class British society's expectations of women. While Nightingale was struggling with decisions about her life, the seeds of modern nursing were being planted in Germany.

Germany was the site of the first organized nursing school. In 1836 Pastor Theodor Fliedner, a protestant pastor in Kaiserswerth, Germany, opened a hospital in a "vacant textile factory with one patient, one nurse, and a cook" (Hegge, 1990, p. 74). When Fliedner realized there was no workforce for the hospital, he designed a school of nursing. The physician for Fliedner's hospital spent an hour a week teaching the nursing students. Gertrude Reichardt, the physician's daughter, taught anatomy and physiology, although her only experience had been gained at her father's side. Reichardt became the first matron of the Deaconess School of Nursing. Local peasant girls were taught hygiene, manners, and ladylike behavior as well as how to read, write, and calculate. There were no textbooks for nursing until 1837, when a German physician prepared a handbook.

Nightingale visited Kaiserswerth for 14 days in 1850 after a trip to Egypt. She applied for admission to the school with a 12-page, handwritten "curriculum" stating her reasons for wanting to be a nurse and entered the nursing program July 6, 1851, as the 134th nursing student to attend the Fliedner School of Nursing. She left Kaiserswerth on October 7, 1851, and was deemed to be educated as a nurse (Hegge, 1990). During the three months she spent studying with the sisters of Kaiserswerth, she developed skills in both nursing care and management, which she took back to England.

When Nightingale returned to England, she used the information from Kaiserswerth to champion her cause as a reformer for the health and well-being of the citizens. Her reform efforts occurred in part because she was frustrated with the conditions in England that limited women's life choices to "indolence, marriage, or servitude" as well as with the two existing social conditions of most of England's citizens: abject poverty or affluence (Nightingale, 1860).

In 1854 Nightingale went to the front of the Crimean War at the request of her friend, Sir Sidney Herbert, secretary at war. She arrived in Scutari on November 5, 1854, accompanied by 38 nurses. Nightingale's 19-month stay at Scutari was difficult. The idea of women being involved in the affairs of the military was difficult for many to accept. The hospital barracks were infested with fleas and rats, and sewage flowed under the wards. The mortality rate at the hospital was 42.7% of those treated, a mortality rate that was higher from disease than from war injuries (Cohen, 1984). Six months after Nightingale came to Scutari, the mortality rate at the hospital dropped to 2.2%. Nightingale achieved this drop in mortality by attending to the environment of the soldiers. A year and nine months after she landed at Scutari, on August 5, 1856, Nightingale returned from the Crimea. She sneaked into England to avoid a hero's welcome.

After her return to England, Nightingale used her knowledge of data concerning the health and well-being of soldiers to influence the decisions of the War Department by providing information to Sir Sidney Herbert. Many of the position papers and reports, although officially submitted by Sir Sidney Herbert, secretary at war, were virtually intact manuscripts written by Nightingale. Because of the position of women *in Victorian England, she was not permitted to submit her findings under her own name. Nightingale's role as a social reformer and contribution to public health has been recognized by sociologist McDonald (2006). Nightingale's contributions to the broader health and well-being of the British have often gone unrecognized.*

Nightingale was also a skilled statistician who used statistics to present her case for hospital reform. According to Cohen, "the idea of using statistics for such a purpose—to analyze social conditions and the effectiveness of public policy—is commonplace today, but at that time it was not" (Cohen, 1984, p. 132). Nightingale was regarded as a pioneer in the graphic display of statistics and was elected a fellow of the Royal Statistical Society in 1858. In 1874 an honorary membership in the American Statistical Association was bestowed on her (Agnew, 1958; Nightingale, 1859/1992). Given her reliance on observable data to support her position, it can be said that Nightingale was the first nurse researcher.

NIGHTINGALE'S APPROACH TO NURSING

Nightingale used her broad base of knowledge, her understanding of the incidence and prevalence of disease, and her acute powers of observation to develop an approach to nursing as well as to the management and construction of hospitals. Nightingale's main focus was the control of the environment of individuals and families, both healthy and ill. She discussed the need for ventilation and light in sickrooms, proper disposal of sewage, and appropriate nutrition. Her most frequently cited work, *Notes on Nursing*, was written not as a nursing text but to "give hints for thought to women who have personal charge of the health of others" (Nightingale, 1859/1992, preface). She did not intend for *Notes on Nursing* to become a manual for teaching nurses to nurse. Rather, *Notes on Nursing* is a thought-provoking essay on the organization and manipulation of the environment of those persons requiring nursing care. Nightingale stated that her purpose was "everyday sanitary knowledge, or the knowledge of nursing, or in other words, of how to put the constitution in such a state as that it will have no disease, or that it can recover from disease" (Nightingale, 1859/1992, preface). She wanted women to teach themselves to nurse and viewed *Notes on Nursing* as hints to enable them to do this. Nightingale viewed disease as a reparative process, a thought that is reflected in the American Nurses Association initial *Social Policy Statement* that nursing is the diagnosis and treatment of human responses to actual or potential health problems (American Nurses Association, 1980).

Although *Notes on Nursing* is Nightingale's most accessible work, she also wrote *Notes on Hospitals* and *Introductory Notes on Lying-in Institutions* (the first maternity centers) as well as numerous letters (Vicinus & Nergaard, 1990). In her volumes of writing she provided much information on the influence of the environment on the human being and the critical nature of balance between the human and his or her environment.[1] For example, Nightingale did not view pregnancy as a disease and recommended facilities away from those treating diseases in which women could bear

---

[1]The complete works of Florence Nightingale are being published by Wilfrid Laurier University Press, University of Guelph; information about the project can be found at http://www.sociology.uoguelph.ca/fnightingale/review/index.htm.

their babies. She analyzed data from the Midwifery Department of King's College Hospital concerning the mortality rate in childbearing and recommended environmental changes and hand washing to decrease puerperal fever, then the leading cause of maternal death (Nightingale, 1871).

NIGHTINGALE'S ENVIRONMENTAL MODEL

Webster's (1991) defines environment as the surrounding matters that influence or modify a course of development. According to Miller (1978), the system must interact and adjust to its environment. Nightingale viewed the manipulation of the physical environment as a major component of nursing care. She identified health of houses, ventilation and warmth, light, noise, variety, bed and bedding, cleanliness of rooms and walls, personal cleanliness, and nutrition ("taking food" and "what food") as major areas of the environment the nurse could control. When one or more aspects of the environment are out of balance, the client must use increased energy to counter the environmental stress. These stresses drain the client of energy needed for healing. These aspects of the physical environment are also influenced by the social and psychological environment of the individual. Nightingale addressed these aspects of the environment in chapters titled "Chattering Hopes and Advices," "Petty Management," "Variety," and "Observation of the Sick." Although Nightingale did not address political activism in *Notes on Nursing*, her life was a model of political involvement. She was very knowledgeable about current affairs and wrote many letters attempting to influence the health of individuals, families, and communities.

Health of Houses

In *Notes on Nursing* Nightingale discussed the importance of the health of houses as being closely related to the presence of pure air, pure water, efficient drainage, cleanliness, and light. To support the importance of hospital-based nursing attending to these, Nightingale (1859/1992) said, "Badly constructed houses do for the health what badly constructed hospitals do for the sick. Once insure that the air is stagnant and sickness is certain to follow" (p. 15). Nightingale also noted that the cleanliness outside the house affected the inside. Just as Nightingale noted that dung heaps affected the health of houses in her time, so too can modern families be affected by toxic waste, contaminated water, and polluted air.

Ventilation and Warming

In her chapter on ventilation and warming, Nightingale (1859/1992) stated it was essential to "keep the air he breathes as pure as the external air, without chilling him" (p. 8). She urged the caregiver to consider the source of the air in the patient's room. The air might be full of fumes from gas, mustiness, or open sewage if the source was not the freshest. Nightingale believed that the person who repeatedly breathed his or her own air would become sick or remain sick. In the 21st century we have buildings that are sealed in such a manner that fresh air is difficult to receive, and a new problem, labeled *building sickness*, has evolved.

Nightingale (1859/1992) was very concerned about "noxious air" or "effluvia"—foul odors that came from excrement. In many public places, as well as hospitals, raw sewage could be found next to patients, in ditches under or near the house, or contaminating drinking water. Her concerns about "effluvia" also included bedpans, urinals, and other utensils used to discard excrement. She also criticized "fumigations," for she believed that the offensive source, not the smell, must be removed.

The importance of room temperature was stressed by Nightingale. The patient should not be too warm or too cold. The temperature could be controlled by appropriate balance between burning fires and ventilation from windows. Today buildings often are constructed to be climate-controlled in such a manner that the client or the nurse cannot control the temperature of the individual room. In shared rooms the climate control may not satisfy either patient, with one wanting the room colder and another wanting it warmer, as each individual interacts with the environment.

Light

Nightingale (1859/1992) believed that second to fresh air the sick needed light. She noted that direct sunlight was what patients wanted. Although acknowledging a lack of scientific information, she noted that light has "quite real and tangible effects upon the human body" (pp. 47–48). She noted that people do not consider the difference between light needed in a bedroom (where individuals sleep at night) and light needed in a sick-room. To a healthy sleeper it does not matter where the light is because he or she is usually in this room only during hours of darkness. She noted that the sick rarely lie with their face toward the wall but are much more likely to face the window, the source of the sun. Again, modern hospitals may be constructed in such a manner that daylight is rarely available. This is particularly the case in neonatal intensive care units, and for many years was also true in the construction of adult intensive care units. The lack of appropriate environmental stimuli can lead to intensive care psychosis or confusion related to the lack of the accustomed cycling of day and night.

Noise

Noise was also of concern to Nightingale, particularly those noises that could jar the patient. She stated that patients should never be wakened intentionally or accidentally during the first part of sleep. She asserted that whispered or long conversations about patients are thoughtless and cruel. She viewed unnecessary noise, including noise from female dress, as cruel and irritating to the patient. Nurses today do not wear crinoline petticoats, but they do wear jewelry and carry keys that jingle and make other noises. Other more modern noises include the snapping of rubber gloves, the clank of a stethoscope against metal bed rails, and radios and televisions. Modern health care facilities contain much equipment that issue alarms, beeps, and other noises that startle or jar a patient from sleep to wakefulness. Nightingale was very critical of noises that annoyed the patient, such as a window shade blowing against the window frame. She viewed it as the nurse's responsibility to assess and stop this kind of noise. While specific testing of the effects of noise has been done, it has not been under the framework of Nightingale. The exception is the work by McCarthy, Ouimet, and Daun (1991), who extrapolated data from animal studies to support Nightingale's assertion that noise affects healing.

Variety

Nightingale believed that variety in the environment was a critical aspect affecting the patient's recovery. She discussed the need for changes in color and form, including bringing the patient brightly colored flowers or plants. She also advocated rotating

10 or 12 paintings and engravings each day, week, or month to provide variety for the patient. She wrote that "volumes are now written and spoken upon the effect of the mind upon the body. Much of it is true" (Nightingale, 1859/1992, p. 34). The increasing research being done on the interaction between mind and body has supported this observation. Nightingale also advocated reading, needlework, writing, and cleaning as activities to relieve the sick of boredom.

Bed and Bedding

Nightingale (1859/1992) viewed bedding as an important part of the environment. Although her view has not been substantiated by data, she noted that an adult in health exhales about three pints of moisture through the lungs and skin in a 24-hour period. This organic matter enters the sheets and stays there unless the bedding is changed and aired frequently. She believed that the bed should be placed in the lightest part of the room and placed so the patient could see out of a window. She reminded the caregiver never to lean against, sit upon, or unnecessarily shake the bed of a patient. In modern hospitals mattresses are usually covered with plastic or other materials that can be washed to remove drainage, excreta, or other matter. These mattresses often cause the patient to perspire, leading to damp bed clothing. Sheets also do not fit tightly on these mattresses, leading to wrinkles that can result in pressure points on the skin of the patient lying in bed. Modern technology may also interfere with providing a comfortable bed environment for the patient. Multiple intravenous pumps, ventilators, and monitors attached to a patient may impede comfort. It remains important for the nurse to keep bedding clean, neat, and dry and to position the patient for maximum comfort.

Cleanliness of Rooms and Walls

Nightingale (1959/1992) indicated that "the greater part of nursing consists in preserving cleanliness" (p. 49). She points out that even the best ventilation cannot freshen a room that is not first of all clean. She urges the removal of, rather than the relocation of, dust. This means using a damp cloth, not a feather duster. Floors should be easily cleaned rather than being covered with dust-trapping carpets. Furniture and walls should be easily washed and not damaged by coming in contact with moisture. Some of Nightingale's restrictions against carpet, fabrics, and wallpaper can be offset today with current cleaning mechanisms, including vacuum cleaners. However, the concept that a clean room is a healthy room continues to be true.

Personal Cleanliness

Nightingale viewed the function of the skin as important, believing that many diseases "disordered," or caused breaks in, the skin. She thought this was particularly true of children and that the excretion that comes from the skin must be washed away. She believed that unwashed skin poisoned the patient and noted that bathing and drying the skin provided great relief to the patient, saying, "Just as it is necessary to renew the air round a sick person frequently, to carry off morbid effluvia from the lungs and skin, by maintaining free ventilation, so is it necessary to keep pores of the skin free from all obstructing excretions" (Nightingale, 1859/1992, p. 53). She also believed that personal cleanliness extended to the nurse and that "every nurse ought to wash her hands very frequently during the day" (p. 53).

Nutrition and Taking Food

Nightingale addressed the food presented to the patient and discussed the importance of variety in the food presented. She found that attention provided to the patient affected how the patient ate. She noted that individuals desire different foods at different times of the day and that frequent small servings may be more beneficial to the patient than a large breakfast or dinner. She observed that patients may desire a different pattern of taking foods, such as eating breakfast foods at lunch, and that chronically ill patients may be starved to death because their incapacitation can make them unable to feed themselves and attention may not be given to what will enhance their ability to eat. She urged that no business be done with patients while they are eating because this was distraction. She also urged that the right food be brought at the right time and "be taken away, eaten or uneaten, at the right time" (p. 37).

Chattering Hopes and Advices

Nightingale did not speak to the social and psychological environment of the patient to the same degree that she addressed the physical environment. However, she included the chapter "Chattering Hopes and Advices," which discussed what is said to the patient. She wrote that the chapter heading might seem "odd" but that to falsely cheer the sick by making light of their illness and its danger is not helpful. She considered it stressful for a patient to hear opinions after only brief observations had been made. False hope was depressing to patients, she felt, and caused them to worry and become fatigued. Nightingale encouraged the nurse to heed what is being said by visitors, believing that sick persons should hear good news that would assist them in becoming healthier.

Social Considerations

Nightingale was an excellent manager. She demonstrated her management skills at Scutari and wrote about them in many of her nursing-related books. In *Notes on Nursing* (1859/1992), she discussed "petty management" or ways to assure that "what you do when you are there, shall be done when you are not there" (p. 20). She believed that the house and the hospital needed to be well managed—that is, organized, clean, and with appropriate supplies.

Nightingale (1859/1992) also emphasized the importance of observing the sick. She stated that "the most important practical lesson that can be given to nurses is to teach them what to observe—how to observe—what symptoms indicate improvement—what is the reverse—which are of importance—which are of none—which are evidence of neglect—and what kind of neglect" (p. 59). She felt so strongly about the importance of obtaining complete and accurate information about patients that she said that "if you cannot get the habit of observation one way or other, you had better give up being a nurse, for it is not your calling, however kind and anxious you may be" (p. 63).

Nightingale (1859/1992) supported the importance of looking beyond the individual to the social environment in which he or she lived. She was an epidemiologist who looked at not only the numbers of people who died but also what was unique about a given house or street. She observed that generations of families lived and died in poverty. Using her statistical data, she wrote letters and position papers and sent them to her acquaintances in the government in an effort to improve undesirable living conditions. Nightingale was a role model for political activism by nurses.

NIGHTINGALE'S ENVIRONMENTAL MODEL AND NURSING'S METAPARADIGM

Nightingale did not invent or define the four major concepts used to organize nursing theory. They evolved from an analysis of nursing curricula (Falco, 1989). Although we have applied our modern conventions to her framework, not all the concepts were addressed specifically by Nightingale. This is not a criticism of Nightingale's thinking but a reality of the development of nursing thought. Therefore, Nightingale's writings were analyzed to identify her definitions of these concepts.

NURSING   "What nursing has to do . . . is to put the patient in the best condition for nature to act upon him" (Nightingale, 1859/1992, p. 74). Nightingale viewed medicine and surgery as removing obstructions to health to allow nature to return the person to health. Nightingale stated that nursing "ought to signify the proper use of fresh air, light, warmth, cleanliness, quiet, and the proper selection and administration of diet—all at the least expense of vital power to the patient" (p. 6). She reflected the art of nursing in her statement that "the art of nursing, as now practised, seems to be expressly constituted to unmake what God had made disease to be, viz., a reparative process" (p. 6).

   Based on her definition of nursing, the following definitions of human beings, environment, and health can be deduced.

HUMAN BEINGS   Human beings are not defined by Nightingale specifically. They are defined in relationship to their environment and the impact of the environment upon them.

ENVIRONMENT   The physical environment is stressed by Nightingale in her writing. As noted, she focused on ventilation, warmth, noise, light, and cleanliness. Nightingale's writings reflect a community health model in which all that surrounds human beings is considered in relation to their state of health. She synthesized immediate knowledge of disease with the existing sanitary conditions in the environment.

HEALTH   Nightingale (1859/1992) did not define health specifically. She believed, however, that pathology teaches the harm disease has done and nothing more. She stated, "We know nothing of health, the positive of which pathology is the negative, except from observation and experience" (p. 74). She believed "nature alone cures" (p. 74). Given her definition that of the art of nursing is to "unmake what God had made disease to be" (p. 6), the goal of all nursing activities should be client health. She believed that nursing should provide care to the healthy as well as the ill and discussed health promotion as an activity in which nurses should engage.

   One way of organizing Nightingale's environmental model can be seen in Figure 3-1. Note that the client, the nurse, and the major environmental concepts are in balance; that is, the nurse can manipulate the environment to compensate for the client's response to it. The goal of the nurse is to assist the patient in staying in balance. If the environment of a client is out of balance, the client expends unnecessary energy. In Figure 3-2 the client is experiencing stress because of noise in the environment. Nursing observations focus on the client's response to noise; nursing interventions focus on reducing the noise and decreasing the client's unnecessary energy expenditure. The nurse's role is to place the client in the best position for nature to act upon him, thus encouraging healing.

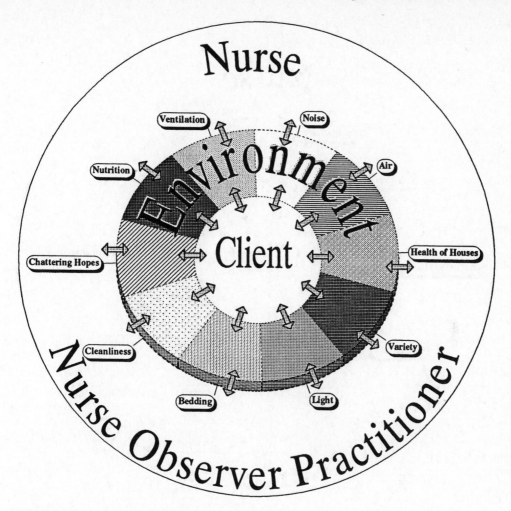

FIGURE 3-1 Client and environment in balance

NIGHTINGALE AND THE NURSING PROCESS

In the *assessment* of clients Nightingale (1859/1992) advocated two essential behaviors by the nurse. The first is to ask the client what is needed or wanted. If the patient is in pain, ask where the pain is located. If the patient is not eating, ask *when* he or she would like to eat and *what* food is desired. Find out what the patient believes is wrong. Nightingale warned against asking leading questions and advocated asking precise questions. She recommended asking questions such as "How many hours' sleep has ___ had? and at what hours of the night?" (p. 61) instead of "Has he had a good night?" Nightingale also warned that the individual asking the questions needed to be concerned about the shyness of the patient in answering questions.

The second area of assessment that Nightingale (1859/1992) advocated was the use of observation. She used precise observations concerning all aspects of the client's physical health and environment. Nurses must make the observations because clients

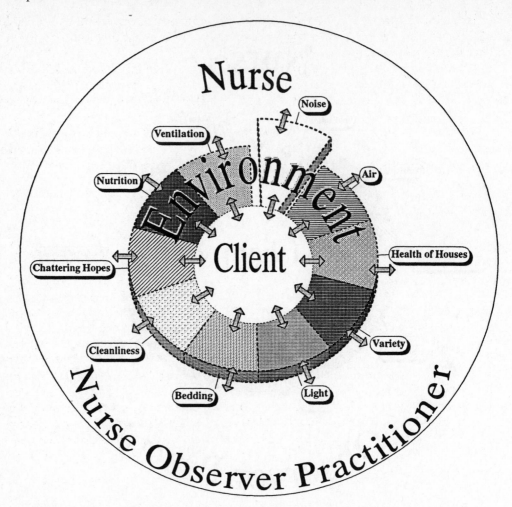

FIGURE 3-2   Client expending unnecessary energy by being stressed by environment (noise)

may be too weak or shy to make them. Observations revolve around Nightingale's environmental model, that is, the impact of the environment on the individual. For example, how do light, noise, smells, and bedding affect the client?

An assessment guide can be structured from Nightingale's environmental model. The major environmental concepts guide the structure of the assessment tool, leading to examining the impact of the environment on clients and integrating the expanding body of scientific knowledge concerning the effects of a balanced or unbalanced environment.

Nursing diagnoses are based on an analysis of the conclusions gained from the information in the assessment. Nightingale believed data should be used as the basis for forming any conclusion. It is important that the diagnosis be the clients' response to their environment and not the environmental problem. Nursing diagnoses reflect the importance of the environment to the health and well-being of the client.

Planning includes identifying the nursing actions needed to keep clients comfortable, dry, and in the best state for nature to work on. "The value of informed action, based on extensive knowledge is well illustrated by the Nightingale personality" (Palmer, 1977, p. 85). Planning is focused on modifying the environment to enhance the client's ability to respond to the disease process.

Implementation takes place in the environment that affects the client and involves taking action to modify that environment. All factors of the environment should be considered, including noise, air, odors, bedding, cleanliness, light, and variety—all the factors that place clients in the best position for nature to work upon them.

Evaluation is based on the effect of the changes in the environment on the clients' ability to regain their health at the least expense of energy. Observation is the primary method of data collection used to evaluate the client's response to the intervention. Some have proposed using Nightingale to guide their practice (e.g., Gillette, 1996); however, these reviews are not data based, nor has any testing of the efficacy of using Nightingale's framework been done.

APPLICATION OF NIGHTINGALE'S WORK IN THE NURSING PROCESS

ASSESSMENT   Nancy Smith, a 10-year-old African American female from a rural area, was injured in an accident related to farm machinery. She had a head injury, and although she was "conscious," she was not oriented to place and time. She had multiple abrasions, multiple bruises, and a deep leg wound containing dirt and debris from the farm equipment that injured her. She was transported to the regional children's hospital by helicopter. After triage in the emergency department and surgery, she was admitted to a crowded pediatric intensive care unit (PICU). In the PICU the lights were on 24 hours a day, noises from equipment permeated the unit, and visits by her parents were restricted. Today, after two days and nights of interrupted sleep, Nancy has become increasingly confused but does not have physiological evidence of increased intracranial pressure. Her leg has become infected, requiring increased intravenous antibiotics and dressing changes twice a day.

ANALYSIS OF DATA   Data gaps include information about family structure; who lives in the household; who was present when the injury occurred; Nancy's school performance; economic resources available to the family, including insurance; Nancy's nutritional status; and evaluation of her growth and development in relation to developmental standards. Of primary concern are Nancy's lack of sleep and the infected wound.

NURSING DIAGNOSIS   Sleep disruption related to environmental light and noise and separation from family.

PLANNING AND IMPLEMENTATION   Nursing actions focus on changing the environment to support more normal sleep patterns, that is, being awake during the day and sleeping at night. During the day, both natural and artificial light is plentiful around Nancy's bed. She also is encouraged to listen to her favorite music or watch her favorite television show to expose her to normal sounds. Her parents are encouraged to visit more often and to talk with her about the future when she will return to home and school. The nurse teaches Nancy about her dressing change and encourages her to participate as much as possible to help her become more comfortable in this new environment. At night, sleep is supported by dimming the lights, reducing noise (including turning down the volume of alarms), and keeping to a minimum activities and procedures that would awaken Nancy.

EVALUATION   Criteria for evaluation: After two nights of uninterrupted sleep, normal sounds, and parental encouragement, Nancy will demonstrate increased orientation to place by being able to identify that she is in the hospital. Nancy will begin participating in her dressing changes by the third day of the care plan.

NIGHTINGALE AND THE CHARACTERISTICS OF A THEORY

1. *What is the historical context of the theory?*   Florence Nightingale is the founder of modern nursing. Her work in the mid-1800s provided the basis for much of modern nursing. Her work in the Crimea led to the development of an epidemiological approach to improving the quality of the environment for the injured and ill at Scutari. Nightingale's work has had a worldwide influence, including the Far East as well as North America and England. Her historical influence has been discussed by authors from England (Ellis, 2008), Australia (Stanley, 2007) and the United States (Kudzma, 2006; Miracle, 2008).

      Nightingale's environmental model fits neither the totality nor the simultaneity paradigms. Primarily, the model is a view of the relationship between the health of human beings and the environments in which they function. It views neither the human as a sum of parts (totality paradigm) nor the human and environment as part of the same whole (simultaneity paradigm).

2. *What are the basic concepts and relationships presented by the theory?*   Nightingale presented her ideas not as a theory but as strategies to help women care for the ill in the home and in hostels for the ill. The major concepts covered in *Notes on Nursing* include ventilation, noise, air, health of houses, variety in the environment, light, bedding, cleanliness, "chattering hopes" or talking over patients, and nutrition. Nightingale never articulates clearly the relationships or interrelationships of her ideas. However, she presents her ideas in a clear manner, and the use of all of her ideas in caring for individuals puts those individuals in the best place to become healthy. When nursing situations are viewed from a Nightingale perspective, using the basic concepts she presents, new insights into phenomena of interest to nursing can be identified. Examining environmental aspects, such as light, noise, or warmth, can provide new insight into human response to health and illness. For example, when a client in an isolation room becomes disoriented, obvious things to consider would be medical pathology and fluid and electrolyte balance. From Nightingale's perspective, the impact of the environment would be an initial concern. Thus, the nurse would examine patterns of light, noise, ventilation, and interaction with other humans as potential sources of environmental stress to the client.

3. *What major phenomena of concern to nursing are presented? (These phenomena may include* **but are not limited to** *human beings, environment, health, interpersonal relations, caring, goal attainment, adaptation, and energy fields.)*   Nightingale's major focus is the environment and the manipulation of the environment by the nurse to put the patients in the best place for nature to act upon them and assist them in getting to maximum health. Nightingale does not address interpersonal relations specifically but does talk about the need for the nurse to consider what she says when talking around the patient. Also the nurse must consider the noise level of the environment, especially sources of unnecessary noise. Cleanliness is also of major importance, as it is discussed in 4 of the 13 canons—health of houses,

personal cleanliness, cleanliness of rooms and walls, and bed and bedding. The nurse is to consider all of these factors in applying the information to the patient.

4. *To whom does this theory apply? In what situations? In what way?* Nightingale's writings are simple, as is the articulation of her model. Nightingale's theory applies in all situations in which nursing care is provided. All care is provided in some type of environmental interface. Structuring the environment to provide the best care for the patient is essential whether in the home, the intensive care unit, a day care center, or the community at large. At times Nightingale uses words that are no longer in common use to describe aspects of her model; however, the elegance of Nightingale's model is its generalizability, including its continued applicability today. Nightingale's model can be applied in the most complex hospital intensive care environment, the home, a work site, or the community at large. Concepts related to pure air, light, noise, and cleanliness can be applied across specific environments.

For example, noise, or noxious sound can be found in any environment. The hospital has carts, monitors, and other machines that disrupt sleep and rest. The intensive care unit is noted for its number of staff members, machines, and alarms, all adding to the noise in the environment. A home may be near an interstate highway with loud truck noises or an airport with planes taking off and landing day and night, or a home may be isolated in the country with outside noises being rare. A work site may be filled with machine noises, computer whine, or large machine alarms. Finally, in our modern society, a community may be involved in a war, with shelling, bombing, and gunfire disrupting sleep, making it difficult to study or do other work.

Reading her work raises a consciousness in the nurse about how the environment influences client outcomes. Considering the effect of noise may make staff more aware of sounds that can be controlled. For example, the noise of placing a clipboard or other equipment on the top of an incubator is disruptive of an infant's sleep. Or, after reading Nightingale's discussion of the importance of light to the well-being of clients and examining the scientific information on light waves, such as the importance of light and darkness in sleep–rest cycles and the release of growth hormone, the neonatal intensive care nurse may begin to turn the lights down at night to encourage a normal sleep–wake cycle in the developing premature infant. Nightingale's theory has directed interventions toward modulating the environment. Noise, light, and ventilation should be controlled to maximize the patient's response to interventions.

Others have proposed Nightingale as a model for the clinical nurse specialist role (Sparacino, 1994). Sparacino noted that Nightingale also lived in tumultuous times where she was required to make major changes in the manner in which care was delivered. The changes in care that she made in the Crimean War front resulted in a dramatic reduction of the mortality rate. She defined the issues and goals for her day. Such definition is a responsibility of the advanced practice nurse in the 21st century.

Nightingale's theory works well with ecological, systems, adaptation, and interpersonal theories. Systems theory discusses the relationships between various layers of the individual and the environment. This is precisely what Nightingale did in her discussions of the effects of the physical environment on the individual. She also discussed how individuals respond to their disease process and viewed nursing's role as putting the client in the best position possible for nature to act upon. This allows clients to adapt or change to their diseased state and maximize their state of health.

Nightingale's work has had a direct impact on critical thinking in nursing practice through the requirement to structure the environment to optimize the patient's health. Nightingale's work is often cited in discussions of the current political climate that affects nursing practice. Her focus on the environment has relevance to practitioners in today's global health care climate. Nurses are approaching care from a more scholarly perspective that includes manipulation of the environment to place the patient in the best place possible for nature to work on him. Nurses exposed to Nightingale's concepts have begun looking at their environment in a broader context.

5. *By what method or methods can this theory be tested?*   While direct testing of Nightingale's theory has not been done, she has stimulated the development of nursing science with her work. For example, Nightingale did not believe in the germ theory; however, the practices she recommended were not inconsistent with the scientific knowledge we have today. In fact, many of her suggestions, which she based on observations of client responses to their environment, have been documented as scientifically sound when tested with rigorous application of modern research methods.

Both quantitative and qualitative methods of research could be used to test relationships in the environmental model. For example, qualitative methods could be used to investigate patient satisfaction in relation to continuity of care as a result of petty management. Nightingale herself supported the use of quantitative data in her use of statistics to demonstrate positive outcomes at Scutari.

6. *Does this theory direct nursing actions that lead to favorable outcomes?* Nightingale's work has not been tested in a manner that nursing actions are proscribed. However, her writings have helped nurses develop interventions that result in restructuring the environment. By structuring the environment to provide an optimum place for patients to improve their health, the result is positive outcomes for the patient. Research on the intensive care unit environment and the effects of noise and light on the patient supports the recommendations made by Nightingale in *Notes on Nursing*. Nightingale's theory has not directly resulted in the development of those interventions.

7. *How contagious is this theory?*   Examples of how Nightingale continues to influence both modern nursing and health care can be seen in a number of articles. In a discussion on perinatal lessons from the past, Dunn (1996) discussed her impact on maternal mortality and the training of midwives. Her writings have influenced those who have written about the effects of noise on wound healing (McCarthy et al., 1991). Others have written about the application of her theory to perioperative nursing (Gillette, 1996). Whall, Shin, and Colling (1999) used Nightingale to guide a model for dementia care in Korea.

Nightingale's work has also been used by individuals in management and leadership positions to influence the stances they have taken about issues affecting nursing today around the world. Hisama (1996) examined Nightingale's influence on the development of professional nursing in Japan. Modern nursing was brought to Japan by a physician who had studied at St. Thomas Hospital in London and was impressed with Nightingale's training school.

Nightingale has stimulated the development of nursing science with her influence on knowledge development in modern nursing. Many nursing theorists have used environment as a part of their theory. She has had a profound effect on many of the other nursing theorists cited in this book. These individuals have indicated the influence of Nightingale by citing her in their work or commenting on her influence in a commemorative edition of *Notes on Nursing*. For example, Leinginger (1992) analyzed what Nightingale did and did not say about caring, noting that although Nightingale never defined human care, she did make inferences about treating the sick. Levine (1992) first wrote about Nightingale in 1962 and discussed the excitement she felt at holding notes written in Nightingale's own hand. Newman (1992) spoke of the timelessness of *Notes on Nursing* and the impact it has had on her work. The research related to the impact of the environment on client health has been influenced by Nightingale. Hypotheses based on her work continue to be generated, although they are often embedded within the context of other theories.

Summary

Nightingale has been called timeless by many of the individuals who have written about her. That Nightingale's writings are as meaningful in the early 21st century as they were in the 19th century is an indication of her genius. The example in this chapter applies Nightingale's concepts to a child in an intensive care unit, but they can also be applied to the senior citizen in a nursing home, the family in their inner-city home, or the child in school. Although Nightingale spoke specifically to the health of human beings, she acknowledged that the health of the home and the community are critical components of the individual's health.

Nightingale continues to inspire nurses and non-nurses to write about her as well as reflect upon what she has written. She continues to influence nurse editors who incorporate her words into editorials (Bliss-Holtz, 2002; Gourlay, 2004). She has also inspired a song, by Country Joe McDonald, "Lady with the Lamp," although the song has been criticized by some as overly romantic and not reflective of the incredible difference she made in the lives of the soldiers at Scutari. Nightingale was a leader and reformer who led the way for the development of science-based practice in the 21st century.

Thought Questions

1. Develop an analogy or a metaphor for Nightingale's model.
2. Identify a clinical situation in which you did not like the outcome, analyze that situation using Nightingale's model, and determine, if you had taken her approach, how the outcome would have been different.
3. In today's health care environment, buildings are often built so windows cannot open. How would you ensure an adequate supply of fresh air in such buildings?
4. How do the "fumes" (effluvia) emitted by modern plastics and other synthetics affect our health? What would Nightingale have done about those "fumes"?

EXPLORE **PEARSON mynursingkit™**

MyNursingKit is your one stop for online chapter review materials and resources. Prepare for success with additional NCLEX®-style practice questions, interactive assignments and activities, web links, animations and videos, and more!

Register your access code from the front of your book at
www.mynursingkit.com.

References

Agnew, L. R. C. (1958). Florence Nightingale—statistician. *American Journal of Nursing, 58,* 644–646.

American Nurses Association. (1980). *Nursing: A social policy statement.* Kansas City, MO: Author.

Bliss-Holtz, J. (2002). Editorial: Nightingale revisited. *Issues in Comprehensive Pediatric Nursing, 25,* i–iv.

Cohen, I. B. (1984, March). Florence Nightingale. *Scientific American, 250,* 131–132.

Dunn, P. M. (1996). Florence Nightingale (1820–1910): Maternal mortality and the training of midwives. *Archives of Disease in Childhood, 74,* F219–F220.

Ellis, H. (2008). Florence Nightingale: Creator of modern nursing and public health pioneer. *Journal of Perioperative Practice, 18,* 404, 406.

Falco, S. M. (1989). Major concepts in the development of nursing theory. *Recent Advances in Nursing, 24,* 1–17.

Gillette, V. A. (1996). Applying nursing theory to perioperative nursing practice. *AORN Journal, 64,* 261–270.

Gourlay, J. (2004). Florence Nightingale: Still lighting the way for nurses. *Nursing Management, 11*(2), 14–15.

Hegge, M. (1990, April/May). In the footsteps of Florence Nightingale: Rediscovering the roots of nursing. *Imprint,* 74–75.

Hisama, K. K. (1996). Florence Nightingale's influence on the development of professionalization of modern nursing in Japan. *Nursing Outlook, 44,* 284–288.

Kudzma, E. C. (2006). Florence Nightingale and health care reform. *Nursing Science Quarterly, 19,* 61–64.

Leininger, M. M. (1992). Reflections on Nightingale with a focus on human care theory and leadership. In F. Nightingale, *Notes on nursing: What it is and what it is not* (Com. ed., pp. 28–38). Philadelphia: Lippincott.

Levine, M. (1992). Nightingale redux. In F. Nightingale, *Notes on nursing: What it is and what it is not* (Com. ed., pp. 39–43). Philadelphia: Lippincott.

McCarthy, D. O., Ouimet, M. E., & Daun, J. M. (1991). Shades of Florence Nightingale: Potential impact of noise stress on wound healing. *Holistic Nursing Practice, 5,* 39–48.

McDonald, L. (2006). Florence Nightingale as social reformer. *History Today, 56*(1), 9–15.

Miller, J. G. (1978). *Living systems.* New York: McGraw-Hill.

Miracle, V. A. (2008). The life and impact of Florence Nightingale. *Dimensions of Critical Care Nursing, 27*(1), 21–23.

Newman, M. A. (1992). Nightingale's vision of nursing theory and health. In F. Nightingale, *Notes on nursing: What it is and what it is not* (Com. ed., pp. 44–47). Philadelphia: Lippincott.

Nightingale, F. (1860). Vol. II, cited in Palmer, I. S. (1977). Florence Nightingale: Reformer, reactionary, researcher. *Nursing Research, 26,* 84–89.

Nightingale, F. N. (1871). *Introductory notes on lying-in institutions.* London: Longman, Green.

Nightingale, F. N. (1992). *Notes on nursing: What it is and what it is not* (Com. ed.). Philadelphia: Lippincott. (Original work published 1859)

Palmer, I. S. (1977). Florence Nightingale: Reformer, reactionary, researcher. *Nursing Research, 26,* 84–89.

Sparacino, P. S. A. (1994). Florence Nightingale: A CNS role model. *Clinical Nurse Specialist*, *8*(2), 64.

Stanley, D. (2007). Lights in the shadows: Florence Nightingale: Selected letters. *Contemporary Nurse, 24*, 45–51.

Vicinus, M., & Nergaard, B. (Eds.). (1990). *Ever yours, Florence Nightingale: Selected letters*. Cambridge, MA: Harvard University Press.

Webster's ninth new collegiate dictionary. (1991). Springfield, MA: Merriam.

Whall, A. L., Shin, Y. H., & Colling, K. B. (1999). A Nightingale-based model for dementia care and its relevance for Korean nursing. *Nursing Science Quarterly, 12*, 319–323.

Selected Sources About Nightingale

Cook, E. (1913). *The life of Florence Nightingale* (Vols. 1 & 2). London: The Macmillan Co. [out of print]

Dossey, B. M. (2000). *Florence Nightingale: Mystic, visionary, reformer.* Philadelphia: Lippincott Williams & Wilkins.

Dossey, B. M., Selanders, L. C., Beck, D-M., & Attewell, A. (2005). *Florence Nightingale today: Healing, leadership, global action.* Silver Spring, MD: American Nurses Association.

Gill, G. (2004). *Nightingales: The extraordinary upbringing and curious life of Miss Florence Nightingale.* New York: Ballantine.

Goldie, S. M. (Ed.). (1997). *Florence Nightingale: Letters from the Crimea.* New York: Palgrave McMillan.

Small, H. (1999). *Florence Nightingale: Avenging angel.* New York: Palgrave McMillan.

Woodham-Smith, C. (1951). *Florence Nightingale.* New York: McGraw-Hill. [out of print]

CHAPTER 4

Interpersonal Relations in Nursing

Hildegard E. Peplau[*][**]

Janice Ryan Belcher

Throughout her career, Dr. Hildegard Peplau was a pioneer in nursing. Born in Reading, Pennsylvania, Peplau (1909–1999) began her career in nursing in 1931 after graduating from a diploma nursing program in Pottstown, Pennsylvania. In 1943, Peplau received a B.A. degree in interpersonal psychology from Bennington College. This was followed in 1947 with an M.A. in psychiatric nursing and in 1953 an Ed.D. in curriculum development from Columbia University in New York. Peplau's nursing experience included private and general duty hospital nursing, the U.S. Army Nurse Corps, nursing research, and a private practice in psychiatric nursing. She taught the first classes in graduate psychiatric nursing at Columbia University before moving to Rutgers University, where she continued to teach for 20 years and held the title of Professor Emeritus. Peplau influenced the development of many nursing programs, including the creation of the first postbaccalaureate nursing program in Belgium.

Peplau published the book Interpersonal Relations in Nursing *in 1952. Although the manuscript was completed in 1949, it was not published until 1952 because it was initially considered to be too radical—it was the first theoretical textbook written by a nurse without having a physician as coauthor. She also published numerous articles in professional journals on topics ranging from interpersonal concepts to current issues in nursing. Her work on anxiety, hallucinations, and the nurse as an individual therapist was especially groundbreaking. Her pamphlet "Basic Principles of Patient Counseling" was derived from her research and workshops ("Profile," 1974).*

Dr. Peplau long held national and international recognition as a nurse and leader in health care. She participated in the development of the National Mental Health Act of 1946 and served with many organizations, including the World Health Organization, the National Institute of Mental Health, and the Nurse Corps. In 1954, Dr. Peplau

[*] *Interpersonal relations in nursing,* Peplau, 1988, Springer Publishing Company, Inc., New York 10012. Used with permission.

[**] Gratitude is expressed to Lois B. Fish for her contributions to this chapter in earlier editions.

created the first clinical nurse specialist program for graduate-prepared nurses in psychiatric-mental health. She was past executive director and past president of the American Nurses Association and in 1998 was inducted into its Hall of Fame. A fellow of the American Academy of Nursing, Peplau was also a board member of the International Council of Nurses, receiving in 1997 its highest honor, the Christianne Reimann Prize, for outstanding contributions in health care. She served as a nursing consultant to various foreign countries as well as to the surgeon general of the U.S. Air Force. Although Peplau "retired" in 1974, she continued professional journal and book publications. Her 1952 book was reissued in 1988 by Springer, New York. Regretfully, Peplau died March 17, 1999. This chapter is dedicated to this nurse, educator, and administrator who was such a remarkable person.

—**J.R.B.**

Hildegard Peplau (1952/1988) published *Interpersonal Relations in Nursing,* referring to her book as a "partial theory for the practice of nursing" (p. 261). It is quite remarkable that in 1952 Peplau referred to her book as a partial theory for nursing since this was before the thrust of nursing theory development. In her book, Peplau discussed the phases of the interpersonal process, roles for nursing, and methods for studying nursing as an interpersonal process. Today, authors continue to debate the utility of her theory, which is central to nursing practice, with its focus on interpersonal relations between the nurse and patient. This chapter defines the crux of Peplau's nursing theory as the phases of the interpersonal process and links her other concepts to this central core.

According to Peplau (1952/1988), nursing is therapeutic because it is a healing art, assisting an individual who is sick or in need of health care. Nursing can be viewed as an interpersonal process because it involves interaction between two or more individuals with a common goal. In nursing, this common goal provides the incentive for the therapeutic process in which the nurse and patient[#] respect each other as individuals, both of them learning and growing as a result of the interaction. An individual learns when she or he selects stimuli in the environment and then reacts to these stimuli.

The attainment of this goal, or any goal, is achieved through a series of steps following a sequential pattern. As the relationship of the nurse and patient develops in these steps, the nurse can choose how she or he practices nursing by using different skills and technical abilities and by assuming various roles.

When the nurse and patient first identify a problem, they begin to develop a course of action to solve the problem. They approach this course of action from diverse backgrounds and with individual uniqueness. Each individual may be viewed as a unique biological-psychological-spiritual-sociological structure, one that will not react in the same way as any other individual. Both the nurse and the patient have learned their perceptions from the different environments, mores, customs, and beliefs of that individual's given culture. Each person comes with preconceived ideas that influence perceptions, and it is these differences in perception that are so important in the interpersonal process. Furthermore, Peplau (1994b) states that these

---

[#] *Patient* will be used throughout this chapter since it is Peplau's definition of the individual who is in need of health care.

"perceptions vary with time, place, and experience" (p. 11). In addition, the nurse has a broad range of nursing knowledge such as stress–crisis management and developmental theories, which leads to a greater understanding of the nurse's professional role in the therapeutic process. Peplau (1992) states, "In all encounters with patients, nurses observe, interpret what they notice, and then decide what needs to be done. This sequence occurs over and over again in any given nurse-patient interaction" (p. 16). As nurse and patient continue the relationship, they begin to understand one another's roles and the factors surrounding the problem. From this understanding, both the nurse and the patient collaborate and share in mutual goals until the problem is resolved.

As the nurse and the patient work together, they become more knowledgeable and mature throughout the process. Peplau (1952/1988) views nursing as a "maturing force and an educative instrument" (p. 8). She believes nursing is a learning experience of oneself as well as of the other individual involved in the interpersonal action. This concept was supported by Genevieve Burton, another nursing author from the 1950s, who stated, "Behavior of others must be understood in light of self understanding" (Burton, 1958, p. 7). Thus, persons who are aware of their own feelings, perceptions, and actions are also more likely to be aware of another individual's reactions.

Each therapeutic encounter influences the nurse's and the patient's personal and professional development. As the nurse works with the patient to resolve problems in everyday life, the nurse's practice becomes increasingly more effective. Thus, the kind of person the nurse is and becomes has a direct influence on her skill in the therapeutic, interpersonal relationship. In fact, Peplau (1992) believes "the behavior of the nurse-as-a-person interacting with the patient-as-a-person has significant impact on the patient's well-being and the quality and outcome of nursing care" (p. 14).

Peplau initially identified four sequential phases in interpersonal relationships: (1) orientation, (2) identification, (3) exploitation, and (4) resolution. Each of these phases overlaps, interrelates, and varies in duration as the process evolves toward a solution. However, in 1997, Peplau wrote that the nurse–patient relationship is composed of three phases: *orientation phase, working phase,* and *termination phase*—thus combining her two original phases, identification and exploitation, into the working phase. In this chapter, Peplau's original four phases will be discussed within the framework of the later three phases. Different nursing roles are assumed during the various phases. These roles can be broadly described as follows:

- *Teacher*   One who imparts knowledge concerning a need or interest
- *Resource*   One who provides specific, needed information that aids in understanding a problem or a new situation
- *Counselor*   One who, through the use of certain skills and attitudes, aids another in recognizing, facing, accepting, and resolving problems that are interfering with the other person's ability to live happily and effectively
- *Leader*   One who carries out the process of initiation and maintenance of group goals through interaction
- *Technical expert*   One who provides physical care by displaying clinical skills and operating equipment in this care
- *Surrogate*   One who takes the place of another

PEPLAU'S PHASES IN NURSING

Orientation

In the initial phase, *orientation*, the nurse and patient meet as two strangers. The patient and/or the family has a "felt need" (Peplau, 1952/1988, p. 18); therefore, professional assistance is sought. However, this need may not be readily identified or understood by the individuals who are involved. For example, a 16-year-old girl may call the community mental health center just because she feels "very down." It is in this phase that the nurse needs to assist the patient and family to realize what is happening to the patient. Peplau (1994b) states, "Interpersonal relationships are important throughout the entire life span. The problems of adolescents, of young adults, and of the elderly are most often psychosocial or interpersonal" (p. 13).

Peplau (1995) emphasizes that "psychiatric nurses who practice in either hospital or community settings need to pay more attention to families" (p. 94). It is of the utmost importance that the nurse work collaboratively with the patient *and* family in analyzing the situation, so that together they can recognize, clarify, and define the existing problem. In the previous example the nurse, in the counselor's role, helps the teenaged girl who feels "very down" to realize that these feelings stem from an argument with her mother over last evening's date. As the nurse listens, a pattern evolves: The girl argues with her mother and then feels depressed. As these feelings are discussed, the girl recognizes that the arguing is the precipitating factor leading to the depression. Thus, the nurse and the patient have defined the problem. Later, the girl and her parents agree to discuss the issue with the nurse. Therefore, by mutually clarifying and defining the problem in the orientation phase, the patient can direct the accumulated energy from her anxiety about unmet needs and begin working with the presenting problem. Nurse–patient rapport is established and continues to be strengthened while concerns are being identified.

While the patient and family are talking to the nurse, a mutual decision needs to be made regarding what type of professional assistance the patient and family need. The nurse, as a resource person, may work with them. As an alternative, the nurse might, with the mutual agreement of all parties involved, refer the family to another source such as a nurse practitioner, psychologist, psychiatrist, family counselor, or social worker. In the orientation phase, the nurse, patient, and family decide what types of services are needed. Even though the nurse may work with the patient and family only a short time, Peplau (1994a) believes that "every professional contact with a patient, however brief, is an opportunity for educative input by nurses" (p. 5).

The orientation phase is directly affected by the patient's and nurse's attitudes about giving or receiving aid from a reciprocal person. In this beginning phase, the nurse needs to be aware of her personal reactions to the patient. For example, the nurse may react differently to the 40-year-old man with abdominal pain who enters the emergency department quietly in contrast to the 40-year-old man with abdominal pain who enters the emergency department boisterously after a few alcoholic drinks. The nurse's, as well as the patient's, culture, religion, race, educational background, experiences, and preconceived ideas and expectations all influence the nurse's reaction to the patient. In addition, the same factors influence the patient's reaction to the nurse (see Figure 4-1). For example, the patient may have stereotyped the nurse as being able to perform only technical skills, such as giving medications or taking blood pressures, and therefore may not perceive the nurse as a resource person who can help define the

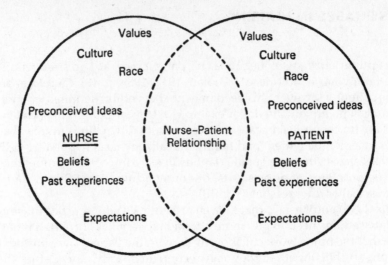

FIGURE 4-1   Factors influencing the blending of the nurse–patient relationship.

problem. Nursing is an interpersonal process, and both the patient and the nurse have an equally important part in the therapeutic interaction.

The nurse, the patient, and the family work together to recognize, clarify, and define the existing problem. Peplau (1995) discusses the need for the nurse to give not only "support but health teaching [to family members]. . . . They need time to talk with staff about their concern about the patient" (p. 94). This in turn decreases the tension and anxiety associated with the felt need and the fear of the unknown. Decreasing tension and anxiety prevents future problems that might arise as a result of repressing or not resolving significant events. Stressful situations are identified through therapeutic interaction. It is imperative that the patient recognize and begin to work through feelings connected with events before an illness.

In summary, in the beginning of the orientation phase, the nurse and the patient meet as strangers. At the end of the orientation phase, they are concurrently striving to identify the problem and are becoming more comfortable with one another. In addition, the patient becomes more comfortable in the helping environment. The nurse and the patient are now ready to logically progress to the next phase—the working phase.

Working Phase

The *working phase* encompasses the activities described in Peplau's early works as the identification and exploitation phases. As this working phase begins, in what was formerly the identification phase, the patient responds selectively to people who can meet his needs. Each patient responds differently in this phase. For example, the patient might actively seek out the nurse or stoically wait until the nurse approaches. The response to the nurse is threefold: (1) participate with and be interdependent with the nurse, (2) be autonomous and independent from the nurse, or (3) be passive and dependent on the nurse (Peplau, 1952/1988). An example is that of a 70-year-old man who wants to plan his new 1,600-calorie diabetic diet. If the relationship is interdependent, the nurse and patient collaborate on the meal planning. Should the relationship be independent, the patient plans the diet himself with minimal input from the nurse. In a dependent relationship, the nurse does the meal planning for the patient.

Throughout the working phase, both the patient and the nurse must clarify each other's perceptions and expectations (Peplau, 1952/1988). Past experiences of both the patient and the nurse will influence their expectations during this interpersonal process. As mentioned in the orientation phase, the initial attitudes of the patient and nurse are important in building a working relationship for identifying the problem and choosing appropriate assistance.

Psychiatric home care nurses need to progress to the working phase quickly because of their limited time with their clients. Peplau (1995) refers to psychiatric home care as "hands-on care, health teaching, coordination of care, and supervision of home health aides are all nursing functions in psychiatric home care. Careful recording of nursing observations and services rendered is required" (p. 94). A broader scope includes these functions for all home health nurses. In home care, the patient responds to the nurse who can provide therapeutic support and individual counseling.

In the working phase, the perception and expectations of the patient and nurse are even more complex than in the orientation phase. The patient is now responding to the helper selectively. This requires a more intense therapeutic relationship.

To illustrate, a patient who has had a mastectomy may express to the home health nurse her conflict in understanding the importance of exercising the arm following surgery. The nurse observes that the affected arm is edematous (swollen). While the nurse is exploring possible reasons for the edema, the patient admits she is not doing her arm exercises because a friend told her that exercising after surgery delays healing. To facilitate the patient's understanding and subsequent resumption of the exercises, the nurse can identify additional professional people, such as the physical therapist and the physician, who will clarify the patient's misconceptions. Generally, it is best if the nurse objectively discusses each professional's role with the patient so that she will be aware of the advantages and disadvantages of consulting with each professional. However, in this case, the patient states that she does not care to discuss the exercises with the nurse or physical therapist because she perceives her physician to be the only one who has the appropriate information. Thus, previous perceptions of nursing and physical therapy can influence the patient's current decision on the selection of the professional person.

While moving through the working phase, the patient begins to have feelings of belonging and a capacity for dealing with the problem. These changes begin to decrease feelings of helplessness and hopelessness, creating an optimistic attitude from which inner strength ensues.

As the working phase continues, the patient moves into what was the exploitation phase, in which the patient takes advantage of all services available. The degree to which these services are used is based on the needs and interests of the patient. The individual starts to feel as though he or she is an integral part of the helping environment and begins to take control of the situation by extracting help from the services offered. In the previous example of the woman with an edematous arm, the patient begins to understand the information regarding the arm exercises. She reads pamphlets and watches videotapes describing the exercises, she discusses concerns with the nurse, and she may inquire about joining an exercise group through the physical therapy department.

During this phase some patients may make more demands than they did when they were seriously ill. They may make many minor requests or may use other attention-getting techniques, depending on their individual needs. These actions may often be difficult, if not impossible, for the health care provider to completely understand. The nurse may need to deal with the subconscious forces causing the patient's actions and may need to use interviewing techniques as tools to explore, understand, and adequately deal with underlying patient problems. The nurse must convey an attitude of acceptance, concern, and trust in order to maintain a therapeutic relationship and prevent damage to the nurse–patient rapport that has been established to this point. Furthermore, she must encourage the patient to recognize and explore feelings, thoughts, emotions, and behaviors by providing a nonjudgmental atmosphere and a therapeutic emotional climate.

Peplau (1994a) states, "There is a significant difference between taking responsibility for the care of patients and being therapeutically responsive to each patient. In taking responsibility, it is the scope of activities that can keep nurses busy, feeling important, and having a sense of some accomplishment at the day's end. However, the purpose of professional services and the expectation—indeed the need—is for patients to come to terms with their problems" (p. 5). Some patients may take an active interest in, and become involved in, self-care. Such patients become self-sufficient and demonstrate initiative by establishing appropriate behavior for goal attainment. In fact, patients may wish to join a self-help group as described by Peplau (1997) when she says that "many lay-oriented helping-each-other health related groups are forming" (p. 222). Through self-determination, patients progressively develop responsibility for self, belief in potentialities, and adjustment toward self-reliance and independence. These patients realistically begin to establish their own goals toward improved health status. They strive to achieve a direction in their lives that promotes a feeling of well-being. Patients who develop self-care become productive, they trust and depend on their own capabilities, and they also become responsible for their own actions. As a result of this self-determination, they develop sources of inner strength that allow them to face new challenges.

While sick, most patients fluctuate between dependence on others and independent functioning approaching an optimal health level. This point is illustrated by using the previous example of the woman who had an edematous arm after surgery. Some days she wants to actively exercise on schedule; however, on other days she states she is too tired to exercise at all. When the patient does not exercise, the nurse needs to intervene by reminding the patient of her scheduled exercises.

This type of inconsistent behavior can be compared to the adjustment reaction of the adolescent in a dependency–independency conflict. The patient may temporarily be in a dependent role while having the simultaneous need for independence. Various stressors may trigger the onset of this psychological disequilibrium. The patient vacillates unpredictably between the two behaviors and appears confused and anxious, protesting dependence while fearing independence. In caring for patients who fluctuate between dependence and independence, the nurse must approach the specific behavior that is presented rather than trying to handle the composite problem of inconsistency. The nurse should provide an atmosphere of acceptance and support, one in which the person can become more self-aware and begin to use his strengths to minimize weaknesses. It is the nurse's responsibility to create a climate for the patient that is conducive to responsible self-growth.

Peplau (1994c) states, "Conversations are too often serial monologues rather than interactions" (p. 58). In this phase, the nurse uses communication tools such as clarifying, listening, accepting, teaching, and interpreting to offer services to the patient. The patient then takes advantage of the services offered based on his needs and interests. Throughout this phase, the patient works collaboratively with the nurse to meet challenges and work toward maximum health. Thus, in the working phase, the nurse aids the patient in using services to help solve the problem. Progress is made toward the final step—the termination phase.

Termination

The last phase in Peplau's interpersonal process is *termination*. The patient's needs have already been met by the collaborative efforts between the patient and nurse. The patient and nurse now need to terminate their therapeutic relationship and dissolve the links between them.

Sometimes the nurse and patient have difficulty dissolving these links. Dependency needs in a therapeutic relationship often continue psychologically after the physiological needs have been met. The patient may feel that it "is just not time yet" to end the relationship. For example, a new mother has a desire to learn infant care. Readiness is one of the most important factors in the learning process, and learning is initiated by a need or purpose. During the first home visit, the community health nurse and the new mother set their goal of having the mother properly demonstrate various facets of infant care by the third visit. The setting of these goals is important in order to evaluate whether the desired outcome has been achieved. After instruction and demonstration by the community health nurse on the first visit, the mother takes a more active role during the next home visits. In order for learning to become relatively permanent, it must be used in actual practice. By the third visit the mother demonstrates correctly all facets of infant care. Their goal is met. The relationship is ended because the mother's problem was solved. However, one week after the resolution, the mother telephones the community health nurse five times with minor questions on infant care. The mother has not dissolved the dependency link with the community health nurse.

The final resolution may also be difficult for the nurse. In the previous example, the mother may be willing to terminate the relationship; however, the community health nurse may continue to visit the home to watch the baby develop. The nurse may be unable to free herself or himself from this bond in their relationship. This may be, in part, due to the nurse's knowledge of the importance of the parent–child relationship. Peplau (1994b) refers to the "enormous influence which parents and significant caretakers have on the early development of infants, and in the shaping of behavior of growing children" (p. 11). In termination, as in the other phases, anxiety and tension increase in the patient and the nurse if there is unsuccessful completion of the phase.

During successful termination, the patient drifts away from identifying with the helping person, the nurse. The patient then becomes independent from the nurse as the nurse becomes independent from the patient. As a result of this process, both the patient and the nurse become stronger maturing individuals. The patient's needs are met, and movement can be made toward new goals. Termination occurs only with the successful completion of the previous phases. Table 4-1 indicates the focus of each phase.

TABLE 4-1 Phases of the Nurse–Patient Relationship	
Phases	**Focus**
Orientation	Problem definition
Working	Selection of appropriate professional assistance and use of professional assistance for problem-solving alternatives
Termination	Termination of the professional relationship

PEPLAU'S THEORY AND NURSING'S METAPARADIGM

Nursing's metaparadigm includes the four concepts of human beings, health, society/ environment, and nursing. Peplau (1952/1988) defines *man* (used in generic terms) as an organism that "strives in its own way to reduce tension generated by needs" (p. 82). *Health* is defined as "a word symbol that implies forward movement of personality and other ongoing human processes in the direction of creative, constructive, productive, personal, and community living" (p. 12).

Although Peplau (1952/1988) does not directly address *society/environment*, she does encourage the nurse to consider the patient's culture and mores when the patient adjusts to hospital routine. Today, the nurse reviews the patient's environment and examines many more factors, such as cultural background and home and work environments, rather than considering only a patient's adjustment to the hospital. Peplau has a narrow perception of the environment, which is a major limitation of her theory.

Peplau (1952/1988) considers *nursing* to be a "significant, therapeutic, interpersonal process" (p. 16). She defines it as a "human relationship between an individual who is sick, or in need of health services, and a nurse especially educated to recognize and to respond to the need for help" (pp. 5–6). The nurse assists the patient in this interpersonal process. Major concepts within this process are nurse, patient, therapeutic relationship, goals, human needs, anxiety, tension, and frustration.

RELATIONSHIP BETWEEN PEPLAU'S PHASES AND THE NURSING PROCESS

When Peplau's continuum of the three phases of *orientation, working,* and *termination* is compared to the nursing process, similarities are apparent (see Table 4-2). Both Peplau's phases and the nursing process are sequential and focus on therapeutic interactions. Both stress that the nurse and patient should use problem-solving techniques collaboratively, with the end purpose of meeting the patient's needs. Both emphasize assisting the patient to define general complaints more specifically so that specific patient needs can be identified. Both use observation, communication, and recording as basic tools for nursing practice.

Peplau's orientation phase parallels the beginning of the *assessment phase* in that both the nurse and the patient come together as strangers. This meeting is initiated by the patient, who expresses a need, although the need is not always understood. Conjointly, the nurse and patient begin to work through recognizing, clarifying, and gathering facts important to this need. This step is presently referred to as data collection in the assessment phase of the nursing process.

In the nursing process the patient's need is not necessarily a felt need. For example, the nurse may be currently working in the community by assessing people who perceive themselves to be healthy. A school nurse screens for hearing impairment in school-aged children. A referral is initiated by the nurse if a deficit is found. Children do not usually seek out the nurse for this problem. In this situation, the need must be identified in order to persuade the parents to seek assistance for the child's hearing deficit. The nurse may send home a note about the hearing deficit so that the parents and child become aware of the problem. The nurse may also have to follow up the note with a telephone call or home visit. The nurse is actively helping the child and family to identify a need.

TABLE 4-2   Comparison of Nursing Process and Peplau's Process

Nursing Process	Peplau's Interpersonal Process
Assessment Data collection and analysis Need not necessarily be a "felt need"; may be nurse initiated	Orientation Nurse and patient come together as strangers; meeting initiated by patient who expresses a "felt need"; work together to recognize, clarify, and define facts related to need. (Note: Data collection is continuous.)
Nursing Diagnosis Summary statement based on nurse analysis, with possible patient involvement	Patient clarifies "felt need."
Outcomes and Planning Mutually set outcomes and goals	Working Interdependent goal setting. Patient has feeling of belonging and selectively responds to those who can meet his needs. Patient initiated.
Implementation Plans initiated that move toward achievement of mutually set goals May be accomplished by patient, health care professional, or patient's family	Patient actively seeking and drawing on knowledge and expertise of those who can help. Patient initiated.
Evaluation Based on mutually established expected behaviors May lead to termination of relationship or initiation of new plans	Termination Occurs after other phases are successfully completed. Leads to termination of the relationship.

Orientation and assessment are not synonymous and must not be confused. Collecting data is continuous throughout Peplau's phases. In the nursing process, the initial collection of data is the nursing assessment, and further collection of data becomes an integral part of reassessment.

In the nursing process, the *nursing diagnosis* evolves once the health problems or deficits are identified. The nursing diagnosis is a summary statement of the data collected and analyzed. Peplau (1952/1988) writes that "during the period of orientation the patient clarifies his first, whole impression of his problem" (p. 30), whereas in the nursing process, the nurse's judgment forms the diagnosis from the data collected. The nurse and the patient may or may not be mutual partners in identifying the nursing diagnosis.

Mutually set outcomes and goals evolve from the nursing diagnosis in the nursing process. These outcomes and goals give direction to the plan and indicate the appropriate helping resources. When the nurse and patient discuss helping resources, the patient can selectively identify with the resource persons. According to Peplau, the patient is then viewed as being in the working phase. While collaborating on mutual outcomes and goals, the nurse and patient may have conflicts based on preconceptions and expectations of each person, as described earlier. The nurse and patient must resolve any discrepancies before mutual outcomes can be developed and mutual goals can be set. These decisions should be an interdependent activity between the patient and nurse.

The next phase in the nursing process is the *planning* phase. In this phase, the nurse must specifically formulate how the patient is going to achieve the mutually set outcomes and goals. The nurse actively seeks patient input so that the patient feels like an integral part of the plan. When the patient feels involved in the plan, outcomes are more likely to be achieved. The nurse is the facilitator, but the planning is a sharing process, a two-directional process of intercommunication with reciprocal feedback by which continuous responses are made between the nurse and the patient. In this phase, the nurse considers the patient's own skills for handling his problems. The planning phase of the nursing process gives direction and meaning to the nursing actions to be taken toward resolving the patient's problems. Using nursing education, the nurse bases the nursing plan on scientific knowledge. In addition, the nurse incorporates the patient's individual strengths and weaknesses into the plan. Peplau (1952/1988) stresses that the nurse wants to develop a therapeutic relationship so that the patient's anxiety will be constructively channeled into seeking resources, thus leading to decreased feelings of hopelessness and helplessness. Planning can be considered to be within Peplau's working phase.

The patient also begins to have a feeling of belonging within the therapeutic relationship because both patient and nurse must have mutual respect, communication, and interest. This feeling of belonging must be analyzed and should assist the patient to develop a healthier personality rather than imitative behavior. Peplau (1952/1988) states, "Some patients identify too readily with nurses, expecting that all of their wants will be taken care of and nothing will be expected of them" (p. 32). In Peplau's working phase, the patient selectively responds to people who can meet his personal needs. Therefore, Peplau's working phase is initiated by the patient, while the planning phase of the nursing process may be initiated by the nurse or the patient.

In the *implementation* phase, as in Peplau's working phase, the patient is finally reaping benefits from the therapeutic relationship by drawing on the nurse's knowledge and expertise. The individualized plans have already been formed, based on the patient's interest and needs. Similarly, the plans are geared toward completion of desired goals. However, there is a difference between the working phase and implementation. In the working phase, the patient is the one who actively seeks varying types of services to obtain the maximum benefits available, whereas in implementation there is a prescribed plan or procedure, holistic in nature, used to achieve predetermined goals or objectives based on nursing assessment. Thus, the working phase is oriented to patient action, and, in contrast, implementation can be accomplished by the patient or by other persons, including health professionals and the patient's family.

In Peplau's termination phase, all other phases have been successfully accomplished, the needs have been met, and resolution and termination are the end result. Although Peplau does not discuss *evaluation* per se, evaluation is an inherent factor in determining the readiness of the patient to proceed through the termination phase. In the nursing process, evaluation is a separate step, and mutually established expected end behaviors (goals) are used as evaluation tools. Time limits on attaining the goals are set for evaluation purposes, although these limits may change with reassessment. In evaluation, if the situation is clear-cut, the problem moves toward termination. If the problem is unresolved, outcomes, goals, and objectives are not met; if outcomes are not achieved or nursing care is ineffective, a reassessment must be done. New goals, planning, implementation, and evaluation are then established. An example of the application of Peplau's work in clinical practice is shown in Table 4-3.

TABLE 4-3   **Application of Interpersonal Relationships in Clinical Practice**

Orientation

You are a staff nurse on the chemical dependency unit of your hospital. You note that Cecilia Bell, 32 years old, is assigned to you today. In reviewing her chart you note that she is admitted for alcohol abuse and that this is her third admission for this diagnosis in the last nine months. Her first admission nine months ago occurred after she was found by the police wandering in the street. She had been drinking heavily and had lost her purse. Three months ago, she requested readmission after drinking heavily and feeling depressed. You remember her from that admission. She had attended all group therapy meetings and all Alcoholic Anonymous (AA) meetings and seemed interested in her treatment and excited about being ready for discharge.

When Ms. Bell sees you, she recognizes you as a nurse whom she had seen during her previous admission. As you discuss why she is here now (seeking to identify her felt need), she reports she has been drinking a fifth of vodka and a "few" beers daily for the past several weeks. In tears, she says, "I'm a failure." Further discussion reveals that she attended AA regularly for about six weeks after her last discharge from the hospital. She returned to her employment as a high school English teacher and felt she did not have time to continue to go to daily meetings. She states she had too many papers to grade and that her friends at work did not understand why she needed to go to meetings every day. She also says that her chemical dependency counselor never listened to her, so she quit meeting with him. Her family lives in another state. The only friends she feels close to abuse alcohol and drugs. She agrees that she needs to once again feel in control of herself and her ability to not abuse alcohol.

Working

Over the next few days, you explore with Ms. Bell what sources of help she believes will be most useful to her. She identifies that group therapy and AA really helped during her last admission and elects to participate in these activities again. The two of you also identify that she would feel more comfortable with a female chemical dependency counselor as a support person after she is discharged. She asks you to investigate if there is a counselor who works in the outpatient service who could meet with her while she is still hospitalized. She recognizes that she would feel better about meeting with someone in outpatient sessions whom she has gotten to know while in the security of the inpatient environment. She also requests help with how to share her needs for support with her fellow teachers in an effort to develop friends who are not abusing substances.

Termination

As Ms. Bell's inpatient therapist and outpatient counselor agree with her that she has developed skills that will help her function without abusing alcohol, she prepares to be discharged from the chemical dependency unit to outpatient care. It is time to terminate the interpersonal relationship you have developed with Ms. Bell. You verify with her that she has practiced how to share her needs with her fellow teachers and that she has selected two teachers to be the first people she will approach. She has also contacted her AA counselor, who has made arrangements to pick her up at the hospital and provide her transportation home. She states she has made a commitment to attend AA meetings and has an appointment for tomorrow with her outpatient counselor. She shares with you that this counselor really listens to her and that she believes she will receive the support she needs. They have begun discussing how she can use time management skills to meet the demands of her job and still have the time she needs to attend AA meetings and counseling sessions. You congratulate Ms. Bell on her progress and say "Good-bye" as she is leaving.

CRITIQUE OF PEPLAU'S INTERPERSONAL RELATIONS

Peplau's work is now critiqued as a theory using the questions in this book's first chapter. Generally, Peplau's work is a theory of nursing.

1. *What is the historical context of the theory?* Peplau's theory was published in 1952, before the major thrust of nursing theory development, and is generally classified as being in the totality paradigm. Her work is a keystone in nursing practice focusing on the therapeutic relationship and theory development. Peplau identifies needs, frustration, conflict, and anxiety as important concepts in nursing situations. Furthermore, she states that these concepts must be addressed for patient and nurse growth to occur. These concepts can readily be identified as having been influenced by some theories of the time, especially Harry S. Sullivan's (1947) and Fromme's (1947) interpersonal theory and Sigmund Freud's (1936) theory of psychodynamics. Interpersonal theorists believe that behavior directly evolves from interpersonal relationships. Similar to Freudian theorists, interpersonal theorists believe that psychological development is critical in the evolution of a person. Even the name of two of her initial phases, identification and exploitation, were strongly influenced by interpersonal and psychodynamic theory.

   Because Peplau focuses on the psychological tasks within the person, her theory does not examine the broad range of environmental influences on the person, a view that was timely in 1949 when the book was written (Sills, 1977, p. 202). In examining the historical trends in psychiatric nursing, this view is categorized as being "within the person," as later contrasted to views of "within the relationship" and "within the social system," both of which consider a broader range of environmental influences on the person (Sills, 1977). Today's nurse evaluates many concepts, such as intrafamily dynamics, socioeconomic forces (e.g., financial resources), personal space considerations, and community social service resources, for each patient. These concepts provide a broader perspective for viewing the patient in his environment than do Peplau's concepts of needs, frustration, conflict, and anxiety.

   Nurses have a broader perspective on nursing roles than that represented in Peplau's original 1952 publication. Nursing now assists the patient to reach a fuller health potential through health maintenance and promotion. As long ago as 1970, Martha Rogers wrote, "Maintenance and promotion of health, prevention of disease, nursing diagnosis, intervention, and rehabilitation encompass the scope of nursing's goals" (p. 86). Today, nurses actively seek to identify health problems in a variety of community and institutional settings.

   Peplau's 1952 view does not support the current viewpoint of independent functioning by advanced practice nurses. Peplau (1952/1988) wrote that the physician's primary function was "recognizing the full import of the nuclear problem and the kind of professional assistance that is needed," which results, for the physician, in "the task of evaluating and diagnosing the emergent problem" (p. 23). Nursing functions, according to Peplau (1952/1988), include clarification of the information the physician gives the patient as well as collection of data about the patient that may point out other problem areas. In contrast, given today's expanded roles in nursing, advanced practice nurses may or may not refer the patient to the physician, depending on the patient's needs. Through expanded roles, nursing is becoming more accountable and responsible, giving professional nursing greater independence than previously. Peplau's view of nursing's role may well be an artifact of the era in which her book was originally published.

2. *What are the basic concepts and relationships presented by the theory?*   The phases of orientation, working, and termination interrelate the various components of each phase. This interrelationship creates a different perspective from which to view the nurse–patient interaction and the transaction of health care. The nurse–patient interaction can apply the concepts of human being, health, society/environment, and nursing. For example, in the phase of orientation there are the components of nurse, patient, strangers, problem, and anxiety.

   Peplau's theory provides a logical and systematic way of viewing nursing situations. The three progressive phases in the nurse–patient relationship are logical, beginning with initial contact in the orientation phase and ending with the termination phase. Key concepts in the theory, such as anxiety, tension, goals, and frustration, are clearly defined with explicit relationships between them and the progressive phases.

   The phases provide simplicity regarding the natural progression of the nurse–patient relationship. This simplicity leads to adaptability in any nurse–patient interaction, thus providing generalizability. The basic nature of nursing is still considered an interpersonal process even though Peplau and Forchuk have debated whether the interpersonal process should be four or three phases. Peplau (1992) refers to this when she states that Forchuk "has redefined the sometimes overlapping phases of the nurse–patient relationship as (a) the orientation phase, (b) the working phase, and (c) the resolution phase" (p. 14). In 1997, Peplau reduced her four phases to (1) orientation phase, (2) working phase, and (3) termination phase.

3. *What major phenomena of concern to nursing are presented? (These phenomena may include* **but are not limited to** *human beings, environment, health, interpersonal relations, caring, goal attainment, adaptation, and energy fields.)*   As discussed in the section of this chapter on nursing's metaparadigm, Peplau's early work defines *man* in the generic use for human beings, health, and nursing. In later writings she emphasized the importance of including the family in the plan of care. However, with her interest in, and emphasis on, interpersonal relations, she presented many more phenomena of interest to nursing. These include tension, anxiety, goals, frustration, therapeutic relationships, human needs, and mutual growth. All of these are defined and discussed by Peplau.

4. *To whom does this theory apply? In what situations? In what ways?*   Peplau's work has contributed greatly to nursing's body of knowledge, not only in psychiatric-mental health nursing but also in nursing in general. An example is the contributions made by her work on anxiety. Nursing is still defined as an interpersonal process built on the progressive nurse–patient phases. As Peplau proposed, communication and interviewing skills remain fundamental nursing tools. Peplau (1992) refers to several interrelated theoretical constructs such as "concepts, processes, patterns, and problems" that the nurse uses in the interpersonal process (p. 16). Also, her anxiety continuum is still used for nursing interventions in working with anxious patients. In applying Peplau's theory in clinical practice, the focus is on assisting the patient to identify psychological and growth needs. This theory is not as useful for working with a patient with many physiological needs. Another limitation of this theory is in working with the

unconscious patient. A major assumption in the theory is the ability of the nurse and patient to interact. For example, the phase of orientation begins when the patient has a felt need and initiates interaction between the nurse and the patient. This viewpoint is extremely limited in working with the unconscious patient.

In 2004, Davidson, Cockburn, Daly, and Fisher discussed the development of a needs assessment instrument for heart failure patients. Their patient-centered needs assessment provides information about health status, expectations, and perceptions and can help plan care. They cite Peplau to support that quality of life is a need related personal perception. They agree with Peplau that it is not safe to assume that relationships between health care providers and patients will be constructive and enhance quality of life and warn about the potential negative impacts of patriarchal models of care and inequity in power relationships.

Hrabe (2005) analyzed the utility of Peplau's theory in cyberspace. Can this theory apply to computer-mediated communication in nurse–patient interaction? With patients in an online relationship, nurses will still be in the roles of stranger, resource person, teacher, leader, surrogate, and counselor. Hrabe stated that the four phases of Peplau's therapeutic relationship apply to online communication. His conclusion is that Peplau's theory retains applicability in a computer-mediated environment; however, research is needed support this premise.

5. *By what method or methods can this theory be tested?*   Peplau's theory has generated both research questions and testable hypotheses. Various methods have been used, including descriptive, content analysis, experimental, and instrument development studies (see Table 4-4).

Early researchers focused on the concept of anxiety and used small samples. Hays (1961) examined teaching the concept of anxiety to six female patients in a group setting. Burd (1963) used Peplau's work on anxiety to develop a framework and to conduct a study of 25 nursing students who worked with anxious patients. Early research was mostly descriptive.

Some studies focused on Peplau's nurse–patient relationship. In 1989, Forchuk and Brown created an instrument to assess Peplau's nurse–client relationship and tested the instrument on 132 clients in Canada. Later, Forchuk (1994a) used a prospective design with 124 newly formed nurse–client dyads to examine the orientation phase and found that preconceptions were an important factor. In 1998, Forchuk et al. studied 10 client–nurse dyads to identify factors influencing the movement from the orientation phase to the working phase. The investigators found that nurses can help the clients move to the working phase by being available and consistent and by promoting trust.

6. *Does this theory direct nursing actions that lead to favorable outcomes?*   Peplau's theory does direct nursing actions that lead to favorable outcomes. Her interpersonal process directly improves communication, and interviewing skills remain fundamental nursing tools. Peplau focused on observing a patient and using communication techniques based on patient needs. The thrust of her theory is improving the nurse–patient communication. The timelessness of Peplau's theory is the focus on the patient and adjusting nursing interventions based on the patient's needs. When nurses continuously assess and refine nursing actions to focus on meeting the the patient's needs, there will be favorable outcomes.

Peplau's theory also provides a framework for nurse self-assessment. Self-assessment is important to all nurses who interact with patients, regardless of the

TABLE 4-4   Selected Significant Nursing Research Using Peplau's Work as a Framework

Date and Author	Research	Findings
1961 Hays, D.	Provided a description of phases and steps of experiential teaching about anxiety to a patient group. Sample was six female psychiatric patients.	Verbal analysis of the group revealed that when taught by the experiential method the patients were able to apply the concepts of anxiety after the group was terminated.
1963 Burd, S. F.	Developed and tested a nursing intervention framework for working with anxious patients Sample was 25 psychiatric nursing students consisting of 15 freshman and 10 graduate students.	Freshman students can develop beginning competency in interpersonal relationships. The earlier the student gains theoretical knowledge, the more the student is aware of his or her own anxiety. As students work with patients, patients respond by going through sequential phases, including denial, ambivalence, and awareness of anxiety.
1989 Forchuk, C., & Brown, B.	Created an instrument to test Peplau's nurse–client relationship. Sample was 58 case management clients and 74 counseling/treatment clients.	The instrument provided an assessment of the nurse–patient relationship. Chronic long orientation phase.
1994a Forchuk, C.	Tested the orientation phase of Peplau's theory. Sample was 124 newly formed nurse–client dyads.	Client and nurse preconceptions were important in the development of the therapeutic relationship. Client and nurse anxieties were not significant in the relationship. Other interpersonal relationships were important for the clients but not for the nurses.
1996 Beeber, L., & Caldwell, C.	Collected data derived from clinical intervention over four month period with six women.	Behaviors were analyzed constituting pattern integrations for reciprocal interaction of nurses and patients.

(continued)

TABLE 4-4   Continued

Date and Author	Research	Findings
1996 Morrison, E., Shealy, A., Kowalski, C., LaMont, J., & Range, B.	Used content analysis to identify nursing role behaviors with 31 RNs and 62 adult, child, and adolescent patients.	Counselor role was supported as being central to psychiatric nursing.
1998 Forchuk, C., et al.	Interviewed 10 nurse–client dyads until all parties agreed that they were in working phase.	In the working phase the relationship was described as being supportive and powerful. There were factors that enhanced and hindered the progression of the relationship.
2003. Douglass, J. L., Sowell, R. L., & Phillips, K. D.	Tested associations between difficulty taking HIV medications and a woman's relationship with primary health care provider and other variables.	The study found significant associations among the relationship with the primary health care provider, the woman's present life satisfaction, and the HIV-infected women taking prescribed medication.
2004 Beebe, L. H., & Tian, L.	Used a prospective experimental design to examine whether face-to-face meetings to establish rapport with schizophrenia patients had an effect on verbal responses when the nurses used telephone intervention after discharge.	Compared to the control group, the experimental group conversed longer at every measurement point and significantly longer in weeks 1–3, including patient use of more feeling statements.
2005 Shattell, M.	Described active strategies that eight medical-surgical patients used to entice nurses within the context of the nurse–patient relationships.	The patient theme was to "make nurses your friends." Active strategies used included everyday conversation, showing interest, eye contact, and smiling. The patient premise was then the nurses would "be there" when patients need them.
2005 McNaughton, D. B.	Observed and audio-recorded five prenatal clients at home using Forchuk and Brown's Relationship Form.	The study found that, over time, relationships progressed as predicted by Peplau.

clinical setting. Peplau asserts that the interpersonal process is directly affected by the nurse's preconceived ideas, values, culture, religion, race, past experiences, and expectations. By using this theory as a framework, the nurse assesses her thoughts and reactions to the patient and continually focuses on whether the relationship is therapeutic to the patient. This ongoing self-assessment is important to the professional growth of the nurse and enhances critical thinking as well as directs therapeutic nursing interventions. The nurse–patient relationship is initiated by a felt need of the patient, the focus of the relationship is to meet that felt need, and the relationship ends when the need is met. Meeting the need is a favorable outcome.

7. *How contagious is this theory?*   Much of Peplau's theory has become public domain or has been integrated into nursing practice without Peplau being overtly identified as the author. For example, nursing is defined as an interpersonal process and self-awareness is presented as a critical component of being therapeutic with a patient without giving attribution to Peplau for these concepts. In every clinical setting, nurses continue to use Peplau's interventions in dealing with anxious patients.

Peplau's theory has spurred some research; however, research efforts have been sporadic since 1952. For example, two-thirds of the nursing research in the 1950s concentrated on the nurse–patient relationship and Peplau's theory (Sills, 1977). However, with the advent of other nursing theorists in the 1960s and 1970s, there was gap in using Peplau as a theorist in research. In the late 1980s, Forchuk et al. began using Peplau's theory as a model for research on the nurse–patient relationship.

In 2004, Beebe and Tian found that an experimental group of home-based patients with schizophrenia interacted longer in telephone contact with nurses who had face-to-face meetings with patients before discharge as compared to a control group who had no face-to-face contact. Shattell (2005) found medical-surgical patients used active interactive strategies to entice nurses in a effort to mitigate the patient's vulnerability and increase the interpersonal connection. Stockmann (2005) reviewed research on the process of Peplau's therapeutic relationship and found that knowledge was limited. Much of the research using Peplau's work as a theoretical framework was conducted in Canada. However, research has generated evidence of the importance of the nurse–patient relationship in clinical practice and to the patients themselves and of nursing knowledge in the development of the orientation phase.

Peplau's work is used internationally. Published works verify its use in Australia and New Zealand (Doncliff, 1994; Harding, 1995), Belgium (Gastmans, 1998), Canada (Forchuk 1992, 1994a, 1994b; Jewell & Sullivan, 1996; Yamashita, 1997), the United Kingdom and Ireland (Almond, 1996; Barker, 1998; Buswell, 1997; Chambers, 1998; Edwards, 1996; Fowler, 1994, 1995; Jones, 1995; Lambert, 1994; Lego, 1998; Price, 1998; Reynolds, 1997; Ryles, 1998; Vardy & Price, 1998), as well as in the United States. In addition to being used by psychiatric nurses, Peplau's theory has also been documented as useful in many other areas, such as AIDS care, health education, moral issues of practice, palliative care, patients with strokes, pediatric oncology, postpartum care, reflective evaluation of practice, quality of life, and research (Almond, 1996; Edwards, 1996; Fowler, 1994, 1995; Gastmans, 1998; Hall, 1994; Harding, 1995; Jewell & Sullivan, 1996; Jones, 1995; Kelley, 1996; Peden, 1998; Peplau, 1994b).

Summary

Peplau's (1952/1988) *Interpersonal Relations in Nursing* is still applicable in theory and practice. The core of Peplau's theory of nursing focuses on the interpersonal relationship, which is an integral part of present-day nursing. The interpersonal relationship process initially consisted of the sequential phases of orientation, identification, exploitation, and resolution. More recently, Peplau (1997) redefined the phases as the orientation phase, the working phase, and the termination phase. These phases overlap, interrelate, and vary in duration. The nurse and patient first clarify the patient's problems, and mutual expectations and goals are explored while deciding on appropriate plans for improving health status. The interpersonal relationship process is influenced by both the nurse's and the patient's perceptions and preconceived ideas emerging from their individual uniqueness.

Peplau stresses that both the patient and the nurse mature as the result of the therapeutic interaction. When two persons meet in a creative relationship, there is a continuing sense of mutuality and togetherness throughout the experience. Both individuals are involved in a process of self-fulfillment, which becomes a growth experience.

Peplau's nursing theory of interpersonal relationships has as its foundation theories of interaction. It has contributed to nursing in the areas of clinical practice, theory, and research, adding to today's base of nursing knowledge. Thus, Peplau's theory creates a unique view for understanding the nurse–patient relationship.

Thought Questions

1. What were some of Dr. Hildegard Peplau's major contributions to nursing?
2. Describe the phases of the nurse–patient interpersonal process.
3. Give examples of the various roles that a nurse might fulfill in the nurse–patient interpersonal process.
4. In 1952, Peplau wrote that her book was a "partial theory" for the practice of nursing. Do you think her work is a theory? Discuss your rationale.
5. In the orientation phase, why should the nurse examine personal values and reaction to the patient?
6. What types of strategies can the nurse use in the working phase of the nurse–patient relationship?
7. In home visiting, the community health nurse has discharged the patient from the service and will not make any more home visits. If the patient is not ready to terminate the relationship with the nurse, what types of behaviors might the patient show?
8. List two areas of nursing research that originate from Peplau's theory.

References

Almond, P. (1996). How health visitors assess the health of postnatal women. *Health Visitor, 69*, 495–498.

Barker, P. (1998). The future of the Theory of Interpersonal Relations: A personal reflection on Peplau's legacy. *Journal of Psychiatric and Mental Health Nursing, 5*, 213–220.

Beebe, L. H., & Tian, L. (2004). TIPS: Telephone intervention—Problem solving for persons with schizophrenia. *Issues in Mental Health Nursing, 25*, 317–329.

Beeber, L., & Caldwell, C. (1996). Pattern integrations in young depressed women: Part 2. *Archives of Psychiatric Nursing, 10*, 157–164.

Burd, S. (1963). Effects of nursing interventions in anxiety of patients. In S. F. Burd & M. A. Marshall (Eds.), *Some clinical approaches to psychiatric nursing* (pp. 307–320). London: Macmillan [out ot print]

Burton, G. (1958). *Personal, impersonal, and interpersonal: A guide for nurses.* New York: Springer.

Buswell, C. (1997). A model approach to care of a patient with alcohol problems . . . Peplau's model. *Nursing Times, 93*, 34–35.

Chambers, M. (1998). Interpersonal mental health nursing: Research issues and challenges. *Journal of Psychiatric and Mental Health Nursing, 5*, 203–211.

Davidson, R., Cockburn, J., Daly, J., & Fisher, R. S. (2004). Patient-centered needs assessment: Rationale for a psychometric measure for assessing needs in heart failure. *Journal of Cardiovascular Nursing, 19*(3), 164–171.

Doncliff, B. (1994). Putting Peplau to work. *Nursing New Zealand, 2*(1), 20–22.

Douglass, J. L., Sowell, R. L., & Phillps, K. D. (2003). Using Peplau's theory to examine the psychosocial factors associated with HIV-infected women's difficulty in taking their medications. *Journal of Theory Construction and Testing, 7*(1), 10–17.

Edwards, M. (1996). Patient–nurse relationships: Using reflective practice. *Nursing Standard, 10*(25), 40–43.

Forchuk, C. (1992). The orientation phase of the nurse–client relationship: How long does it take? *Perspectives in Psychiatric Care, 28*(4), 7–10.

Forchuk, C. (1994a). Preconceptions in the nurse–client relationship. *Journal of Psychiatric and Mental Health Nursing, 1*, 145–149.

Forchuck, C. (1994b). The orientation phase of the nurse–client relationship: Testing Peplau's theory. *Journal of Advanced Nursing, 20*, 532–537.

Forchuk, C., & Brown, B. (1989). Establishing a nurse–client relationship. *Journal of Psychosocial Nursing, 27*, 30–34.

Forchuk, C., Westwell, J., Martin, M., Azzapardi, W. B., Kosterewa-Tolman, D., & Hux, M. (1998). Factors influencing movement of chronic psychiatric patients from the orientation to the working phase of the nurse–client relationship on an inpatient unit. *Perspectives in Psychiatric Care: The Journal for Nurse Psychotherapists, 34*(1), 36–44.

Fowler, J. (1994). A welcome focus on a key relationship: Using Peplau's model in palliative care. *Professional Nurse, 10*, 194–197.

Fowler, J. (1995). Taking theory into practice: Using Peplau's model in the care of the patient. *Professional Nurse, 10*, 226–230.

Freud, S. (1936). *The problem of anxiety.* New York: Norton.

Fromme, E. (1947). *Man for himself.* New York: Rinehart.

Gastmans, C. (1998). Interpersonal relations in nursing: A philosophical-ethical analysis of the work of Hildegard E. Peplau. *Journal of Advanced Nursing, 28*, 1312–1319.

Hall, K. (1994). Peplau's model of nursing: Caring for a man with AIDS. *British Journal of Nursing, 3*, 418–422.

Harding, T. (1995). Exemplar . . . the essential foundation of nursing lies in the establishment of a therapeutic relationship. *Professional Leader, 2*(1), 20–21.

Hays, D. (1961). Teaching a concept of anxiety. *Nursing Research, 10*, 108–113.

Hrabe, D. P. (2005). Peplau in cyberspace: An analysis of Peplau's interpersonal relations theory and computer-mediated communication, *Issues in Mental Health Nursing, 26*, 397–414.

Jewell, J. A., & Sullivan, E. A. (1996). Application of nursing theories in health education. *Journal of the American Psychiatric Nurses Association, 2*(3), 79–85.

Jones, A. (1995). Utilizing Peplau's psychodynamic theory for stroke patient care. *Journal of Clinical Nursing, 4*(1), 49–54.

Kelley, S. J. (1996). "It's just me, my family, my treatments, and my nurse . . . oh, yeah, and Nintendo": Hildegard Peplau's day with kids with cancer. *Journal of the American Psychiatric Nurses Association, 2*(1), 11–14.

Lambert, C. (1994). Depression: Nursing management, part 2. *Nursing Standard, 8*(48), 57–64.

Lego, S. (1998). The application of Peplau's theory to group psychotherapy. *Journal of Psychiatric and Mental Health Nursing, 5,* 193–196.

McNaughton, D. B. (2005). A naturalistic test of Peplau's theory in home visiting. *Public Health Nursing, 22*(5), 429–438.

Morrison, E. G., Shealy, A. H., Kowalsi, C., LaMont, J., & Range, B. A. (1996). Work roles of staff nurses in psychiatric settings. *Nursing Science Quarterly, 9,* 17–21.

Peden, A. R. (1998). The evolution of an intervention—The use of Peplau's process of practice-based theory development. *Journal of Psychiatric and Mental Health Nursing, 5,* 173–178.

Peplau, H. E. (n.d.). *Basic principles of patient counseling.*

Peplau, H. E. (1988). *Interpersonal relations in nursing.* NY: Springer. (Original work published 1952, New York: G. P. Putnam's Sons)

Peplau, H. E. (1992). Interpersonal relations: A theoretical framework for application in nursing practice. *Nursing Science Quarterly, 5,* 13–18.

Peplau, H. E. (1994a). Psychiatric mental health nursing: Challenge and change. *Journal of Psychiatric and Mental Health Nursing, 1,* 3–7.

Peplau, H. E. (1994b). Quality of life: An interpersonal perspective. *Nursing Science Quarterly, 7,* 10–15.

Peplau, H. E. (1994c). The "Bridges of Madison County" has been on the best-seller list for more than 1 year: From a psycho-social perspective, what is the appeal of this popular book? *Journal of Psychosocial Nursing, 32,* 57–58.

Peplau, H. E. (1995). Some unresolved issues in the era of biopsychosocial nursing. *Journal of the American Psychiatric Nurses Association, 1,* 92–96.

Peplau, H. E. (1997). Peplau's theory of interpersonal relations. *Nursing Science Quarterly, 10,* 162–167.

Price, B. (1998). Explorations in body image care: Peplau and practice knowledge. *Journal of Psychiatric and Mental Health Nursing, 5,* 179–186.

Profile: Hildegard E. Peplau, R.N., Ed.D. (1974). *Nursing '74, 4,* 13.

Reynolds, W. J. (1997). Peplau's theory in practice. *Nursing Science Quarterly, 10,* 168–170.

Rogers, M. E. (1970). *An introduction to the theoretical basis of nursing.* Philadelphia: F. A. Davis. [out of print]

Ryles, S. (1998). Applying Peplau's theory in psychiatric nursing practice. *Nursing Times, 94,* 62–63.

Shattell, M. (2005). Nurse bait: Strategies hospitalized patients use to entice nurse within the context of interpersonal relationship. *Issues in Mental Health, 26,* 205–223.

Sills, G. (1977). Research in the field of psychiatric nursing, 1952–1977. *Nursing Research, 26,* 201–207.

Stockmann, C. (2005). A literature review of the progress of the psychiatric nurse–patient relationship as described by Peplau. *Issues in Mental Health Nursing, 26,* 911–919.

Sullivan, H. S. (1947). *Conceptions of modern psychiatry.* Washington, DC: William Alanson White Psychiatric Foundation.

Vardy, C., & Price, V. (1998). Commentary: The utilization of Peplau's theory of nursing in working with a male survivor of sexual abuse. *Journal of Psychiatric and Mental Health Nursing, 5,* 149–155.

Yamashita, M. (1997). Family caregiving: Application of Newman's and Peplau's theories. *Journal of Psychiatric and Mental Health Nursing, 4,* 401–405.

Bibliography

Beeber, L., Anderson, C. A., & Sills, G. M. (1990). Peplau's theory in practice. *Nursing Science Quarterly, 3,* 6–8.

Forchuk, C. (1991). Peplau's theory: Concepts and their relations. *Nursing Science Quarterly, 4,* 54–60.

Forchuk, C., & Dorsay, J. P. (1995). Hildegard Peplau meets family systems nursing: Innovation in theory-based practice. *Journal of Advanced Nursing, 21,* 110–115.

Peplau, H. E. (1969, March). Theory: The professional dimension. In *Proceedings from the First Nursing Theory Conference.* University of Kansas Medical Center. [Reprinted 1986 in L. H. Nicholl (Ed.), *Perspectives on nursing theory* (pp. 455–466). Boston: Little, Brown]

Peplau, H. E. (1978). Psychiatric nursing: Role of nurses and psychiatric nurses. *International Nursing Review, 25*, 41–47.

Peplau, H. E. (1982). Some reflections on earlier days in psychiatric nursing. *Journal of Psychosocial Nursing and Mental Health Services, 20*, 17–24.

Peplau, H. E. (1985). Is nursing's self-regulatory power being eroded? *American Journal of Nursing, 85*, 140–143.

Peplau, H. E. (1985). The power of the dissociative state. *Journal of Psychosocial Nursing and Mental Health Services, 8*, 31–33.

Peplau, H. E. (1986). The nurse as counselor. *Journal of American College of Health, 35*, 11–14.

Peplau, H. E. (1987). Psychiatric skills, tomorrow's world. *Nursing Times, 83*, 29–33.

Peplau, H. E. (1988). The art and science of nursing: Similarities, differences, and relations. *Nursing Science Quarterly, 1*, 8–15.

Peplau, H. E. (1989). Future directions in psychiatric nursing from the history. *Journal of Psychosocial Nursing, 2*, 18–21, 25–28.

Peplau, H. E. (1990). Evolution of nursing in psychiatric settings. In E. M. Varcarolis (Ed.), *Foundations of psychiatric mental health nursing.* Philadelphia: Saunders.

Peplau, H. E. (1997). Is healthcare a right? *Journal of Nursing Scholarship, 3*, 220–222.

Rust, J. E. (2004). Dr. Hildegard Peplau: Profile. *Clinical Nurse Specialist, 18*(5), 262–263.

Thompson, L. (1980). Peplau's theory: An application to short-term individual therapy. *Journal of Psychosocial Nursing, 24*, 26–31.

Trench, A. S. (Executive producer), Wallace, D. (Producer), & Coberg, T. (Director). (1988). *Hildegard Peplau—The nurse theorists: Portraits of excellence* [Videotape]. Oakland, CA: Studio Three Production, Samuel Merritt College of Nursing.

Annotated Bibliography

Beeber, L., & Caldwell, C. (1996). Pattern integrations in young depressed women: Part 1 and Part 2. *Archives of Psychiatric Nursing, 10*(3), 151–164.

Research in which 42 hours of clinical tapes were analyzed consisting of data derived from clinical interventions over a four-month period with six depressed women. Analysis of clusters of behaviors for nurse/client reciprocal interactions was made identifying four common pattern integrations of complementary, mutual, alternating, and antagonistic patterns as described by Peplau. Clinical illustrations and a model for intervention using the integrations is discussed.

Forchuk, C. (1995). Development of nurse–client relationships: What helps. *Journal of the American Psychiatric Nurses Association, 1*, 146–153.

This secondary analysis of data investigated factors that influence the progress of the therapeutic relationship during Peplau's orientation phase. Factors related to a shorter orientation phase included longer meetings between the nurse and patient, more cumulative time spent in such meetings, and a history of shorter previous hospitalizations. Factors that influenced the progression of the relationship in this phase included those that cannot be altered.

Forchuk, C., Beaten, S., Crawford, L., Ide, L., Voorberg, N., & Bethune, J. (1989). Incorporating Peplau's theory and case management. *Journal of Psychosocial Nursing, 2*, 35–38.

A case management program was established with a target client group of chronic mentally ill individuals who had no connection with the mental health system. Links were identified incorporating Peplau's theory and the case management model to develop a consistent approach. The importance of the interactive interpersonal relationship between the practitioner and the client became the main link. The combined model provided a basis for comprehensive permanent follow-up. Implementation is described in a case study.

Fowler, J. (1995). Taking theory into practice: Using Peplau's model in the care of patient. *Professional Nurse, 10*, 226–230.

The philosophy of palliative care and Peplau's Interpersonal Relations Model were reviewed for compatibility. A case study focused on the care of one terminally ill patient in a hospice setting as the model was applied to clinical practice.

Lego, S. (1998). The application of Peplau's theory to group psychotherapy. *Journal of Psychiatric and Mental Health Nursing, 5*(3), 193–196.

This is a portrayal of the phases of Peplau's interpersonal theory as they pertain to group psychotherapy. Clinical illustrations are discussed. Steps of the learning process are detailed as the patient moves through them in group therapy. Also, the nurse's roles are presented as they arise during group sessions.

Morrison, E. G., Shealy, A. H., Kowalski, C., LaMont, J., & Range, B. A. (1996). Work roles of staff nurses in psychiatric settings. *Nursing Science Quarterly, 9*, 17–21.

This research was conducted to authenticate the work roles of the psychiatric staff nurse as referenced by Peplau. Audiotaped one-to-one interactions were performed between 30 registered nurses and 62 patients. Overlapping behaviors were found between some roles. The most frequently occurring primary work role was that of the counselor, sustaining Peplau's view of the counselor's role.

Peden, A. R. (1998). The evolution of an intervention—The use of Peplau's process of practice-based theory development. *Journal of Psychiatric and Mental Health Nursing, 5*, 173–178.

Reviews Peplau's theories of nursing knowledge/ practice. Peplau is credited for research methodology and is acknowledged as setting precedents in psychiatric nursing.

Peplau, H. E. (1997). Peplau's theory of interpersonal relations. *Nursing Science Quarterly, 10*, 162–167.

Peplau first presents other theories essential to nursing practice before describing her interpersonal relations theory. The remainder of the article's focus is on this interpersonal theory. Participant observation includes the nurse self-analyzing overt and covert behaviors and ability to empathize. The nurse and patient progress through three phases of their relationship in the interpersonal process. These phases are discussed, as are the issues that occur throughout the interactions.

CHAPTER 5

Definition and Components of Nursing
Virginia Henderson*

Marie L. Lobo

Virginia Henderson was born on March 19, 1897, in Kansas City, Missouri, and died on November 30, 1996. She was the fifth child in a family of eight children and lived most of her formative years in Virginia, where the family resided during the period her father practiced law in Washington.

Henderson's interest in nursing evolved during World War I from her desire to help the sick and wounded military personnel. She enrolled in the Army School of Nursing in Washington, D.C., and graduated in 1921. In 1926, Henderson began the continuation of her education at Columbia University Teachers College and completed her B.S. (1932) and M.A. (1934) degrees in nursing education. She taught clinical nursing courses with a strong emphasis on the use of the analytical process from 1934 to 1948 at Teachers College. From 1948 to 1953 she worked with Harmer on an extensive revision of the fifth edition of The Principles and Practice of Nursing. *In 1953 she was appointed as faculty at Yale University School of Nursing. The Yale years were very productive, with a number of Henderson's major publications copyrighted between 1955 and 1978 (McBride, 1996). From 1959 to 1971, Henderson directed the Nursing Studies Index Project, which clearly showed her interest in supporting nursing research (Henderson & Watt, 1983). Also, during 1953–1958, she was on the Survey and Assessment of Nursing Research staff, a project directed by Leo Simmons. In the 1980s Henderson (1982b) supported the idea that nursing must accept the responsibility for conducting investigations on nursing practice and that the focus ought to be on measures of consumer welfare, satisfaction, and cost-effectiveness. Henderson also played an important role in the publication of the* International Nursing Index *in 1966. The* Index *was the result and production of the promotional efforts of the Interagency on Library Resources in Nursing (Henderson, 1991). During retirement, she was Senior Research Associate Emeritus at Yale University.*

* Gratitude is expressed to Chiyoko Yamamoto Furukawa and Joan Swartz Howe for their contributions to this chapter in previous editions.

Henderson was the recipient of numerous recognitions for her outstanding contributions to nursing, including the Sigma Theta Tau International Nursing Library, which bears her name. She received honorary doctoral degrees from Catholic University of America, Pace University, University of Rochester, University of Western Ontario, Yale University, Old Dominion University, Boston College, Thomas Jefferson University, and Emory University.

Her writings are far-reaching and have made an impact on nursing throughout the world. In June 1985, the International Council of Nurses presented her with the first Christianne Reimann Prize in recognition of her influence as nursing consultant to the world (McBride, 1996). Her publications The Nature of Nursing *(1966) and* Basic Principles of Nursing Care *(1960; 1997 [revised]) are widely known, and the latter, published by the International Council of Nurses, has been translated into many languages for the benefit of non-English-speaking nurses. She clarified her beliefs about nursing, nursing education, and nursing practice in view of recent technological and societal advances in publications, interviews, and personal appearances (Henderson, 1978, 1979a, 1979b, 1982a, 1985, 1987). One of her last publications, in 1991, was* The Nature of Nursing: A Definition and Its Implications for Practice, Research, and Education. Reflections After 25 Years. *The addendum to each chapter contains changes in her views and opinions relative to the 1966 first edition of* The Nature of Nursing.

Questions about the exclusive functions of nurses provided the impetus for Virginia Henderson to devote her career to defining nursing practice. Some of these questions were the following: What is the practice of nursing? What specific functions do nurses perform? What are nursing's unique activities? The development of her definition of nursing communicated her thoughts on these questions. She believed that an occupation that affects human life must outline its functions, particularly if it is to be regarded as a profession (Henderson, 1966, 1991). Her ideas about the definition of nursing were influenced by her nursing education and practice, by her students and colleagues at Columbia University School of Nursing, and by distinguished nursing leaders of her time. All these experiences and nursing practice were the dominating forces that gave her insight into nursing: what it is and what its functions are.

THE DEVELOPMENT OF HENDERSON'S DEFINITION OF NURSING

Two events are the basis for Henderson's development of a definition of nursing. First, she participated in the revision of a nursing textbook. Second, she was concerned that many states had no provision for nursing licensure to ensure safe and competent care for the consumer.

In the revision of *Textbook of the Principles and Practice of Nursing*, written with Canadian nurse Bertha Harmer, Henderson recognized the need to be clear about the functions of the nurse (Harmer & Henderson, 1939; Safier, 1977). She believed that a textbook that serves as a main learning source for nursing practice should present a sound and definitive description of nursing. Furthermore, the principles and practice of nursing must be built on and derived from the definition of the profession.

Henderson was committed to the process of regulating nursing practice through state licensure. She believed that to accomplish this, nursing must be explicitly defined in nurse practice acts that would provide the legal parameters for nurses' functions in caring for consumers and safeguard the public from unprepared and incompetent practitioners.

Although official statements on the nursing function were published by the American Nurses Association (ANA) in 1932 and 1937, Henderson (1966, 1991) viewed these statements as nonspecific and unsatisfactory definitions of nursing practice. Then, in 1955, the earlier ANA (1962) definition was modified to read as follows:

> The practice of professional nursing means the performance for compensation of any act in the observation, care, and counsel of the ill, injured, or infirm, or in the maintenance of health or prevention of illness of others, or in the supervision and teaching of other personnel, or the administration of medications and treatment as prescribed by a licensed physician or dentist; requiring substantial specialized judgment and skill and based on knowledge and application of the principles of biological, physical, and social science. The foregoing shall not be deemed to include acts of diagnosis or prescription of therapeutic or corrective measures. (p. 7)

This statement was seen as an improvement because nursing functions were identified, but the definition still was thought to be very general and too vague. In the new statement, the nurse could observe, care for, and counsel the patient and could supervise other health personnel without herself being supervised by the physician. The nurse was to give medications and do treatments ordered by the physician but was prohibited from diagnosing, prescribing treatment for, or correcting nursing care problems. Thus, Henderson viewed the statement as another unsatisfactory definition of nursing.

Henderson's extensive experiences as a student, teacher, practitioner, author, and participant in conferences on the nurse's function contributed to the development of her definition of nursing. She regretted that publications of conference debates and investigations were not widely circulated. Only a few nurses were privy to the information published about the outcomes of these conferences.

In 1955, Henderson's first definition of nursing was published in Bertha Harmer's revised nursing textbook (Harmer & Henderson, 1955). It reads as follows:

> Nursing is primarily assisting the individual (sick or well) in the performance of those activities contributing to health, or its recovery (or peaceful death) that he would perform unaided if he had the necessary strength, will, or knowledge. It is likewise the unique contribution of nursing to help the individual to be independent of such assistance as soon as possible. (p. 4)

This statement on nursing conveys the essence of Henderson's definition of nursing as it is known today. Since there was collaboration, it is instructive to compare Henderson's definition with Harmer's 1922 definition, which follows:

> Nursing is rooted in the needs of humanity and is founded on the ideal of service. Its object is not only to cure the sick and heal the wounded but to bring health and ease, rest and comfort to mind and body, to shelter, nourish, and protect and to minister to all those who are helpless or handicapped, young, aged, or immature. Its object is to prevent disease and to preserve health. Nursing is, therefore, linked with every other social agency which strives for the prevention of disease and the preservation of health. The nurse finds herself not only concerned with the care of the individual but with the health of a people. (p. 3)

Some similarities can be seen between the two definitions of nursing. Henderson's definition abbreviated and consolidated portions of Harmer's beliefs about nursing. Harmer's definition highlighted disease prevention, health preservation, and the need for linkages with other social agencies to strive for preventive care. Harmer stressed that nursing's role in society was oriented toward the community and wellness. Henderson placed more emphasis on the care of sick and well individuals and did not mention nursing's concern for the health and welfare of the aggregate. However, there is brief mention in *Basic Principles of Nursing* that at times nurses do function with families or other aggregates rather than solely with individuals (Henderson, 1997).

Henderson's focus on individual care is evident in that she stressed assisting individuals with essential activities to maintain health, to recover, or to achieve peaceful death. She proposed 14 components of basic nursing care to augment her definition (Henderson, 1966, 1991), as follows:

[The individual can . . .]

1. Breathe normally
2. Eat and drink adequately
3. Eliminate body wastes
4. Move and maintain desirable postures
5. Sleep and rest
6. Select suitable clothes—dress and undress
7. Maintain body temperature within normal range by adjusting clothing and modifying the environment
8. Keep the body clean and well groomed and protect the integument
9. Avoid dangers in the environment and avoid injuring others
10. Communicate with others in expressing emotions, needs, fears, or opinions
11. Worship according to one's faith
12. Work in such a way that there is a sense of accomplishment
13. Play or participate in various forms of recreation
14. Learn, discover, or satisfy the curiosity that leads to normal development and health and use the available health facilities (pp. 16–17)

In 1966 Henderson's ultimate statement on the definition of nursing was published in *The Nature of Nursing*. This statement was viewed as "the crystallization of my ideas":

The unique function of the nurse is to assist the individual, sick or well, in the performance of those activities contributing to health or its recovery (or to peaceful death) that he would perform unaided if he had the necessary strength, will or knowledge. And to do this in such a way as to help him gain independence as rapidly as possible. (p. 15)

Except for slight wording changes, the 1955, 1966, and more recent 1978 definitions are quite similar, indicating that her definition of nursing, conceived earlier, remains intact (Harmer & Henderson, 1955; Henderson, 1966; Henderson & Nite, 1978). Henderson's definition of nursing in itself fails to fully explain her main ideas and views. To appreciate the breadth of her thoughts about nursing functions and the 14 components of basic nursing care, it is necessary to study *Basic Principles of Nursing Care*, a publication of the International Council of Nurses (Henderson, 1960, 1997). This booklet eloquently describes each of the basic nursing care components so that they can be used as a guide to delineate the unique nursing functions. The definition of nursing and the 14 components together outline the functions the nurse can initiate and control. Further understanding of these components can be gained through study of the sixth edition of *Principles and Practice of Nursing*. This edition was organized according to the 14 components and also includes citations from the work of nurses around the world.

Henderson (1966, 1991) expects nurses to carry out the therapeutic plan of the physician as a member of the medical team. The nurse is the prime helper to the ill person in ensuring that the medical prescriptions are instituted. This nursing function is believed to foster the therapeutic nurse–client relationship. As a member of an interdisciplinary health team, the nurse assists the individual to recovery or provides support in dying. The ideal situation for a nurse is full participation as a team member with no interference with the nurse's unique functions. The nurse serves as a substitute for whatever the patient lacks in order to make him "complete," "whole," or "independent," considering his available physical strength, will, or knowledge to attain good health.

The nurse is cautioned about tasks that detract from the professional role and the need to give priority to the nurse's unique functions. However, Henderson encourages the nurse to assume the role and functions of other health workers if the need is apparent and the nurse has expertise. On a worldwide basis, nursing functions differ from country to country or even within countries. The ratio of nurses to physicians and to other health care providers affects what nurses do. Consequently, the public is confused about the nurse's role, particularly since the creation of nurse practitioners.

In one of her last publications, Henderson (1991) acknowledged that the efforts to define nursing had been unsuccessful: "In spite of the fact that generations of nurses have tried to define it, 'the nature of nursing' remains a question" (p. 7). In her opinion, nurses were no closer to consensus on the official definition of nursing than in 1966. She stated the only difference now is that nursing education offers courses in nursing theory and nursing process. If *The Nature of Nursing* were to be written in the 1990s, she felt she would be obliged to include a discussion of both nursing theory and the nursing process.

Furthermore, with respect to a universal definition of nursing, Henderson (1991) concluded that there is difficulty in promoting the notion of universality. She based her view on her numerous visits to countries worldwide where she observed the variations in nursing education coupled with differing nursing practices used to serve the needs of various populations.

HENDERSON'S THEORY AND NURSING'S METAPARADIGM

In viewing the concept of the *human* or individual, Henderson considered the biological, psychological, sociological, and spiritual components. Her 14 components of nursing functions can be categorized in the following manner: The first eight components are physiological, the ninth component is protective, the tenth and fourteenth components are psychological aspects of communicating and learning, the eleventh component is spiritual and moral, and the twelfth and thirteenth components are sociologically oriented to occupation and recreation. She referred to humans as having basic needs that are included in the 14 components. However, she further stated, "It is equally important to realize that these needs are satisfied by infinitely varied patterns of living, no two of which are alike" (Henderson, 1997, p. 27). Henderson (1966, 1991) also believed that mind and body are inseparable. It is implied that the mind and body are interrelated.

Henderson emphasized some aspects of the concept of *society/environment*. In her writings, however, she primarily discussed individuals. She saw individuals in relation to their families but minimally discussed the impact of the community on the individual and family. In the book cowritten with Harmer (Harmer & Henderson, 1955), she supported the tasks of private and public agencies in keeping people healthy. She believed that society wants and expects the nurse's service of acting for individuals who are unable to function independently (Henderson, 1966, 1991). In return she expected society to contribute to nursing education: The nurse needs the kind of education that, in our society, is available only in colleges and universities. "Training programs operated on funds pinched from the budgets of service agencies cannot provide the preparation the nurse needs" (Henderson, 1966, p. 69).

In her chapter on nursing education, Henderson did advocate for nursing education to include experiences in all aspects of the health care continuum. "It is difficult or impossible to offer students an opportunity to see and participate in all phases of rehabilitative and preventive health care within the hospital. Experience in other health agencies and in home care programs therefore is indicated. . . ." (Henderson, 1966, p. 45). While her thoughts on the 14 components of nursing care are very illness oriented, it is clear that she understood the importance of nursing in the context of the greater community. Henderson also advocated a broad education for nurses. She believed this generalized education gave nurses a better understanding of the consumers of nursing care and the various environmental factors that influence people.

Henderson's beliefs about *health* were related to human functioning. Her definition of health was based on the individual's ability to function independently, as outlined in the 14 components. Because good health is a challenging goal for individuals, she argued that it is difficult for the nurse to help the person reach it (Henderson, 1997). She also referred to nurses stressing promotion of health and prevention and cure of disease (Henderson, 1966). Henderson (1997) explained how the factors of age, cultural background, physical and intellectual capacities, and emotional balance affect one's health. These conditions are always present and affect basic needs. Because of her concern for the welfare of people, Henderson (1989) believed that nurses "should be in the forefront of those who work for social justice, for a healthful environment, for access to adequate food, shelter, and clothing, and universal opportunities for education and employment, realizing that all of these as well as preventive and creative health care are essential to the well-being of citizens" (p. 82). By working on various social issues, nurses can have an impact on people's health.

Henderson's concept of nursing is interesting from the perspective of time. She was one of the early leaders who believed nurses need a liberal education, including knowledge of sciences, social sciences, and humanities. Aside from using the definition of nursing and the 14 components of basic nursing care, the nurse is expected to carry out the physician's therapeutic plan. Individualized care is the result of the nurse's creativity in planning for care. Furthermore, the nurse is expected to improve patient care by using the results of nursing research:

> The nurse who operates under a definition that specifies an area of independent practice, or an area of expertness, must assume responsibility for identifying problems, for continually validating her function, for improving the methods she uses, and for measuring the effect of nursing care. In this era research is the name we attach to the most reliable type of analysis. (Henderson, 1966, p. 38)

For Henderson, the nurse must be knowledgeable, have some base for practicing individualized and humane care, and be a scientific problem solver. In her update of *The Nature of Nursing*, Henderson (1991) viewed "research in nursing as *essential* to the validation and improvement of practice" (p. 58). It is important that nursing care be improved by implementing valid research results.

HENDERSON AND THE NURSING PROCESS

Henderson (1980a) viewed the nursing process as "really the application of the logical approach to the solution of the problem. The steps are those of the scientific method" (p. 906). With this approach, each person can receive individualized care. Likewise, with the nursing process, individualized care is the result.

In Henderson's later writings, she raised some issues regarding the nursing process. One of the issues questioned whether the problem-solving approach of the nursing process is peculiar to nursing. She compared the nursing process to the traditional steps of the medical process: "the nursing history parallels the medical history; the nurse's health assessment, the physician's medical examination, the nursing diagnosis corresponds to the physician's diagnosis; nursing orders to the plan of medical management; and nursing evaluation to medical evaluation" (Henderson, 1980a, p. 907). It looks as if the language has been changed to fit nursing's purpose. Could other health care workers use the steps of the nursing process to fit their practice? If so, then what makes the nursing process peculiar to nursing?

Another issue Henderson raised also dealt with problem solving. But now she asked if problem solving is all there is to nursing. Henderson (1987) stated, "This makes it so specific that activities outside those in the problem solving steps of the process cannot be peculiar to or characteristic of nursing" (p. 8). She questioned where intuition, experience, authority, and expert opinion fit into the nursing process since they are not stressed. She further commented, "Expert opinion or authority is also, by implication, discredited as a basis for practice" (Henderson, 1982a, p. 108). Does the "the" in the nursing process make it too limiting for effective practice? (Henderson, 1982a, p. 108).

A third issue Henderson raised flows from the problem-solving approach. She asks where the art of nursing fits into the nursing process. If one views science as objective, with little left undefined, and art as subjective, with some parts hard to define, then where does intuition fit? Henderson (1987) argued that "the nursing process now weighted so heavily on the scientific side, seems to belittle the intuitive, artistic side of nursing" (p. 8). She also claimed, "Nursing process stresses the science of nursing rather than the mixture of science *and art* on which it seems effective health care services of any kind is based" (Henderson, 1987, p. 9). Does the nursing process disregard the subjective and intuitive qualities used in nursing?

The fourth concern Henderson raised about the nursing process deals with the lack of collaboration among health care workers, the patient, and the family. She stated, "As currently defined, nursing process does not seem to suggest a collaborative approach on diagnosis, treatment, *or* care by health care workers, nor does it suggest the essential rights of patients and their families in all of these questions" (Henderson, 1982a, p. 109). Henderson (1987) thought the nursing process stressed an independent function for the nurse rather than a collaborative one with other health professionals, the patient, and the patient's family. Does the nursing process focus more on independent nursing functions than on interdependent functions?

Perhaps it is semantics that is a problem with the nursing process. The real value of the nursing process depends on one's understanding, interpretation, integration, and use of it. The nursing process is now examined with Henderson's definition of nursing.

Even though Henderson's definition and explanation of nursing do not fit directly with the steps of the nursing process, a relationship between them can be demonstrated. Although Henderson did not refer directly to assessment, she implied it in her description of the 14 components of basic nursing care. The nurse uses the 14 components to assess the individual's needs. For example, in assessing the first component, "breathe normally," the nurse gathers all pertinent data about the person's respiratory status. The nurse then moves to the next component and gathers data in that area. The gathering of data about the person continues until all components have been assessed.

To complete the assessment phase of the nursing process, the nurse needs to analyze the data. According to Henderson, the nurse must have knowledge about what is normal in health and disease. Using this knowledge base, then, the nurse compares the assessment data with what was known about the area. For example, if respirations were observed to be 40 per minute in an adult aged 50, the nurse would conclude that this person's respiratory rate is faster than normal. Or if a laboratory report showed that the urine was highly concentrated, the nurse would know this "means that the patient's fluid intake is inadequate, unless he is losing body fluids by other routes" (Henderson, 1997, p. 51). With a scientific knowledge base, the nurse can draw conclusions from the assessment data. Henderson (1997) stated that "the nursing needed by the individual is affected by age, cultural background, emotional balance and the patient's physical and intellectual capacities. All of these should be considered in the nurse's evaluation of the patient's needs for help" (p. 31).

Following the analysis of the data according to these factors, the nurse then determines the nursing diagnosis. Henderson did not specifically discuss nursing diagnosis. She believed that the physician makes the diagnosis, and the nurse acts on that diagnosis, or that both could make the same diagnosis and there was no need for a separate nursing diagnosis. However, if one looks at Henderson's definition, the nursing diagnosis deals with identifying the individual's ability to meet human needs with or without assistance, taking into account that person's strength, will, and knowledge. Given the assessment data and its analysis, the nurse can identify actual problems such as abnormal respirations. In addition, potential problems may be identified. For example, with component 11, about one's faith, a potential problem could develop because of hospitalization and a change in the person's normal activities of daily living. If, based on the nurse's assessment and analysis of the data, a person were unable to meet this need, then a nursing diagnosis regarding an actual problem would be made.

Once the nursing diagnosis is made, the nurse must identify the outcomes that are desired and develop an effective plan of care. Henderson believed that all effective nursing care was planned. She also believed that "a written plan *forces* those who make it to give some thought to the individual's needs—unless the person's regimen is made to fit into the routines of the institution" (Henderson, 1997, p. 37). She advocated for the incorporation of information from family and friends into understanding the patient. She understood that the family was an important part of a patient's well-being, stating, "Her (the nurse) greatest contribution may be to help a member of the family to understand what the patient needs from him or her" (Henderson, 1966, p. 26).

Henderson's belief in the importance of a plan of care is demonstrated in *The Nature of Nursing* by an exemplar that identifies treatment and nursing care needs and then offers suggestions for giving care. She provides an hourly plan of care for an individual from awakening in the morning to sleep. She also encourages the nurse to allow the patient to sleep through the night unless the patient is restless or asks for something.

Implementation follows the planning of nursing care. For Henderson (1966, 1991), nursing implementation was based on helping the patient meet the 14 components. For example, in helping the individual with sleep and rest, the nurse tries known methods of inducing sleep and rest before giving drugs. The plan of care includes the treatment prescribed by the physician. Henderson (1966) summarized, "I see nursing as primarily complementing the patient by supplying what he needs in knowledge, will, or strength to perform his daily activities and to carry out the treatment prescribed by the physician" (p. 21).

Another important aspect of implementation that Henderson (1966, 1991) discussed is the relationship between the nurse and patient. The nurse gets "inside the skin" of the patient to better understand the patient's needs and carry out measures to meet those needs. Henderson (1997) also spoke about the quality of nursing care:

> The danger of turning over physical care of the patient to relatively unqualified nurses is twofold. They may fail to assess the patient's needs adequately but, perhaps more important, the qualified nurse, being deprived of the opportunity while giving physical care to assess the patient's needs, may not find any other chance to do so. In this connection it should also be pointed out that it is easier for any person to develop an emotional supportive role with another if he can perform a tangible service. (p. 36)

This statement clearly supports the idea that the competent nurse uses both the interpersonal process and assessment while giving care.

Henderson (1966, 1991) bases the evaluation of each person "according to the speed with which, or the degree to which, he performs independently the activities that make, for him, a normal day" (p. 27). This notion is outlined in her definition of nursing and description of the unique function of the nurse. For evaluation purposes, changes in a person's level of functioning need to be observed and recorded. A comparison of the data about the person's functional abilities is done pre- and post-nursing care. All changes are noted for evaluation.

To summarize the stages of the nursing process as applied to Henderson's definition of nursing and to the 14 components of basic nursing care, refer to Table 5-1. Also, the case study in Table 5-2 demonstrates the application of the nursing process with Henderson's definition and 14 components.

CRITIQUE OF HENDERSON'S DEFINITION AND COMPONENTS OF NURSING

1. *What is the historical context of the theory?*   Henderson was one of the earliest "theorists" who attempted to describe and define the practice of nursing. She began to develop her definition of nursing prior to 1920 as a student in the Army School of Nursing. This is demonstrated by the analysis she made of each student experience; this analysis continued after her graduation in 1921. The assumptions

TABLE 5-1   Summary of the Nursing Process and of Henderson's 14 Components and Definition of Nursing

Nursing assessment	Assess need of human being based on the 14 components of basic nursing care: 1. Breathe normally 2. Eat and drink adequately 3. Eliminate body wastes 4. Move and maintain posture 5. Sleep and rest 6. Suitable clothing, dress or undress 7. Maintain body temperature 8. Keep body clean and well groomed 9. Avoid dangers in environment 10. Communicate 11. Worship according to one's faith 12. Work accomplishment 13. Recreation 14. Learn, discover, or satisfy curiosity Analysis: Compare data to knowledge base of health and disease.
Nursing diagnosis	Identify individuals' ability to meet own needs with or without assistance.
Outcomes	Establish desired outcomes based on return to independence.
Planning	Document how the nurse can assist the individual, sick or well.
Implementation	Assist the sick or well individual and the family in the performance of activities in meeting human needs to maintain health, recover from illness, or aid in peaceful death. Implementation based on physiological principles, age, cultural background, emotional balance, and physical and intellectual capacities. Carry out treatment prescribed by the physician.
Evaluation	Use the acceptable definition of nursing and appropriate laws related to the practice of nursing—can the person now meet the basic human needs? The quality of care is drastically affected by the preparation and native abilities of the nursing personnel rather than the number of hours of care. Successful outcomes of nursing care are based on the speed with which or the degree to which the patient performs independently the activities of daily living that are normal to him.

for the definition are implicit in the process by which it evolved. Henderson recognized the need to focus on the functions that were exclusive to the domain of nursing and therefore did not rely on any other discipline's philosophy as a basis for nursing. Henderson's (1966, 1991) interpretation of the nurse's function was the synthesis of many positive and negative influences. She was a pioneer in her mission to identify the components of nursing practice. A review of Henderson's educational preparation and nursing practice furnishes the basis on which to examine the history of the development of her definition of nursing.

A major influence was her basic nursing education in a general hospital affiliated with the Army School of Nursing, which emphasized learning by doing, speedy performance, technical competence, and successful mastery of nursing procedures such as catheterizations and making beds. As a result, an impersonal approach to care emerged and was interpreted as professional behavior. Although the importance of ethics in nursing and a compassionate attitude toward humanity were stressed, these were not given as high a priority as were the nursing procedures.

Physician lectures were the major portion of classroom learning for the nursing students. The lectures were a simplified version of the lectures given to medical

TABLE 5-2   The Nursing Process for Mr. Ortiz, Using Henderson's 14 Components

Mr. Ortiz is 28 years old, Hispanic, married, and the father of two school-aged children. His wife is pregnant with their third child. Mr. Ortiz quit school after the ninth grade. His parents spoke only Spanish at home. He was not exposed to English until elementary school. He struggled through school; his parents wanted him to leave school at the end of his freshman year to help with family finances. He has worked multiple menial jobs until four years ago when he got a job as a skilled laborer in a factory. He works a second job in a restaurant five days a week to meet family expenses. Mr. Ortiz smokes and the state has recently banned smoking in all indoor public buildings. Additionally the city has banned smoking on all city properties.

Nursing Process | **Data and Relevant Information**

Assessment—assess the needs of Mr. Ortiz based on the 14 components of basic nursing care

1. Breathe normally — 1. Respiratory rate—18 regular, smokes two packs of cigarettes/day; dry cough in AM; no shortness of breath. (Data about work environment needed.)

2. Eat and drink adequately — 2. Height five feet eight inches; weight 200 lbs; skin turgor good, takes tortillas, beans, and rice for lunch, picks up a soda; eats evening meal at restaurant. (Results of 72-hour recall needed.)

3. Elimination of body wastes — 3. Reports no problems related to elimination.

4. Move and maintain posture — 4. Reports pain in both legs after eight hours of working at the restaurant. Stands on cement floors for both jobs.

5. Sleep and rest — 5. Reports five to six hours of sleep/night. "Feels tired most of the time."

6. Suitable clothing, dress/undress — 6. Wears jeans and shirt to work for both jobs. Owns jacket and boots for cold weather.

7. Maintain body temperature — 7. Temperature 37° C, reports no problem with being hot or cold.

8. Keep body clean and well groomed — 8. Showers and shampoos hair daily.

9. Avoid environmental hazards — 9. Wears clothes to match weather conditions. Lives in subsidized housing. (Home environment safety—need more data.)

10. Communication — 10. Fluent in English and Spanish. Able to speak and be understood in both languages. (Communication with family—need more information.)

11. Worship according to faith — 11. Attends church (Catholic) with family every Sunday. Church has primarily Hispanic parishioners with Mass in both English and Spanish.

12. Work accomplishment — 12. Frustrated that he is not earning more money but likes what he does.

(continued)

TABLE 5-2 Continued	
13. Recreation	**13.** "Need more time to spend with family."
14. Learn, discover, or satisfy curiosity	**14.** Reports interested in finishing high school. Desire to go to community college "to get a better job." Stated, "I don't know when I will find the time to do this."
Analysis	According to Erikson's (1963) developmental theory, Mr. Ortiz is in the intimacy stage. He is able to support his family and take care of most of their needs, except for recreational needs, by working 80 hours a week. Physiologically, Mr. Ortiz is functioning within the normal range except for weight. Concerns include his smoking, pains in his legs, inadequate sleep and rest pattern, and risk for type II diabetes. Mr. Ortiz's plans for the future include returning to school to improve his education to seek better employment. Concerned about allocating time to do this.
Nursing Diagnosis	**1.** Inadequate sleep and rest patterns resulting in feeling tired and no time to spend with family.
	2. Knowledge deficit regarding cigarette smoking resulting in potential health hazard for self and family.
	3. Leg pain resulting from standing for eight or more hours in his jobs.
	4. Risk for developing type II diabetes related to weight and exercise patterns.
Outcomes	Long-range plan for stable family income that will allow for rest and recreation.
	Decreased smoke exposure for himself and family.
	Decreased leg pain.
	Decreased risk for type II diabetes.
Nursing Plan	**1.** Explore with Mr. Ortiz and his wife: a. Alternatives to his working two jobs b. Adjusting schedule to allow for more family recreation
	2. Assure that Mr. Ortiz is fully aware of the hazards of smoking to himself and his family and of resources to help him quit smoking.
	3. Teach Mr. Ortiz isometric exercises for his legs.
	4. Review diet and exercise patterns to begin modification.

TABLE 5-2   Continued

Nursing Implementation	**1.** Discuss with Mr. Ortiz and his wife:
	a. Feasible alternatives to his working two jobs
	b. Schedule changes that would allow for more family recreation
	2. With Mr. Ortiz and his wife:
	a. Discuss pros and cons of smoking
	b. Teach the health hazards of smoking, including the effects of secondhand smoke on the family
	c. Discuss options available to help Mr. Ortiz stop smoking
	3. Teach Mr. Ortiz:
	a. Isometric exercises for his legs
	b. To walk around or march in place instead of standing in one position
	4. Teach Mr. Ortiz and his wife:
	a. Diet strategies—increased fruits and vegetables
	b. Exercise strategies—walking, encourage to walk with family
	c. Discuss precursors to type II diabetes
Evaluation	The outcomes of nursing care were successful because Mr. Ortiz demonstrated his independence in making changes in his activities of daily living.
	Deciding to work toward his GED so he can meet his long-range goal of going to college; a Saturday morning GED preparation course was identified.
	Working with his employers to adjust his work shifts so that, at least two days a week, he works only one job. This allows him to get more sleep and to spend more time with his family. Obtained WIC resources for his pregnant wife and new baby to decrease food expenses.
	Not smoking in the house, accessed the free smoking cessation nicotine products offered by the state health department.
	Doing leg exercises regularly, he reports his legs feel better, and that makes the shift seem faster.
	Taking more fruits and vegetables with his lunch. Walking with his family at least four days per week, once each weekend day and twice on his shorter workdays.

students. The focus was on disease, diagnosis, and treatment regimens. Henderson was discontented with the regimentalized care based on medical practice (Henderson, 1966, 1991). Her dean, Annie W. Goodrich, agreed with this evaluation of nursing education.

Another educational concern for Henderson was a lack of an appropriate role model for students to emulate when they were learning to give nursing care. She yearned to observe patient care given by either her teacher or graduate nurses, which was impossible because students staffed the hospitals in return for their nursing education. Thus, clinical practice was viewed as a self-learned process while students cared for the sick and wounded soldiers. She perceived this atmosphere to be one of indebtedness to the patients for having served the country in a time of war. The nurse–patient relationship was described as warm and generous. The soldiers asked for little, and the nurses wanted to do all they could. This experience was believed to be unique and special, for the opportunity to express indebtedness to military patients did not exist in a civilian hospital.

Henderson's next educational experience, psychiatric nursing, was disappointing because the human relations skills that could have been learned in this setting failed to materialize. As in her previous experiences, the approach to psychiatric patient care continued to focus on disease entities and treatment. There was a lack of understanding about the nurse's role in the prevention of mental illness or the curative aspects of care for the psychiatric patient. Her experience resulted in a sense of failure as a nurse. The only value of the psychiatric affiliation was the opportunity to gain some appreciation of mental illness.

The pediatric experience at the Boston Floating Hospital was more positive and introduced three concepts of care: patient-centered care, continuity of care, and tender, loving care. The task-oriented and regimented approach to care was discarded in this setting. However, other shortcomings were identified, such as the failure to use family-centered care. Parents were not allowed to visit a sick child. Therefore, the child was isolated from parental support when it was most needed. Furthermore, Henderson saw little or no effort to assess the home environment to identify the needs of the child and family.

The final student experience at the Henry Street Visiting Nurse Agency in New York introduced her to community nursing care. The formal approach to patient care learned earlier was replaced with care that considered the sick person's lifestyle. Henderson was concerned about discharging patients to the same environments that originally led them to be hospitalized. She believed that the hospital care only served as a stopgap measure without getting to the cause of the problem. She recognized that this type of care failed to consider the person living outside the behavioral controls of the institutional setting.

As a graduate nurse, Henderson worked for several years in Visiting Nursing Services in Washington, D.C., and New York because she deplored the hospital system of nursing and did not want to be in it. This experience was rewarding and offered the opportunity to try out her ideas about nursing.

Her next position was teaching nursing students at the Norfolk Protestant Hospital diploma program in Virginia. She accepted this five-year responsibility without further education—a situation that was not uncommon because many diploma schools at that time did not require academic credentials for teaching. Despite this, she recognized the need for more knowledge and for clarification of the functions of nursing. Subsequently she enrolled at Columbia University Teachers College to learn about sciences and humanities relevant to nursing. These courses enabled Henderson to develop an inquiring and analytical approach to nursing.

After graduation, she briefly accepted the position of teaching supervisor at Strong Memorial Hospital's clinics in Rochester, New York. Next, she returned to Columbia, where her distinguished teaching career continued until 1948. While at the university, Henderson implemented several ideas about nursing in her medical-surgical nursing courses. The concepts taught were a patient-centered approach, the nursing problem method replacing the medical model, field experience, family follow-up care, and chronic illness care. She also established nursing clinics and encouraged coordinated multidisciplinary care.

With her appointment to the faculty at Yale University School of Nursing, Henderson continued to develop the concepts that supported her evolving definition of nursing. She was influenced by her colleagues, Ernestine Wiedenbach and Ida Orlando, in the areas of observing and interpreting patient behavior and the nurse's role in meeting patients' needs. Henderson acknowledged faculty discussion on these topics, which continued to assist her in clarifying her own notions about nursing. In return, her colleagues also benefited from Henderson's discussion of not only her definition of nursing but also the concepts outlined in her publications *Basic Principles of Nursing Care* and the *Principles and Practice of Nursing*.

2. *What are the basic concepts and relationships presented by the theory?* Henderson used the concepts of fundamental human needs, biophysiology, culture, and interaction–communication. These concepts are borrowed from other disciplines rather than being unique to nursing; it is how they are used that makes them unique to nursing. These concepts are not defined as one now expects in the process of theory development; therefore, the relationships of the concepts as currently known are not presented as based on stated assumptions. Much of Henderson's work may be considered to be descriptive statements to convey the definition and unique function of nursing.

However, Maslow's (1970) hierarchy of human needs fits well with the basic 14 components. The first eight components are physiological, and the ninth is for safety needs. The remaining five components deal with love and belonging, social esteem, and self-actualization needs.

Henderson used the biophysiological concept when she stressed the importance of physiology and physiological balances in making decisions about nursing care. Biological knowledge was deemed to be the basis on which the nurse helped the patient with the necessary activities to get well or to assist in peaceful death. To Henderson, the information provided by physiology, anatomy, and microbiology about how the human body functions was important. This then can be used by the nurse to determine appropriate care to alleviate the illness or injury.

The concept of culture as it affects human needs is learned from the family and other social groups. Because of this, Henderson suggests that a nurse is unable to fully interpret or supply all the requirements for the individual's well-being. At best the nurse can merely assist the individual in meeting human needs.

The concept of interaction–communication can be seen in Henderson's writings. She believed sensitivity to nonverbal communication is essential to encourage the expression of feelings (Henderson, 1966). Henderson supported the findings of her colleagues, Ernestine Wiedenbach and Ida Orlando (Pelletier), in their work on interaction between patients and nurses. Wiedenbach and Orlando clearly identified "what the nurse observes, what she thinks or feels, what she says or does in response to this thought or feeling, and how the patient responds, how he affirms or denies the nurse's interpretation of his problems and needs, and finally how the nurse evaluates her successes in helping the patient to solve his problem or meet his needs" (Henderson, 1991, p. 36). In addition, interaction–communication includes the opportunities to see and talk with the patient's friends and family to increase understanding of needs to be addressed by the nurse. Furthermore, a prerequisite to validate a patient's needs is a constructive nurse–patient relationship. It can be seen that from the social sciences, Henderson believed that understanding the background of the individual was important. An individual's nursing needs must include the context in which the person lives. A person's cultural background, including his or her socioeconomic status, beliefs, and values, must be taken into account to meet nursing care needs.

It is evident that the concepts of human needs, biophysiology, culture, and interaction–communication are interrelated. Put into the context of Henderson's definition of nursing, all of these concepts are identified and incorporated to describe what the nurse is expected to provide to those in need of her services. These concepts are clearly in support of the 14 components of basic nursing. Therefore, one can surmise that the concepts underlying Henderson's components of basic nursing care are interrelated and address the care that nurses ought to provide to their clients/patients.

3. *What major phenomena of concern to nursing are presented?* **(***These phenomena may include* **but are not limited to** *human beings, environment, health, interpersonal relations, caring, goal attainment, adaptation, and energy fields.***)** Henderson's definition of nursing and 14 components of basic nursing provide the basis for identifying the phenomena she believed are of concern to nursing. The phenomena of concern are human being, environment, health, interpersonal relations, caring, goal attainment, and adaptation and are explicit and implicit in these sources.

In terms of concern for human beings, Henderson viewed nursing as helping patients with the necessary activities they are unable to perform to make them "complete," "whole," or "independent." She emphasized that the patient is the central figure to be served or assisted by the nurse. This enables persons to care for themselves as soon as possible and be better off because they have achieved independence (Henderson, 1991).

The phenomenon of environment is the ninth component of basic nursing, "avoid dangers in the environment and avoid injuring others." Early in her experiences as a student, she recognized the importance of assessment of the home environment of sick children and their families to identify their needs after hospitalization. Then again, in her experience with the Henry Street Visiting Nurse Agency, she was concerned about discharging patients to the same environment that precipitated admission to the hospital.

When the 14 components of basic nursing are taken together, all contribute to the health of the individual. Henderson stated, "In talking about nursing, we tend to stress promotion of health and prevention and cure of disease" (1991, p. 25).

Interpersonal relations between the nurse and individual to facilitate care were a key factor in the performance of the unique functions of nursing. Henderson believed the process for the nurse to "get inside the skin" of the patient is always difficult and only relatively successful. However, in the tenth component of nursing functions (communicate with others in expressing emotions, needs, fears or opinions), she stressed there is a need for a "listening ear and constant observation and interpretation of nonverbal behavior" (Henderson, 1991, p. 34). It is also important for the nurse to have a self-understanding and recognition of her own emotions that hinder concentrating on the patient's needs and to respond to these needs appropriately. For a mutual understanding to develop between the patient and the nurse, the nurse must be willing to selectively express what she is feeling and thinking. The nurse who tries to put herself in the patient's position is assisted by the use of unlimited knowledge of the general laws underlying human behavior and specific information about people in different cultures and walks of life. Henderson acknowledged the contributions of Orlando and Wiedenbach in relation to the interactions of patients and nurses. Furthermore, she thought that the involvement of the patient and family to develop an individualized plan required interactions with the health care team as well.

The concept of caring is heavily emphasized in Henderson's definition of nursing. She saw the concept of the nurse as a substitute for what the patient lacks to make him "complete," "whole," or "independent." The nurse is "temporarily the consciousness of the unconscious, love of life for the suicidal, the leg of the amputee, the eyes of the newly blinded, a means of locomotion for the infant, knowledge and confidence for the young mother, the mouth-piece for those too weak or withdrawn to speak and so on" (Henderson, 1991, p. 22).

The phenomenon of goal attainment is quite clearly stated within Henderson's (1991) definition of nursing in the final sentence: "and to do this in such a way as to help him gain independence as rapidly as possible" (p. 21). The nurse is the master to initiate and control the care of individuals and helps the patient carry out the treatment plan ordered by the physician. Also, as a team member, the nurse assists other members who in turn assist the nurse to plan and carry out the total health care plan whether for improvement of health, recovery from illness, or support in death. Henderson (1997) expected all team members to view the recipient of care as the central figure and provide assistance for understanding, acceptance, and participation in the plan of care. Ultimately, the sooner the person can care for himself, find health information, or carry out prescribed treatments, the better off the person is. It is hoped that the recipients of care feel that the choice is their own. "In the last analysis it is the patient's self-understanding and desire to adopt a healthful regimen that is the critical factor" (Henderson, 1997, p. 23). Although Henderson presented the 14 components of basic nursing as the nurses' function, the outcome is to enable patients to achieve the "normal" basic human functions, physiologically, psychologically, sociologically, and spiritually.

Henderson does not explicitly use the concept of adaptation in her definition of nursing or in the 14 components of basic nursing care. However, there is evidence that the adaptation process is an expectation for recipients of nursing care in which the nurse assists. Examples are components 4, move and maintain desirable postures; 6, select suitable clothes; 9, avoid dangers in the environment and avoid injuring others; 12, work in a way that there is a sense of accomplishment; and 14, learn, discover, or satisfy the curiosity that leads to normal development and health. These examples give indication that the individual needs to adjust to changes in response to the environmental, physiological, social, cultural, and educational factors that challenge the human system. Adaptation is a constant phenomenon that humans and other living creatures must face on a daily basis and to adjust for survival. Both sick and well individuals must adapt to daily needs in different ways depending on the degree of illness or health or compromising status.

4. *To whom does this theory apply? In what situations? In what ways?*   The far-reaching impact of Henderson's work, particularly her definition of nursing and the *Basic Principles of Nursing Care*, on nurses throughout the word is well-known and celebrated. McBride (1996) eloquently stated,

> Miss Henderson used her emeritus years to serve as nursing consultant to the world . . . her elegant definition of nursing, with its emphasis on complementing the patient's capabilities, provides a clear direction for what nursing should be—a wonderful counter force to the confusion that surrounds a health care system increasingly preoccupied with bottom line rather than the enduring values. (p. 23)

Basic Principles of Nursing Care was originally published by the International Council of Nurses in 1960 and was reprinted seven times and revised and then reprinted several times, the last time in 2004. Clearly this indicates the acceptance of Henderson's notions about nursing functions.

In 1960, Bridges noted in the forward of *Basic Principles of Nursing Care* that this publication would provide its worldwide membership with a number of diverse activities to assist in maintaining the highest standards of nursing or improve their nursing care by education, by legislation, and through professional organizations. Furthermore, it was hoped that this publication on the fundamentals of nursing would provide a stimulus to further progress for nursing in many countries through the benefits experienced by patients and the encouragement given to nurses to provide the best possible care.

Basically, Henderson was interested in defining nursing, and the 14 components of nursing care were not intended to explain or predict phenomena. Rather, her intent was to describe fully the function of nursing in the care of individuals, families, and communities. Thus, her work applies in any situation where a person lacks the strength, will, or knowledge to perform those activities that contribute to health, its recovery, or a peaceful death.

5. *By what method or methods can this theory by tested?*   Henderson's definition of nursing cannot be viewed as theory, given today's understanding of theories. Therefore, it is challenging to generate testable hypotheses from it. Several investigators in Spain have been examining Henderson's 14 components in relationship to nursing care and nursing diagnosis (Alberdi, Artigas, Cuxart, & Aquera, 2003; Coll et al., 2007; Llamas, 2003; Lopez, Pancorbo, Sanchez, & Sanchez, 2003; Miro et al., 2000; Roca et al., 2000). There are many additional questions that could be generated to investigate the definitions of nursing and the 14 components. Some examples of these questions include the following:

1. Is the sequence of the 14 components followed by nurses in the United States? In other countries?
2. What priorities are evident in the use of the basic nursing functions?
3. Do nurses give care to presenting medical problems initially and then use the unique functions, or do they first use the unique functions?
4. Which clinical specialty areas of nursing practice include or exclude components 10 through 14?

Henderson (1977) was an advocate for conducting research in nursing. She favored studies directed toward improving practice rather than those conducted as an academic or theoretical endeavor.

In one of her last publications, support for the application of research in nursing practice is emphasized and encouraged (Henderson, 1991). Henderson acknowledged that "research is identified as one of the eight processes nurses use in arriving at a valid reason for their actions" (p. 56). However, there are no suggestions made regarding the testing of the concepts that underlie her 1966 definition of nursing. The reason for this may be that Henderson saw the research process as time consuming and inappropriate to use for minute-by-minute life decisions. She believed that research is not a substitute for instinctive and intuitive reactions to situations but that these reactions are influenced by the nurse's knowledge of the sciences that guide human behavior in the society of which nursing is an integral part.

6. *Does this theory direct nursing actions that lead to favorable outcomes?* A search of the literature reveals little research conducted about Henderson's work directing practice to demonstrate favorable client outcomes. What was found has been done in the past 10 years (e.g., Alberdi et al., 2003; Coll et al., 2007; Llamas, 2003; Lopez et al., 2003; Miro et al., 2000; Roca et al., 2000). However, one may deduce that, given the number of reprints of the publication *Basic Principles of Nursing Practice,* used by practicing nurses, educators, and administrators around the world, the possibility exists that anecdotal or other information about improved outcomes on patient care is attributable to using information from this book. While there is a belief that a number of underdeveloped countries use Henderson's book a guide for nursing education and practice, there is a lack of published data to support this belief.

On the other hand, the goal of nursing using Henderson ideas is to do for the person what that person lacks the strength, will, or knowledge to do until that person can return to independence. Nursing actions are directed to do only what the person cannot do, thus supporting the individual in continuing to do as much as possible. The directed outcome is a return to independence. This must be considered a favorable outcome.

Ideally, the nurse would improve nursing practice by using Henderson's definition and 14 components to improve the health of individuals and thus reduce illness. The final desirable outcome would be a measure of recovery rate, health promotion and maintenance, or a peaceful death. With respect to Henderson's (1991) most recent thought on the use of theories, she stated that "application of general principles should be part of any effort to improve or advance a profession" (p. 98). However, she disagreed with the current nursing education practice that encourages students to adopt and practice the theory of others. If she were to write *The Nature of Nursing* today, she would stress to students not only the need to study the existing theories but also the need to recognize that the guiding concepts should be their own, for the reason that the mixture of concepts studied may differ from those concepts uniquely suited to that individual nurse.

7. *How contagious is this theory?*   Those who have used Henderson's work and the extent to which they have used it cannot be precisely determined, as these details have not appeared in publications. It is likely that many nurses have used this work without attribution. However, from the information about the number of reprints by the International Council of Nurses (ICN) for *Basic Principles of Nursing Care*, it may be concluded that nursing practice, nursing education, and nursing administration have benefited by this worldwide publication. ICN resources indicated that the publication has been translated into more than 30 languages since 1960 (S. Patel, personal communication, February 1999). Also, the textbooks written with Harmer (1939, 1955) and with Nite (1978) provide further evidence about the influence of Henderson's notion of nursing functions on nursing education and practice. A recent literature review identified four publications that demonstrate Henderson's worldwide influence.

Miller and Beckett (1980) surveyed randomly elected general practitioners about their support for the extended role of nurses in British primary care. They cited Henderson's contribution to defining the skills of the practice nurse and the need for educational aims of a special training program.

Halloran and Halloran (1985), in their publication on exploring the DRG/nursing equation, discussed Henderson's definition and the American Nurses Association definition of nursing and expressed the opinion that "most nurses' practice today reflects the concepts of both of these definitions" (p. 1093). However, these authors viewed Henderson's definition as being the more eloquent.

Swedish investigators cited Henderson's (1980b) publication on the effects of technology on the essence of nursing. They investigated the elderly intensive care unit (ICU) patient experiences of pain and distress as well as interventions aimed at reducing these conditions by nurse and assistant nurses (Hall-Lord, Larrson, & Steen, 1998). They concluded that Henderson's notion of nursing function about the need for assessing the total needs of ICU patients is desirable.

Authors from Sydney, Australia, in their literature review on the impact of the technological care environment on the nursing role, cite Henderson (1980b) for her contribution to resolve the issue of conflict between the humane and the technological aspects of nursing (Pelletier et al., 1996). Henderson acknowledged that the essence of nursing would be difficult to preserve in the high-technology environment of the health care system. However, if *effective* nursing is to prevail, it is essential to incorporate high technology to successfully treat the most critically ill and to extend the life span of those who are in need of such care. "Nursing has never been more important than in this age when the comforting, caring presence and touch of the nurse enable institutionalized patients to tolerate invasive, often frightening and sometimes painful technology" (Henderson, 1985, p. 7). These four examples support Henderson's worldwide influence on nursing practice. Her original definition of nursing continues to have influence, particularly in the changing nursing practice scene with high technology, expanded roles, and the evolving health care system.

More recently, a number of articles have been published that indicate the use of Henderson's work in Spain. Articles in relation to the influence of Henderson on the delivery of nursing care include case studies (Arboledas Bellón, 2009; Cañones

Castelló, 2008; Díaz Hernández et al., 2009) as well as use in home care (Coll et al., 2007), in assessment in a nursing home (Sánchez, Palma, & Sánchez, 2007), in nursing care planning for care and prevention of pressure ulcers (Arboledas Bellón & Melero López, 2004), and in guiding nursing intervention in situations of domestic violence (González Arroyo, & Macias Garcia, 2006). Research studies have focused on the needs of immigrants (Pallarés Martí, 2004) and the development of the SIPPS (Soins Individualisés à la Personne Soignée) tool for analyzing patient care requirements using Henderson's components (Subirana Casacuberta & Solà Arnau, 2006).

In relation to the use of her name for the Sigma Theta Tau International library, "Virginia Henderson was arguably the most famous nurse of our century. She was only willing to permit use of her name if the electronic networking system to be developed would advance the work of staff nurses by getting to them current and jargon-free information wherever they were based. She was proud of that living testimonial to nursing excellence" (McBride, 1996, p. 23). This attests to Henderson's commitment to disseminate relevant information about nursing practice to the majority of nurses who give day-to-day care in a variety of health care settings. It is important to reiterate here that Henderson was truly a pioneer, following Nightingale to communicate what she believed was the essence of nursing practice to her definition.

LIMITATIONS AND STRENGTHS

Henderson based her ideas about nursing care on fundamental human needs and the physical and emotional aspects of the individual. A major shortcoming in her work is the lack of a conceptual linkage between physiological and other human characteristics. The concept of the holistic nature of human beings does not clearly emerge from her publications. However, it must be kept in mind that Henderson wrote her ideas about nursing before the emergence of the holism concept. If the assumption is made that the 14 components are stated in their order of priority, the relationship among the components is unclear. Each component does affect the next one on the list. In later publications, however, Henderson did indicate her acceptance of the holistic approach to nursing.

If priority according to individual needs is implied in the listing of the components, does a presenting emotional problem take a backseat to physical care? Is the emotional area of care deferred until the physiological needs have been given proper attention? Henderson specifies that the nurse must consider such factors as age, temperament, social or cultural status, and physical and intellectual capacity in the use of the components, thus emphasizing differences among individuals. How these factors interrelate and influence nursing care is vague, except individualized care must emerge when all factors of a person are taken into account in the process of nursing.

In a critique of a major international conference on primary care, Henderson (1989) offered some conclusions about the weaknesses of today's nurses. She thought that the basic sciences (e.g., biophysical sciences) as well as the scientific method and its application to nursing were neglected in the presentations. Other areas in which a lack of knowledge by the presenters was of concern to Henderson included budgeting and financial management, holistic family-centered and community-based approaches to health care, policymaking and planning processes, roles of leaders as change agents, taking risks with unpopular actions, and being assertive. These concerns underscore the currency of Henderson's thinking and views about nursing; many of these concerns were not reflected in her earlier writings.

In fairness to Henderson, her effort to define nursing evolved before the discussions of a theoretical basis for the profession emerged. Therefore, the lack of theory in her definition of nursing should not lessen her contribution to nurses and nursing. Her pioneering spirit to lead nursing toward a profession and accountability to the public for competent care were enormous contributions to society as well as to nursing.

Last, in assisting the individual in the dying process, Henderson contended that the nurse helps, but she gave little explanation of what the nurse does. In her definition of nursing, the placing of parentheses around the words "peaceful death" is curious. It leads one to wonder why the parentheses were used—perhaps it was merely to single out this event as an important one in which nursing has a significant role. However, in her later writings, she provided more information about this process. In 1991 she reflected on her earlier thinking about the role of the nurse in helping people have a good death when death is inevitable. She wrote that she would emphasize the "question of prolonging life beyond the period of usefulness" (p. 33). She supported working with families and the patient over the issues of "right to die" or dying with dignity that have become an increasingly important part of nursing care. Henderson explained that the development of hospice care has influenced the philosophy of care for the dying. This may not have been reflected in her 1966 definition of nursing. Finally, it must be noted that in 1966 she eloquently described the nurse's role in the final stage of life, and this description supported much of the thinking expressed in her 1991 publication.

Summary

The concept of nursing formulated by Henderson in her definition of nursing and the 14 components of basic nursing is uncomplicated and self-explanatory. Therefore, it could be used without difficulty as a guide for nursing practice by most nurses. Many of the ideas she presented continue to be used worldwide in both developed and undeveloped countries to guide nursing curricula and practice, which is validated by the demand for her ICN publication.

If a suggestion can be made to improve Henderson's concept of nursing, it would be to delineate a theoretical basis and to increase the study of its utility. For example, it would be interesting to see how holism or general systems theory might explain the relationship of the components of basic nursing care to each other. Confirmation of whether the list of components is prioritized is needed to clarify what the nurse ought to do if the presenting problem is other than a physical one.

In view of the time in which Henderson published her definition of nursing, she deserves much credit as a leader in the development of nursing practice, education, and licensure. Her work should to be considered a beginning and impetus for nurses to pursue the highest academic degree. This is critical for analyses of nursing in practice and for identifying and testing the theoretical bases for patient care.

In conclusion, Henderson provides the essence of what she believes is a definition of nursing as follows:

I believe that the function the nurse performs is primarily an independent one—that of acting for the patient when he lacks knowledge, physical strength, or the will to act for himself as he would ordinarily act in health, or in carrying out prescribed therapy. This function is seen as complex and creative, as offering unlimited opportunity for the application of the physical, biological, and social sciences, and the development of skills based on them. (Henderson, 1966, p. 68)

Thought Questions

1. Develop an analogy or metaphor for Henderson's definition and 14 components.
2. Identify a clinical problem in your practice and analyze it using Henderson's definition and 14 components. If you had applied Henderson's model from the beginning, how might the outcome have been different?

3. How could Henderson's work be used in a community health situation?
4. Identify research questions that would test Henderson's model. Discuss how you might implement this research.

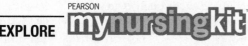

EXPLORE   PEARSON **mynursingkit**™

MyNursingKit is your one stop for online chapter review materials and resources. Prepare for success with additional NCLEX®-style practice questions, interactive assignments and activities, web links, animations and videos, and more!

Register your access code from the front of your book at
www.mynursingkit.com.

References

Alberdi, C. R., Artigas, L. B., Cuxart, A. N., & Aguera, P. A. (2003). Guidelines for nursing methodology implantation [Spanish]. *Revista de Enfermeria, 26*(9), 73–74. Abstract in English retrieved June 19, 2007, through Ovid.

ANA statement on auxiliary personnel in nursing service. (1962). *American Journal of Nursing, 62,* 7.

Arboledas Bellón, J. (2009). Pain and depression: Strategies to improve primary health care, based on a clinical case [Spanish]. *Revista Rol de Enfermería, 32*(6), 55–60. Abstract in English retrieved November 30, 2009, from CINAHL Plus with Full Text database.

Arboledas Bellón, J., & Melero López, Á. (2004). Standarised [sic] nursing care plan for the prevention and treatment of pressure ulcers [Spanish]. *Metas de Enfermería, 7*(4), 13–16. Abstract in English retrieved November 30, 2009, from CINAHL Plus with Full Text database.

Cañones Castelló, M. E. (2008). Case report: A gastrectomized patient under treatment with chemotherapy and radiotherapy [Spanish]. *Enfermeria Clinica, 18,* 216–219. Abstract in English retrieved November 30, 2009, from CINAHL Plus with Full Text database.

Coll, M., Besora, I., Icart, T., Vall, A. F., Manito, I., Ondiviela, A., et al. (2007). Nursing care according to Virginia Henderson in the at home care field [Spanish]. *Revista de Enfermeria, 30*(3), 53–56. Abstract in English retrieved June 19, 2007, through Ovid.

Díaz Hernández, M., Hernández Rodríguez, J. E., Suárez Canino, J. A., Garcia Lázaro, I., Díaz Pérez, R., & Giráldez Macia, F. (2009). Lowerlimb amputation patient nursing care plan from the perspective of the Virginia Henderson model [Spanish]. *Metas de Enfermería, 12*(1), 58–62. Abstract in English retrieved November 30, 2009, from CINAHL Plus with Full Text database.

Erikson, P. H. (1963). *Childhood and society* (2nd ed.). New York: Norton.

González Arroyo, A. A., & Macias Garciá, J. (2006). Domestic violence: A nursery [sic] guideline [Spanish]. *Nure Investigación, 23,* 8 pp. Abstract in English retrieved November 30, 2009, from CINAHL Plus with Full Text database.

Hall-Lord, M. L., Larrson, G., & Steen, B. (1998). Pain and distress among elderly intensive care unit patients: Comparison of patient's experiences and nurses' assessment. *Heart and Lung, 27,* 123–132.

Halloran, B., & Halloran, C. D. C. (1985). Exploring the DRG/nursing equation. *American Journal of Nursing, 85,* 1090–1095.

Harmer, B. (1922). *Textbook of the principles and practice of nursing.* New York: Macmillan.

Harmer, B., & Henderson, V. (1939). *Textbook of the principles and practice of nursing* (4th ed.). New York: Macmillan.

Harmer, B., & Henderson. V. (1955). *Textbook of the principles and practice of nursing* (5th ed.). New York: Macmillan.

Henderson, V. (1960). *Basic principles of nursing care.* Geneva: International Council of Nurses.

Henderson, V. (1966). *The nature of nursing.* New York: Macmillan.

Henderson, V. (1977). We've "come a long way" but what of the direction? *Nursing Research, 26,* 163–164.

Henderson, V. (1978). The concept of nursing. *Journal of Advanced Nursing, 3,* 16–17.

Henderson, V. (1979a). Preserving the essence of nursing in a technological age, part I. *Nursing Times, 75,* 2012–2013.

Henderson, V. (1979b). Preserving the essence of nursing in a technological age, part II. *Nursing Times, 75,* 2056–2058.

Henderson, V. (1980a). Nursing—Yesterday and tomorrow. *Nursing Times, 76,* 905–907.

Henderson, V. (1980b). Preserving the essence of nursing in a technological age. *Journal of Advanced Nursing, 5,* 245–260.

Henderson, V. (1982a). The nursing process—Is the title right? *Journal of Advanced Nursing, 7,* 103–109.

Henderson, V. (1982b). Speech at History of Nursing Museum, Philadelphia, May.

Henderson, V. (1985). The essence of nursing in high technology. *Nursing Administration Quarterly, 9,* 1–9.

Henderson, V. (1987). Nursing process—A critique. *Holistic Nursing Practice, 1,* 7–18.

Henderson, V. (1989). Countdown to 2000: A major international conference for the primary health care team, 21–23 September 1987, London. *Journal of Advanced Nursing, 14,* 81–85.

Henderson, V. (1991). *The nature of nursing: A definition and its implications for practice, research, and education. Reflections after 25 years* (Pub. No. 15-2346). New York: National League for Nursing Press.

Henderson, V. (1997). *Basic principles of nursing care* (Rev. ed.). Geneva: International Council of Nurses.

Henderson, V., & Nite, G. (1978). *Principles and practice of nursing* (6th ed.). New York: Macmillan.

Henderson, V., & Watt, S. (1983). 70+ and going strong. Virginia Henderson: A nurse for all ages. *Geriatric Nursing, 4,* 58–59.

Llamas, R. C. (2003). How is the nursing care process used? [Spanish]. *Revista de Enfermeria, 26*(5), 22–30. Abstract in English retrieved June 19, 2007, through Ovid.

Lopez, M. M., Pancorbo, H. P. L., Sanchez, J. L. I., & Sanchez, C. V. (2003). Nursing diagnosis and reports [Spanish]. *Revista de Enfermeria, 26*(3), 62–66. Abstract in English retrieved June 19, 2007, through Ovid.

Maslow, A. (1970). *Motivation and personality* (2nd ed.). New York: Harper & Row.

McBride, A. B. (1996). In celebration of Virginia Avenuel Henderson. *Reflections, 22*(1), 22–23.

Miller, D. S., & Beckett, F. M. (1980). A new member of the team? Expanding the role of the nurse in British primary care. *The Lancet, 2,* 358–361

Miro, B. M., Amoros, C. S. M., De Juan Sanchez, S., Fortea, C. E., Frau, M. J., Moragues, M. J., et al. (2000). Assessment of the critical patient at admission: An indicator of quality of care [Spanish]. *Revista de Enfermeria, 11*(2), 51–58. Abstract in English retrieved June 19, 2007, through Ovid.

Pallarés Martí, A. (2004). Influence of transcultural factors on immigrants populations' needs and nursing diagnosis [Spanish]. *Cultura de los Cuidados, 8*(16), 62–67. Abstract in English retrieved November 30, 2009, from CINAHL Plus with Full Text database.

Pelletier, O., Duffield, C. M., Adams, A., Crisp, I., Nagy, S., & Murphy, J. (1996). The impact of the technological care environment on the nursing role. *International Journal of Technology Assessment in Health Care, 12,* 358–366.

Roca, R. M., Ubeda, B. I., Fuentelsaz, G. C., Lopez, P. R., Pont, R. A., Garcia, V. L., et al. (2000). Impact of caregiving on the health of family caregivers [Spanish]. *Atencion Primaria, 26*(4), 217–223. Abstract in English retrieved June 19, 2007, through Ovid.

Safier, G. (1977). *Contemporary American leaders in nursing.* New York: McGraw-Hill.

Sánchez, J. M. V., Palma, M. R., & Sánchez, M. M. V. (2007). Geriatric nurse assessment: A model of register in nursing home care. *Gerokomos, 18*(2), 72–76. Abstract in English retrieved November 30, 2009, from CINAHL Plus with Full Text database.

Subirana Casacuberta, M., & Solà Arnau, I. (2006). Instruments based on direct measures II: SIIPS and SIGN II [Spanish]. *Metas de Enfermería, 9*(8), 50–53. Abstract in English retrieved November 30, 2009, from CINAHL Plus with Full Text database.

Bibliography

Campbell, C. (1985). Virginia Henderson: The definitive nurse. *Nursing Mirror, 160,* 12.

Fulton J. S. (1987). Virginia Henderson: Theorist, prophet, poet. *Advances in Nursing Science, 10,* 1–9.

Halloran, E. J. (1996). Virginia Henderson and her timeless writings. *Journal of Advanced Nursing, 23W,* 17–24.

Halloran, E. J., & Wald, F. S. (1996). Professionally speaking: Virginia Henderson, the nursing profession and the reform of health services. *Nursing Leadership Forum, 2*(2), 58–63.

Henderson, V. (1977). *Reference resource for research and continuing education in nursing.* Kansas City, MO: American Nurses Association Publication No. 6125.

Henderson, V. (1982). Is the study of history rewarding for nurses? *Society for Nursing History Gazette, 2,* 1–2.

Henderson, V. (1986). Some observations on health care by health services or health industries (editorial). *Journal of Advanced Nursing, 1,* 1–2.

Henderson, V., & Watt, S. (1983). Epidermolysis bullosa. *Nursing Times, 79,* 43–46.

McCarty, P. (1987). How can nurses prepare for year 2000? (A response from Virginia Henderson). *The American Nurse, 19,* 3, 6.

Shamansky, S. L. (1964). CHN revisited: A conversation with Virginia Henderson. *Public Health Nursing, 1,* 193–201.

Shamansky, S. L. (1984). Virginia Henderson: A national treasure. *Focus on Critical Care, 11,* 60–61.

Annotated Bibliography

Fulton, J. S. (1987). Virginia Henderson: Theorist, prophet, poet. *Advances in Nursing Science, 10*(1), 1–9. A journey, using nursing's metaparadigm as guideposts, that looks at the aesthetics and character of Virginia Henderson's work. The major work considered is *The Nature of Nursing.* Unique in the translation of selected materials into poetry.

Halloran, E. J. (1995). *A Virginia Henderson reader: Excellence in nursing.* New York: Springer. A compilation of 22 of Henderson's works, spanning a 30-year period. This volume organizes these into the categories of patient care, nursing education, nursing research, and nursing in society. Included are 12 chapters from the 1978 edition of *Principles and Practice of Nursing.*

Hardin, S. R. (1997). Virginia Henderson: Universality and individuality. *Journal of Multicultural Nursing and Health, 3*(3), 6–9. This article summarizes Henderson's definition of nursing and her thoughts on culture. It addresses Henderson's work in relation to culturally competent care.

Hargrove-Huttel, R. A. (1988). Virginia Henderson's nature of nursing theory and quality of life for the older adult. *Dissertation Abstracts International, 49*(08B), 3104. A descriptive study that investigated the relationship between Henderson's basic care needs and the quality of life for 174 older adults living in rural area. Findings supported that meeting the basic care needs is positively associated with the quality of life for older adults.

Lindell, M. E., & Olsson, H. M. (1989). Lack of care givers' knowledge causes unnecessary suffering in elderly patients. *Journal of Advanced Nursing, 14,* 976–979. This study investigated the personal hygiene of women over the age of 65; 35 of these women were healthy, and 28 were residents of long-term care wards.

Those in long-term care required assistance with daily hygiene activities. Results indicated that those who required assistance with personal hygiene were likely to have abnormal genital problems. It was concluded that their caregivers lacked knowledge about the normal physiological aging process in women and thus were hindered in carrying out basic component 8, "Keep the body clean and well groomed and protect the integument."

Smith, J. P. (1989). *Virginia Henderson: The first ninety years.* Harrow, Middlesex, England: Scutari.

This biography is based on information obtained during interviews with Virginia Henderson and several of those who knew her well. James Smith spent several weeks as Henderson's guest in New Haven, Connecticut, with the support of Trevor Clay, Royal College of Nursing, United Kingdom, and Vernice Ferguson, deputy assistant medical director for nursing programs, Veterans Administration, Washington, D.C. This volume adds to our information about who Virginia Henderson was as well as what she did.

CHAPTER 6

Self-Care Deficit Nursing Theory

Dorothea Elizabeth Orem

Peggy Coldwell Foster

Dorothea Elizabeth Orem (1914–July 22, 2007) was born in Baltimore, Maryland, the younger of two sisters. She received her diploma in nursing from Providence Hospital School of Nursing, Washington, D.C., in 1934 and her bachelor of science in nursing education (1939) and master of science in nursing education (1945) from Catholic University of America, Washington, D.C. Her clinical practice included staff nurse in the operating room, pediatrics, and adult medical surgical units. She also did private-duty nursing in private homes and the hospital and was an emergency room supervisor. She taught biological sciences and later served as director of nursing service and director of the school of nursing at Providence Hospital, Detroit, Michigan, and served as an assistant to the director of Providence Hospital–Catholic University, Washington, D.C. In 1949, Orem went to the Indiana State Board of Health, Hospital Division, where she worked to help upgrade the nursing services in general hospitals.

Orem received several honorary degrees, including doctor of science from Georgetown University, Washington, D.C., in 1976; doctor of science from the Incarnate Word College, San Antonio, Texas, in 1980; doctor of humane letters from Illinois Western University, Bloomington, in 1988; and an honorary doctorate of nursing from the University of Missouri, Columbia, in 1998. Other national awards she received include Catholic University of America's Alumni Association Award for Nursing Theory, 1980; National League of Nursing Linda Richards Award, 1991; Honorary Fellow of Nursing from the American Academy of Nursing, 1992; and the Edith Moore Copeland Award for Creative Excellence, Sigma Theta Tau, International Honor Society of Nursing, 1997. Dr. Orem was a member of Sigma Theta Tau and of Pi Gamma Mu.

As part of her master's work, Dorothea E. Orem had to formulate a definition of nursing. Then, during 1958–1959, as a consultant to the Office of Education, Department of Health, Education, and Welfare, Orem participated in a project to improve practical (vocational) nurse training. This work stimulated her to seek to identify the condition or circumstance under which a decision is made that nursing care is needed or desirable (Orem, 2001, p. 20). Her answer encompassed the idea that a nurse is "another self." This idea evolved into her nursing concept of "self-care" and later into the "self-care deficit nursing theory." Self-care implies that when they are able, individuals care for themselves. When the person is unable to care for himself, the nurse provides the assistance needed. For children, nursing care is needed when the parents or guardians are unable to provide the amount and quality of care needed.

Orem's concept of nursing as the provision of self-care was first published in 1959. She joined with several faculty members from the Catholic University of America in 1965 to form a Nursing Model Committee. In 1968, a portion of the Nursing Model Committee, including Orem, continued their work through the Nursing Development Conference Group (NDCG). This group was formed to produce a conceptual framework for nursing and to establish the discipline of nursing. The NDCG published *Concept Formalization in Nursing: Process and Product* in 1973 and 1979.

Orem continued to develop her nursing concepts and her self-care deficit theory of nursing. In 1971 she published *Nursing: Concepts of Practice*. The second, third, fourth, fifth, and sixth editions of this book were published in 1980, 1985, 1991, 1995, and 2001, respectively. The first edition focused on the individual. The second edition was expanded to include multiperson units (families, groups, and communities). The third edition presented Orem's general theory of nursing, comprised of three related theoretical constructs: self-care, self-care deficits, and nursing systems. The fourth edition more fully developed the ideas presented in earlier editions. The fifth edition (with a chapter contributed by Susan Taylor and Kathie McLaughlin Renpenning) provided an increased emphasis on multiperson situations—family and community groups in our society. The sixth edition continued the development of Orem's ideas, provided a prologue to understanding nursing, organized and outlined Orem's key concept components, emphasized the interpersonal aspects of nursing, and included a discussion of the importance of positive mental health.

OREM'S GENERAL THEORY OF NURSING

Orem (2001) states her general theory as follows:

> Nursing has as its special concern man's need for self-care action and the provision and maintenance of it on a continuous basis in order to sustain life and health, recover from disease and injury, and cope with their effects. (p. 22)
>
> . . . The condition that validates the existence of a **requirement for nursing** in an adult is *the health-associated absence of the ability to maintain continuously that amount and quality of self-care that is therapeutic in sustaining life and health, in recovering from disease or injury, or in coping with their effects.* With children, the condition is the *inability of the parent (or guardian) associated with the child's health state to maintain continuously for the child the amount and quality of care that is therapeutic.* (p. 82)

TABLE 6-1   Relationship of Orem's Concepts to the Three Theories

Theory of Self-Care	Theory of Self-Care Deficit	Theory of Nursing Systems
Self-care	When therapeutic self-care	Nursing agency
Self-care agency	demand exceeds self-care	Nursing systems
Self-care requisites	agency, a self-care deficit	Wholly compensatory
Universal	exists and nursing is needed	Partly compensatory
Developmental		Supportive–educative
Health deviation		
Therapeutic self-care demand		

←———————————— Basic conditioning factors ————————————→

From Julia B. George, California State University, Fullerton, 1997. Used with permission.

Orem developed the Self-Care Deficit Nursing Theory, her general theory, which is composed of three interrelated theories: (1) the theory of self-care, (2) the theory of self-care deficit, and (3) the theory of nursing systems. Incorporated within these three theories are six central concepts and one peripheral concept. Understanding these central concepts of self-care and dependent care, self-care agency and dependent care agency, therapeutic self-care demand, self-care deficit, nursing agency, and nursing systems, as well as the peripheral concept of basic conditioning factors, is essential to understanding her general theory. See Table 6-1 for the relationship of these concepts to the three interrelated theories.

The Theory of Self-Care

To understand the theory of self-care one must first understand the concepts of self-care, self-care agency, basic conditioning factors, and therapeutic self-care demand. *Self-care* is the performance or practice of activities that individuals initiate and perform on their own behalf to maintain life, health, and well-being. When self-care is effectively performed, it helps to maintain structural integrity and human functioning and contributes to human development (Orem, 2001, p. 43). Self-care is learned through interpersonal relations and communications. "Self-care is action that I perform for myself, for my own sake, for my life, health, and well-being" (Renpenning & Taylor, 2003, p. 304).

Self-care agency is the human's acquired powers and capabilities to engage in self-care. The ability to engage in self-care is affected by basic conditioning factors. These *basic conditioning factors* are age, gender, developmental state, health state, sociocultural orientations, health care system factors (i.e., diagnostic and treatment modalities), family system factors, patterns of living (e.g., activities one regularly engages in), environmental factors, and resource adequacy and availability (Orem, 2001, p. 328). Under usual circumstances, adults care for themselves. However, those who are young, aged, ill, or disabled need either help with self-care or complete assistance in those activities necessary to meet self-care needs (p. 43). The *therapeutic self-care demand* is the total of care activities needed, either at an identified moment or over a period of time, to meet a person's known requirements for self-care (p. 523). The therapeutic self-care demand is modeled on deliberate action—that is, actions intentionally performed by some members of a society to benefit themselves or others.

An additional concept incorporated within the theory of self-care is *self-care requisites*. Self-care requisites are the reasons self-care activities occur and are an expression of the hoped-for results (Orem, 2001, p. 522). Orem presents three categories of self-care requisites, or requirements: (1) universal, (2) developmental, and (3) health deviation. *Universal self-care requisites* are found in every human being, across all stages of life, and are involved with the maintenance of both structure and function as well as with general well-being (p. 48). They should be viewed as interrelated factors, each affecting the others. A common term for these requisites is *activities of daily living*. Orem identifies self-care requisites as follows:

1. The maintenance of a sufficient intake of air.
2. The maintenance of a sufficient intake of water.
3. The maintenance of a sufficient intake of food.
4. The provision of care associated with elimination processes and excrements.
5. The maintenance of a balance between activity and rest.
6. The maintenance of a balance between solitude and social interaction.
7. The prevention of hazards to human life, human functioning, and human well-being.
8. The promotion of human functioning and development within social groups in accord with human potential, known human limitations, and the human desire to be normal. *Normalcy* is used in the sense of that which is essentially human and that which is in accord with the genetic and constitutional characteristics and the talents of individuals. (p. 225)

In contrast with universal self-care requisites, *developmental self-care requisites* are more specific to the processes of growth and development and are influenced by what is happening during the life cycle stages; such influence may be positive or negative (Orem, 2001, p. 48). Examples would be adjusting to a new job or adjusting to body changes such as facial lines, changes in body shape, or hair loss. Orem identifies the life cycle stages with developmental events as intrauterine life and the process of birth; neonatal; infancy; childhood, including adolescence and entry into adulthood; adulthood; and pregnancy, whether in childhood or adulthood (p. 230).

Health deviation self-care requisites are related to changes in human structure and function, out of the range of normal, and may be associated with genetic variations or other defects (Orem, 2001, p. 48). They may be performed when there are medical measures used to diagnose and/or correct a certain condition (e.g., right upper quadrant abdominal pain when foods with a high fat content are eaten or learning to walk using crutches following the casting of a fractured leg) and may deal with the effects of defects or deviations and the effects of efforts to diagnose and treat them. The health deviation self-care requisites are as follows:

1. Seeking and securing appropriate medical assistance . . .
2. Being aware of and attending to the effects and results of pathologic conditions and states . . .
3. Effectively carrying out medically prescribed diagnostic, therapeutic, and rehabilitative measures . . .
4. Being aware of and attending to or regulating the discomforting or deleterious effects of medical care measures . . .
5. Modifying the self-concept (and self-image) in accepting oneself as being in a particular state of health and in need of specific forms of health care
6. Learning to live with the effects of pathologic conditions and states and the effects of medical diagnostic and treatment measures in a life-style that promotes continued personal development (Orem, 2001, p. 235)

In the theory of self-care, Orem explains *what* is meant by self-care and lists the various factors that affect its provision. In the self-care deficit theory, she specifies *when* nursing is needed to assist individuals in the provision of self-care.

The Theory of Self-Care Deficit

The theory of self-care deficit is the basic element of Orem's (2001) general theory of nursing because it delineates when nursing is needed. Nursing is required when adults (or, in the case of a dependent, the parent or guardian) are incapable of or limited in their ability to provide continuous effective self-care. Nursing may be provided if the capacity to provide care is less than what is needed for an identified self-care demand or when the ability to provide care is currently adequate but a deficit is predicted for the future due to predictable decreases in the ability to provide care, increases in the care demands, or both (p. 147). Nursing may be necessary when individuals need to carry out new and complex measures of self-care, particularly when these new measures require specialized knowledge or skill that must be obtained through instruction and practice (p. 283), or when an individual needs help in dealing with an illness or injury, either to recover from or to cope with changes that result from the illness or injury (p. 82). It is important to note that the first category includes universal, developmental, and health-deviation self-care needs, whereas the other categories focus on health-deviation self-care.

Orem (2001) identifies the following five methods of helping that nurses may use:

1. Acting for or doing for another
2. Guiding and directing
3. Providing physical or psychological support
4. Providing and maintaining an environment that supports personal development
5. Teaching (p. 56)

The nurse may help the individual by using any or all of these methods to provide assistance with self-care.

The relationship between Orem's concepts is demonstrated in Figure 6-1. From this model it can be seen that at any given time an individual has specific self-care abilities (self-care agency) as well as therapeutic self-care demands. If there are more demands than abilities, nursing is needed. The activities in which nurses engage when they provide nursing care can be used to describe the domain of nursing. Orem (2001) has identified work operations of nurses in clinical nursing practice:

• Entering into and maintaining nurse–patient relationships with individuals, families, or groups
• Designing, planning for, instituting, and managing systems of nursing care
• Responding to patients' requests, desires, and needs for nurse contact and assistance
• Coordinating nursing care
• Establishing the kind and amount of immediate and continuing care needed
• Coordinating the care with other services, such as other health care, social, or educational services, needed or being received
• Discharging patients from nursing care when they have regained their abilities to perform their own self-care needs (p. 19)

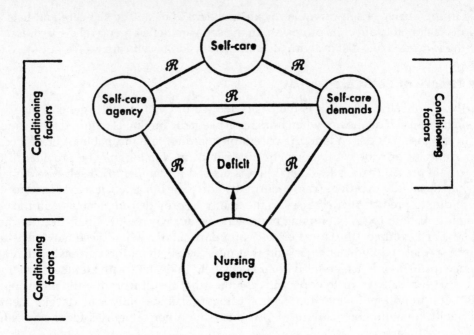

FIGURE 6-1. A conceptual framework for nursing. (R = relationship; < = deficit relationship, current or projected.) *(From Orem, D. E. (1991). Nursing: Concepts of practice (4th ed.), St. Louis: Mosby, p. 64. Used with permission.)*

Self-care has been defined and the need for nursing explained in the first and second theories (self-care and self-care deficit theories). In Orem's third theory of nursing systems, she outlines *how* the patient's self-care needs will be met by the nurse, the patient, or both.

The Theory of Nursing Systems

The nursing system, designed by the nurse, is based on the assessment of an individual's self-care needs and on the assessment of the abilities of the patient to perform self-care activities. If there is a self-care deficit—that is, if there is a difference between what the individual can do (self-care agency) and what needs to be done to maintain optimum functioning (therapeutic self-care demand)—nursing is required.

Nursing agency is a complex property or attribute of mature or maturing people educated and trained as nurses that enables them to act, to know, and to help others meet their therapeutic self-care demands. Nursing agency is similar to self-care agency in that both symbolize characteristics and abilities for specific types of deliberate action. They differ in that nursing agency is carried out for the benefit and well-being of others, and self-care agency is employed for one's own benefit (Orem, 2001, p. 289). Nursing agency is power that the nurse has to engage in effective nursing practice. It has been developed by the nurse and enables the nurse to compose and manage a system of nursing (Renpenning & Taylor, 2003, p. 106).

Self-care agency, self-care demand, and nursing agency may be affected by conditioning factors. These conditioning factors are human or environmental factors that affect self-care agency, self-care demand, and nursing agency at points in time (Renpenning & Taylor, 2003). An example of this would be if the nursing system were being implemented in an environment of 100° F because the air conditioner has broken down; the self-care demand, the self-care agency, and the nursing agency might all be affected.

Orem (2001) has identified three classifications of nursing systems to meet the self-care requisites of the patient (see Figure 6-2). These systems are the wholly compensatory system, the partly compensatory system, and the supportive–educative system.

The design and elements of the nursing system make clear four elements: the extent of the responsibility of the nurse in the health care situation, the various roles of the players (nurse, patient, and others) in the situation, the reason for there being a nurse–patient relationship, and the actions to be carried out by the nurse and the patient to enable the self-care agency of the patient and to meet the therapeutic self-care demand (Orem, 2001, p. 348). All nurses must have some skills in designing or in making adjustments in the design of nursing systems.

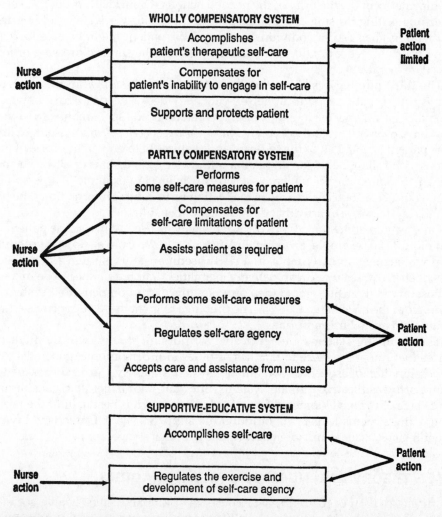

FIGURE 6-2 Basic nursing systems. *(Adapted from Orem, D. E. (1991). Nursing: Concepts of practice (4th ed.), St. Louis: Mosby, p. 288. Used with permission.)*

The *wholly compensatory nursing system* is represented by a situation in which the individual is unable to carry out needed self-care actions (including ambulation and other movement), either through inability to be self-directed or due to a medical prescription. Those who have such limitations are dependent upon others for their well-being and even their very existence (Orem, 2001, p. 352). Subtypes of the wholly compensatory system are nursing systems for those who are not able to perform any kind of deliberate action, for those who are aware and can make decisions but either cannot or should not be physically active, and for those who can be physically active but who must have supervision due to their inability to make rational decisions (p. 352). Examples of persons in the first subtype could include those in a coma or under anesthesia, the second subtype could include those with C3–C4 vertebral fractures, and the third subtype could include persons who are severely mentally impaired.

The *partly compensatory nursing system* is represented by a situation in which the patient and nurse are both physically active in meeting the patient's self-care needs and either may perform the majority of the needed actions (Orem, 2001, p. 354). An example of a person needing nursing care in the partly compensatory system would be an individual who has had recent abdominal surgery. This patient might be able to wash his face and brush his teeth but needs the nurse to change the surgical dressing or for help to ambulate or bathe.

The third nursing system is the *supportive–educative system*. In this system, the person is fully capable of performing self-care activities or needs to learn how to meet therapeutic self-care needs; in either case, the person needs some manner of assistance (Orem, 2001, p. 354). This is also known as a *supportive–developmental* system. In this system the patient is doing all of the self-care and requires help only in the areas of making decisions, controlling behavior, and gaining knowledge and skills (p. 354). The nurse's role, then, is to promote the patient as a self-care agent. An example of a person in this system would be a 16-year-old who is requesting birth control information. The nurse's role in this system is primarily that of a teacher or consultant.

One or more of the three types of systems may be used with a single patient over a period of time. For example, a woman in labor may move from a supportive–educative system while she is in early labor to a partly compensatory system as her labor advances. If she requires a cesarean delivery, her care might require her to be in a wholly compensatory system. She would then progress to a partly compensatory system as she recovers from the anesthetic. Later, as she prepares to go home, a supportive–educative system would again be appropriate.

These nursing systems are applicable for nursing care with individuals. Orem indicates that nursing service to families or other mutiperson units generally requires some combination of aspects of two nursing systems, namely, the partly compensatory and supportive–educative nursing systems. She states her belief that, considering the current stage of the development of nursing knowledge, it is best to limit the use of the three nursing systems to the care of individuals (pp. 350–351). Obviously, Taylor and Renpenning (1995, 2001) are not in agreement with this stance.

OREM'S THEORY AND NURSING'S METAPARADIGM

Orem discusses each of the four major concepts of human beings, health, society, and nursing in her work. *Human beings* are different from other living things in that they have the ability to think about themselves and their interactions with their environment, to create symbols relating to their experiences, and to use symbols such as words and concepts to think, communicate, and act in efforts to be useful to themselves and to others (Orem, 2001, p. 182). Integrated human functioning includes physical, psychological, interpersonal, and social aspects. Orem believes that individuals have the potential for learning and developing. The way an individual meets self-care needs is not instinctual but is a learned behavior. Factors that affect learning include age, mental capacity, culture, society, and the emotional state of the individual. If the individual cannot learn self-care measures, others must learn the care and provide it.

In the sixth edition of *Nursing: Concepts of Practice*, Orem (2001) considers human beings from two different perspectives. The first is as persons viewed as maturing and seeking to achieve each one's unique potential as a human (p. 187). Orem stresses that this development is a dynamic, ever-changing concept. She indicates that the terms self-realization and personality development are sometimes used to refer to this developmental process (p. 188). In the second view the focus is on the differences in human structure and function; the information for this view can be found in various sciences such as biochemistry, biophysics, genetics, anatomy, physiology, and various aspects of psychology (p. 188). Orem emphasizes, however, that both perspectives need to be integrated for effective nursing care.

Orem (2001) supports the World Health Organization's definition of *health* as "a state of physical, mental, and social well-being and not merely the absence of disease or infirmity" (p. 184) as well as speaking to the relationship between health, well-being, and being whole or sound. However, she acknowledges that a person's definition of health will change as the person's physical and mental characteristics change (p. 182). Orem recognizes that the various aspects of health (physical, psychological, interpersonal, and social) cannot be separated within the individual (p. 182). Orem also presents health based on the concept of preventive health care. This health care includes the promotion and maintenance of health (primary prevention), the treatment of disease or injury (secondary prevention), and the prevention of complications (tertiary prevention). Orem also discusses the mental health of individuals. She indicates that over the course of a lifetime, an individual will continue to seek to gain and maintain positive mental or psychic health as part of the process of maturing (p. 383).

About *nursing*, Orem (2001) states,

> In modern society, adults are expected to be self-reliant and responsible for themselves and for the well-being of their dependents. Most societies accept that persons who are helpless, sick, aged, handicapped, or otherwise deprived should be helped in their immediate distress and helped to attain or regain responsibility within their existing capacities. Thus both self-help and help to others are valued by society as desirable activities. Nursing as a specific type of human service is based on both values. In most communities people see nursing as a desirable and necessary service. (p. 81) . . . Nursing is required whenever the maintenance of continuous self-care requires the use of special techniques and the application of scientific knowledge in providing care or in designing it. (p. 83)

Orem speaks to several factors related to the concept of nursing. These are the art and prudence of nursing, nursing as a service, role theory related to nursing, and technologies in nursing. Orem defines the art of nursing as an intellectual quality of the individual nurse; this quality is related to creativity as well as analysis and synthesis of information (in her terms, the variables and conditioning factors in the situation), all of which contribute to development of nursing systems to assist individuals or multiperson units (p. 293). These decisions require a theoretical base in the discipline of nursing and in the sciences, arts, and humanities. This base directs decisions when designing nursing systems within the nursing process. Nursing prudence leads the nurse to seek the help of others when needed (as in a new or very challenging situation), to come to appropriate conclusions, to make decisions about what actions to take, and to take those actions (p. 293). Unique life and nursing experiences affect the development of the individual nurse's art and prudence.

Orem (2001) further defines nursing as a human service. Nursing is distinguished from other human services by its focus on persons with inabilities to maintain the continuous provision of health care. Nursing is needed when the adult cannot continually carry out the efforts (either in quantity or in quality) needed to sustain life, sustain health, recover from disease or injury, or cope with the effects of disease or injury (p. 82). With children, nursing is needed when the parent or guardian associated with the child's health state is unable to continuously provide the quantity and quality of needed care (p. 82). For children, nursing may be needed to assist with development or maturation.

The nurse's and the patient's roles define the expected behaviors for each in the specific nursing situation. Various factors that influence the expected role behaviors are culture, environment, age, sex, the health setting, and finances. The roles of nurse and patient are complementary. That is, a certain behavior of the patient elicits a certain response in the nurse and vice versa. Both work together to accomplish the goal of self-care.

In the nurse–patient relationship, the nurse or patient may experience role conflict because each is performing concurrent roles. For example, the patient has expected behaviors from his roles as father, husband, Cub Scout leader, soccer coach, and librarian. The nurse has expected behaviors from her roles as wife, mother, daughter, choir director, and PTA president. Thus, the conflict in the behaviors required for the various roles may affect the performance of self-care by the patient and by the nurse.

It is important to note that although Orem (2001) recognizes that specialized technologies are usually developed by members of the health professions, she emphasizes the need for social and interpersonal dimensions in nursing. The effective integration of social and interpersonal technologies with regulatory technologies promotes quality professional nursing. She describes what she calls "treatment or regulatory" activities as the ways in which prescriptions are carried out so that the identified problem or conditions are treated; the goal of such activities is to eliminate the problem, or control it or keep it within limits that allow for life, health, or well-being (p. 308).

OREM'S THEORY AND THE NURSING PROCESS

Orem (2001) describes *nursing process* as the phrase used by nurses to describe what she terms the "professional-technologic" aspects of the practice of nursing (p. 309). Other activities associated with nursing process are planning and evaluation. A process is a continuous and regular sequence of goal-achieving, deliberately performed actions taking place or carried out in a definite manner.

TABLE 6-2   Comparison of Orem's Nursing Process and the Nursing Process

Nursing Process	Orem's Nursing Process
1. Assessment	Step 1. Diagnosis and prescription; determine why
2. Nursing diagnosis	nursing is needed. Analyze and interpret—make
3. Outcomes	judgments regarding care.
4. Plans with scientific rationale	Step 2. Design of a nursing system and plan for delivery
5. Implementation	of care.
6. Evaluation	Step 3. Production and management of nursing systems.

Orem (2001) discusses a three-step nursing process that she labels the professional-technologic operations of nursing practice. These steps are shown in Table 6-2 as follows:

Step 1 Nursing diagnosis and prescription—that is, determining why nursing is needed; analysis and interpretation—making judgments regarding care, also labeled case management operations.

Step 2 Designing the nursing system and planning for delivery of care.

Step 3 The production and management of nursing systems, also labeled planning and controlling.

Orem (2001) states that the nursing process is represented by a nurse carrying out the activities associated with diagnostic, prescriptive, regulatory, and treatment operations and includes evaluation as an aspect of control (p. 309).

Nursing Diagnosis and Prescription (Step 1)

Nursing diagnosis requires the nurse to acquire data about the patient's self-care agency and therapeutic self-care demand and to identify current and predicted future relationships between the agency and demand (Orem, 2001, p. 310). The goal defines the direction and nature of the actions. Prescriptive operations specify the means (course of actions and care measures) to be used to meet particular self-care requisites or to meet all components of the therapeutic self-care demand. Orem emphasizes that, in nursing's diagnostic and prescriptive operations and in the regulatory or treatment operations, patients' and families' abilities and interests in collaboration affect what nurses can do.

Designs for Regulatory Operation (Step 2)

Designing an effective and efficient system of nursing involves choosing suitable ways to help the patient. This design includes nurse and patient roles in relation to which self-care tasks will be performed when modifying the therapeutic self-care demands, controlling the implementation of self-care agency, shielding the already developed powers of self-care agency, and assisting with new developments in self-care agency (Orem, 2001, p. 319).

Planning is the movement from designing the nursing systems to identifying the mechanisms of their production. Orem (2001) indicates that the plan organizes those tasks that must be carried out in relation to the responsibilities of the nurse and the patient (p. 321). The plan will also include a time line for when the nurse will be with the patient and when necessary equipment and materials will be needed (p. 322).

Production/Management of Nursing Systems (Step 3)

A regulatory nursing system is created through the nurse's interaction with the patient with the result that the nurse's actions consistently strive to meet unmet and prescribed therapeutic self-care demands and to help the patient carry out or develop self-care agency (Orem, 2001, p. 322). In this, the third step of the professional-technologic nursing process, nurses act to produce and manage nursing systems.

During the interactions of nurses and patients, nurses do the following:

1. Perform and regulate the performance of self-care tasks for patients or assist patients with their performance of self-care tasks
2. Coordinate self-care task performance so that a unified system of care is produced and coordinated with other components of health care
3. Help patients, their families, and others bring about systems of daily living for patients that support the accomplishment of self-care and are, at the same time, satisfying in relation to patients' interest[s], talents, and goals
4. Guide, direct, and support patients in their exercise of, or in withholding the exercise of, their self-care agency
5. Stimulate patients' interest in self-care by raising questions and promoting discussions of care problems and issues when conditions permit; be available to patients at times when questions are likely to arise
6. Support and guide patients in learning activities and provide cues for learning as well as instructional sessions
7. Support and guide patients as they experience illness or disability and the effects of medical care measures and as they experience the need to engage in new measures of self-care or change their ways of meeting ongoing self-care requisites
8. Monitor patients and assist patients to monitor themselves to determine if self-care measures were effectively performed and to determine the effects of self-care, the results of efforts to regulate the exercise or development of self-care agency, and the sufficiency and efficiency of nursing action directed to these ends
9. Make characterizing judgments about the sufficiency and efficiency of self-care, the regulation of the exercise or development of self-care agency, and nursing assistance
10. Make judgments about the meaning of the results derived from nurses' performance of the preceding two operations for the well-being of patients and make or recommend adjustments in the nursing care system through changes in nurse and patient roles (Orem, 2001, pp. 322–323)

The first seven operations constitute direct nursing care. The last three are for the purpose of deciding if the care provided should be continued in the present form or be changed. This comprises the evaluation component of the nursing process.

The case study demonstrates the use of Orem's theory and the nursing process (see Table 6-3 and Table 6-4).

STEP 1   Orem defines step 1 as the diagnosis and prescription phase, determining if nursing is needed. In this assessment phase, the nurse collects data in six areas:

1. The person's health status
2. The physician's perspective of the person's health

TABLE 6-3 Application of Orem's Theory to Nursing Process

Basic Conditioning Factors	Universal Self-Care	Developmental Self-Care	Health Deviations	Medical Problem and Plan	Self-Care Deficits
Age Sex Height Weight Culture Race Marital status Religion Occupation	Air, water, food Excrements Activity and rest Solitude and social interaction Hazards to life and well-being Promotion of human functioning and development	Specialized needs for developmental processes New requisites from a condition Requisites associated with an event	Conditions of illness or Injury Treatments to correct the condition	Physician's perspective of condition Medical diagnosis Medical treatment	Difference between self-care needs and self-care capabilities

Nursing Diagnosis	Outcomes and Plan	Implementation
Based on self-care deficits	Outcomes, nursing goals, and objectives: a. Congruent with nursing diagnosis b. Based on self-care demands c. Promote patient as self-care agent Designing the nursing system: a. Wholly compensatory b. Partly compensatory c. Supportive–educative Appropriate methods of helping: a. Guidance b. Support c. Acting or doing for d. Providing developmental environment	Nurse–patient actions to: a. Promote patient as self-care agent b. Meet self-care needs c. Decrease self-care deficit Effectiveness of nurse–patient actions to: a. Promote patient as self-care agent b. Meet self-care needs c. Decrease self-care deficits

Adapted from Pinnell, N. N., & de Meneses, M. (1986). *The nursing process—Theory, application and related processes.* Norwalk, CT: Appleton-Century-Crofts, p. 66. Used with permission.

TABLE 6-4 Application of Orem's Theory Using Ms. M.'s Case Study Within the Nursing Process

Assessment

Basic Conditioning Factors	Universal Self-Care	Developmental Self-Care	Health Deviations	Medical Problem and Plan	Self-Care Deficits
48 years old Female 5'2'' 175 lbs. Italian White Widowed for six months after 25 years of happy marriage Catholic University faculty	Smokes 1.5 packs/day Frequently eats fast food; high-fat diet; drinks 48 oz. of water daily Largest meal of day is late evening No difficulties with elimination No regular exercise Sleeps six to seven hours nightly Decreased social interaction × six months—no longer plays bridge with group she and her husband played with	Loss of husband Loss of social activity Finds work as university faculty fulfilling Works 12-hour days Well groomed	Family history: F—heart attack, age 50 M—died of stroke, age 53 Cholesterol 260 mg; other lab values WNL Lacks knowledge of risk factors and cardiovascular functioning B/P 142/88 T 98.4° F P 92 R 26, not SOB Potential for cardiac disease related to obesity, smoking, elevated cholesterol, lack of exercise, and family history	Diagnoses of obesity with potential for cardiac disease and low motivation for weight loss Prescription to: Monitor cholesterol levels and vital signs Decrease cholesterol and fat intake Increase exercise Decrease or stop smoking Reevaluate and if needed prescribe medication to lower cholesterol	Difference between healthy lifestyle and Ms. M.'s knowledge base and lifestyle, which increases her risk of heart attack or stroke

Nursing Diagnosis	Outcomes and Plan	Implementation	Evaluation
Potential for impaired cardiovascular functioning related to lack of knowledge about relationship between current lifestyle and risk of heart attack or stroke	Outcome: Lowered cholesterol Healthier lifestyle with regular exercise, decreased smoking, and balanced nutrition Nursing Goals and Objectives: Goal: To decrease risk for cardiac impairment Objectives: Ms. M. will state that high cholesterol levels increase her risk for cardiac impairment Ms. M. will recognize the relationship between smoking and cardiovascular risk Design of Nursing System: Supportive-educative Methods of Helping: Guidance, support, teaching, and provision of a developmental environment	Jointly develop contract related to: 1. Cholesterol Reduction Ms. M. will keep a three-day food diary Ms. M. will learn about cholesterol and its effects on cardiovascular functioning Ms. M. will request/obtain cholesterol and fat content of fast foods Ms. M. will learn about low-cholesterol and fast foods, foods that decrease cholesterol, and restaurants that serve low-cholesterol and fat-free foods Jointly analyze food diary and decide how to decrease cholesterol/fat intake to reduce Ms. M.'s weight Jointly determine Italian foods that are low in cholesterol and fat and how recipes may be adapted Ms. M.'s accomplishments will be reinforced Ms. M. will seek advice from her physician re: medication to reduce cholesterol 2. Reduction of Smoking Ms. M. will identify when she smokes and what initiates the desire for a cigarette Ms. M. will plan ways to replace smoking with other activities (exercising, chewing gum)	Does Ms. M. understand that, with her present lifestyle, her risk of heart attack or stroke is high? Did Ms. M. select low-cholesterol, low-fat foods? Did Ms. M.'s self-care deficit decrease? Is Ms. M.'s cholesterol lower? Did Ms. M. lose weight? Has Ms. M. decreased the number of cigarettes smoked daily? Was the supportive-educative system effective in promoting Ms. M. as a self-care agent?

3. The person's perspective of his health
4. The health goals within the context of life history, lifestyle, and health status
5. The person's requirements for self-care
6. The person's capacity to perform self-care

Specific data are gathered in the areas of the individual's universal, developmental, and health-deviation self-care needs and their interrelationship. Data are also collected about the individual's knowledge, skills, motivation, and orientation. Orem is careful to point out that the data to be collected should be limited to those needed to come to legitimate conclusions about the person's needs (Orem, 2001, p. 310).

Within step 1, the nurse seeks answers to the following questions:

1. What is the patient's therapeutic care demand? Now? At a future time?
2. Does the patient have a deficit for engaging in self-care to meet the therapeutic self-care demand?
3. If so, what is its nature and the reasons for its existence?
4. Should the patient be helped to refrain from engagement in self-care or to protect already developed self-care capabilities for therapeutic purposes?
5. What is the patient's potential for engaging in self-care at a future time period? Increasing or deepening self-care knowledge? Learning techniques of self-care? Fostering willingness to engage in self-care? Effectively and consistently incorporating essential self-care measures (including new ones) into the systems of self-care and daily living? (Orem, 1985, pp. 225–226)

Once the assessment data have been gathered, they must be analyzed. In the category of universal self-care needs, Ms. M. demonstrates a deficit in adequate air, water, and food intake because she is 5 feet 2 inches, weighs 175 pounds, and consumes excessive calories, fat, and cholesterol from fast-food and late-night meals. Ms. M. shows an imbalance between activity and rest because she has minimal exercise. There is also an imbalance between her solitude and social interaction since her husband's death, which is a significant loss for her in the midlife developmental needs category. Ms. M.'s elevated cholesterol levels, when interrelated with her family history of stroke and heart attack, present a hazard to her life, functioning, and well-being. The physician's perspective is that Ms. M. needs to lose 40 pounds because of her family history and elevated blood cholesterol but that she has limited nutritional knowledge. However, Ms. M. has a motivational deficit to lose weight because her Italian cultural tradition associates food with family and love.

Based on the analysis of Ms. M.'s data, she has potential hazards to her health related to obesity, high cholesterol, smoking, social isolation, and decreased exercise. The analysis of the collected data leads to the nursing diagnosis and enables the nurse to prioritize self-care deficits. The nursing diagnosis must include the response and etiology pattern. Within Orem's framework, the nursing diagnosis would be stated as an inability to meet the self-care demand (the response) related to the self-care deficit (etiology) (Ziegler, Vaughn-Wrobel, & Erlen, 1986). For Ms. M. the response pattern would be "potential for impaired cardiovascular functioning," and the etiology would be "lack of knowledge about how her current life style increases her risk for heart attack and stroke."

STEP 2   Orem defines step 2 as designing the nursing systems and planning for the delivery of nursing. The nurse designs a system that is wholly compensatory, partly compensatory, or supportive–educative. The specific design of the nursing system develops as the nurse and patient interact, move to identify and meet the patient's therapeutic self-care demands, offset or overcome any identified limitations, and control the patient's development and use of self-care abilities (Orem, 2001, p. 348).

Using Orem's model, the outcomes and goals are congruent with the nursing diagnosis to enable the patient to become an effective self-care agent. Outcomes and goals are directed by the response statement of the nursing diagnosis and are focused on health. The outcome for Ms. M. would be to decrease her risk of cardiovascular impairment. The goals would be lowered blood cholesterol level and a healthier lifestyle that includes regular exercise, decreased smoking, and balanced nutrition.

Once the outcomes and goals have been determined, the objectives can be stated. An example of an objective for Ms. M. would be that Ms. M. will state that high cholesterol levels increase her risk for cardiac impairment. Other objectives might relate to the risk factors of obesity, lack of exercise, smoking, and family history. The designed nursing system for Ms. M. would be the supportive–educative nursing system.

STEP 3   Within Orem's (2001) nursing process, step 3 includes the production and management of the nursing system. In this step, the nurse performs and regulates the patient's self-care tasks or assists the patient in doing so; coordinates the performance of self-care with other components of health care; helps patients, families, and others create and use systems of daily living that meet self-care needs in a satisfying way; guides, directs, and supports patients in exercising or not exercising self-care agency; stimulates the patient's interest in care problems; supports learning activities; supports and guides the patient in adapting to the needs arising from medical measures; monitors and assists in self-monitoring the performance and effects of self-care measures; judges the sufficiency and efficiency of self-care, self-care agency, and nursing agency; and adjusts the nursing care system as needed.

The nurse and patient actions are directed by the etiology component of the nursing diagnosis. "Lack of knowledge about how her current lifestyle increases her risk for heart attack and stroke" is the etiology component of Ms. M.'s nursing diagnosis. When the nurse and patient implement this supportive–educative system, each has specific roles. Examples of these roles might be that together they would develop a contract relating to the goal of blood cholesterol reduction. Ms. M. would keep a three-day food diary. The nurse would provide information about cholesterol and its effects on cardiovascular function. Ms. M. would request and obtain the fat and cholesterol content of the fast-food menu items from the restaurants she frequents. The nurse would provide information about specific foods that are low in fat and cholesterol, those food items that help reduce cholesterol, and a list of fast-food restaurants that offer low-fat and low-cholesterol food items. Together they would analyze the three-day food diary and decide how Ms. M. might modify her diet to reduce her fat and cholesterol intake. They would determine which Italian dishes are low in fat and cholesterol or how these recipes can be adapted. As her blood cholesterol levels decrease, Ms. M. would be praised for her accomplishments. During this implementation, the nurse would teach, guide, and support Ms. M. while providing a developmental environment.

Step 3 includes evaluation. The nurse and patient together do the evaluation. Questions they might ask are the following: When evaluating some of Ms. M.'s plans, does she understand that her present lifestyle may increase her risk of developing a heart attack or stroke? Did she select low-fat and low-cholesterol fast foods? Did she attain her goal of reducing her blood cholesterol levels? Did she lose weight? The results must then be communicated with the physician and any further medical interventions needed then obtained. Were the plans effective in decreasing the self-care deficit? Was the nursing system effective in promoting the patient as a self-care agent?

Evaluation is an ongoing process. It is essential that the nurse and patient continually evaluate any changes in the data that would affect the self-care deficit, the self-care agency, and the nursing system.

CRITIQUE OF OREM'S SELF-CARE DEFICIT THEORY OF NURSING

Orem first presented a conceptual framework (Orem, 1959). Since then her work has continued to evolve. Orem's general theory of nursing was formulated and expressed in 1979–1980. This Self-Care Deficit Theory of Nursing is comprised of three interrelated theories: the theory of self-care, the theory of self-care deficit, and the theory of nursing systems. These three interrelated theories are the basis of the following discussion.

1. *What is the historical context of the theory?*   Orem began her work in the late 1950s while working with licensed practical nurses. She continued the development of her theory throughout the 20th century and into the 21st century. Her work initially focused on the individual inpatient but in her fifth and sixth editions (1995, 2001) discusses the multiperson unit, the person at home, and positive mental health. She has indicated that the theory is derived from clinical practice and that its evaluation is dependent on continued contact and exchange with clinicians (Trench, Wallace, & Cobert, 1988). In an interview with Susan Taylor, Orem stated, "My goal from the very beginning has been to have a nursing literature. A structured body of knowledge for consumption by nursing students" (Taylor, 2007, p. 25).

2. *What are the basic concepts and relationships presented by the theory?*   Orem discusses persons as those needing to have self-care needs met in order to live and develop. When persons are unable to care for themselves (self-care needs are greater than self-care abilities or self-care agency), then someone else must provide that care, and nursing is needed. The basic concepts are "self-care," "universal, developmental, and health deviation self-care requisites," "basic conditioning factors," "therapeutic self-care demand" "self-care deficit," "supportive–educative, partly compensatory, and wholly compensatory nursing systems," "self-care agency," and "nursing agency." When a person's self-care agency is adequate to meet the therapeutic self-care demand created by the self-care requisites and basic conditioning factors, then self-care needs are met by that individual. When the therapeutic self-care demand is greater than the self-care agency, then a self-care deficit exists and nursing is needed. Nursing agency supports the person in meeting self-care needs through the design and delivery of supportive–educative, partly compensatory, and wholly compensatory nursing systems.

3. *What major phenomena of concern to nursing are presented?* (*These phenomena may include* **but are not limited to** *human beings, environment, health, interpersonal relations, caring, goal attainment, adaptation, and energy fields.*)   Orem (2001) discusses human beings as differentiated from other living beings in three ways: the ability to reflect both upon self and upon environment, the ability to create symbols from experiences, and the ability to use symbols in thought and communication as well as in efforts to create improvements both for self and others (p. 182).

   Within Orem's theory, the environment directly influences the patient. Orem (2001) discusses the individual's needs for air, water, and food as well as preventing hazards to living, the importance of both function and well-being in maintaining integrity, and promoting the function and development of the human (p. 226).

Orem's discussion of health and the supportive–educative system is relevant in today's society because she supports health promotion and health maintenance. Self-care in Orem's theory likewise supports the premises of holistic health in that both promote the individual's responsibility for health care.

Orem's discussion of interpersonal relations would involve the nurse acting for or doing for the patient but also relying on the other (patient or nurse) in the partly compensatory and wholly compensatory systems. She incorporates the care of the patient with the abilities of the family members and recognizes that they may be the ones providing the "self-care" for the patient. She also discusses the need to determine what the physician's perspective is of the patient's illness.

Nursing is needed, according to Orem, whenever the maintenance of continuous self-care requires the use of special techniques and the application of scientific knowledge to provide or design care. These are required when there is a self-care deficit. The design of nursing systems involves consideration of the areas in which and the degree to which support is needed.

Orem (2001) states, "The interpersonal features of nursing are based on existent contractual relationships of nurses and patients" (p. 99). She recognizes that in the ideal situation, the relationship between the nurse and the patient will help decrease the patient's stress as well as that of the patient's family. The reduction in stress will help both the patient and the family to do what is best in relation to health and health care (p. 101). Orem's theory refers to "care" from a more physical provision of nursing care with the interpersonal relationships discussed rather than feeling the emotional perspective of "caring."

4. *To whom does this theory apply? In what situations? In what ways?* Orem's theory applies to all persons who need nursing care. The theory applies to situations in which individuals (including children) cannot meet all of their self-care needs. One of the unique characteristics of Orem's theory is that she recognizes that normal life and human development necessitates adjustments, which might be improved by supportive–educative care from the nurse. Orem's theory has been expanded by Taylor and Renpenning (1995, 2001) to include multiperson units, families, and communities. However, Orem recommended in 2001 that, based on knowledge at that time, the nursing systems be limited to use with individuals as units of service.

A search of the literature supports the use of this theory in a wide variety of settings and with a variety of patients. A partial list includes the following:

Multiperson units (Chevannes, 1997; DeMoutigny, 1995; Geden & Taylor, 1999; Logue, 1997; Shum, McGonigal, & Biehler, 2005; Taylor & McLaughlin, 1991; Taylor & Renpenning, 2001)

Caregivers (Baker, 1997; Carlson, Kotzé, & Van Rooyen, 2005; Fawdry, Berry, & Rajacich, 1996; Schott-Baer, Fisher, & Gregory, 1995)

Culture (Grubbs & Frank, 2004; Hadley & Roques, 2007; Hartweg & Berbiglia, 1996; Hurst, Montgomery, Davis, Killion, & Baker, 2005; Lee, 1999; Roberson & Kelley, 1996; Sonderhamm, Evers, & Hamrin, 1996; Villarruel & Denyes, 1997; Wang, 1997)

Health education (Jewell & Sullivan, 1996)

Multiple age-groups (Anderson & Olnhausen, 1999; Brock & O'Sullivan, 1985; Callaghan, 2005, 2006a, 2006b; Chang, Cuman, Linn, Ware, & Kane, 1985; Chang, Hancock, Hickman, Glasson, & Davidson, 2007; Chang, Liu, & Chang, 2007; Clark, 1998; Dahlen, 1997; Denyes, 1982; Fan, 2008; Faulkner & Chang, 2007; Foote, Holcombe, Piazza, & Wright, 1993; Harper, 1984; Reed, 1986; Roy & Collin, 1994; Smith, 1996; Vesely, 1995; Villarruel & Denyes, 1991)

Framework for inpatient care (Laurie-Shaw & Ives, 1988a, 1988b)

Various clinical areas (Ailinger & Dear, 1997; Aish, 1996; Aish & Isenberg, 1996; Anastasio, McMahan, Daniels, Nicholas, & Paul-Simon, 1995; Beach et al., 1996; Becker, Teixeira, & Zanetti, 2008; Campbell & Weber, 2000; Chen, Li, & Gong, 2009; Conway, McMillan, & Solman, 2006; Ferraz, de Almeida, Girardi, & Soares, 2007; Fitzgerald, 1980; Frey & Denyes, 1989; Fujita & Dungan, 1994; Graham, 2006; Grando, 2005; Gulick, 1987; Hagopian, 1996; Jaarsma, Halfens, Senten, AbuSaad, & Dracup, 1998; Keohane & Lacey, 1991; Kline, Scott, & Britton, 2007; Logue, 1997; Mack, 1992; Magnan, 2004; Manzini & Simonetti, 2009; Norris, 1991; Orem & Vardiman, 1995; Ramos, Chagas, Freitas, Monteiro, & Leite, 2007; Sampai, Aquino, de Araujo, & Galvao, 2008; Simmons, 2009; Tseng, 2007; Tolentino, 1990; Zinn, 1986)

Concepts of the theory that have received specific focus include:
Self-care deficit (Gaffney & Moore, 1996; Timmins & Horan, 2007)
Self-care agency (Akyol, Çetinkaya, Bakan, Yaral, & Akkus, 2007; Allan, 1990; Allison, 2007; Baker, 1997; Brillhart, 2007; Denyes, 1988; Gast et al., 1989; Hart & Foster, 1998; Hines et al., 2007; Jirovic & Kasno, 1990, 1993; Kearney & Fleischer, 1979; McDermott, 1993; Tokem, Akyol, & Argon, 2007; Ulbrich, 1999; Utz, Shuster, Merwin, & Williams, 1994; Zrínyi & Zékányné, 2007)

Dependent-care agency (Moore & Gaffney, 1989)

Basic conditioning factors (Ailinger & Dear, 1997; Anatasio et al., 1995; Callaghan, 2006a, 2006b; Carroll, 1995; Conner-Warren, 1996; Freston et al., 1997; Frey & Denyes, 1989; Gaffney & Moore, 1996; Geden & Taylor, 1991; Hanucharurnkul, 1989; Jirovec & Kasno, 1990; Lawrence & Schank, 1995; Mapanga & Andrews, 1995; Marz, 1988; Moore, 1993; Moore & Mosher, 1997; Zadinsky & Boyle, 1996)

Therapeutic self-care demand (Kubricht, 1984)

5. *By what method or methods can this theory be tested?* Orem's theory is one of the most readily applied theories. In an electronic search, Taylor, Geden, Isaramalai, and Wongvatunyu (2000) found 143 journal articles (unpublished dissertations are not included) that used Orem's theory. The search was limited to those written in English and identified as being research articles. Of these, 66 were identified as clearly testing relationships within the theory. The others used Orem's work as part of the organizing framework or to provide a definition of self-care. The studies reviewed included both quantitative and qualitative research methods. Taylor et al. identified several instruments that have been developed and validated to measure aspects of Orem's theory. Self-care agency was the focus in the Denyes Self-Care Agency Instrument (Denyes, 1982), the Exercise of Self-Care Agency (Kearney & Fleischer, 1979), and the Assessment of Self-Care Agency (Evers, Isenberg, Philipsen, Senten, & Brouns, 1989; Lorensen, Holter, Evers, Isenberg, & Van Achterberg, 1993; Van Achterberg, Lorensen, Isenberg, Evers, & Phillipsen,

1991). Geden and Taylor (1991) developed the Self-as-Carer Inventory, and Shum, McGonigal, and Biehler (2005) developed the Community Care Deficit Nursing Model for use with multiperson units in a community care setting.

6. *Does this theory direct nursing actions that lead to favorable outcomes?*   Orem's theory definitely directs nursing actions that lead to favorable outcomes. The individual is recognized as having self-care needs that the person (if a healthy adult) has the ability or self-care agency to meet. These needs develop and change as the person grows, develops, and experiences life events. Orem's theory recognizes that if there are more self-care needs present than there are abilities to meet them, then there is a self-care deficit. Nursing would then be needed. A nursing system can be designed to help the person meet those needs. When the nurse and patient work together in that designed system, the patients' self-care needs can be met, and the outcomes are favorable.

7. *How contagious is this theory?*   Orem's theory is extremely contagious. The easily understood concepts are simple yet complex and may be used by practitioners at all levels (beginning through advanced) and in all areas of practice. Taylor et al. (2000) found 143 research-related journal articles published in English. There is an additional body of literature related to application of the theory in practice, unpublished dissertation reports, and articles published in languages other than English. In 2009, several nurse scholars presented their views on her influence, both during her life and for the future of nursing and healthcare (Clarke, Allison, Berbiglia, & Taylor, 2009).

Orem's work is used internationally. Its use in Australia, Bangladesh, Brazil, Canada, Hungary, India, The Netherlands, Norway, Pakistan, Sweden, Switzerland, Thailand, and Turkey is also supported by reports in the literature (Aish, 1996; Aish & Isenberg, 1996; Akyol et al., 2007; Chang et al., 2007; Conway et al., 2006; Dahlen, 1997; Hadley & Roques, 2007; Hanucharurnkul, 1989; Hanucharurnkul, Wittayasooporn, Luecha, & Maneesriwongul, 2003; Jewell & Sullivan, 1996; Laurie-Shaw & Ives, 1988a, 1988b; Lee, 1999; Moser, Houtepen, & Widdershoven, 2007; Shaini, Venkatesan, & Ben, 2007; Soderhamm et al., 1996; Spirig & Willhelm, 1995; Tokem et al., 2007; Weimers, Svensson, Dumas, Navér, & Wahlberg, 2007; Wing & Cartana, 2007; Zŕinyi & Zékányné, 2007). Further support is demonstrated by the 1991 founding and ongoing activity of the International Orem Society, which was established to advance nursing science and scholarship through the use of Dorothea E. Orem's nursing conceptualizations in nursing education, practice, and research, and also the publishing of *Self-Care, Dependent Care, and Nursing Journal* begun in 2002. Her work has also provided a basis for numerous master's theses and doctoral dissertations. A partial listing of these is provided at the end of this chapter.

STRENGTHS AND LIMITATIONS

In the preface to the sixth edition of *Nursing: Concepts of Practice*, Orem (2001) outlines the following six broad themes: why persons need and can be helped by nursing, the relationship between persons needing and producing nursing, the unitary nature of humans, the selection and performance of deliberate actions to achieve desired results, assistive methods, and nursing as a practical science. In the text she describes her general theory, which is supported by three interrelated theories. Within these theories, six central concepts and one peripheral concept are identified. These provide the learner with a blueprint for the structure of Orem's Self-Care Deficit Theory of Nursing.

The development of the theory was influenced by collaboration among clinicians, scholars, and educators. The fifth and sixth editions of Orem's text include a chapter by Taylor and Renpenning focusing on the position of family involvement within the self-care deficit nursing theory (Orem, 1995, 2001). Also, the Self-Care Deficit Theory of Nursing has been supported by clinical case-study data (Orem & Taylor, 1986).

Orem's theory of nursing provides a comprehensive base for nursing practice. It has utility for professional nursing in the areas of education, clinical practice, administration, research, and nursing information systems. A major strength of Orem's theory is that it is applicable for nursing by the beginning practitioner as well as the advanced clinician. The terms *self-care, nursing systems,* and *self-care deficit* are easily understood by the beginning nursing student and can be explored in greater depth as the nurse gains more knowledge and experience.

Another strength of Orem's (2001) theory is that she specifically defines when nursing is needed: Nursing is needed when the individual cannot maintain continuously that amount and quality of self-care necessary to sustain life and health, recover from disease or injury, or cope with their effects. Nursing is also required when special techniques and scientific knowledge are needed to maintain continuous self-care (p. 83).

Orem (2001) promotes the concepts of professional nursing. She defines the roles of vocational, technical, and professional nurses and recognizes the importance of each. She indicates that "thinking nursing" and conceptualizing the dynamics and structure of nursing situations is distinct from viewing nursing as the skilled performance of tasks.

Her self-care premise is contemporary with the concepts of health promotion and health maintenance. Self-care in Orem's theory is comparable to holistic health in that both promote the individual's responsibility for health care. This is especially relevant with today's emphasis on early hospital discharge, home care, and outpatient services. Orem (2001) recognizes the term *client* as a regular seeker of services but prefers the term *patient* for a person during the time that person is receiving care from a health care professional (p. 70).

Orem (2001) indicates that nurses should identify one type of nursing system, or a sequence of nursing systems, to achieve the optimum effect in regulating the patient's self-care agency and meeting the patient's self-care requisites (p. 355). Some practitioners have found Orem's theory to be more clinically applicable when more than one system is used concurrently (Knust & Quarn, 1983).

Another strength is Orem's delineation of three identifiable nursing systems. These are easily understood by the beginning nursing student. Orem's use of the term *system* has developed to include entities that behave as a whole and in which a change in a part affects the whole (Orem, 2001, p. 155). This definition is congruent with the general system theory view of a system as a dynamic, flowing process.

Orem (2001) has expanded her initial focus of individual self-care to include multiperson units (families, groups, and communities). She notes that when multiperson units are served by nurses, the resulting nursing systems combine the features of partly compensatory and supportive–educative nursing systems. However, an incongruence is present because she suggests that "it is advisable at this stage of the development of nursing knowledge to confine the use of the three nursing systems to situations in which individuals are the units of care or service" (p. 351).

Orem's theory is simple yet complex. However, the essence is clouded by ancillary descriptions. The term *self-care* is used with numerous configurations. This multitude of terms, such as self-care agency, self-care demand, self-care premise, self-care deficit, self-care requisites, and universal self-care, can be very confusing initially until the essence of each concept is understood. Orem's sixth edition is much more readable than the previous editions; however, some of her terminology remains confusing. An example is in relation to the science of self-care, where she states, "Speculatively practical with practically practical content elements" (p. 177).

Other limitations include her discussion of health. Health is often viewed as dynamic and ever changing. Orem's model of the boxed nursing systems (see Figure 6-2) implies three static conditions of health. She refers to a "concrete nursing system," which connotes rigidity. Another impression from the model of nursing systems is that a major determining factor for placement of a patient in a system is the individual's capacity for physical movement. Throughout her work there is limited acknowledgment of the individual's emotional needs.

Summary

Orem presents her general theory of nursing, the self-care deficit theory of nursing, which is composed of the three interrelated theories of self-care, self-care deficit, and nursing systems. Incorporated within and supportive of these theories are the six central concepts of self-care—self-care agency, therapeutic self-care demand, self-care deficit, nursing agency, and nursing system, as well as the peripheral concept of basic conditioning factors.

Nursing is needed when the self-care demands are greater than the self-care abilities. The nurse designs nursing systems when it has been determined that nursing care is needed. The systems of wholly compensatory, partly compensatory, and supportive–educative specify the roles of the nurse and the patient.

Throughout Orem's work, she interprets nursing's metaparadigm of human beings, health, nursing, and society. She defines three steps of nursing process as (1) diagnosis and prescription, (2) design of a nursing system and planning for the delivery of care, and (3) production and management of nursing systems. This process parallels the nursing process of assessment, diagnosis, outcomes, planning, implementation, and evaluation.

Orem's theory of self-care has pragmatic application to nursing practice. It has been applied by nursing clinicians in a variety of settings. The theory has been used as the basis for nursing school curricula and the base for a nursing information system.

Orem's Self-Care Deficit Theory of Nursing continues to evolve, and its impact is international. The widespread use of this theory reflects its utility for professional nursing. Orem's theory offers a unique way of looking at the phenomenon of nursing. Her work contributes significantly to the development of nursing theories for this generation and the next. Perhaps one of the best commentaries on her impact on nursing theory was made by Kathleen Jones, an RN who left a notation in Dr. Orem's memorial service guest book. Dr. Dorothea E. Orem made "nursing theory exciting, realistic and usable in practice. She will live on through her work" (DeLorme, 2007, p. 3).

Thought Questions

1. Describe what you believe to be the most useful features of Orem's work.
2. How might nursing systems be used with a healthy adult?
3. Design a nursing system to be used with a four-year-old hospitalized for an emergency appendectomy.
4. Does Orem's work lead you to include the parents or guardian of the four-year-old in question 3? Why or why not?

References

Ailinger, R. L., & Dear, M. R. (1997). An examination of the self-care needs of clients with rheumatoid arthritis. *Rehabilitation Nursing, 22*(3), 13–14.

Aish, A. (1996). A comparison of female and male cardiac patients' responses to nursing care promoting nutritional self-care. *Canadian Journal of Cardiovascular Nursing, 7*(3), 4–13.

Aish, A. E., & Isenberg, M. (1996). Effects of Orem-based nursing intervention on nutritional self-care of myocardial infarction patients. *International Journal of Nursing Studies, 33,* 259–270.

Akyol, A. D., Çetinkaya, Y., Bakan, G., Yaral, S., & Akkus, S. (2007). Self-care agency and factors related to this agency among patients with hypertension. *Journal of Clinical Nursing, 16,* 679–687.

Allan, J. D. (1990). Focusing on living, not dying: A naturalistic study of self-care among seropositive gay men. *Holistic Nursing Practice, 4*(2), 56–63.

Allison, S. E. (2007). Self-care requirements for activity and rest: An Orem nursing focus. *Nursing Science Quarterly, 20,* 68–76.

Anastasio, D., McMahan, T., Daniels, A., Nicholas, P. K., & Paul-Simon, A. (1995). Self-care burden in women with human immunodeficiency virus. *Journal of the Association of Nurses for AIDS Care, 6*(3), 31–42.

Anderson, J. A., & Olnhausen, K. S. (1999). Adolescent self-esteem: A foundational disposition. *Nursing Science Quarterly, 12,* 62–67.

Baker S. (1997). The relationships of self-care agency and self-care actions to caregiver strain as perceived by female family caregivers of elderly parents. *Journal of New York State Nurses Association, 28*(1), 7–11.

Beach, E. K., Smith, A., Luthringer, L., Utz, S. K., Ahrens, S., & Whitmire, V. (1996). Self-care limitations of persons after acute myocardial infarction. *Applied Nursing Research, 9*(1), 24–28.

Becker, T. A. C., Teixeira, C. R., & Zanetti, M. L. (2008). Nursing diagnoses for diabetic patients using insulin [Portuguese]. *Revista Brasileira de Enfermagem, 61,* 847–852. Abstract in English retrieved November 30, 2009, from CINAHL Plus with Full Text database.

Brillhart, B. (2007). Internet education for spinal cord injury patients: Focus on urinary management. *Rehabilitation Nursing, 32,* 214–219.

Brock, A. M., & O'Sullivan, P. (1985). A study to determine what variables predict institutionalization of the elderly. *Journal of Advanced Nursing, 10,* 533–537.

Callaghan, D. (2005). Healthy behaviors, self-efficacy, self-care, and basic conditioning factors in older adults. *Journal of Community Health Nursing, 22,* 169–178.

Callaghan, D. (2006a). Basic conditioning factors' influences on adolescents' healthy behaviors, self-efficacy, and self-care. *Issues in Comprehensive Pediatric Nursing, 29*(4), 191–204.

Callaghan, D. (2006b). The influence of basic conditioning factors on healthy behaviors, self-efficacy, and self-care in adults. *Journal of Holistic Nursing, 24*(3), 178–185.

Campbell, J. C., & Weber, N. (2000). An empirical test of a self-care model of women's response to battering. *Nursing Science Quarterly, 13,* 45–53.

Carlson, S., Kotzé, W. J., & Van Rooyen, D. (2005). A self-management model towards professional maturity for the practice of nursing. *Curationis, 28*(5), 44–52.

Carroll, D. (1995). The importance of self-efficacy expectations in elderly patients recovering from coronary artery bypass. *Heart & Lung, 24*(1), 50–59.

Chang, B. L., Cuman, G., Linn, L. S., Ware, J. E., & Kane, R. L. (1985). Adherence to health care regimens among elderly women. *Nursing Research, 34,* 27–31.

Chang, E., Hancock, K., Hickman, L., Glasson, J., & Davidson, P. (2007). Outcomes of acutely ill older hospitalized patients following implementation of tailored models of care: A repeated measures (pre- and post-intervention) design. *International Journal of Nursing Studies, 44,* 1079–1092.

Chen, Y., Li, Y., & Gong, S. (2009). Application of Orem's self-care theory in postoperative nursing care of patients accepting artificial stapes implantation assisted by CO2 laser [Chinese]. *Chinese Nursing Research, 23,* 1731–1732. Abstract in English retrieved November 30, 2009, from CINAHL Plus with Full Text database.

Chevannes, J. (1997). Nurses caring for families— Issues in a multiracial society. *Journal of Clinical Nursing, 6*(2), 161–167.

Chiang, H., Liu, Y., & Chang, S. (2007). Applying Orem's Theory to the care of a diabetes patient with a foot ulcer [Chinese]. *Tzu Chi Nursing Journal, 6*(6), 127–135. Abstract in English retrieved November 30, 2009, from CINAHL Plus with Full Text database.

Clark, C. C. (1998). Wellness self-care by healthy older adults. *Image: Journal of Nursing Scholarship, 30,* 351–355.

Conner-Warren, R. (1996). Pain intensity and home pain management of children with sickle cell disease. *Issues in Comprehensive Pediatric Nursing, 19,* 183–195.

Conway, J., McMillan, M. A., & Solman, A. (2006). Enhancing cardiac rehabilitation nursing through aligning practice to theory: Implications for nursing education. *Journal of Continuing Education in Nursing, 37,* 233–238.

Dahlen, A. (1997). Health status of elderly— 67 years and older in a community—and their need of nursing care. A survey [Norwegian]. *Nordic Journal of Nursing Research and Clinical Studies, 17*(3), 36–42. Abstract in English retrieved December 26, 2007, from CINAHL Plus Full Text database.

DeLorme, R. H. (2007). Dorothea Elizabeth Orem made nursing theory exciting, realistic and usable. *Southern Cross Diocese Newsletter, 87*(37), 3.

De Moutigny, F. (1995). Family nursing interventions during hospitalization. *Canadian Nurse, 91*(10), 38–42 .

Denyes, M. J. (1982). Measurement of self-care agency in adolescents (abstract). *Nursing Research, 31,* 63.

Denyes, M. J. (1988). Orem's model used for health promotion: Directions from research. *Advances in Nursing Science, 11*(1), 13–21.

Evers, G. C., Isenberg, M. A., Philipsen, H., Senten, M., & Brouns, G. (1993). Validity testing of the Dutch translation of the appraisal of the self-care agency A.S.A. scale. *International Journal of Nursing Studies, 30,* 331–342.

Fan, L. (2008). Self-care behaviors of school-age children with heart disease. *Pediatric Nursing, 34*(2), 131–140.

Faulkner, M. S., & Chang, L. (2007). Family influence on self-care, quality of life, and metabolic control in school-age children and adolescents with type I diabetes. *Journal of Pediatric Nursing, 22*(1), 59–68.

Fawdry, M. K., Berry, M. L., & Rajacich, D. (1996). The articulation of nursing systems with dependent care systems of intergenerational caregivers. *Nursing Science Quarterly, 9,* 22–26.

Ferraz, L., de Almeida, F. M., Girardi, F., & Soares, S. C. (2007). Nursing assistance for the promotion of self-care for people with special needs [Portuguese]. *Revista Engermagem, 15,* 597–600. Abstract in English retrieved November 30, 2009, from CINAHL Plus with Full Text.

Fitzgerald, S. (1980). Utilizing Orem's self-care model in designing an educational program for the diabetic. *Topics in Clinical Nursing, 2,* 57–65.

Foote, A., Holcombe, J., Piazza, D., & Wright, P. (1993). Orem's theory used as a guide for the nursing care of an eight-year-old child with leukemia. *Journal of Pediatric Oncology Nursing, 10*(1), 26–32.

Freston, M., Young, S., Calhoun, S., Fredericksen, T., Salinger, L., Malchodi, C., et al. (1997). Responses of pregnant women to potential preterm labor symptoms. *Journal of Obstetric, Gynecologic, and Neonatal Nursing, 26,* 35–41.

Frey, M. A., & Denyes, M. J. (1989). Health and illness self-care in adolescents with IDDM: A test of Orem's theory. *Advances in Nursing Science, 12*(1), 67–75.

Fujita, L. Y., & Dungan, J. (1994). High risk for ineffective management of therapeutic regimen: A protocol study. *Rehabilitation Nursing, 19,* 75–79, 126.

Gaffney, K. F., & Moore, J. B. (1996). Testing Orem's theory of self-care deficit: Dependent care agent performance for children. *Nursing Science Quarterly, 9,* 160–164.

Gast, H. L., Denyes, M. J., Campbell, J. C., Hartweg, D. L., Schott-Baer, D., & Isenberg, M. (1989). Self-care agency: Conceptualizations and operationalizations. *Advances in Nursing Science, 12*(1), 26–38.

Geden, E., & Taylor, S. G. (1991). Construct and empirical validity of the Self-as-Carer Inventory. *Nursing Research, 40,* 47–50.

Geden, E. A., & Taylor, S. G. (1999). Theoretical and empirical description of adult couples' collaborative self-care systems. *Nursing Science Quarterly, 12,* 329–334.

Graham, J. (2006). Nursing theory and clinical practice: How three nursing models can be incorporated into the care of patients with end stage kidney disease. *CANNT Journal, 16*(4), 28–31.

Grando, V. T. (2005). A self-care deficit nursing theory practice model for advanced practice psychiatric/mental health nursing. *Self-Care, Dependent-Care and Nursing, 13*(1), 4–8.

Grubbs, L., & Frank, D. (2004). Self-care practices related to symptom responses in African-American and Hispanic adults. *Self-Care, Dependent-Care and Nursing, 12*(1),10–14.

Gulick, E. E. (1987). Parsimony and model confirmation of the ADL Self-Care Scale for Multiple Sclerosis persons. *Nursing Research, 36,* 278–283.

Hadley, M. B., & Roques, A. (2007). Nursing in Bangladesh: Rhetoric and reality. *Social Science and Medicine, 64,* 1153–1165.

Hagopian, G. A. (1996). The effects of informational audiotapes on knowledge and self-care behaviors of patients undergoing radiation therapy. *Oncology Nursing Forum, 23,* 697–700.

Hanucharurnkul, S. (1989). Predictors of self-care in cancer patients receiving radiotherapy. *Cancer Nursing, 12*(1), 21–27.

Hanucharurnkul, S., Wittayasooporn, J., Luecha, Y., & Maneesriwongul, W. (2003). An integrative review and meta-analysis of self-care research in Thailand: 1988–1999. In K. M. Renpenning & S. Taylor (Eds.), *Self-care theory in nursing, Selected papers of Dorothea Orem* (pp. 339–354). New York: Springer.

Harper, D. C. (1984). Application of Orem's theoretical constructs to self-care medication behaviors in the elderly. *Advances in Nursing Science, 6*(3), 29–46.

Hart, J. A., & Foster, S. N. (1998). Self-care agency in two groups of pregnant women. *Nursing Science Quarterly, 11,* 167–171.

Hartweg, D. L., & Berbiglia, V. A. (1996). Determining the adequacy of a health promotion self-care interview guide with healthy, middle-aged, Mexican-American women: A pilot study. *Health Care for Women International, 17*(1), 57–68.

Hines, S. H., Sampselle, C. M., Ronis, D. L., Yeo, S., Fredrickson B. L., & Boyd, C. J. (2007). Women's self-care agency to manage urinary incontinence: The impact of nursing agency and body experience. *Advances in Nursing Science, 30*(2), 175–188.

Hurst, C., Montgomery, A. J., Davis, B. L., Killion, C., & Baker, S. (2005). The relationship between social support, self-care agency, and self-care practices of African American Women who are HIV-positive. *Journal of Multicultural Nursing and Health, 11*(3), 11–22.

Jaarsma, T., Halfens, R., Senten, M., AbuSaad, H. H., & Dracup, K. (1998). Developing a supportive–educative program for patients with advanced heart failure within Orem's General Theory of Nursing. *Nursing Science Quarterly, 11,* 79–85.

Jewell, J. A., & Sullivan, E. A. (1996). Application of nursing theories in health education. *Journal of the American Psychiatric Nurses Association, 2*(3), 79–85.

Jirovec, M., & Kasno, J. (1990). Self-care agency as a function of patient-environmental factors among nursing home residents. *Research in Nursing and Health, 13,* 303–309.

Jirovec, M. M., & Kasno, J. (1993). Predictors of self-care abilities among the institutionalized elderly. *Western Journal of Nursing Research, 15,* 314–326.

Kearney, B., & Fleischer, B. (1979). Development of an instrument to measure self-care agency. *Research in Nursing and Health, 2,* 25–34.

Keohane, N. S., & Lacey, L. A. (1991). Preparing the woman with gestational diabetes for self-care. *Journal of Obstetric, Gynecologic, and Neonatal Nursing, 20,* 189–193.

Kline, K. S., Scott, L. D., &. Britton, A. S. (2007). The use of supportive–educative and mutual goal-setting strategies to improve self-management for patients with heart failure. *Home Healthcare Nurse, 25*, 502–510.

Knust, S. J., & Quarn, J. M. (1983). Integration of self-care theory with rehabilitation nursing. *Rehabilitation Nursing, 8*(4), 26–28.

Kubricht, D. W. (1984). Therapeutic self-care demands expressed by outpatients receiving external radiation therapy. *Cancer Nursing, 7*, 43–52.

Laurie-Shaw, B., & Ives, S. M. (1988a). Implementing Orem's self-care deficit theory . . . part I. *Canadian Journal of Nursing Administration, 1*(1), 9–12.

Laurie-Shaw, B., & Ives, S. M. (1988b). Implementing Orem's self-care deficit theory . . . part 2. *Canadian Journal of Nursing Administration, 1*(2), 16–19.

Lawrence, D., & Schank, M. (1995). Health care diaries of young women. *Journal of Community Health Nursing, 12*(3), 171–182.

Lee, M. B. (1999). Power, self-care and health in women living in urban squatter settlements in Karachi, Pakistan: A test of Orem's theory. *Journal of Advanced Nursing, 30*(1), 248–259.

Logue, G. A. (1997). An application of Orem's Theory to the nursing management of pertussis. *Journal of School Nursing, 13*(4), 20–25.

Lorensen, M., Holter, I. M., Evers, G. C. M., Isenberg, M. A., & Van Achterberg, T. (1993). Cross-cultural testing of the "Appraisal of Self-care Agency: ASA scale" in Norway. *International Journal of Nursing Studies, 30*(1), 15–23.

Mack, C. J. (1992). Assessment of the autologous bone marrow transplant patient according to Orem's self-care model. *Cancer Nursing, 15*, 429–436.

Magnan, M. A. (2004). The effectiveness of fatigue-related self-care methods and strategies used by radiation oncology patients. *Self-Care, Dependent-Care and Nursing, 12*(3), 12–21.

Manzini, F. C., & Simonetti, J. P. (2009). Nursing consultation applied to hypertensive clients: Application of Orem's self-care theory. *Revista Latino-Americana de Enfermagem, 17*(1), 113–119.

Mapanga, K., & Andrews, C. (1995). The influence of family and friends' basic conditioning factors and self-care agency on unmarried teenage primiparas' engagement in contraceptive practice. *Journal of Community Health Nursing, 12*(2), 89–100.

Marz, M. S. (1988). Effect of differentiated practice, conditioning factors and nursing agency on performance and strain of nurses in hospital settings. *Dissertation Abstracts International, 50*(05B),

1856. Abstract retrieved December 26, 2007, from Dissertation Abstracts Online database.

McDermott, M. A. N. (1993). Learned helplessness as an interacting variable with self-care agency: Testing a theoretical model. *Nursing Science Quarterly, 6*, 28–38.

Moore, J. B. (1993). Predictors of children's self-care performance: Testing the theory of self-care deficit. *Scholarly Inquiry for Nursing Practice: An International Journal, 7*, 199–212.

Moore, J. B., & Gaffney, K. F. (1989). Development of an instrument to measure mother's performance of self-care activities for children. *Advances in Nursing Science, 12*(1), 76–84.

Moore, J. B., & Mosher, R. (1997). Adjustment responses of children and their mothers to cancer: Self-care and anxiety. *Oncology Nursing Forum, 24*, 519–525.

Moser, A., Houtepen, R., & Widdershoven, G. (2007). Patient autonomy in nurse-led shared care: A review of theoretical and empirical literature. *Journal of Advanced Nursing, 57*, 357–365.

Norris, M. K. G. (1991). Applying Orem's theory to the long-term care of adolescent transplant recipients. *American Nephrology Nurses Association Journal, 18*(1), 45–47, 53.

Nursing Development Conference Group. (1973). *Concept formalization in nursing: Process and product*. Boston: Little, Brown.

Nursing Development Conference Group. (1979). *Concept formalization in nursing: Process and product* (2nd ed.). Boston: Little, Brown.

Orem, D. E. (1959). *Guides for developing curricula for the education of practical nurses*. Washington, DC: Government Printing Office.

Orem, D. E. (1971). *Nursing: Concepts of practice*. New York: McGraw-Hill. [out of print]

Orem, D. E. (1980). *Nursing: Concepts of practice* (2nd ed.). New York: McGraw-Hill. [out of print]

Orem, D. E. (1985). *Nursing: Concepts of practice* (3rd ed.). New York: McGraw-Hill. [out of print]

Orem, D. E. (1991). *Nursing: Concepts of practice* (4th ed.). St. Louis: Mosby.

Orem, D. E. (1995). *Nursing: Concepts of practice* (5th ed.). St. Louis: Mosby.

Orem, D. E. (2001). *Nursing: Concepts of practice* (6th ed.). St. Louis: Mosby.

Orem, D. E., & Taylor, S. G. (1986). Orem's General Theory of Nursing. In P. Winstead-Fry (Ed.), *Case studies in nursing theory* (pp. 37–71) (Pub. No. 15-2152). New York: National League for Nursing.

Orem, D. E., & Vardiman, E. M. (1995). Orem's nursing theory and positive mental health: Practical considerations. *Nursing Science Quarterly, 8*, 165–173.

Ramos, I. C., Chagas, N. R., Freitas, M. C., Monteiro, A. R. M., & Leite, A. C. S. (2007). Orem's Theory and the chronic kidney patient [Portuguese]. *Revista Enfermagem, 15*, 444–449. Abstract in English retrieved November 30, 2009, from CINAHL Plus with Full Text database.

Reed, P. G. (1986). Developmental resources and depression in the elderly. *Nursing Research, 35*, 368–374.

Renpenning, K. M., & Taylor, S. G. (Eds.). (2003). *Self-care theory in nursing: Selected papers of Dorothea Orem.* New York: Springer.

Roberson, M. R., & Kelley, J. H. (1996). Using Orem's theory in transcultural settings: A critique. *Nursing Forum, 31*(3), 22–28.

Roy, O., & Collin, F. (1994). The aged patient with dementia. *Canadian Nurse, 90*(1), 39–42.

Sampaio, F. A. A., Aquino, P. S., de Araujo, T. L., & Galvao, M. T. G. (2008). Nursing care to an ostomy patient: Application of the Orem's theory. *Acta Paulista de Enfermagem, 21*(1), 94–100.

Schott-Baer, D., Fisher, L., & Gregory, C. (1995). Dependent care, caregiver burden, hardiness, and self-care agency of caregivers. *Cancer Nursing, 18*, 299–305.

Shaini, G. S., Venkatesan, L., & Ben, A. (2007). Effectiveness of structured teaching on home care management of diabetes mellitus. *Nursing Care of India, 98*(9), 197–199.

Shum, S., McGonigal, R., & Biehler, B. (2005). Development and application of the Community Care Deficit Nursing Model (CCDNM) in two populations. *Self-Care, Dependent-Care and Nursing, 13*(1), 22–25.

Simmons, L. (2009). Dorthea Orem's self care theory as related to nursing practice in hemodialysis. *Nephrology Nursing Journal, 36*, 419–421.

Smith, C. (1996). Care of the older hypothermic patient using a self-care model. *Nursing Times, 92*(3), 29–31.

Soderhamm, O., Evers, G., & Hamrin, E. (1996). A Swedish version of the Appraisal of Self-Care Agency (ASA) Scale. *Scandinavian Journal Caring Science, 10*(1), 3–9.

Spirig, R., & Willhelm, A. B. (1995). Bibliography on the subject of Dorothea Orem's nursing theory [German]. *Pflege, 9*, 213–220. Abstract in English retrieved January 21, 2008, from CINAHL Plus Full Text online.

Taylor, S. G. (2007). The development of Self-care Deficit Nursing Theory: An historical analysis. *Self-Care, Dependent-Care and Nursing, 15*(1), 22–25. Abstract in English retrieved December 26, 2007, from CINAHL Plus Full Text database.

Taylor, S. G., Geden, E., Isaramalai, S., & Wongvatunyu, S. (2000). Orem's Self-Care Deficit Nursing Theory: Its philosophic foundation and the state of the science. *Nursing Science Quarterly, 13*, 104–110.

Taylor, S. G., & McLaughlin, K. (1991). Orem's General Theory of Nursing and community nursing. *Nursing Science Quarterly, 4*, 153–160.

Taylor, S. G., & Renpenning, K. M. (1995). The practice of nursing in multiperson situations, family and community. In D. E. Orem, *Nursing: Concepts of practice* (5th ed., pp. 348–380). St. Louis: Mosby.

Taylor, S. G., & Renpenning, K. M. (2001). The practice of nursing in multiperson situations, family and community. In D. E. Orem, *Nursing: Concepts of practice* (6th ed., pp. 394–433). St. Louis: Mosby.

Timmins, F., & Horan, P. (2007). A critical analysis of the potential contribution of Orem's (2001) Self-Care Deficit Nursing Theory to contemporary coronary care nursing practice. *European Journal of Cardiovascular Nursing, 6*(1), 32–39.

Tokem, Y., Akyol, A. D., & Argon, G. (2007). The relationship between disability and self-care agency of Turkish people with rheumatoid arthritis. *Journal of Clinical Nursing, 16*(3a), 44–50.

Tolentino, M. B. (1990). The use of Orem's self-care model in the neonatal intensive-care unit. *Journal of Obstetric, Gynecologic, and Neonatal Nursing, 19*, 496–500.

Trench, A. S. (Executive producer), Wallace, D. (Producer), & Coberg, T. (Director). (1988). *Dorothea E. Orem—The nurse theorists: Portraits of excellence.* Oakland, CA: Studio Three Production, Samuel Merritt College of Nursing.

Tseng, S. (2007).Nursing a diabetes patient undergoing amputation surgery [Chinese]. *Tzu Chi Nursing Journal, 6*(3), 117–127. Abstract in English retrieved November 30, 2009, from CINAHL Plus with Full Text database.

Ulbrich, S. L. (1999). Nursing practice theory of exercise as self-care. *Image—The Journal of Nursing Scholarship, 31*, 65–70.

Utz, S. W., Shuster, G. F., Merwin, E., & Williams, B. (1994). A community based smoking cessation program: Self-care behaviors and success. *Public Health Nursing, 11*, 291–299.

Van Achterberg, T., Lorensen, M., Isenberg, M. A., Evers, G. C. M., Levine, E., & Phillipsen, H. (1991). The Norwegian, Danish, and Dutch version of the Appraisal of Self-Care Agency scale: Comparing reliability aspects. *Scandinavian Journal of Caring Sciences, 5*(2), 101–108.

Vesely, C. (1995). Pediatric patient-controlled analgesia: Enhancing the self-care construct. *Pediatric Nursing, 21*(2), 124–128.

Villarruel, A. M., & Denyes, M. J. (1991). Pain assessment in children: Theoretical and empirical validity. *Advances in Nursing Science, 14*, 32–41.

Villarruel, A. M., & Denyes, N. J. (1997). Testing Orem's theory with Mexican Americans. *Image—The Journal of Nursing Scholarship, 29*, 283–288.

Wang, C. Y. (1997). The cross cultural applicability of Orem's conceptual framework. *Journal of Cultural Diversity, 4*(2), 44–48.

Weimers, L., Svensson, K., Dumas, L., Navér L., & Wahlberg, V. (2007). Hands-on approach during breastfeeding support in a neonatal intensive care unit: A qualitative study of Swedish mothers' experiences. *Neonatal Intensive Care, 20*(2), 20–27.

Wing, S., & do Horto Fontoura Cartana, M. (2007). Promoting self-care to patients suffering headache through the oriental perspective of health [Portuguese]. *Revista Brasileira de Enfermagem, 60*, 225–226. Abstract in English retrieved December 12, 2007, from CINAHL Plus with Full Text database.

Zadinsky, J., & Boyle, J. (1996). Experiences of women with chronic pelvic pain. *Healthcare of Women International, 17*, 223–232.

Ziegler, S. M., Vaughn-Wrobel, B. C., & Erlen, J. A. (1986). *Nursing process, nursing diagnosis, nursing knowledge—Avenues to autonomy.* Norwalk, CT: Appleton-Century-Crofts.

Zinn, A. (1986). A self-care program for hemodialysis patients based on Dorothea Orem's concepts. *Journal of Nephrology Nursing, 3*, 65–77.

Zrínyi, M., & Zékányné, R. I. (2007). Does self-care agency change between hospital admission and discharge? An Orem-based investigation. *International Nursing Review, 54*, 256–262.

THESES AND DISSERTATIONS
Theses
Barbel, L. L. (1988). Perceived learning needs of cardiac patients. *Masters Abstracts International, 27*(01), 90. Abstract retrieved December 12, 2007, from Dissertation Abstracts Online database.

Buti, R. L. (1998). The effects of meditation on global and factor scores on the BSI: A secondary analysis. *Masters Abstracts International, 36*(04), 1060. Abstract retrieved December 12, 2007, from Dissertation Abstracts Online database.

Cipolla, R. M. (1992). Retrospective record review of lost work days and a cumulative trauma disorders abatement program in a clothing manufacturer: Implications for nursing. *Masters Abstracts International, 31*(01), 268. Abstract retrieved December 12, 2007, from Dissertation Abstracts Online database.

Esterhuysen, A. E. C. (1997). Orem's theory applied in the community health practice [Afrikaans]. *Masters Abstracts International, 36*(03), 781. Abstract in English retrieved December 12, 2007, from Dissertation Abstracts Online database.

Grachek, M. K. (1987). The relationship between loneliness and self-care practices of elderly residents of a senior housing complex. *Masters Abstracts International, 26*(01), 105. Abstract retrieved December 12, 2007, from Dissertation Abstracts Online database.

Harter, J. W. (1988). Self-care action demands identified by female myocardial infarction patients. *Masters Abstracts International, 27*(02), 254. Abstract retrieved December 12, 2007, from Dissertation Abstracts Online database.

Hendershott, S. M. (1994). Attitudes of seniors with diabetes: Reliability and validity of the English version of the semantic differential in diabetes. *Masters Abstracts International, 33*(06), 1838. Abstract retrieved December 12, 2007, from Dissertation Abstracts Online database.

Kozy, M. A. (1993). The relationship of hardiness and self-care agency in persons with HIV infection. *Masters Abstracts International, 32*(03), 939. Abstract retrieved December 12, 2007, from Dissertation Abstracts Online database.

Ludlow, M. D. (1997). The relationship between basic conditioning factors and the self-care practice of meditation in HIV-seropositive persons. *Masters Abstracts International, 35*(06), 1775. Abstract retrieved December 12, 2007, from Dissertation Abstracts Online database.

Palyo, K. A. (1995). Lived experiences of women with HIV within a self-care framework. *Masters Abstracts International, 33*(06), 1642. Abstract retrieved December 12, 2007, from Dissertation Abstracts Online database.

Price, H. J. (1987). Variables influencing burden in spousal and adult child primary caregivers of persons with Alzheimer's disease in the home setting. *Masters Abstracts International, 27*(01), 90. Abstract retrieved December 12, 2007, from Dissertation Abstracts Online database.

Reynolds, C. S. (1999). Health beliefs and medication compliance with clients at high risk for cardiovascular events. *Masters Abstracts International, 37*(04), 1182. Abstract retrieved December 12, 2007, from Dissertation Abstracts Online database.

Sullivan, C. A. (1994). Description of homeless men's perceptions of relevant life experiences within a self-care framework. *Masters Abstracts International, 32*(04), 1172. Abstract retrieved December 12, 2007, from Dissertation Abstracts Online database.

Thompson, M. E. (1997). Self-care agency in adults with diabetes mellitus. *Masters Abstracts International, 36*(03), 784. Abstract retrieved December 12, 2007, from Dissertation Abstracts Online database.

Ward, S. T. (1990). Physical restraint use on the confused elderly patient in an acute care setting: A retrospective study. *Masters Abstracts International, 29*(04), 653. Abstract retrieved December 12, 2007, from Dissertation Abstracts Online database.

Wiebe, V. M. (1999). Examining self-care among the elderly using Orem's self-care framework. *Masters Abstracts International, 38*(03), 685. Abstract retrieved December 12, 2007, from Dissertation Abstracts Online database.

Dissertations

Baiardi, J. M. (1997). The influence of health status, burden, and degree of cognitive impairment on the self-care agency and dependent-care agency of caregivers of elders. *Dissertation Abstracts International, 58*(11B), 5885. Abstract retrieved December 12, 2007, from Dissertation Abstracts Online database.

Banfield, B. E. (1997). A philosophical inquiry of Orem's Self-Care Deficit Nursing Theory. *Dissertation Abstracts International, 58*(11B), 5885. Abstract retrieved December 12, 2007, from Dissertation Abstracts Online database.

Beauchesne, M. F. (1989). An investigation of the relationship between social support and the self care agency of mothers of developmentally disabled children. *Dissertation Abstracts International, 50*(01B), 121. Abstract retrieved December 12, 2007, from Dissertation Abstracts Online database.

Carroll, D. L. (1993). Recovery in the elderly after coronary bypass surgery. *Dissertation Abstracts International, 54*(06B), 2992. Abstract retrieved December 12, 2007, from Dissertation Abstracts Online database.

Denyes, M. J. (1980). Development of an instrument to measure self-care agency in adolescents. *Dissertation Abstracts International, 41*(05B), 1716. Abstract retrieved December 12, 2007, from Dissertation Abstracts Online database.

Dodd, M. J. (1980). Enhancing self-care behaviors through informational interventions in patients with cancer who are receiving chemotherapy. *Dissertation Abstracts International, 42*(02B), 565. Abstract retrieved December 12, 2007, from Dissertation Abstracts Online database.

Eith, C. A. (1983). The nursing assessment of readiness for instruction of breast self-examination instrument (NARIB): Instrument development. *Dissertation Abstracts International, 44*(06B), 1780. Abstract retrieved December 12, 2007, from Dissertation Abstracts Online database.

Emerson, E. A. (1992). Playing for health: The process of play and self-expression in children who have experienced a sexual trauma. *Dissertation Abstracts International, 53*(06B), 2784. Abstract retrieved December 12, 2007, from Dissertation Abstracts Online database.

Fernsler, J. R. (1983). A comparison of patient and nurse perceptions of patients' self-care deficits associated with cancer chemotherapy. *Dissertation Abstracts International, 45*(03B), 827. Abstract retrieved December 12, 2007, from Dissertation Abstracts Online database.

Ford, D. C. (1987). Complications and referrals of patients with protein-calorie malnutrition. *Dissertation Abstracts International, 49*(04B), 1089. Abstract retrieved December 12, 2007, from Dissertation Abstracts Online database.

Fuller, F. J. (1992). Health of elderly male dependent-care agents for a spouse with Alzheimer's disease. *Dissertation Abstracts International, 53*(09B), 4589. Abstract retrieved December 12,

2007, from Dissertation Abstracts Online database.

Gallegos, E. C. (1997). The effect of social, family and individual conditioning factors on self-care agency and self-care of adult Mexican women. *Dissertation Abstracts International, 55*(11B), 5889. Abstract retrieved December 12, 2007, from Dissertation Abstracts Online database.

Garde, P. P. (1987). Orem's "Self-Care Model" of nursing practice: Implications for program development in continuing education in nursing. *Dissertation Abstracts International, 48*(02A), 284. Abstract retrieved December 12, 2007, from Dissertation Abstracts Online database.

Hehn, D. M. (1985). Hospice care: Critical role behaviors related to self-care and role supplementation. *Dissertation Abstracts International, 46*(08B), 2623. Abstract retrieved December 12, 2007, from Dissertation Abstracts Online database.

Hines, S. J. H. (2006). An exploratory study of the relationship between body experience and self-care agency to manage urinary incontinence. *Dissertation Abstracts International, 67*(07B), 3701. Abstract retrieved December 12, 2007, from Dissertation Abstracts Online database.

Horsburgh, M. E. (1994). The contribution of personality to adult well-being: A test and explication of Orem's theory of self-care. *Dissertation Abstracts International, 56*(03B), 1346. Abstract retrieved December 12, 2007, from Dissertation Abstracts Online database.

Hurst, J. D. (1991). The relationship among self-care agency, risk-taking, and health risks in adolescents. *Dissertation Abstracts International, 52*(03B), 1352. Abstract retrieved December 12, 2007, from Dissertation Abstracts Online database.

Jesek-Hale, S. R. (1994). Self-care agency and self-care in pregnant adolescents: A test of Orem's theory. *Dissertation Abstracts International, 56*(01B), 173. Abstract retrieved December 12, 2007, from Dissertation Abstracts Online database.

Kain, C. D. (1985). Dorothea E. Orem's self-care model of nursing: Implications for program development in associate degree nursing education. *Dissertation Abstracts International, 47*(03B), 994. Abstract retrieved December 12, 2007, from Dissertation Abstracts Online database.

Keatley, V. M. (1998). Critical incident stress in generic baccalaureate nursing students. *Dissertation Abstracts International, 59*(05B), 969.

Abstract retrieved December 12, 2007, from Dissertation Abstracts Online database.

Kennedy, L. M. (1990). The effectiveness of a self-care medication education protocol on the home medication behaviors of recently hospitalized elderly. *Dissertation Abstracts International, 51*(08B), 3779. Abstract retrieved December 12, 2007, from Dissertation Abstracts Online database.

Kleinbeck, S. V. M. (1995). Postdischarge surgical recovery of adult laparoscopic outpatients. *Dissertation Abstracts International, 57*(02B), 989. Abstract retrieved December 12, 2007, from Dissertation Abstracts Online database.

Klymko, K. L. (2006). African American hypertensives: Cognition and self care. *Dissertation Abstracts International, 67*(05B), 2474. Abstract retrieved December 12, 2007, from Dissertation Abstracts Online database.

Koster, M. K. (1995). A comparison of the relationship among self-care agency, self-determinism, and absenteeism in two groups of school-age children. *Dissertation Abstracts International, 56*(10B), 5418. Abstract retrieved December 12, 2007, from Dissertation Abstracts Online database.

McDermott, M. A. N. (1989). The relationship between learned helplessness and self-care agency in adults as a function of gender and age. *Dissertation Abstracts International, 50*(08B), 3403. Abstract retrieved December 12, 2007, from Dissertation Abstracts Online database.

Magnan, M. A. (2001). Self-care and health in persons with cancer-related fatigue: Refinement and evaluation of Orem's self-care framework. *Dissertation Abstracts International, 62*(12B), 5664. Abstract retrieved December 12, 2007, from Dissertation Abstracts Online database.

Marten, M. L. C. (1982). The relationship of level of depression to perceived decision-making capabilities of institutionalized elderly women. *Dissertation Abstracts International, 43*(09B), 2855. Abstract retrieved December 12, 2007, from Dissertation Abstracts Online database.

Metcalfe, S. A. (1996). Self-care actions as a function of therapeutic self-care demand and self-care agency in individuals with chronic obstructive pulmonary disease. *Dissertation Abstracts International, 57*(12B), 7453. Abstract retrieved December 12, 2007, from Dissertation Abstracts Online database.

Monsen, R. B. (1988). Autonomy, coping, and self-care agency in healthy adolescents and in adolescents with spina bifida. *Dissertation Abstracts International, 50*(06B), 2340. Abstract retrieved December 12, 2007, from Dissertation Abstracts Online database.

Neuman, B. M. (1996). Relationships between children's descriptions of pain, self-care and dependent-care, and basic conditioning factors of development, gender, and ethnicity: "Bears in my throat." *Dissertation Abstracts International, 57*(04B), 2482. Abstract retrieved December 12, 2007, from Dissertation Abstracts Online database.

Nicholas, P. K. (1989). Hardiness, self-care practices, and perceived health status in the elderly. *Dissertation Abstracts International, 52*(04B), 1957. Abstract retrieved December 12, 2007, from Dissertation Abstracts Online database.

Nicholson, L. L. (2002). Self-care activities and quality of life in ovarian cancer survivors. *Dissertation Abstracts International, 63*(03B), 1272. Abstract retrieved December 12, 2007, from Dissertation Abstracts Online database.

Olson, G. P. (1985). Perceived opportunity for and preference in decision-making of hospitalized men and women. *Dissertation Abstracts International, 47*(02B), 572. Abstract retrieved December 12, 2007, from Dissertation Abstracts Online database.

Ortiz-Martinez, M. A. (1994). The self-care model for nursing in Puerto Rico: A crosscultural study of the implementation of change [Spanish]. *Dissertation Abstracts International, 56*(07B), 3696. Abstract in English retrieved December 12, 2007, from Dissertation Abstracts Online database.

Renker, P. R. (1997). Physical abuse, social support, self-care agency, self-care practices, and late adolescent pregnancy outcome. *Dissertation Abstracts International, 58*(11B), 5891. Abstract retrieved December 12, 2007, from Dissertation Abstracts Online database.

Robinson, M. K. (1995). Determinants of functional status in chronically ill adults. *Dissertation Abstracts International, 56*(10B), 5424. Abstract retrieved December 12, 2007, from Dissertation Abstracts Online database.

Slusher, I. L. (1994). Self-care agency and self-care practice of adolescent primiparas during the in-hospital postpartum period. *Dissertation Abstracts International, 55*(08B), 3240. Abstract retrieved December 12, 2007, from Dissertation Abstracts Online database.

Sonninen, A. L. (1997). Testing reliability and validity of the Finnish version of the appraisal of self-care agency (ASA) with elderly Finns. *Dissertation Abstracts International, 60*(03C), 604. Abstract retrieved December 12, 2007, from Dissertation Abstracts Online database.

Wells-Biggs, A. J. (1985). Hermeneutic interpretation of the work of Dorothea E. Orem: A nursing metaphor. *Dissertation Abstracts International, 47*(02B), 576. Abstract retrieved December 12, 2007, from Dissertation Abstracts Online database.

White, M. A. M. (2000). Predictors of self-care agency among community-dwelling older adults. *Dissertation Abstracts International, 61*(03B), 1332. Abstract retrieved December 12, 2007, from Dissertation Abstracts Online database.

ANNOTATED BIBLIOGRAPHY

Aish, A. (1996). A comparison of female and male cardiac patients' responses to nursing care promoting nutritional self-care. *Canadian Journal of Cardiovascular Nursing, 7*(3), 4–13.

This study investigated gender-based response to an Orem-based nursing care plan that focused on nutrition. The care was provided to 62 men and 42 women who had suffered myocardial infarctions in the patients' homes within a week of discharge from the hospital. A three-day diet record was obtained seven weeks after discharge. Both men and women in the treatment group had changed their dietary habits by lowering the intake of both total and saturated fat.

Aish, A. E., & Isenberg, M. (1996). Effects of Orem-based nursing intervention on nutritional self-care of myocardial infarction patients. *International Journal of Nursing Studies, 33*, 259–270.

This study investigated the effect of an Orem-based nursing care measure on the nutrition of patients who had experienced myocardial infarction. The major variables of interest were the impact of self-care agency and self-efficacy on healthy eating. The treatment took place during the first six weeks after discharge for 104 patients who were randomly assigned to treatment and control groups. Findings supported that the nursing care influenced self-care agency but did not have an impact on self-efficacy in healthy eating.

Anderson, J. A., & Olnhausen, K. S. (1999). Adolescent self-esteem: A foundational disposition. *Nursing Science Quarterly, 12*, 62–67.

After conducting a concept synthesis and concept derivation, the authors argue that self-esteem is a foundational disposition within the self-care deficit theory. As such, self-esteem is also a component of self-care agency.

Baker, S. (1997). The relationships of self-care agency and self-care actions to caregiver strain as perceived by female family caregivers of elderly parents. *Journal of the New York State Nurses Association, 28*(1), 7–11.

This descriptive correlational study investigated caregiver strain in 131 primary caregivers. Findings included an inverse relationship between self-care agency and caregiver strain; mediation effects of self-care actions on the relationships between household tasks, emotional support, and caregiver strain; that multiple roles increased caregiver strain and that personal care tasks had a moderator effect on self-care actions that decreased caregiver strain. The author suggests that nurses need to educate caregivers of the importance of self-care.

Callaghan, D. (2005). Healthy behaviors, self-efficacy, self-care, and basic conditioning factors in older adults. *Journal of Community Health Nursing, 22*(3), 169–173.

This study, a secondary statistical analysis, focused on selected basic conditioning factors in relation to healthy behaviors, self-efficacy beliefs, and ability for self care. Subjects were 235 older adults. Findings included that the basic conditioning factors of education, income, health insurance, race, support system, routine religious practice, medical problems, marital status, gender, age, and number of children had statistically significant relationships with healthy behaviors, self-efficacy, and self-care.

Chang, E., Hancock, K., Hickman, L., Glasson, J., & Davidson, P. (2007). Outcomes of acutely ill older hospitalized patients following implementation of tailored models of care: A repeated measures (pre- and post-intervention) design. *International Journal of Nursing Studies, 44*, 1079–1092.

The purpose of this study was to evaluate the use of tailored models of care for older patients in an aged care ward and a medical ward in two Sydney, Australia, teaching hospitals. The efficacy of care was evaluated through patient and nurses' satisfaction with the provided care, increase in activities of daily living, reduction of unplanned readmissions, and knowledge of medications. The groups of patients, aged 65 and older and admitted for an acute illness with the exclusion of those with moderate or severe dementia, included 232 admitted before the implementation of the care models and 116 admitted during the implementation. There were 90 nurses in the pre-model group and 22 in the implementation group. The implementation of the ward-specific models resulted in statistically significant increased satisfaction for both patients and nurses, increased participation in activities of daily living, and increased knowledge of medication.

Dennis, C. M. (1997). *Self-care deficit theory of nursing: Concepts and applications.* St. Louis: Mosby.

This text provides a basic introduction to Orem's theory, based on work done by faculty at Illinois Wesleyan University. It seeks to define the concepts and terminology associated with the theory in ways that are useful to beginning students of nursing and aid them in the practical application of the theory.

Taylor, S. G., Geden, E., Isaramalai, S., & Wongvatunyu, S. (2000). Orem's Self-Care Deficit Nursing Theory: Its philosophic foundation and the state of the science. *Nursing Science Quarterly, 13*, 104–110.

Reviews the published research relating to Orem's theory, using the five stages of theory development identified by Orem. Most of the studies reviewed were descriptive research and served to increase the knowledge base about self-care but provided little indication of sustained research programs based on the theory. The authors conclude that "the bricks are piling up around the framework, but only a few scholars are working on building the walls" (p. 108).

CHAPTER 7

Behavioral System Model
Dorothy E. Johnson

Marie L. Lobo

Dorothy Johnson was born in Savannah, Georgia, in 1919, the last of seven children. She earned her bachelor of science in nursing from Vanderbilt University, Nashville, Tennessee, and her master's in public health from Harvard. She began publishing her ideas about nursing soon after graduation from Vanderbilt. Most of her teaching career was in pediatric nursing at the University of California, Los Angeles. She retired as Professor Emeritus, January 1, 1978, and died in Florida in 1999.

Dorothy Johnson has influenced nursing through her publications since the 1950s. Throughout her career, Johnson stressed the importance of research-based knowledge about the effect of nursing care on clients. Johnson was an early proponent of nursing as a science as well as an art. She also believed nursing had a body of knowledge reflecting both the science and the art. From the beginning, Johnson (1959) proposed that the knowledge of the science of nursing necessary for effective nursing care included a synthesis of key concepts drawn from basic and applied sciences.

In 1961, Johnson proposed that nursing care facilitated the client's maintenance of a state of equilibrium. Johnson proposed that clients were "stressed" by a stimulus of either an internal or an external nature. These stressful stimuli created such disturbances, or "tensions," in the patient that a state of disequilibrium occurred. Johnson identified two areas of foci for nursing care that are based on returning the client to a state of equilibrium. First, nursing care should reduce stimuli that are stressors, and, second, "nursing care should provide support of the client's 'natural' defenses and adaptive processes" (p. 66).

In 1992, Johnson articulated that much of her thinking was influenced by Florence Nightingale. Johnson related that she was first exposed to Nightingale in the mid-1940s. While reading Nightingale's (1859/1992) *Notes on Nursing*, she found that Nightingale focused on the "fundamental needs" of people rather than on the disease process. She also noted that Nightingale focused on the relationship of the person to the environment rather than of the disease to the person. In the 1950s and 1960s, as Johnson developed her model, an increasing number of observational studies on child and adult behavior patterns were published. During these same years, general system theory was also discussed frequently. All these experiences influenced Johnson (1992) in the development of her Behavioral System Model.

Johnson first proposed her model of nursing care as the fostering of "the efficient and effective behavioral functioning in the patient to prevent illness" (1968, April, p. 2). The patient is identified as a behavioral system with multiple subsystems. At this point Johnson began to integrate concepts related to systems models into her work. Johnson's (1968) integration of systems concepts into her work was further illustrated by her statement of belief that nursing was "concerned with man as an integrated whole and this is the specific knowledge of order we require" (p. 207). Not only did nurses need to care for the "whole" client, but the generation of nursing knowledge needed to take a course in the direction of concern with the entire needs of the client.

In the mid- to late 1970s several nurses published conceptualizations of nursing based on Johnson's Behavioral System Model. Some of these were revised in the 1980s. Auger (1976), Damus (1980), Grubbs (1980), Holaday (1980), and Skolny and Riehl (1974) are authors who have interpreted Johnson. Roy (1989), Wu (1973), and others were sharing their beliefs about nursing at the same time, and Johnson's influence, as their professor, is clearly reflected in their works. In 1980, Johnson published her conceptualization of the Behavioral System Model for Nursing. This is the first work published by Johnson that explicates her definitions of the Behavioral System Model. The evolution of this complex model is clearly demonstrated in the progression of Johnson's ideas from works published in the 1950s to her latest available work published in 1990.

DEFINITION OF NURSING

Johnson (1980) developed her Behavioral System Model for nursing from a philosophical perspective "supported by a rich, sound, and rapidly expanding body of empirical and theoretical knowledge" (p. 207). From her early beliefs, which focused on the impaired individual, Johnson evolved a much broader definition of nursing. By 1980, she defined nursing as "an external regulatory force which acts to preserve the organization and integration of the patient's behavior at an optimal level under those conditions in which the behavior constitutes a threat to physical or social health, or in which illness is found" (p. 214). Based on this definition, the following four goals of nursing are to assist the patient to become a person:

1. Whose behavior is commensurate with social demands
2. Who is able to modify his behavior in ways that support biologic imperatives
3. Who is able to benefit to the fullest extent during illness from the physician's knowledge and skill
4. Whose behavior does not give evidence of unnecessary trauma as a consequence of illness (p. 207)

ASSUMPTIONS OF THE BEHAVIORAL SYSTEM MODEL

Johnson makes several layers of assumptions in the development of her conceptualization of the Behavioral System Model. Assumptions are made about the system as a whole as well as about the subsystems. Another set of assumptions deals with the knowledge base necessary to practice nursing.

As with Rogers (1970) and Roy (1989), Johnson believes that nurses need to be well grounded in the physical and social sciences. Particular emphasis should be placed on knowledge from both the physical and the social sciences that is found to influence behavior. Thus, Johnson believes it would be of equal importance to have information available about endocrine influences on behavior as well as about psychological influences on behavior.

In developing assumptions about behavioral systems, Johnson was influenced by Buckley, Chin, and Rapport, early leaders in the development of systems concepts. Johnson (1980) cites Chin (1961) as the source for her first assumption about systems. In constructing a behavioral system, the assumption is made that there is "'organization, interaction, interdependency, and integration of the parts and elements' (Chin, 1961) of behavior that go to make up the system" (p. 208). It is the interrelated parts that contribute to the development of the whole.

The second assumption about systems also evolves from the work of Chin. A system "'tends to achieve a balance among the various forces operating within and upon it' (1961), and that man strives continually to maintain a behavioral system balance and steady states by more or less automatic adjustments and adaptations to the 'natural' forces impinging upon him" (Johnson, 1980, p. 208). The individual is continually presented with situations in everyday life that require adaptation and adjustment. These adjustments are so natural that they occur without conscious effort by the individual. Johnson says,

> The third assumption about a behavioral system is that a behavioral system, which both requires and results in some degree of regularity and constancy in behavior, is essential to man; that is to say, it is functionally significant in that it serves a useful purpose both in social life and for the individual. (p. 208)

The patterns of behavior characteristic of the individual have a purpose in the maintenance of homeostasis by the individual. The development of behavioral patterns that are acceptable to both society and the individual foster the individual's ability to adapt to minor changes in the environment.

The final assumption about the behavioral system is that the "system balance reflects adjustments and adaptations that are successful in some way and to some degree" (Johnson, 1980, p. 208). Johnson acknowledges that the achievement of this balance may and will vary from individual to individual. At times this balance may *not* be exhibited as behaviors that are acceptable or meet society's norms. What may be adaptive for the individual in coping with impinging forces may be disruptive to society as a whole. Most individuals are flexible enough, however, to be in some state of balance that is "functionally efficient and effective" for them (p. 209).

The integration of these assumptions by the individual provides the behavioral system with the patterns of action to form "an organized and integrated functional unit that determines and limits the interaction between the person and his environment and establishes the relationship of the person to the objects, events, and situations in his environment" (Johnson, 1980, p. 209). The function of the behavioral system, then, is to regulate the individual's response to input from the environment so that the balance of the system can be maintained.

Four assumptions are made about the structure and function of each subsystem. These four assumptions are the "structural elements" common to each of the seven subsystems. The first assumption is "from the form the behavior takes and the conse-quences it achieves can be inferred what *drive* has been stimulated or what *goal* is being sought" (Johnson, 1980, p. 210). The ultimate goal for each subsystem is expected to be the same for all individuals. However, the methods of achieving the goal may vary depending on culture or other individual variations.

The second assumption is that each individual has a "predisposition to act, with ref-erence to the goal, in certain ways rather than in other ways" (Johnson, 1980, pp. 210–211). This predisposition to act is labeled "set" by Johnson. The concept of "set" implies that despite having only a few alternatives from which to select a behavioral response, the individual will rank those options and choose the option considered most desirable.

The third assumption is that each subsystem has available a repertoire of choices or "scope of action" alternatives from which choices can be made. Johnson (1980) subsumes under this assumption that larger behavioral repertoires are available to more adaptable individuals. As life experiences occur, individuals add to the number of alternative actions available to them. At some point, however, the acquisition of new alternatives of behavior decreases as the individual becomes comfortable with the available repertoire. The point at which the individual loses the desire or ability to acquire new options is not identified by Johnson.

The fourth assumption about the behavioral subsystems is that they produce ob-servable outcomes—that is, the individual's behavior (Johnson, 1980). The observable behaviors allow an outsider—in this case the nurse—to note the actions the individual is taking to reach a goal related to a specified subsystem. The nurse can then evaluate the effectiveness and efficiency of these behaviors in assisting the individual in reaching one of these goals.

In addition, each of the subsystems has three functional requirements. First, each subsystem must be "*protected* from noxious influences with which the system cannot cope" (Johnson, 1980, p. 212). Second, each subsystem must be "*nurtured* through the input of appropriate supplies from the environment" (p. 212). Finally, each subsystem must be "*stimulated* for use to enhance growth and prevent stagnation" (p. 212). As long as the subsystems are meeting these functional requirements, the system and the sub-systems are viewed as self-maintaining and self-perpetuating. The internal and external environments of the system need to remain orderly and predictable for the system to maintain homeostasis or remain in balance. The interrelationships of the structural ele-ments of the subsystem are critical for each subsystem to function at a maximum state. The interaction of the structural elements allows the subsystem to maintain a balance that is adaptive to that individual's needs.

An imbalance in a behavioral subsystem produces tension, which results in disequilibrium. The presence of tension resulting in an unbalanced behavioral system requires the system to increase energy use to return the system to a state of balance (Johnson, 1968, April). Nursing is viewed as a part of the external environment that can assist the client to return to a state of equilibrium or balance.

Johnson's Behavioral System Model

Johnson (1980) believes each individual has patterned, purposeful, repetitive ways of acting that comprise a behavioral system specific to that individual. These actions or be-haviors form an "organized and integrated functional unit that determines and limits the interaction between the person and his environment and establishes the relationship of the person to the objects, events, and situations in his environment" (p. 209). These behaviors are "orderly, purposeful and predictable . . . [and] sufficiently stable and recurrent to be amenable to description and explanation" (p. 209). Johnson identifies seven subsystems within the Behavioral System Model, an identification that is at variance with others who have published interpretations of Johnson's model. Johnson (1990) states that the seven subsystems identified in her 1980 publication are the only ones to which she subscribes, and she recognizes they are at variance with Grubbs. These seven subsystems were originally identified in Johnson's 1968 paper presented at Vanderbilt University. The seven subsystems are considered to be interrelated, and changes in one subsystem affect all the subsystems.

Johnson has never produced a schematic representation of her system. Conner, Harbour, Magers, and Watt (1994); Loveland-Cherry and Wilkerson (1989); and Torres (1986) have produced similar schematic representations of Johnson's model (see Figure 7-1).

Johnson's Seven Behavioral Subsystems

The *attachment* or *affiliative* subsystem is identified as the first response system to develop in the individual. The optimal functioning of the affiliative subsystem allows "social inclusion, intimacy, and the formation and maintenance of a strong social bond" (Johnson, 1980, p. 212). Attachment to a significant caregiver has been found to be critical for the survival of an infant. As the individual matures, the attachment to the caretaker continues and there are additional attachments to other significant individuals as they enter both the child's and the adult's network. These "significant others" provide the individual with a sense of security.

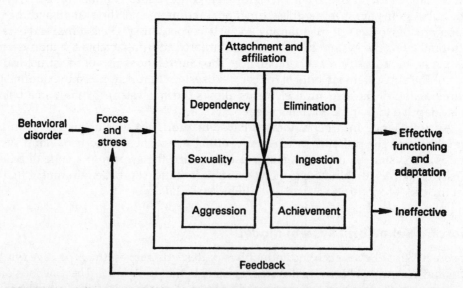

FIGURE 7-1   Johnson's model. (*From Torres, G. (1986). Theoretical foundations of nursing. Norwalk, CT: Appleton-Century-Crofts, p. 121. Used with permission.*)

The second subsystem identified by Johnson is the *dependency* subsystem. Johnson (1980) distinguishes the dependency subsystem from the attachment or affiliative subsystem. Dependency behaviors are "succoring" behaviors that precipitate nurturing behaviors from other individuals in the environment. The result of dependency behavior is "approval, attention or recognition, and physical assistance" (p. 213). It is difficult to separate the dependency subsystem from the affiliative or attachment subsystem because without someone invested in or attached to the individual to respond to that individual's dependency behaviors, the dependency subsystem has no animate environment in which to function.

The *ingestive* subsystem relates to the behaviors surrounding the intake of food. It is related to the biological system. However, the emphasis for nursing, from Johnson's (1980) perspective, is the meanings and structures of the social events surrounding the occasions when food is eaten. Behaviors related to the ingestion of food may relate more to what is socially acceptable in a given culture than to the biological needs of the individual.

The *eliminative* subsystem relates to behaviors surrounding the excretion of waste products from the body. Johnson (1980) admits this may be difficult to separate from a biological system perspective. However, as with behaviors surrounding the ingestion of food, there are socially acceptable behaviors for the time and place for humans to excrete waste. Human cultures have defined different socially acceptable behaviors for excretion of waste, but the existence of such a pattern remains from culture to culture. Individuals who have gained physical control over the eliminative subsystem control this subsystem rather than behave in a socially unacceptable manner. For example, biological cues are often ignored if the social situation dictates that it is objectionable to eliminate wastes at a given time.

The *sexual* subsystem reflects behaviors related to procreation (Johnson, 1980). Both biological and social factors affect behaviors in the sexual subsystem. Again, the behaviors are related to culture and vary from culture to culture. Behaviors also vary according to the gender of the individual. The key is that the goal in all societies has the same outcome—behaviors acceptable to society at large.

The *aggressive* subsystem relates to behaviors concerned with protection and self-preservation. Johnson (1980) views the aggressive subsystem as one that generates defensive responses from the individual when life or territory is threatened. The aggressive subsystem does not include those behaviors with a primary purpose of injuring other individuals but rather those whose purpose is to protect and preserve self and society.

Finally, the *achievement* subsystem provokes behaviors that attempt to control the environment. Intellectual, physical, creative, mechanical, and social skills are some of the areas that Johnson (1980) recognizes. Other areas of personal accomplishment or success may also be included in this subsystem.

JOHNSON'S BEHAVIORAL SYSTEM MODEL AND NURSING'S METAPARADIGM

Johnson views *human beings* as having two major systems: the biological system and the behavioral system. It is the role of medicine to focus on the biological system, whereas nursing's focus is the behavioral system. There is recognition of the reciprocal actions that occur between the biological and behavioral systems when some type of dysfunction occurs in one or the other of the systems.

Society relates to the environment in which an individual exists. According to Johnson, an individual's behavior is influenced by all the events in the environment.

Cultural influences on the individual's behavior are viewed as profound. However, it is felt that there are many paths, varying from culture to culture, that influence specific behaviors in a group of people, although the outcome for all the groups or individuals is the same.

Health is an elusive state that is determined by psychological, social, biological, and physiological factors (Johnson, 1978). Johnson's behavioral model supports the idea that the individual is attempting to maintain some balance or equilibrium. The individual's goal is to maintain the entire behavioral system efficiently and effectively but with enough flexibility to return to an acceptable balance if a malfunction disrupts the original balance.

Nursing's primary goal is to foster equilibrium within the individual, which allows for the practice of nursing with individuals at any point in the health–illness continuum. Nursing implementations may focus on alterations of a behavior that is not supportive to maintaining equilibrium for the individual. In earlier works, Johnson focused nursing on impaired individuals. By 1980, she stated that nursing is concerned with the organized and integrated whole but that the major focus is on maintaining a balance in the behavioral system when illness occurs in the individual.

JOHNSON'S BEHAVIORAL SYSTEM AND THE NURSING PROCESS

Johnson's Behavioral System Model easily fits the nursing process model. Grubbs (1980) developed an assessment tool based on Johnson's seven subsystems, plus a subsystem she labeled "restorative," which focused on activities of daily living. Activities of daily living are considered to include such areas as patterns of rest, hygiene, and recreation. A diagnosis can be made related to insufficiencies or discrepancies within a subsystem or between subsystems. Planning for the implementation of nursing care should start at the subsystem level, with the ultimate goal of effective behavioral functioning of the entire system. Implementations by the nurse present to the client an external force for the manipulation of the subsystem back to the state of equilibrium. Evaluation of the result of this implementation is readily possible if the state of balance that is the goal has been defined during the planning phase before the implementation.

Assessment

In the assessment phase of the nursing process, questions related to specific subsystems are developed. Holaday (1980), Damus (1980), and Small (1980) propose that the assessment focus on the subsystem related to the presenting health problem. An assessment based on the behavioral subsystems does not easily permit the nurse to gather detailed information about the biological system. Assessment questions related to the affiliative subsystem might focus on the presence of a significant other or on the social system of which the individual is a member. In the assessment of the dependency subsystem, attention is placed on understanding how the individual makes needs known to significant others so that the significant others in the environment can assist the individual in meeting those needs. Assessment of the ingestive subsystem examines patterns of food and fluid intake, including the social environment in which the food and fluid are ingested. The eliminative subsystem generates questions related to patterns of defecation and urination and the social context in which the patterns occur. The sexual subsystem assessment includes information about sexual patterns and behaviors. The aggressive subsystem generates questions about how individuals protect themselves from perceived threats to safety. Finally, the achievement subsystem allows for assessment of how the individual changes the environment to facilitate the accomplishment of goals.

There are many gaps in information about the whole individual if only Johnson's Behavioral System Model is used to guide the assessment. There are few physiological data on the individual's present or past health status. The exception might be when an impaired health state is demonstrated in the ingestive or eliminative subsystems. Family interaction and patterns are touched on only in the affiliative and dependency subsystems. Basic information relating to education, socioeconomic status, and type of dwelling is tangentially related to most of the subsystems. However, these factors are not clearly identified as an important aspect of any of the subsystems.

Diagnosis

Diagnosis using Johnson's Behavioral System Model becomes cumbersome. Diagnosis tends to be general to a subsystem rather than specific to a problem. Grubbs (1980) has proposed four categories of nursing diagnoses derived from Johnson's Behavioral System Model, as follows:

1. *Insufficiency*   a state which exists when a particular subsystem is not functioning or developed to its fullest capacity due to inadequacy of functional requirements, . . .
2. *Discrepancy*   a behavior that does not meet the intended goal. The incongruity usually lies between the action and the goal of the subsystem, although the set and choice may be strongly influencing the ineffective action, . . .
3. *Incompatibility*   the goals or behaviors of two subsystems in the same situation conflict with each other to the detriment of the individual, . . .
4. *Dominance*   the behavior in one subsystem is used more than any other subsystem regardless of the situation or to the detriment of the other subsystems. (pp. 240–241)

Since Johnson never wrote about the use of nursing diagnosis with her model, it is difficult to know to what degree these diagnostic classifications are Johnson's or if they are an extension of Johnson's work by Grubbs.

Planning and Implementation

Planning for implementation of the nursing care related to the diagnosis may be difficult because of the lack of client input into the plan. The plan focuses on the nurse's action to modify client behavior. These plans, then, have a goal: to bring about homeostasis in a subsystem that is based on the nurse's assessment of the individual's drive, set, behavioral repertoire, and observable behavior. The plan may include protection, nurturance, or stimulation of the identified subsystem.

Planning and implementation for clients that are based on Johnson's Behavioral System Model focus on maintaining or returning an individual's subsystem to a state of equilibrium. Implementation focuses on achieving the goals of nursing as identified by Johnson (1980). Although Johnson refers to the biological system in her goals of nursing, it is not included in her Behavioral System Model and can and does produce incongruities for the planning and implementation of nursing care in relation to a specific diagnosis.

Evaluation

Evaluation is based on the attainment of a goal of balance in the identified subsystem(s). If baseline data are available for the individual, the nurse may have a goal for the individual to return to the baseline behavior. If the alterations in behavior that are planned do occur, the nurse should be able to observe the return to previous behavior patterns.

There is little or no recognition by either Johnson (1980) or Grubbs (1980) of the client's input into plans for nursing implementation. They use the term *nursing intervention*. Holaday's (1980) example of implementation also does not contain strong client input. Using Johnson's Behavioral System Model with the nursing process is a nurse-centered activity, with the nurse determining the client's needs and the state of behavior appropriate to those needs.

Holaday (1980) demonstrates the flexibility available in the use of the Johnson Behavioral System Model with the nursing process by using a very specific assessment tool to determine appropriate interventions. Holaday uses tests of cognitive development developed by Piaget to determine the level of information to present to a child during a preoperative teaching session.

SITUATION   An example of the use of the nursing process with Johnson's Behavioral System Model is demonstrated with Johnny Smith, age six weeks, brought into the clinic for a routine checkup. He presents with no weight gain since his checkup at age two weeks. His mother states that she feeds him but that he does not seem to eat much. He sleeps four to five hours between feedings. His mother holds him in her arms without making trunk-to-trunk contact. As the assessment is made, the nurse notes that Mrs. Smith never looks at Johnny and never speaks to him. She states that he was a planned baby but that she never "realized how much work an infant could be." She says her mother has told her she is not a good mother because Johnny is not gaining weight as he should. She states that she has not called the nurse when she knew Johnny was not gaining weight because she thought the nurse would think she is a "bad mother" just as her own mother thinks she is a "bad mother."

Based on the information available and using the Johnson Behavioral System Model, assessment focuses on the affiliative and dependency subsystems between mother and Johnny. Further assessment of Mrs. Smith's relationship with her own mother needs to be done. The critical need is for Johnny to begin gaining weight. The secondary need is for Mrs. Smith to resolve her conflict with her own mother. The assessment of the affiliative subsystem focuses on the specific behaviors manifested by Johnny to indicate attachment to his mother. The assessment of the dependency subsystem focuses on the specific behaviors manifested by Johnny to cue his mother to his needs. Because of the nature of his problem, a decision is made to use a tool that specifically focuses on parent–infant interaction during a feeding situation. Thus, the Nursing Child Assessment Feeding Scale (Barnard, 1978) is used during a feeding that takes place at a normal feeding time for Johnny. Johnny cries at the beginning of the feeding and turns toward his mother's hand when she touches his cheek. Mrs. Smith does not speak to Johnny or in any verbal way acknowledge his hunger. When Johnny slightly chokes on some formula, she does not remove the bottle from his mouth. Mrs. Smith does not describe any of the environment to Johnny, nor does she stroke his body or make eye contact with him. Johnny does not reach out to touch his mother, nor does he make any vocalizations. The assessment scale indicates that both mother and baby are not cuing each other at a level at which they can respond appropriately.

The diagnoses based on this assessment, using Johnson's Behavioral System Model, are "insufficient development of the affiliative subsystem" and "insufficient development of the dependency subsystem." Based on these diagnoses, nursing implementation focuses on increasing Mrs. Smith's awareness of the meaning of Johnny's infrequent cues. By increasing her awareness of the meaning of his cues, she can begin to reinforce them so that he begins to know there is someone in the environment who cares about him, thus fostering his attachment to her. Further assistance needs to be given in helping Mrs. Smith in communicating with her infant. If further assessment indicates Mrs. Smith is uncomfortable talking with an infant who does not respond with words, it may be suggested that she read to Johnny from a book, thus providing him with needed verbal stimulation. Another implementation may include the nurse placing herself in Johnny's role and "talking" for him to his mother. The nurse may sit, watching Mrs. Smith hold Johnny, and say such things as "I like it when you pat me," "It feels good when you cuddle me," or "When I turn my head like this, I'm hungry."

Evaluation of these implementations are based on two criteria. First, Johnny's weight gains or losses are carefully assessed. Not gaining weight places him in a life-threatening situation; therefore, it is critical that a pattern of weight gain be initiated. Second, the mother–infant interaction can be reassessed, again using the Nursing Child Assessment Feeding Scale (Barnard, 1978), which allows for comparison of the first observation with a series of subsequent observations.

JOHNSON'S WORK AND THE CHARACTERISTICS OF A THEORY

Johnson states that she is presenting a model related to subsystems of the human being that have observable behaviors leading to specific outcomes, although the method of attaining the specific outcomes may vary according to the culture of the individual. Using the characteristics of a theory discussed in Chapter 1 as a guide, it is clear that Johnson has indeed developed a model. Johnson's Behavioral System Model is based on general system concepts. However, the definitions related to the terms used to label her concepts have not been made explicit by Johnson. Grubbs (1980) presented her definitions of Johnson's terms, and those are the definitions most often reflected in the literature of other investigators claiming to use Johnson's model.

1. *What is the historical context of the theory?*   Johnson developed her model in the 1950s while teaching at the University of California, Los Angeles (UCLA). At that time increasing numbers of observational studies on child and adult behavior patterns were being published, and general system theory was generating much discussion. All of these experiences influenced Johnson in the development of her Behavioral System Model. In the 1960s and 1970s Johnson taught many of the nursing leaders of today in her nursing theory classes at UCLA. In 1974 she spoke to the need for theory development in nursing.
2. *What are the basic concepts and relationships presented by the theory?*   The basic concepts are the seven behavioral subsystems of affiliative, dependency, ingestive, eliminative, sexual, aggressive, and achievement; the four structural characteristics of drive, set, choices, and observable behaviors; and the three

functional requirements of protection, nurturance, and stimulation as well as tensions and balance. Johnson does not clearly interrelate her concepts of subsystems that make up the Behavioral System Model. The lack of clear interrelationships among the concepts creates difficulty in following the logic of Johnson's work. The definitions of the concepts are so abstract that they are difficult to use. For example, intimacy is identified as an aspect of the affiliative subsystem, but the concept is not defined or described. An advantage of the abstract definition is that individuals using the model may identify an assessment tool that most specifically fits a problem and use it in their work. There are two major disadvantages. First, the abstract level and multiplicity of definitions make it difficult to compare the same subsystem across studies. Second, the lack of clear definitions for the interrelationships among and between the subsystems makes it difficult to view the entire behavioral system as an entity.

In general, the Johnson Behavioral System Model does not meet the criteria for a theory. However, it must be stressed that Johnson does not suggest that she developed a theory, although other nurse scholars have identified and used Johnson as a theorist.

3. *What major phenomena of concern to nursing are presented? (These phenomena may include* **but are not limited to** *human beings, environment, health, interpersonal relations, caring, goal attainment, adaptation, and energy fields.)* Johnson's Behavioral System Model provides a framework for organizing human behavior that is different from that provided by other nursing theorists, such as Roy (1989) or Rogers (1970). Johnson believed that she was the first person to view "man as a behavioral system." Others have viewed the behavioral subsystem as just one piece of the biopsychosocial human being. Johnson's framework does contribute to the general body of nursing knowledge but needs further development. Johnson's Behavioral System Model is based on principles of general system theory. Her statements on the multiple modes of attaining the same subsystem goal, regardless of culture, are an example of the principle of "equifinality." As with Rogers, this allows individuals to develop and change through time at unique rates but with the same outcomes at the end of the process: mature, adult behaviors that are culturally acceptable.

Johnson's Behavioral System Model is not as flexible as Rogers's (1970) concept of homeodynamics or Roy's (1989) adaptation model. Rogers's concepts are so broadly applicable that nursing care can take place at any level: individual, family, or community. All systems within the human being can be considered for the focus of nursing implementations. With Roy's model, the focus is still at the individual level, but the total human being can be considered. Roy's assumptions include that the human being is a biopsychosocial being, which allows for all the subsystems of a human being to be included for nursing assessment and implementation.

Johnson's Behavioral System Model is congruent with many of the nursing models in the belief that the individual is influenced by the environment. Since Nightingale (1859/1992) first presented her beliefs about nursing, nurses have been concerned with the individual's relationship with the environment. In practice, nurses often have the necessary control over the environment to promote a healthier state for the individual.

4. *To whom does this theory apply? In what situations? In what way?*   Johnson's behavioral model can be generalized across the life span and across cultures. However, the focus on the behavioral system may make it difficult for nurses working with physically impaired individuals to use the model. Johnson's model is also very oriented to the individual, so that nurses working with groups of individuals with similar problems would have difficulty using the model. The subsystems in Johnson's Behavioral System Model are individually oriented to such an extent that the family can be considered only as the environment in which the individual presents behaviors and not as the focus of care. The model has been used to guide psychiatric nursing practice (Dee, 1990; Dee, van Servellen, & Brecht, 1998; Grice, 1997; Poster, Dee, & Randell, 1997; Puntil, 2005; Talerico, 1999). Derdiarian and Schobel (1990) used the model as a strategy to measure, describe, and classify major changes related to a diagnosis of acquired immune deficiency syndrome. Herbert (1989) used the model to guide the nursing care of a 75-year-old stroke patient. Colling, Owen, McCreedy, and Newman (2003) used the model in investigating the effects of a continence program with frail elderly persons, and Benson (1997) used the model to provide the context for a study of the older adult and fear of crime. Several authors have reported use of the model in caring for persons with cancer (Coward & Wilkie, 2000; Deridiarian, 1988; Martha, Bhaduri, & Jain, 2004; Wilkie, Lovejoy, Dodd, & Tesler, 1988). Ma and Gaudet (1997) discussed its use in caring for persons with end-stage renal disease. D'Huyvetter (2000) presented trauma as a disease within the context of the Behavioral System Model. However, a greater amount of rigorous research is needed to validate the premises or the findings presented in these publications.

Dee (1990) reported on the practical issues that arose in the course of implementing the Johnson Behavioral System Model at a psychiatric institution. They revised the definitions of the subsystems and included a restorative subsystem. Others have used Johnson's model to assist in the understanding of the family member's adjustment to Alzheimer's disease (Freuhwirth, 1989) and extended childhood illnesses (Holaday, Turner-Henson, & Swan, 1996; Lovejoy, 1981; Turner-Henson, 1992). Riegel (1989) used the model to guide the review of literature related to social support of individuals with coronary heart disease. It is unclear whether others have used the information they have shared to further develop their practice.

5. *By what method or methods can this theory be tested?*   It is difficult to test Johnson's model by the development of hypotheses. Subsystems of the model can be examined because relationships within the subsystems can be identified. The lack of definitions and connections between the subsystems creates a barrier for stating relationships in the form of hypotheses to be tested. Although such relationships may be predicted, the lack of definitions in the original work makes it impossible to identify whether it is Johnson's work or someone's interpretation of her work that is being tested.

However, several dissertations have been conducted using the Behavioral System Model. Lovejoy (1981) constructed and tested the Johnson Model First-Level Family Assessment Tool in an outpatient allergy clinic with asthmatic children and their families. She found the tool to be clinically useful but recommended revision and further testing. Reigel (1991) investigated the role of inappropriate social support in cardiac invalidism and found a significant negative relationship between social support and interpersonal dependency at one month following a first acute myocardial infarction. Turner-Henson (1992) found that the interaction of environmental variables was predictive of the mothers' perception of the environment as resourceful, safe, and accessible but was not predictive of their perception of the environment as supportive. Turner-Henson indicated that the Behavioral System Model provided a framework helpful to nurses in identifying mothers' needs upon which nursing care could be based. Grice (1997) used the Behavioral System Model with attribution theory to study the causes identified by nurses for giving psychiatric patients medication for agitation. Results indicate that the patients' behavior was unstable at the time of the administration of the medication, but no specific subsystem is discussed. Talerico (1999) investigated the role of various resources and control-based care in aggressive behavioral actions in older residents with dementia in nursing homes and found that control-based care not only does not work well but may actually cause aggressive behavioral actions.

None of the reported research using the Behavioral System Model has been experimental. A variety of methods have been used: descriptive (Coward & Wilkie, 2000; Turner-Henson, 1992), quasi-experimental (Colling et al. 2003; Derdiarian, 1990a), secondary analysis (Turner-Henson, 1992), correlational methods (Grice, 1997; Wilkie et al., 1988), instrument development (Derdiarian, 1988, 1991; Holaday, 1988; Lovejoy, 1981), and exploratory methodology (Derdiarian, 1990b).

6. *Does this theory direct nursing actions that lead to favorable outcomes?* Johnson does not clearly define the expected outcomes when one of the subsystems is being affected by nursing implementation. An implicit expectation is made that all humans in all cultures will attain the same outcome—homeostasis. Because of the lack of definitions, the model does not allow for control of the areas of interest, so it is difficult to use the model to guide practice. The authors reportedly using the model to guide practice have not integrated the subsystems to the degree necessary to label this model a theory. In fact, Reynolds and Cormack (1991) reported that there was an inability to prescribe specific nursing interventions using this model. In contrast, Dee (1990) reported that using the Johnson model provided "a comprehensive and systematic method of assessing patient behavior" (p. 38). Dee found that the Johnson model could be used to "explain, predict, and control clinical phenomena for the purpose of achieving desired patient outcomes" (p. 41). The implementation of the Johnson model to guide practice in one specific institution is unusual in that few clinical institutions select just one theory or model to guide the practice in their institution.

7. *How contagious is this theory?* Johnson's Behavioral System Model has a limited following when compared to Callista Roy and Martha Rogers. There is a limited body of literature on the use of the Behavioral System Model in clinical practice or to provide the framework for nursing research. Its use in a variety of clinical areas has been discussed. There is some evidence of use internationally in India (Dhasaradhan, 2001; Martha et al., 2004), Canada (Ma & Gaudet, 1997), Australia (Orb & Reilly, 1991), and Slovenia (Urh, 1998).

Summary

Although Johnson's Behavioral System Model has many limitations, she does provide a frame of reference for nurses concerned with specific client behaviors. It must also be noted that Johnson, through her work at UCLA, has had a profound influence on the development of nursing models and nursing theories. Through her position as a faculty member she influenced Roy, Grubbs, Holaday, and others. As a peer, she influenced Riehl, Neuman, Wu, and others, scholars who have generated many ideas about nursing concepts and theories.

Johnson's Behavioral System Model is a model of nursing care that advocates the fostering of efficient and effective behavioral functioning in the patient to prevent illness. The patient is identified as a behavioral system composed of seven behavioral subsystems: affiliative, dependency, ingestive, eliminative, sexual, aggressive, and achievement. Each subsystem is composed of four structural characteristics: drive, set, choices, and observable behaviors. The three functional requirements for each subsystem include protection from noxious influences, provision for a nurturing environment, and stimulation for growth. An imbalance in any of the behavioral subsystems results in disequilibrium. It is nursing's role to assist the client to return to a state of equilibrium.

Thought Questions

1. Develop an analogy or metaphor for Johnson's model.
2. Identify a clinical problem in your practice and analyze it using Johnson's model. If you had applied Johnson's model from the beginning, how might the outcomes have been different?
3. How do you see the physical, social, and psychological systems of your patients affecting each other?
4. How could you integrate Johnson's theory with other nursing theories to create a unique approach to your patient?

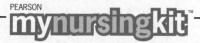

EXPLORE

References

Auger, J. R. (1976). *Behavioral systems and nursing.* Upper Saddle River, NJ: Prentice Hall.

Barnard, K. E. (1978). *Nursing Child Assessment Feeding Scale.* Seattle: University of Washington.

Benson, S. (1997). The older adult and fear of crime. *Journal of Gerontological Nursing, 23*(10), 24–31.

Chin, R. (1961). The utility of system models and developmental models for practitioners. In K. Benne, W. Bennis, & R. Chin (Eds.), *The planning of change.* New York: Holt.

Colling, J., Owen, T. R., McCreedy, M. & Newman, D. (2003). The effects of a continence program on frail community-dwelling elderly persons. *Urologic Nursing, 23*(2), 117–122, 127–131.

Conner, S. S., Harbour, L. S., Magers, J. A., & Watt, J. K. (1994). Dorothy E. Johnson: Behavioral System

Model. In A. Marriner-Tomey (Ed.), *Nursing theorists and their work* (3rd ed., pp. 231–245). St. Louis: Mosby.

Coward, D. D., & Wilkie, D. J. (2000). Metastatic bone pain: Meanings associated with self-report and self-management decision making. *Cancer Nursing, 23*(2), 101–108.

Damus, K. (1980). An application of the Johnson Behavioral System Model for nursing practice. In J. P. Riehl & C. Roy (Eds.), *Conceptual models for nursing practice* (2nd ed., pp. 274–289). New York: Appleton-Century-Crofts.

Dee, V. (1990). Implementation of the Johnson Model: One hospital's experience. In M. E. Parker (Ed.), *Nursing theories in practice* (pp. 33–44) (Pub. No. 15-2350). New York: National League for Nursing.

Dee, V., van Servellen, G., & Brecht, M. (1998). Managed behavioral health care patients and their nursing care problems, level of functioning, and impairment on discharge. *Journal of the American Psychiatric Nurses Association, 4*(2), 57–66.

Derdiarian, A. K. (1988). Sensitivity of the Derdiarian Behavioral System Model instrument to age, site, and stage of cancer: A preliminary validation study. *Scholarly Inquiry for Nursing Practice, 2*(2), 103–121.

Derdiarian, A. K. (1990a). Effects of using systematic assessment instruments on patient and nurse satisfaction with nursing care. *Oncology Nursing Forum, 17*(1), 95–101.

Derdiarian, A. K. (1990b). The relationships among the subsystems of Johnson's Behavioral System Model. *Image: Journal of Nursing Scholarship, 22*, 219–224.

Derdiarian, A. K. (1991). Effects of using a nursing model-based assessment instrument on quality of nursing care. *Nursing Administration Quarterly, 15*(3), 1–16.

Derdiarian, A. K., & Schobel, D. (1990). Comprehensive assessment of AIDS patients using the behavioural systems model for nursing practice instrument. *Journal of Advanced Nursing, 15*, 436–446.

Dhasaradhan, I. (2001). Application of nursing theory into practice. *Nursing Journal of India, 92*(10), 224, 236.

D'Huyvetter, C. (2000). The trauma disease. *Journal of Trauma Nursing, 7*(1), 5–12.

Freuhwirth, S. E. S. (1989). An application of Johnson's Behavioral Model: A case study. *Journal of Community Health Nursing, 6*, 61–71.

Grice, S. L. (1997). Nurses' use of medication for agitation for the psychiatric inpatient (as needed). *Dissertation Abstracts International, 58*(02B), 631.

Grubbs, J. (1980). An interpretation of the Johnson Behavioral System Model for nursing practice. In J. P. Riehl & C. Roy (Eds.), *Conceptual models for nursing practice* (2nd ed., pp. 217–254). New York: Appleton-Century-Crofts.

Herbert, J. (1989). A model for Anna. *Nursing—Oxford, 3*(42), 30–34.

Holaday, B. (1980). Implementing the Johnson Model for Nursing Practice. In J. P. Riehl & C. Roy (Eds.), *Conceptual models for nursing practice* (2nd ed., pp. 255–263). New York: Appleton-Century-Crofts.

Holaday, B. (1988). Response to "Sensitivity of the Derdiarian Behavioral System Model instrument to age, site, and stage of cancer: A preliminary validation study." *Scholarly Inquiry for Nursing Practice, 2*(2), 123–127.

Holaday, B., Turner-Henson, A., & Swan, J. (1996). The Johnson Behavioral System Model: Explaining activities of chronically ill children. In P. H. Walker & B. Neuman (Eds.), *Blueprint for use of nursing models: Education, research, practice, and administration* (pp. 33–63). New York: National League for Nursing.

Johnson, D. E. (1959). The nature of a science of nursing. *Nursing Outlook, 7*, 291–294.

Johnson, D. E. (1961). The significance of nursing care. *American Journal of Nursing, 61*, 63–66.

Johnson, D. E. (1968, April). *One conceptual model of nursing*. Paper presented at Vanderbilt University, Nashville, TN.

Johnson, D. E. (1968). Theory in nursing: Borrowed and unique. *Nursing Research, 17*, 206–209.

Johnson, D. E. (1974). Development of theory: A requisite for nursing as a profession. *Nursing Research, 23*, 372–377.

Johnson, D. E. (1978). State of the art of theory development in nursing. In *Theory development: What, why, how?* (pp. 1–10) (Pub. No. 15-1708). New York: National League for Nursing.

Johnson, D. E. (1980). The Behavioral System Model for Nursing. In J. P. Riehl & C. Roy (Eds.), *Conceptual models for nursing practice* (2nd ed., pp. 207–216). New York: Appleton-Century-Crofts.

Johnson, D. E. (1990). The Behavioral System Model for nursing. In M. E. Parker (Ed.), *Nursing theories in practice* (pp. 23–32) (Pub. No. 15-2350). New York: National League for Nursing.

Johnson, D. E. (1992). The origins of the Behavioral System Model. In F. Nightingale, *Notes on nursing: What it is, and what it is not* (Com. ed.). Philadelphia: Lippincott. (Original work published 1859)

Lovejoy, N. C. (1981). An empirical verification of the Johnson Behavioral System Model for Nursing. *Dissertation Abstracts International, 42*(07B), 2781.

Loveland-Cherry, C., & Wilkerson, S. A. (1989). Dorothy Johnson's Behavioral System Model. In J. Fitzpatrick & A. Whall (Eds.), *Conceptual models of nursing: Analysis and application* (2nd ed., pp. 147–164). Norwalk, CT: Appleton & Lange.

Ma, T., & Gaudet, D. (1997). Assessing the quality of life of our end-stage renal disease client population. *CANNT Journal, 7*(2), 13–16.

Martha, L., Bhaduri, A., & Jain, A. G. (2004). Impact of oral cancer and related factors on the quality of life of patients. *Nursing Journal of India, 95*(6), 129–131.

Nightingale, F. (1992). *Notes on nursing: What it is, and what it is not* (Com. ed.). Philadelphia: Lippincott. (Original work published 1859)

Orb, A., & Reilly, D. E. (1991). Changing to a conceptual base curriculum. *International Nursing Review, 38*(2), 56–60.

Poster, E. C., Dee, V., & Randell, B. P. (1997). The Johnson Behavioral System Model as a framework for patient outcome evaluation. *Journal of the American Psychiatric Nurses Association, 3*, 73–80.

Puntil, C. (2005). New graduate orientation program in a geriatric psychiatric inpatient setting. *Issues in Mental Health Nursing, 26*(1), 65–80.

Reynolds, W., & Cormack, D. F. S. (1991). An evaluation of the Johnson Behavioral System Model for nursing. *Journal of Advanced Nursing, 16*, 1122–1130.

Riegel, B. (1989). Social support and psychological adjustment to chronic coronary heart disease: Operationalization of Johnson's Behavioral System Model. *Advances in Nursing Science, 11*(2), 74–84.

Riegel, B. (1991). Social support and cardiac invalidism following acute myocardial infarction. *Dissertation Abstracts International, 52*(04B), 1959.

Rogers, M. (1970). *The theoretical basis for nursing.* Philadelphia: F. A. Davis.

Roy, C. (1989). The Roy Adaptation Model. In J. Riehl-Sisca (Ed.), *Conceptual models for nursing practice* (3rd ed., pp. 105–114). Norwalk, CT: Appleton & Lange.

Skolny, M. A., & Riehl, J. P. (1974). Hope: Solving patient and family problems by using a theoretical framework. In J. P. Riehl & C. Roy (Eds.), *Conceptual models for nursing practice* (pp. 206–217). New York: Appleton-Century-Crofts.

Small, B. (1980). Nursing visually impaired children with Johnson's Model as a conceptual framework. In J. P. Riehl & C. Roy (Eds.), *Conceptual models for nursing practice* (2nd ed., pp. 264–273). New York: Appleton-Century-Crofts.

Talerico, K. A. (1999). Correlates of aggressive behavioral actions of older adults with dementia. *Dissertation Abstracts International, 60*(12B), 6026.

Torres, G. (1986). *Theoretical foundations of nursing.* Norwalk, CT: Appleton-Century-Crofts.

Turner-Henson, A. (1992). Chronically ill children's mothers' perceptions of environmental variables. *Dissertation Abstracts International, 53*(07B), 3405.

Urh, I. (1998). Dorothy Johnson's theory and nursing care of a pregnant woman [Slovene]. *Obzornik Zdravstvene Nege, 32*(5/6), 199–203.

Wilkie, D., Lovejoy, N., Dodd, M., & Tesler, M. (1988). Cancer pain control behaviors: Description and correlation with pain intensity. *Oncology Nursing Forum, 15*, 723–731.

Wu, R. (1973). *Behavior and illness.* Upper Saddle River, NJ: Prentice Hall.

CHAPTER 8

Nursing Process Discipline
Ida Jean Orlando

Julia B. George

Ida Jean Orlando Pelletier (1926–November 28, 2007) had a varied career as a practitioner, educator, researcher, and consultant in nursing. During the early part of her career, she worked as a staff nurse in such areas as obstetrics, medicine, surgery, and the emergency room. She also held supervisory positions and the title of second assistant director of nurses. She received a diploma in nursing from New York Medical College, Flower Fifth Avenue Hospital School of Nursing in 1947, and a B.S. in public health nursing from St. John's University in Brooklyn, New York, in 1951. In 1954, she received her M.A. in mental health consultation from Teachers College, Columbia University, New York. She then went to Yale University as a research associate and principal investigator on a project studying the integration of mental health concepts into the basic nursing curriculum. This led to the publication of her first book, The Dynamic Nurse–Patient Relationship: Function, Process, and Principles, *in 1961 (reprinted 1990). She also served as director of the graduate program in mental health and psychiatric nursing at Yale.*

In 1962, Orlando married Robert Pelletier and moved to Massachusetts. She became a clinical nursing consultant to a psychiatric hospital, McLean Hospital, in Belmont, Massachusetts, and at a veterans' hospital. At McLean Hospital, she carried out the research that led to the publication in 1972 of her second book, The Discipline and Teaching of Nursing Process.

Orlando was associated intermittently with the Boston University School of Nursing, where she taught nursing theory and supervised graduate students in the clinical area. She served as a project consultant for the New England Board of Higher Education in its Mental Health Project for Associate Degree Faculties. She also served as a nurse educator at Metropolitan State Hospital in Waltham, Massachusetts. In 1992 she retired from active nursing practice and in 2006 was recognized by the Massachusetts Registered Nurse Association as a Nursing Living Legend.

Throughout her career, Orlando was active in a variety of organizations, including the Massachusetts Nurses' Association and the Harvard Community Health Plan. She also lectured and offered workshops and consultation to a wide variety of agencies.

Ida Jean Orlando Pelletier describes a nursing process based on the interaction between a patient and a nurse. Her nursing process discipline was developed through research and presented in two books. Her initial work, *The Dynamic Nurse–Patient Relationship: Function, Process and Principles*, was originally published in 1961 and reprinted in 1990. *The Discipline and Teaching of Nursing Process*, showing further testing and refinement of her work, appeared in 1972.

Orlando's educational background and the work that led to her publications provide insight into the content of her theory. Her advanced nursing preparation and area of teaching responsibility and practice were in mental health and psychiatric nursing. Although she applied her ideas to many nursing specialty areas, the focus of her work is interaction.

The Dynamic Nurse–Patient Relationship was written to report the results of a five-year project at Yale University during the mid-1950s. The purpose of this project, supported by a grant from the National Institute of Mental Health, was "to identify the factors which enhanced or impeded the integration of mental health principles in the basic nursing curriculum" (Orlando, 1961/1990, p. vii). This research resulted in the identification that a nurse's statement of her perception, thought, or feeling about the patient's behavior differentiated between effective and ineffective communication. The book describes the curriculum content developed from the study. Its stated purpose is "to offer the professional nursing student a theory of effective nursing practice" (p. viii). This book was completed in 1958 and was initially rejected for publication as not being marketable in nursing. Finally, in 1961, it was recognized as making an important contribution to the practice of nursing.

Orlando refined her ideas and put them into practice at a private psychiatric facility, McLean Hospital, in Belmont, Massachusetts. Again with a National Institute of Mental Health grant, she studied an objective means to evaluate her process and training in its discipline. The discipline variable was found to make a statistically significant difference in patient outcomes. This work, done during the 1960s, led to *The Discipline and Teaching of Nursing Process* (1972), in which she was concerned with the specific definition of nursing function and with incorporating nursing activities beyond the nurse–patient relationship into a total nursing system. She also developed more readily measured criteria to guide the nurse in her reaction to patient behavior.*

Orlando's work spans a fertile period of nursing thinking. She was influenced by, as well as an influence on, other nursing theorists. For example, Orlando is similar to Nightingale when she states, "It is important for the nurse to concern herself with the patient's distress because the treatment and prevention of disease proceed best when conditions extraneous to the disease itself and its management do not cause the patient additional suffering" (Orlando, 1961/1990, pp. 22–23). Another nursing theorist, Peplau (1952/1988), published her highly interpersonal theory two years before Orlando began her first study. Henderson was refining her definition of nursing during Orlando's first study. Henderson's 1955 definition is consistent with Orlando when she states, "Nursing is primarily assisting the individual . . . in the performance of those activities . . . that he

---

* In this chapter, the feminine pronoun is used when referring to the nurse and the masculine pronoun when referring to the patient. This is consistent with Orlando's use of these pronouns and terms.

would perform unaided if he had the necessary strength, will, or knowledge" (Harmer & Henderson, 1955, p. 4). Ernestine Wiedenbach's interest in the initial study led to an increased concentration of data collection about nursing practice in the maternal/newborn area (Trench, Wallace, & Coberg, 1987).

ORLANDO'S KEY CONCEPTS

Certain major concepts are evident in Orlando's theory of nursing. She believes that nursing is *unique* and *independent* because it concerns itself with an *individual's need for help*, real or potential, in an *immediate* situation. The process by which nursing resolves this helplessness is *interactive* and is pursued in a *disciplined* manner that requires *training*. She believes one's actions should be based on rationale, not protocols.

Throughout her career, Orlando has been concerned with identifying that which is *uniquely* nursing. In her first book, she presents principles related to patient behavior, need for help, nurse reaction, and nursing action to guide nursing practice (Orlando, 1961/1990). She believes that the use of general principles from other fields is not sufficient to help the nurse in her interaction with patients. She identifies nursing's role as follows: "It is the nurse's direct responsibility to see to it that the patient's needs for help are met either by her own activity or by calling in the help of others" (p. 22).

Orlando (1972) also suggests that nursing's failure to establish its uniqueness is a result of the lack of a clearly identifiable function, which leads to inadequate care and insufficient attention to the patient's reactions to his immediate experiences. Thus, she identifies nursing's function as being "concerned with providing direct assistance to individuals in whatever setting they are found for the purpose of avoiding, relieving, diminishing, or curing the individual's sense of helplessness" (p. 12). She also indicates that policies and practices developed for the purposes of institutional bureaucracy or the aims of medicine place nurses in a dependent position (Orlando, 1987).

It is the unique function of nursing and the license held by the individual nurse that gives nurses the authority to work *independently* (Orlando, 1987). Orlando recommends that "nurses . . . must radically shift their focus from assistance to physicians and institutions to assisting patients with what they cannot do alone" (Pelletier, 1967, p. 28). Physicians' orders are directed to patients, not to nurses. Moreover, at times nurses may even assist patients in *not* complying with medical orders when such orders are in conflict with the patient's need for help. Nurses must also resolve conflicts between the patient's need for help and institutional policies. Nursing's unique function allows nurses to work in any setting where persons experience a need for help that they cannot resolve themselves. Thus, nurses may practice with well or ill persons in an independent practice or in an institutional setting.

Orlando's theory focuses on the patient as an *individual*. Each person, in each situation, is different. To be appropriate, nursing actions for two patients with the same presenting behavior, or the same patient at different times, are to be individualized. Nurses cannot automatically act only on the basis of principles, past experience, or physicians' orders. They must first ascertain that their actions will meet the patient's specific need for help.

Nursing is concerned with "individuals who suffer or anticipate a sense of helplessness" (Orlando, 1961/1990, p. 12). Orlando (1972) defines need as "a requirement of the patient which, if supplied, relieves or diminishes his immediate distress or improves his immediate sense of adequacy or well-being" (p. 5). In many instances, people can meet their own needs do so and do not require the help of professional nurses. When they cannot do so or do not clearly understand these needs, a *need for help* is present. The nurse's function is to correctly identify and relieve this need.

The *immediacy* of the nursing situation is a vital concept in Orlando's theory. Each patient's behavior must be assessed to determine whether it expresses a need for help. Furthermore, identical behaviors by the same patient may indicate different needs at different times. The nursing action must also be specifically designed for the immediate encounter. Long-term planning has no part in Orlando's theory except as it pertains to providing adequate staff coverage for a job setting.

Orlando describes a nursing process discipline that is totally *interactive*. It describes, step-by-step, what goes on between a nurse and a patient in a specific encounter. A patient behavior causes the process discipline to begin. The process discipline involves the nurse's reaction to this behavior and the nurse's consequent action. The nurse shares her reaction with the patient to identify the need for help and the appropriate action. The nurse also verifies that the action met the need for help. Orlando's principles are meant to guide the nurse at various stages of the interaction. She emphasizes the importance of interaction when she writes, "Learning how to understand what is happening between herself and the patient is the central core of the nurse's practice and comprises the basic framework for the help she gives to patients" (Orlando, 1961/1990, p. 4).

The actual *process* of a nurse–patient interaction may be the same as that of any interaction between two persons. When nurses use this process to communicate their reactions in caring for patients, Orlando calls it the "nursing process discipline." It is the tool that nurses use to fulfill their function to patients. In an attempt to extend her theory to encompass all nursing activities, Orlando (1972) broadens the use of the process discipline beyond the individual nurse–patient relationship in her book *The Discipline and Teaching of Nursing Process*. She applies the process discipline to contacts between a nurse leader and those she supervises or directs. When it is used in this manner, she refers to the process discipline as the "directive or supervisory job process in nursing" (p. 29).

If the nursing process is the same as the interactive process between any two individuals, how can nursing call itself a profession? The key is *discipline* in use of the process. Orlando (1972) provides three criteria to evaluate this discipline. These criteria differentiate an "automatic personal response" from a "disciplined professional response" (p. 31). Only the latter leads to effective nursing care, that is, relief of the patient's sense of helplessness. Learning to employ the process discipline requires *training*. This justifies the need for specific education in nursing. Orlando's nursing process discipline and the criteria for its use are discussed in more detail in the next section.

ORLANDO'S NURSING PROCESS DISCIPLINE

Orlando's (1972) nursing process discipline is based on the "process by which any individual acts" (p. 24). The purpose of the process discipline, when it is used between a nurse and a patient, is to meet the patient's immediate need for help. Improvement in the patient's behavior that indicates resolution of the need is the desired result. The process discipline is also used with other persons working in a job setting. The purpose here is to understand how the professional and job responsibilities of each affect the other. This understanding allows each nurse to effectively fulfill her professional function for the patient within the organizational setting.

Patient Behavior

The nursing process discipline is set in motion by *patient behavior*. All patient behavior, no matter how seemingly insignificant, must be considered an expression of need for help until its meaning to a particular patient in the immediate situation is understood. Orlando (1961/1990) stresses this in her first principle: "The presenting behavior of the patient, regardless of the form in which it appears, may represent a plea for help" (p. 40).

Patient behavior may be verbal or nonverbal. Inconsistency between verbal and nonverbal behaviors may be the factor that alerts the nurse that the patient needs help. Verbal behavior encompasses all the patient's use of language. It may take the form of "complaints . . . , requests . . . , questions . . . , refusals . . . , demands . . . , and . . . comments or statements" (Orlando, 1961/1990, p. 11). Nonverbal behavior includes physiological manifestations such as heart rate, perspiration, edema, and urination and motor activity such as smiling, walking, and avoiding eye contact. Nonverbal patient behavior may also be vocal, including such actions as sobbing, laughing, shouting, and sighing.

When the patient experiences a need that he cannot resolve, a sense of helplessness occurs. The patient's behavior reflects this distress. In *The Dynamic Nurse–Patient Relationship*, Orlando (1961/1990) describes some categories of patient distress: "physical limitations, . . . adverse reactions to the setting and . . . experiences which prevent the patient from communicating his needs" (p. 11). Feelings of helplessness caused by physical limitations may result from incomplete development, temporary or permanent disability, or restrictions of the environment, real or imagined. Adverse reactions to the setting, on the other hand, usually result from incorrect or inadequate understanding of an experience there. Patients may become distressed by a negative reaction to any aspect of the setting, despite its helpful or therapeutic intent. A need for help may also arise from the patient's inability to communicate effectively. This inability may be due to such factors as ambivalence concerning dependency brought on by illness, embarrassment related to the need, lack of trust in the nurse, and inability to state the need precisely.

Although all patient behavior may indicate a need for help, the behavior may not effectively communicate that need. When the behavior does not communicate the need, problems in the nurse–patient relationship can arise. Ineffective patient behavior "prevents the nurse from carrying out her concerns for the patient's care or from maintaining a satisfactory relationship to the patient" (Orlando, 1961/1990, p. 78). Ineffective patient behavior may also indicate difficulties in the initial establishment of the nurse–patient relationship, inaccurate identification of the patient's need by the nurse, or negative patient reaction to automatic nursing action. Resolution of ineffective patient behavior deserves high priority, for the behavior usually becomes worse over time if the need for help that it expresses remains unresolved. The nurse's reaction and action are designed to resolve ineffective patient behaviors as well as to meet the immediate need.

Nurse Reaction

The patient behavior stimulates a *nurse reaction*, which marks the beginning of the nursing process discipline. This reaction is comprised of three sequential parts (Orlando, 1972). First, the nurse perceives the behavior through any of her senses. Second, the perception leads to automatic thought. Finally, the thought produces an automatic feeling. For example, the nurse sees a patient grimace, thinks he is in pain, and feels concern. The nurse then shares her reaction with the patient to ascertain that she has correctly identified the need for help and to identify the nursing action appropriate to resolve it. Orlando (1961/1990) offers a principle to guide the nurse in her reaction to patient behavior: "The nurse does not assume that any aspect of her reaction to the patient is correct, helpful, or appropriate until she checks the validity of it in exploration with the patient" (p. 56).

Perception (sees the grimace), thought (thinks he is in pain), and feeling (feels concern) occur automatically and almost simultaneously. Therefore, the nurse must learn to identify each part of her reaction. This helps her to analyze the reaction to determine why she responded as she did. With this analysis, the process becomes logical rather than intuitive and thus disciplined rather than automatic. The nurse is able to use her reaction for the purpose of helping the patient.

The discipline in the nursing process prescribes how the nurse shares her reaction with the patient. Orlando (1961/1990) offers a principle to explain the usefulness of this sharing: "Any observation shared and explored with the patient is immediately useful in ascertaining and meeting his need or finding out that he is not in need at that time" (pp. 35–36).

Orlando (1972) also provides three criteria to ensure that the nurse's exploration of her reaction with the patient is successful:

1. What the nurse says to the individual in the contact must match (*be consistent with*) any or all of the items contained in the immediate reaction, and what the nurse does nonverbally must be verbally expressed and the expression must match one or all of the items contained in the immediate reaction; 2. The nurse must clearly communicate to the individual that the item being expressed belongs to herself; 3. The nurse must ask the individual about the item expressed in order to obtain correction or verification from that same individual. (pp. 29–30)

Which aspect of her reaction the nurse shares with the patient is not as important as that it be shared in the manner described in the criteria. From a practical standpoint, it may be more expeditious to share a perception than a thought or feeling. "You are grimacing" contains less assumption than "Are you in pain?" In this way the patient can more easily express his need for help without having to correct the nurse's misconception.

Feelings can and should be shared even when they are negative. The nonverbal actions of the nurse will usually show her feelings even if they are not verbally expressed. Thus, the nurse's verbal and nonverbal behavior may be inconsistent. Proper sharing of feelings can effectively help the patient to express his need for help. For example, a nurse may react to a patient's refusal of a medication with anger. If she says, "I am angry with your refusal of your medication. Could you explain to me why you have refused?" she invites the patient to explain the need for help that his refusal expressed. Her expression meets the three criteria, and the patient's need for help can be identified and resolved.

This example shows the importance of the nurse sharing her reaction as a fact about herself. She states, "I am angry," rather than, "You make me angry." This clear identification of the reaction as her own reduces the chance of misinterpretation by the patient. The sharing of the nurse's immediate reaction creates a climate in which the patient is more able to share his own reaction.

Adequate identification of the three aspects of the nurse's reaction helps to resolve extraneous feelings that may interfere with the patient's care. The nurse may find that her feelings come from her personal belief of how people should act or from stresses in the organizational setting or in her personal life. These feelings or stresses are unrelated to meeting the patient's need. If they are not resolved, the nurse's verbal and nonverbal behavior will again be inconsistent. This same process should be employed with nurses or other professionals in the job setting to resolve any conflicts that interfere with the nurse's fulfilling her professional function for the patient.

Orlando (1972) used her three criteria in the study described in *The Discipline and Teaching of Nursing Process* and found that use of the process discipline is positively related to improvement in patient behavior. The study also showed a positive relationship between the nurse's use of the process discipline and its use by the patient. Thus, use of the process discipline alone can help the patient communicate his need more effectively.

Orlando (1972) offers a diagram depicting open sharing of the nurse's reaction versus keeping the reaction secret (see Figure 8-1 and Figure 8-2). The nurse action that results from the reaction becomes a behavior that stimulates a reaction by the patient. Only openness in sharing of the nurse's reaction ensures that the patient's need will be effectively resolved. This sharing, in the manner prescribed, differentiates professional nursing practice from automatic personal response.

Nurse's Action

Once the nurse has validated or corrected her reaction to the patient's behavior through exploration with him, she can complete the nursing process discipline with the *nurse's action*. Orlando (1961/1990) includes "only what she [the nurse] says or does with or for

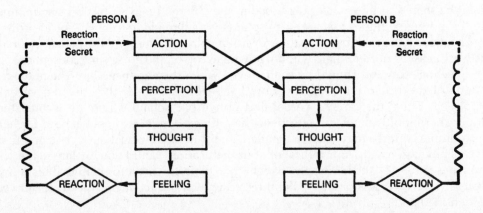

FIGURE 8-1 The action process in a person-to-person contact functioning in secret. The perceptions, thoughts, and feelings of each individual are not directly available to the perception of the other individual through the observable action. *(From Orlando, I. J. (1972). The discipline and teaching of nursing process. New York: G. P. Putnam's Sons, p. 26. Used with permission.)*

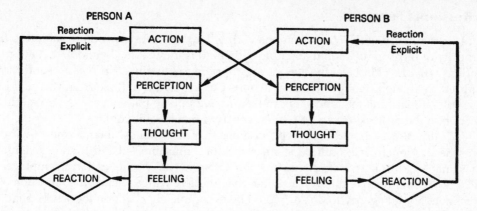

FIGURE 8-2   The action process in a person-to-person contact functioning in open disclosure. The perceptions, thoughts, and feelings of each individual are directly available to the perception of the other individual through the observable action. (*From Orlando, I. J. (1972). The discipline and teaching of nursing process. New York: G. P. Putnam's Sons, p. 26. Used with permission.*)

the benefit of the patient" as professional nursing action (p. 60). The nurse must be certain that her action is appropriate to meet the patient's need for help. Orlando's principle for guiding nursing action states, "The nurse initiates a process of exploration to ascertain how the patient is affected by what she says or does" (p. 67).

The nurse can act in two ways: automatic or deliberative. Only the second manner fulfills her professional function. Automatic actions are "those decided upon for reasons other than the patient's immediate need," whereas deliberative actions ascertain and meet this need (Orlando, 1961/1990, p. 60). There is a distinction between the purpose an action actually serves and its intention to help the patient. For example, a nurse administers a sleeping pill because the physician orders it. Carrying out the physician's order is the purpose of the action. However, the nurse has not determined that the patient is having trouble sleeping or that a pill is the most appropriate way to help him sleep. Thus, the action is automatic, not deliberative, and the patient's need for help is unlikely to be met. The following list identifies the criteria for deliberative actions:

1. Deliberative actions result from the correct identification of patient needs by validation of the nurse's reaction to patient behavior.
2. The nurse explores the meaning of the action with the patient and its relevance to meeting his need.
3. The nurse validates the action's effectiveness immediately after completing it.
4. The nurse is free of stimuli unrelated to the patient's need when she acts.

Automatic actions fail to meet one or more of these criteria. Automatic actions are most likely to be done by nurses concerned primarily with carrying out physicians' orders, routines of patient care, or general principles for protecting health or by nurses who do not validate their reactions to patient behaviors. Although any nursing action may be purported to have occurred with the intention of helping the patient, deliberation is needed to determine if the action achieved its purpose and to identify if the patient was helped.

Professional Function

Nurses often work within organizations with other professionals and are subject to the authority of the organization that employs them. It is inevitable, therefore, that at times conflicts will arise between the actions appropriate to the nurse's profession and those required by the job. Nonprofessional actions can prevent the nurse from carrying out her professional function, and this can lead to inadequate patient care. A well-defined function of the profession can help to prevent and resolve this conflict.

Ideally, nurses should not accept positions that do not allow them to meet their patients' needs for help. If a conflict does arise, the nurse must present data to show that nursing is unable to fulfill its professional function. Orlando (1972) believes that an employer is unlikely to continue to require job activities that interfere with a well-defined function of a profession. For an agency to do so "would be to completely abandon the whole point of having enlisted the services of that profession in the agency or institution" (p. 16).

Nurses must be constantly aware that their "activity is professional only when it deliberately achieves the purpose of helping the patient" (Orlando, 1961/1990, p. 70). Some automatic activities may be necessary to the running of an institution. These should, however, be kept to a minimum and should be carried out as much as possible by support personnel. The nurse must attend to helping patients resolve any conflict between these routines and their needs for help.

In many health care institutions the potential demand for nursing skill and judgment exceeds the availability of such qualities. As a result, nursing care delivery systems may be evaluated and revised to enable the nurse to practice in those situations or areas where she is most needed. Some of these situations are reflected in the accreditation standards of the Joint Commission (formerly the Joint Commission on Accreditation of Healthcare Organizations). These include nursing assessment at the time of admission (identify the need for help), planning and delivery of patient education based on patient needs (deliberative action to meet the need), and preparation for discharge (verifying that the need has been met). In each of these situations, the use of Orlando's theory would guide the nurse in expeditiously meeting the patient's need. Nurses in acute care facilities are expected to use their professional skills and knowledge to recognize and resolve the patient's need for help. Some of this recognition of the nursing contribution may be related to the situational pressures arising out of the prospective payment reimbursement system in place in health care institutions. Under this system, emphasis is placed on the patient being treated and discharged within a predetermined number of days or cost of care. Nursing can capitalize on this situation and use it to the patient's and profession's best interests. Orlando's theory, although simple in nature, provides direction and focus for identifying, understanding, and meeting the patient's need in a potentially cost-effective manner. If the needs identified by the patient are met, then less nursing time should be involved than if the nurse uses primarily automatic actions and must provide additional care when the need has not been met.

Thus, the nursing process discipline is set in motion by a patient behavior that may indicate a need for help. The nurse reacts to this behavior with perceptions, thoughts, and feelings. She shares an aspect of her reaction with the patient, making sure that her verbal and nonverbal actions are consistent with her reaction, that she identifies the reaction as her own, and that she invites the patient to comment on the validity of her reaction. A properly shared reaction by the nurse helps the patient to use the same process to more effectively communicate his need. Next, an appropriate action to resolve the need is mutually decided on by the patient and nurse. After the nurse acts, she immediately asks the patient if the action has been effective. Throughout the interaction, the nurse makes sure that she is free of any extraneous stimuli that interfere with her reaction to the patient.

ORLANDO'S THEORY AND NURSING'S METAPARADIGM

Orlando includes material specific to three of the four major concepts: the human, health, and nursing. The fourth concept, environment or society, is not included in her theory.

She uses the concept of *human* as she emphasizes individuality and the dynamic nature of the nurse–patient relationship. For Orlando, humans in need are the focus of nursing practice.

Although *health* is not specified by Orlando, it is implied. In her initial work, Orlando focused on illness. Later, she indicated that nursing deals with the individual whenever there is a need for help. Thus, a sense of helplessness replaces the concept of health or illness as the initiator of a need for nursing.

Orlando largely ignores *society*. She deals only with the interaction between a nurse and a patient in an immediate situation and speaks to the importance of individuality. She does discuss the overall nursing system in an institutional setting. However, she does not discuss how the patient is affected by the society in which he lives, nor does she use society as a focus of nursing action. It is possible the immediate need could involve persons other than the patient. However, Orlando does not discuss nursing action with families or groups.

Nursing is, of course, the focus of Orlando's work. She speaks of nursing as unique and independent in its concerns for an individual's need for help in an immediate situation. The efforts to meet the individual's need for help are carried out in an interactive situation and in a disciplined manner that requires proper training.

COMPARISON OF ORLANDO'S PROCESS DISCIPLINE AND THE NURSING PROCESS

Orlando's nursing process discipline may be compared with the nursing process. Certain overall characteristics are similar in both processes. For example, both are interpersonal in nature and require interaction between patient and nurse. The patient is asked for input throughout the process. Both processes also view the patient as a total person. He is not merely a disease process or body part. Orlando does not use the term *holistic*, but she effectively describes a holistic approach. Both processes are also used as a method to provide nursing care and as a means to evaluate that care. Finally, both are deliberate intellectual processes.

The *assessment* phase of the nursing process corresponds to the sharing of the nurse reaction to the patient behavior in Orlando's process discipline. Patient behavior initiates the assessment. The collection of data includes only information relevant to identifying the patient's need for help. An ongoing database is not useful to the immediate situation of the patient. The nurse's reaction, however, is probably influenced by her past experiences with the patient and other patients.

Orlando (1961/1990) discusses data collection in her first book, *The Dynamic Nurse–Patient Relationship*. She defines observation as "any information pertaining to a patient which the nurse acquires while she is on duty" (p. 31). Direct data are comprised of "any perception, thought, or feeling the nurse has from her own experience of the patient's behavior at any or several moments in time" (p. 32). Indirect data come from sources other than the patient, such as records, other health team members, or the patient's significant others. Both types of data require exploration with the patient to determine their relevance to the specific situation. Both verbal and nonverbal patient behaviors are important. Their consistency or inconsistency is a data piece in itself. This corresponds somewhat with subjective and objective data in the nursing process.

The sharing of the nurse's reaction in Orlando's process discipline has components similar to the analysis in the nursing process. Although the nurse's reaction is automatic, her awareness of it and the way she shares it is a deliberate intellectual activity. Orlando's sharing of the reaction, however, is a process of exploration with the patient. The nursing process, on the other hand, intentionally makes use of nursing's theoretical base and principles from the physical and behavioral sciences.

The product of the analysis in the nursing process is the *nursing diagnosis.* Exploration of the nurse's reaction with the patient in Orlando's process discipline leads to identification of his need for help. The statement of the nursing diagnosis is a more formal process than that of need. Many nursing diagnoses may be made, given priority ratings, and resolved over time. Orlando deals with immediate nurse–patient interaction; only one need is dealt with at a time.

The *outcomes and planning* phases of the nursing process involve writing outcomes, goals, and objectives and deciding on appropriate nursing action. This corresponds to the nurse's action phase of Orlando's process discipline. Any outcome beyond the immediate situation is not likely in Orlando's process discipline. Her goal is always relief of the patient's immediate need for help; the objective relates to improvement in the patient's behavior. The nursing process mandates a more formal action of writing and giving priority to goals and objectives.

Both processes require patient participation in determining the appropriate action. In the nursing process this participation occurs mostly in identification of outcomes and goal setting. Outcomes are based on mutual decision making of what the patient wants to change. This is similar in both processes and begins the nurse action phase. Orlando's process discipline sees the patient as an active participant in determining the actual nurse action. The nursing process, on the other hand, relies more heavily on scientific principles and nursing theories in deciding how the nurse will act.

Implementation involves the final selection and carrying out of the planned action and is also part of the nurse's action phase of Orlando's process discipline. Both processes mandate that the action be appropriate for the patient as a unique individual. The nursing process expects the nurse to consider all possible effects of the action on the patient. Orlando's process discipline is concerned only with the effectiveness of the action in resolving the immediate need for help.

Evaluation is inherent in Orlando's action phase of her process discipline. For an action to be deliberative, the nurse must evaluate its effectiveness when it is completed. Failure to evaluate can result in a series of ineffective actions, including failure to meet the patient's need and an increase in the cost of nursing care and materials.

Evaluation in both processes is based on objective criteria. In the nursing process, evaluation asks whether the outcome was achieved. In Orlando's process discipline, the nurse observes patient behavior to see whether the patient has been helped. Thus, both processes evaluate in terms of outcomes of care.

Both the nursing process and Orlando's process discipline are described as a series of sequential steps. The steps do not actually occur discretely and in order in either process. As new information becomes available, earlier steps may be repeated. Thus, new assessment data may alter the nursing diagnosis or the plan. Orlando's process discipline is almost a continuous interchange in which patient behavior leads to nurse reaction, which leads to nurse behavior, which leads to patient reaction (see Figure 8-2). Thus, both processes are dynamic and responsive to changes in the patient's situation.

The nursing process and Orlando's process discipline have many similarities. They do, however, have important differences. The nursing process is far more formal and has more detailed phases than does Orlando's process discipline. The nursing process requires the nurse to use her knowledge of scientific principles and nursing theory to guide her behavior. Orlando demands only that the nurse follow the principles she lays down to guide nursing care. Long-term planning is part of the nursing process but is not relevant to Orlando's process discipline. Although both processes call for patient involvement in his care, Orlando's demands this participation more comprehensively.

An example of Orlando's process is as follows:

Case Situation: One of your patients is Jeremy Isaac, a 20-year-old college senior. This is Jeremy's first postoperative day after exploratory abdominal surgery that resulted in a splenectomy. He is an athlete and has been having abdominal muscle spasms. These spasms have been well controlled with his pain medication and a muscle relaxant. His vital signs have been stable, and he does not yet have bowel sounds. He has expressed a clear preference for the room temperature to be no greater than 72° F. He has been resting comfortably at this temperature. Within the last hour, a new admission has been placed in the other bed in Jeremy's room. This patient is an 80-year-old man who has noisily and frequently complained since his admission that the room is too cold. You have just entered the room.

Patient behavior: Jeremy is moving restlessly in his bed. Previously, he was sleeping.

Nurse's reaction: You perceive that Jeremy is now restless, think that this is a change in his behavior, and feel that he may be in pain. You say to him, "It appears to me that you are uncomfortable. Do you need pain medication?" His response is, "No, I'm not in pain. I just want to sleep." At this moment, the roommate once again yells out that the room is too cold. You quietly ask Jeremy if that is what is keeping him awake, and Jeremy nods yes, thus validating your perception that the most recent dose of pain medication is still effective and the disturbance is the noisy roommate.

Nurse's action: You arrange for the roommate to be moved into another room with a patient closer to his age. Within 30 minutes of taking this deliberative action, you note that Jeremy is once again resting quietly, thus validating that the action was effective.

CRITIQUE OF ORLANDO'S NURSING PROCESS DISCIPLINE

1. *What is the historical context of the theory?* Orlando's disciplined nursing process was developed from research conducted on nursing practice, as discussed earlier in this chapter. Orlando's research was being conducted during the same time that Henderson was developing her components and definition of nursing and Wiedenbach was developing her prescriptive theory of nursing. All of these theorists were at Yale. The observations from the original research were divided into "good" and "bad" nursing, and the disciplined sharing of the nurse's reaction was identified as the primary difference between good and bad nursing. Orlando's nursing process discipline is easy to understand and is needs based.

2. *What are the basic concepts and relationships presented by the theory?* Nursing is presented as a unique, independent, and disciplined profession. Nursing functions to meet the immediate need that is demonstrated by the patient's behavior. The nurse's reaction (perception, thought, feeling) to the patient's behavior is shared with patient in order to validate, or correct, the accuracy of that reaction. This disciplined nursing process leads to deliberative nursing actions taken to meet the patient's need. Automatic actions may be taken for reasons other than meeting the patient's immediate need. This interactive process requires training for the nurse to be effective.

3. *What major phenomena of concern to nursing are presented? (These phenomena may include but are not limited to human beings, environment, health, interpersonal relations, caring, goal attainment, adaptation, and energy fields.)* The phenomena of concern to nursing presented in Orlando's theory include the human being, interactive communication, immediate need, validation, and deliberative actions. She also describes nursing as unique, independent, and disciplined. These have been discussed within this chapter.

4. *To whom does it apply? In what situations? In what ways?* This theory applies to anyone with an immediate need who is in contact with a nurse. The situations are limited only by the requirements of the presence of a nurse and a person with an immediate need. The requirement for the need to be immediate does limit the application for long-term needs, anticipatory guidance, or education when the need is not recognized by the person and for most planning situations. This means not that Orlando's work cannot be used in long-term care settings but that the focus would be on the patient's immediate need rather than on long-term goals. Rosenthal (1996) has described the beneficial use of this theory in the perioperative setting, and Faust (2002) spoke of its use in an extended care facility.

   Other situations in which the theory may be used are those in which the nurse is functioning as a leader or manager. In these situations, another nurse or staff member will be the person in need. The effectiveness of this theory in nursing leadership has been supported by Schmeiding (1988, 1990a, 1990c, 1991), Sheafor (1991), and Laurent (2000).

5. *By what method or methods can this theory be tested?* This theory was derived from initial research that used a qualitative, observational methodology. Orlando's second research project was quantitative in nature, as it used statistical analysis. However, this second study focused on the effects on nursing outcomes of teaching the disciplined process to nurses rather than on manipulating nurse–patient interactions. With the strong support received for the effectiveness

of the disciplined nursing process, it would not be ethical to use a true experimental model in which one group of patients was assigned to receive only nursing care that has been delivered based solely on the nurse's reaction rather than on the validation of that reaction with the patient.

Research studies reported in the literature have used a variety of quasi- and nonexperimental methods to study this theory. Potter and Bockenhauer (2000) used a quasi-experimental method to support positive outcomes in decreasing patients' levels of distress. Ellis (1999) used a quantitative survey to identify barriers experienced by registered nurses in the emergency department in relation to screening for domestic violence. Haggerty (1987), using videotaped patient situations, found that the type of patient distress was more predictive of the response of senior nursing students than was the type of educational program in which the students were enrolled (associate degree or baccalaureate). Ponte (1988) investigated the relationship between nurses' empathy skills and patient distress in adult cancer patients. Ponte found a positive relationship between empathy skills and use of Orlando's deliberative process. However, she also found that while nurses scored low in the use of empathy skills as well as in the use of the deliberative nursing process, the patients demonstrated low levels of distress.

The most common research methodology has been descriptive correlational. Olson (1993) and Olson and Hanchett (1997) investigated the relationships between nurse-expressed empathy and the outcomes of patient perception of empathy and patient distress. They found a statistically significant negative relationship between nurse-expressed empathy and patient distress as well as between patient-perceived empathy and patient distress. The relationship between nurse-expressed empathy and patient perception of empathy was moderately positive and statistically significant. Schmieding (1987, 1988, 1990a, 1990b, 1990c, 1991) has proposed a model for exploring the relationship between the responses of nurse administrators and the actions of staff nurses and reported several descriptive correlational studies conducted using the model. She has found that administrators often respond in ways that prevent staff participation in problem solving, which may limit the development of inquiry skills in staff nurses, but that many staff nurses preferred not being included in the identification of problems (Schmieding, 1990a, 1990c). In studying the relationship between the responses of head nurses and staff responses to patients, she found a positive relationship with little influence from the characteristics of the nurses or the size of the hospital (Schmieding, 1991). The primary mode of response was the one termed nonexploratory by Schmieding. This response parallels Orlando's automatic actions.

6. *Does this theory direct nursing actions that lead to favorable outcomes?*   The purpose of the nursing process discipline is for deliberative nursing actions to be taken to meet the patient's immediate need. If the need is met, the nursing interventions were therapeutic and the patient outcomes are positive. Potter and Bockenhauer (2000) and Rosenthal (1996) speak to the positive effect of the use of the nursing process discipline on patient outcomes. Deliberative nursing actions are taken for the purpose of meeting the patient's identified immediate need. The outcomes of these actions must be favorable or the need has not been met and new actions must be selected. Automatic nursing actions may or may not lead to favorable

outcomes and do not require that the nurse validate the effectiveness of the actions. Orlando's disciplined nursing process indicates that nursing actions should not be taken until the patient's need has been validated and the planned actions are agreed on between the nurse and the patient as being appropriate to meet the need. The intent of this deliberative process is to achieve favorable outcomes. Allen, Bockenhauer, Egan, and Kinnaird (2006) applied Orlando's theory in a study that focused on relating excellent nursing practice and clinical outcomes; Potter, Williams, and Costanzo (2004) report that the use of Orlando's theory led to improved patient response in using a structured psychoeducational curriculum with inpatient groups. Potter, Vitale-Nolen, and Dawson (2005) also reported positive effects when using Orlando's theory in designing and using a form of contracting with patients in an acute psychiatric facility.

7. *How contagious is this theory?*   This use of this theory has been documented in clinical practice, nursing administration, and nursing education. It has been used primarily in the United States. An electronic search did locate two references each from Japan (Ikeda, 1975; Kawakami, Kawashima, Hirao, Yamane, & Kosaka, 1972), Brazil (Prá & Picoli, 2004; Toniolli & Pagliuca, 2002), and the United Kingdom (Tutton & Seers, 2003; Wadensten & Carlsson, 2003). Also, Olson and Hanchett (1977) have reported its use in Canada. Thus, the theory is contagious as to the areas of nursing in which it can be used, but the literature does not support that it has been widely contagious in any particular area of practice or throughout the world.

STRENGTHS AND LIMITATIONS

Orlando's theory has much to offer to nursing. The predominant strength of her work is its usefulness in nursing practice. It guides nurses through their interactions with patients. Use of her theory virtually ensures that patients will be treated as individuals and that they will have an active and constant input into their own care. The nurse's focus must remain on the patient rather than on the demands of the work setting. Use of the process discipline helps the nurse deal with her personal reactions and leads her to value her own individuality as a thinking person.

The nurse can keep Orlando in mind while applying the nursing process. Use of her theory prevents inaccurate diagnosis or ineffective plans because the nurse has to constantly explore her reactions with the patient. No nurse, following Orlando's principles, could fail to evaluate the care she has given.

Another of Orlando's strengths is her assertion of nursing's independence as a profession and her belief that this independence must be based on a sound theoretical framework. She bases this belief on her definition of nursing function. She believes that this clearly defined function will assist nursing in establishing its independence and in structuring the work setting so that nurses can effectively meet their patients' needs for help. The function of finding and meeting the patient's immediate need for help is broad enough to encompass nurses practicing in all settings and in all specialty areas. It allows nursing to evolve over time by avoiding a rigid list of nursing activities.

Orlando guides the nurse to evaluate her care in terms of objectively observable patient outcomes. It is not the structure of the setting or the number of nurses on duty that determines effective care. Orlando and others have found a positive relationship between the use of her process and favorable outcomes of patient behavior. The immediate and interactive nature of her process does, however, make evaluation a time-consuming process.

The nursing profession's input into accreditation standards for health care organizations has placed great emphasis on the evaluation of interventions in terms of patient outcomes. Consistent use of Orlando's theory by nurses could make evaluation a less time-consuming and more deliberate function, the results of which would be documented in patient charts. Such documentation of patient needs, planned interventions, and evaluation of interventions would provide data for analysis that would contribute to the general body of knowledge within the field of nursing.

Orlando's testing of her theory in the practice setting lends further support to its usefulness. Her first study, published in *The Dynamic Nurse–Patient Relationship*, provided a basis for future work. For a second study, described in *The Discipline and Teaching of the Nursing Process*, she developed specific criteria amenable to statistical testing. Nursing can pursue Orlando's work by retesting and further developing her work.

Orlando's mental health background is probably responsible for the highly interactive nature of her theory. Although this interactive nature is one of the theory's strengths, it also provides limitation in her ideas. Nurses deal extensively with monitoring and controlling the physiological processes of patients to prevent illness and restore health. Orlando scarcely mentions this aspect of the nurse's role other than to question if monitoring machines is practicing nursing. The decidedly interactive nature of Orlando's theory makes it hard to include the highly technical and physical care that nurses give in certain settings, such as intensive care units. Her theory does, however, prevent the nurse from forgetting the patient in her efforts to fulfill the technical aspects of her job.

Orlando's theory is also limited by its focus on interaction with an individual, whereas the patient should be viewed as a member of a family and within a community. Often it is vital to deal with the family as a whole to help the patient. Orlando does not deal with these areas.

Long-term care and planning are not applicable to Orlando's focus on the immediate situation. She views long-term planning only as it is relates to adequate staffing within an institution. Orlando herself recognizes this problem. In *The Dynamic Nurse–Patient Relationship,* she speculated that "repeated experiences of having been helped undoubtedly culminate over periods of time in greater degrees of improvement" (p. 90). She also identified the cumulative effect of nursing as an area for further study.

In *The Discipline and Teaching of Nursing Process*, Orlando sought to define the entire nursing system. She described the system as the "regularly, interacting parts of a nursing service" (p. 18). This part of her theory attempts to incorporate nurses' relationships with other nurses and with members of different professions in the job setting. Her theory struggles with the authority derived from the function of the profession and that of the employing institution's commitment to the public. The same process is offered for dealing with others as for working with an individual patient.

When a nurse manager deals with staff, Orlando's theory provides a framework for an interaction that leads to a positive result. As the nurse executive listens to the needs of the staff, she must decide if deliberate action is needed; such action may take the form of a policy or procedure change, staffing variation, or institutional policy change. The nurse executive may need to influence another department, group, or level within the organization to effect a positive intervention with staff. On the administrative level, Orlando's theory is used, but the time span needed to complete all components varies depending on the situations. An organization that consistently and methodically uses Orlando's theory can positively respond to all issues that need to be confronted. In such an environment, needs can be met and emphasis placed on the present rather than the past or the way it has always been done. Thus, the organization is able to maintain its competitive edge.

Orlando should be considered a nursing theorist who made a significant contribution to the advancement of nursing practice. She helped nurses to focus on the patient rather than on the disease or institutional demands. The nurse is firmly viewed as in service for the patient, not as handmaiden to the physician. Nurses must base their practice on logical thinking rather than on intuition. Orlando's nursing process discipline continues to be useful to nurses in their interactions with patients, although an additional limitation is the lack of current publications about her nursing process discipline and its utility.

Summary

Orlando's nursing process discipline is rooted in the interaction between a nurse and a patient at a specific time and place. A sequence of interchanges involving patient behavior and nurse reaction takes place until the patient's need for help, as he perceives it, is clarified. The nurse then decides, in cooperation with the patient, on an appropriate action to resolve the need. This action is evaluated after it is carried out. If the patient behavior improves, the action was successful, the desired outcomes were achieved, and the process is completed. If there is no change or the behavior gets worse, the process recycles with new efforts to clarify the patient's behavior or the appropriate nursing action.

Orlando (1961/1990) summarizes her process as follows:

> A deliberative nursing process has elements of continuous reflection as the nurse tries to understand the meaning to the patient of the behavior she observes and what he needs from her in order to be helped. Responses comprising this process are stimulated by the nurse's unfolding awareness of the particulars of the individual situation. (p. 67)

Thought Questions

1. In the case study in this chapter, the nurse used deliberative action. Name at least two automatic actions the nurse might have taken.
2. Consider a clinical situation of interest to you and identify/define what the three parts of the nurse reaction would be for you.
3. You are assigned to care for a comatose patient. Since this patient is not speaking, how might you be able to use the nursing process discipline?
4. How would you go about assisting another nurse in learning to use the nursing process discipline?

References

Allen, D. E., Bockenhauer, B., Egan, C., & Kinnaird, L. S. (2006). Relating outcomes to excellent nursing practice. *Journal of Nursing Administration, 36*(3), 140–147.

Ellis, J. M. (1999). Barriers to effective screening for domestic violence by registered nurses in the emergency department. *Critical Care Nursing Quarterly, 22*(1), 27–41.

Faust, C. (2002). Clinical outlook. Orlando's Deliberative Nursing Process Theory: A practice application in an extended care facility. *Journal of Gerontological Nursing, 28*(7), 14–18.

Haggerty, L. A. (1987). An analysis of senior nursing students' immediate response to distressed patients. *Journal of Advanced Nursing, 12*, 451–461.

Harmer, B., & Henderson, V. (1955). *Textbook of the principles and practice of nursing* (5th ed.). New York: Macmillan.

Ikeda, S. (1975). Ms. Ida Jean Orlando's nursing theory and my own concepts [Japanese]. *Kango (KUI), 27*(10), 30–35.

Kawakami, T., Kawashima, M., Hirao, H., Yamane, M., & Kosaka, F. (1972). Nursing theory for nurses. 8. On Orlando's "Nursing Research" [Japanese]. *Kangogaku Zasshi (KNM), 36*, 1018–1022.

Laurent, C. L. (2000). A nursing theory for nursing leadership. *Journal of Nursing Management, 8*, 83–87.

Olson, J. K. (1993). Relationships between nurse expressed empathy, patient perceived empathy and patient distress. *Dissertation Abstracts International, 55–02B*, 0369. (University Microfilms No. AAG9418218)

Olson, J., & Hanchett, E. (1997). Nurse-expressed empathy, patient outcomes, and development of a middle-range theory. *Image: Journal of Nursing Scholarship, 29*, 71–76.

Orlando, I. J. (1972). *The discipline and teaching of nursing process.* New York: G. P. Putnam's Sons. [out of print]

Orlando, I. J. (1987). Nursing in the 21st century: Alternate paths. *Journal of Advanced Nursing, 12*, 405–412.

Orlando, I. J. (1990). *The dynamic nurse–patient relationship: Function, process and principles.* New York: National League for Nursing. (Reprinted from 1961, New York: G. P. Putnam's Sons)

Pelletier, I. O. (1967). The patient's predicament and nursing function. *Psychiatric Opinion, 4*, 25–30.

Peplau, H. E. (1988). *Interpersonal relations in nursing.* London: Macmillan Education. (Original work published 1952, New York: G. P. Putnam's Sons)

Ponte, P. A. R. (1988). The relationships among empathy and the use of Orlando's deliberative process by the primary nurse and the distress of the adult cancer patient. *Dissertation Abstracts International, 50–07B*, 2848. (University Microfilms No. AAG8916380)

Potter, M. L., & Bockenhauer, B. J. (2000). Implementing Orlando's nursing theory: A pilot study. *Journal of Psychosocial Nursing and Mental Health Services, 38*(3), 14–21.

Potter, M. L., Vitale-Nolen, R., & Dawson, A. M. (2005). Implementation of safety agreements in an acute psychiatric facility. *Journal of the American Psychiatric Nurses Association, 11*(3), 144–155.

Potter, M. L., Williams, R. B., & Costanzo, R. (2004). Using nursing theory and a structured psychoeducational curriculum with inpatient groups. *Journal of the American Psychiatric Nurses Association, 10*(3), 122–128.

Prá, L. A., & Piccoli, M. (2004). Perioperative nursing: Nursing diagnosis based on the theory of Orlando [Portuguese]. *Revista Electronica de Enfermagem, 6*(2), 234–253. Abstract in English retrieved May 18, 2007, from CINAHL Plus with Full Text database.

Rosenthal, B. C. (1996). An interactionist's approach to perioperative nursing. *Association of Operating Room Nurses Journal, 64*, 254–260.

Schmieding, N. J. (1987). Analysing managerial responses in face-to-face contacts . . . Orlando's theory. *Journal of Advanced Nursing, 12,* 357–365.

Schmieding, N. J. (1988). Action process of nurse administrators to problematic situations based on Orlando's theory. *Journal of Advanced Nursing, 13,* 99–107.

Schmieding, N. J. (1990a). A model for assessing nurse administrators' actions. *Western Journal of Nursing Research, 12,* 293–306.

Schmieding, N. J. (1990b). An integrative nursing theoretical framework. *Journal of Advanced Nursing, 15,* 463–467.

Schmieding, N. J. (1990c). Do head nurses include staff nurses in problem-solving? *Nursing Management, 21*(3), 58–60.

Schmieding, N. J. (1991). Relationship between head nurses responses to staff nurses and staff nurse responses to patients. *Western Journal of Nursing Research, 13,* 746–760.

Sheafor, M. (1991). Productive work groups in complex hospital units: Proposed contributions of the nurse executive. *Journal of Nursing Administration, 21*(5), 25–30.

Toniolli, A. C. S., & Pagliuca, L. M. F. (2002). Analysis of Orlando's theory applied in the Barsiliens' nursing magazines [Portuguese]. *Revista Brasileira de Enfermagem, 55*(5), 489–494. Abstract in English retrieved May 18, 2007, from CINAHL Plus with full text database.

Trench, A. S. (Executive producer), Wallace, D. (Producer), & Coberg, T. (Director). (1987). *Ida Jean Orlando—The nurse theorists: Portraits of excellence* [Videotape]. Oakland, CA: Studio Three Production, Samuel Merritt College of Nursing.

Tutton, E., & Seers, K. (2003). An exploration of the concept of comfort. *Journal of Clinical Nursing, 12,* 689–696.

Wadensten, B., & Carlsson, M. (2003). Nursing theory views on how to support the process of ageing. *Journal of Advanced Nursing, 42*(2), 118–124.

CHAPTER 9

Other Theories from the 1950s and 1960s*

Julia B. George

Peggy Coldwell Foster

In addition to Peplau, Henderson, Orem, Johnson, Orlando, and Levine, Lydia E. Hall, Faye Glenn Abdellah, Ernestine Wiedenbach, and Joyce Travelbee also published nursing theories in the 1950s/1960s. Hall's care, core, and cure theory; Abdellah's patient-centered approaches; Wiedenbach's prescriptive theory; and Travelbee's Human-to-Human Relationship Model will be reviewed.

CARE, CORE, AND CURE

Lydia E. Hall

Lydia Eloise Hall (1906–1969) received her basic nursing education at York Hospital School of Nursing in York, Pennsylvania, and graduated in 1927. Both her B.S. in public health nursing (1937) and her M.A. in teaching natural sciences (1942) are from Teachers College, Columbia University, New York, New York. She was the first director of the Loeb Center for Nursing and Rehabilitation and continued in that position until her death in 1969. Her experience in nursing spans the clinical, educational, research, and supervisory components. Her publications include several articles on the definition of nursing and quality of care. Lydia Hall articulated what she considered a basic philosophy of nursing upon which the nurse may base patient care.

LOEB CENTER FOR NURSING AND REHABILITATION As a nurse theorist, Lydia Hall is unique in that her beliefs about nursing were demonstrated in practice with relatively little documentation in the literature. Hall originated the philosophy of care of Loeb Center at Montefiore Hospital, Bronx, New York. Loeb Center opened in January 1963 to provide professional nursing care to persons past the acute stage of illness. The center's functioning concept was that the need for professional nursing care increases as the need for medical care decreases.

---

* The theorists in this chapter used the term *patient* and *he* for the recipient of nursing care and *she* for the nurse, at least in their initial publications. This approach will be used in this chapter.

Those in need of continued professional care who were 16 years of age or older and who were no longer experiencing an acute biological disturbance were transferred from the acute care hospital to Loeb Center. Good candidates for care at Loeb were those who had a desire to come to Loeb, were recommended by their physicians, and possessed a favorable potential for recovery and return to the community.

As physically designed by Hall, Loeb Center had a capacity of 80 beds and was attached to Montefiore Hospital. The rooms were arranged with patient comfort and maneuverability as the first priority. The patients also had access to a large communal dining room. The primary caregivers were registered professional nurses. Nonpatient care activities were supplied by messenger–attendants and ward secretaries. The center's philosophy, as stated by Bowar-Ferres (1975), was as follows:

> Loeb's primary purpose was and is to demonstrate that high quality nursing care given by registered nurses, in a non-directive setting, offers a supportive setting to people in the post-acute phase of their illness that enables them to recover sooner, and to leave the center able to cope with themselves and what they must face in the future. (p. 810)

To create a nondirective setting, there were very few rules or routines, no schedules, and no dictated mealtimes or specified visiting hours at Loeb Center (Bower-Ferres, 1975). The nurses at Loeb strove to help the patient determine and clarify goals and, with the patient, to work out ways to achieve the goals at the individual's pace, consistent with the medical treatment plan and congruent with the patient's sense of self. At Loeb Center, the nurses were in charge, and Hall, as director of the center, hired and fired the physicians who were employed there (Hall, 1955, 1969).

LYDIA HALL'S THEORY OF NURSING   Lydia Hall presented her theory of nursing by drawing three interlocking circles, each circle representing a particular aspect of nursing: *care, core,* and *cure.*

The Care Circle   The care circle (Figure 9-1) represents the nurturing component and is exclusive to nursing. Nurturing involves using the factors that make up the concept of mothering (care and comfort of the person) and provide for teaching–learning activities. The professional nurse provides bodily care for the patient and helps the patient to complete such basic daily biological functions as eating, bathing, elimination, and dressing. When providing this care, the nurse's goal is the comfort of the patient.

Providing care for a patient at the basic needs level presents the nurse and patient with an opportunity for closeness. As closeness develops, the patient can share and explore feelings with the nurse. This opportunity to explore feelings represents the teaching–learning aspect of nurturing.

When functioning in the care circle, the nurse applies knowledge of the natural and biological sciences to provide a strong theoretical base for nursing implementations. In interactions with the patient the nurse's role needs to be clearly defined. A strong theory base allows the nurse to maintain a professional status rather than a mothering status while at the same time incorporating closeness and nurturance in giving care. The patient views the nurse as a potential comforter, one who provides care and comfort through the laying on of hands.

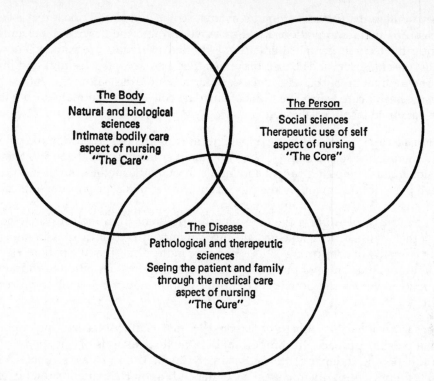

FIGURE 9-1   The care-core-cure circles. (*Adapted from Hall, L. Nursing—What is it? P. 1. Publication of the Virginia State Nurses' Association, Winter 1959. Used with permission.*)

The Core Circle   The core circle (Figure 9-1) of patient care is based in the social sciences, involves the therapeutic use of self, and is shared with other members of the health team. The professional nurse, by developing an interpersonal relationship with the patient, is able to help the patient verbally express feelings regarding the disease process and its effects as well as discuss the patient's role in recovery. Through such expression the patient is able to gain self-identity and further develop maturity. As Hall (1965) says,

> To look at and listen to self is often too difficult without the help of a significant figure (nurturer) who has learned how to hold up a mirror and sounding board to invite the behaver to look and listen to himself. If he accepts the invitation, he will explore the concerns in his acts and as he listens to his exploration through the reflection of the nurse, he may uncover in sequence his difficulties, the problem area, his problem, and eventually the threat which is dictating his out-of-control behavior.

The professional nurse, by use of the reflective technique (acting as a mirror for the patient), helps the patient look at and explore feelings regarding his current health status and related potential changes in lifestyle. The nurse uses a freely offered closeness to help the patient bring into awareness the verbal and nonverbal messages being sent to others. Motivations are discovered through the process of bringing into awareness the feelings being experienced. With this awareness the patient is now able to make conscious decisions based on understood and accepted feelings and motivations. The motivation and energy necessary for healing exist within the patient rather than in the health care team. The focus of any data collection is on that which will benefit the patient to increase self-healing.

The Cure Circle   The cure circle of patient care (Figure 9-1) is based in the pathological and therapeutic sciences and is shared with other members of the health team. The professional nurse helps the patient and family through the medical, surgical, and rehabilitative prescriptions made by the physician. During this aspect of nursing care, the nurse is an active advocate of the patient.

The nurse's role during the cure aspect is different from the care circle because many of the nurse's actions take on a negative quality of avoidance of pain rather than a positive quality of comforting. This is negative in the sense that the patient views the nurse as a potential cause of pain, one who is involved in such actions as administering injections, versus the potential comforter who provides care and comfort in the care circle.

Interaction of the Three Aspects of Nursing   Because Hall emphasizes the importance of a total person approach, it is important that the three aspects of nursing be viewed not as functioning independently but as interrelated. The three aspects interact, and the circles representing them change size, depending on the patient's total course of progress.

In observing what happened during hospitalization, Hall became convinced that as persons moved past the acute stage of illness, the need for professional nursing care increased, while the need for medical care decreased. It is important to note that this was during the time of retrospective payment systems when patients typically remained hospitalized until they were nearly ready to fully resume their usual activities. Thus, patients who were past the acute stage of their illness had access to 24 hours of nursing care and the full services of a hospital setting as needed. Hall's underlying assumption was that the person who had an increased need for professional nursing care could be best served in a setting that focused on his needs and encouraged participation.

In the philosophy of Loeb Center, the professional nurse functions most therapeutically when patients have entered the second stage of their hospital stay (i.e., they arerecuperating and are past the acute stage of illness). During this recuperation stage, the care and core aspects are the most prominent, and the cure aspect is less prominent. The size of the circles represents the degree to which the patient is progressing in each of the three areas. The professional nurse at this time is able to help the patient reach the core of his problem through the closeness provided by the care aspect of nursing. Unfortunately, in today's managed care environment, all too often this stage occurs post-hospitalization, and the patients' access to nursing care is limited.

Five questions have been identified to assist in evaluating the patient's progress toward meeting health goals:

1. Is the patient learning "who he is, where he wants to go, and how he wants to get there"? (Bowar-Ferres, 1975, p. 813)
2. Is the patient learning to understand and explore the feelings that underlie behavior?

3. Is the nurse helping the patient see motivations more clearly?
4. Are the patient's goals congruent with the medical regime? Is the patient successful in meeting the goals?
5. Is the patient physically more comfortable?

METAPARADIGM, RESEARCH, AND PRACTICE WITH CARE, CORE, AND CURE   Hall did not speak directly to each of the concepts in nursing's metaparadigm of human being, health, society, and nursing. However, there is content relevant to each concept in her work. See Table 9-1.

Hall tested her theory through demonstrating its use in a practice setting and conducting quantitative research to evaluate the effectiveness of Loeb Center. This research was conducted at Hall's insistence, in spite of the enthusiastic acceptance of her philosophy by those in the Montefiore health care community (Brown, 1970). This research is evidence that hypotheses can be developed and tested. In addition, the sharing of a report about the Loeb Center in a congressional hearing is evidence of an increase in the general body of knowledge (Loeb Center, 1963). Quantitative methods can be used to test the impact of the use of Hall's theory on length of stay, readmission rates, and other quantitative measures of the outcomes of health care. Qualitative measures could be used to investigate the quality of life achieved by those who received care from those practicing Hall's theory as compared to those who received care in another manner.

After Hall's death in 1969, the Loeb Center continued to function at Montefiore Hospital, under the direction of Genrose Alfano, and served as the primary demonstration of Hall's theory. Loeb Center became a nursing home in 1985; in 2004 the nursing home closed, and the space reverted to acute care.

An electronic search of CINAHL and Medline found a very limited number of articles related to Hall or Loeb Center. One of these discusses Hall's induction into the ANA Hall of Fame (Loose, 1994). Others are those listed in the reference list of this chapter that discuss Loeb Center. A third grouping is discussion by Griffiths (1997) and Griffiths and Willis-Barnett (1998) about nurse-led centers in the United Kingdom.

TABLE 9-1   Hall's Care, Core, Cure Theory and Nursing's Metaparadigm

Metaparadigm Concept	Hall's Care, Core, Cure Theory
Human	Not directly defined. Focus in on the individual, 16 or older, past the acute stage of illness, who is unique, is capable of growth and learning, and is the source of energy and motivation for healing
Health	Inferred to be a state of self-awareness with conscious selection of optimal behaviors
Society/environment	Dealt with in relation to the individual and providing a setting that is conducive to self-development; family is included in the cure circle
Nursing	Participation in the care, core, and cure aspects with other members of the health care team; the major purpose of care is to achieve an interpersonal relationship that will facilitate development of the core

Hall's theory of nursing has several areas that limit its application to general patient care. The first of these areas is the stage of illness. Hall applies her ideas of nursing to a patient who has passed the acute stage of biological stress—that is, the patient who is experiencing the acute stage of illness is not included in Hall's approach to nursing care. However, it is possible to apply the care, core, and cure ideas to the care of those who are acutely ill. The acutely ill individual often needs care in relation to basic needs as well as core awareness of what is going on and, in cure, understanding of the plan of medical care.

A second limiting factor is age. Hall refers only to adult patients in the second stage of their illness, thus eliminating all younger patients. On the basis of this theory, Loeb Center admitted only patients 16 years of age and older. However, it would be possible to apply Hall's theory with younger individuals. Certainly adolescents younger than 16 are capable of seeking self-identity.

A third limiting factor is the description of how to help a person toward self-awareness. The only tool of therapeutic communication Hall discusses is reflection. By inference, all other techniques of therapeutic communication are eliminated. This emphasis on reflection arises from the belief that both the problem and the solution lie in the individual and that the nurse's function is to help the individual find them. But reflection is not always the most effective technique to be used. Other techniques, such as active listening and nonverbal support, may be used to facilitate the development of self-identity.

Fourth, the family is mentioned only in the cure circle. This means that the nursing contact with families is used only in regard to the patient's own medical care. It does not allow for helping a family increase awareness of the family's self and limits the use of the theory to the individual as the unit of care.

Finally, Hall's theory relates only to those who are ill. This would indicate no nursing contact with healthy individuals, families, or communities, and it negates the concept of health maintenance and health care to prevent illness.

Basically, Hall's theory can be readily applied within the confines of the definition of adults past the acute stage of illness. However, this is too confining for a total view of nursing, which includes working with individuals, families, and communities throughout the life cycle and in varying states of health.

However, it should be noted that the nurse who uses Hall's theory functions in a manner similar to the method of assignment that became known as primary nursing. Considering that Hall instituted Loeb Center in the early 1960s, her ideas certainly provided leadership and innovation in nursing practice. She also deserves praise not only for having the courage to create a new environment in which to put her ideas into practice but also for insisting that research be conducted to document the effects of that environment.

PATIENT-CENTERED APPROACHES

Faye Glenn Abdellah

Faye Glenn Abdellah was born in New York City in 1919. She graduated magna cum laude from Fitkin Memorial Hospital School of Nursing (now Ann May School of Nursing) in Neptune, New Jersey, in 1942. She attended Teachers College, Columbia University, New York, New York, and received her B.S. in 1945, M.A. in 1947, and Ed.D.

in 1955. As a new graduate, she taught at Yale. The frustrations that arose from this teaching experience led to the beginnings of her pursuit of the scientific basis of nursing practice (Abdellah, 1998).

Dr. Abdellah was the first nurse and woman to serve as deputy surgeon general. She also served as chief nurse officer for the U.S. Public Health Service (USPHS), Department of Health and Human Services, Washington, D.C. She retired from the USPHS with the rank of rear admiral. In 1993 she became founding dean of the newly formed Graduate School of Nursing, Uniformed Services University of the Health Sciences, Bethesda, Maryland. She is the author of more than 150 publications related to nursing care, education for advanced practice in nursing, health care administration, and nursing research. Some of these have been translated into six languages.

She has been granted 11 honorary doctorates by various institutions, including Case Western Reserve, Cleveland, Ohio; Rutgers, New Brunswick, New Jersey; University of Akron, Ohio; Catholic University of America, Washington, D.C.; and Eastern University, St. Davids, Pennsylvania. These honors recognized her work in nursing research, development of the first nurse scientist training program, expertise in health policy, as well as her outstanding contributions to the health of the nation.

Her international service includes delegation member to the Soviet Union, Yugoslavia, France, and the People's Republic of China; coordinator of the U.S.–Argentina Cooperation in Health and Medicine Research Project; consultant to Portugal for program development for the disabled and the elderly; consultant to Tel Aviv University on long-term care and nursing research; consultant to the Japanese Nursing Association in relation to nursing education and research; and consultant in Australia and New Zealand in relation to nursing home care, nursing education, and research. She has also been a research consultant to the World Health Organization.

Dr. Abdellah is a Charter Fellow of the American Academy of Nursing, has served as this organization's vice president and president, and received its Living Legend Award. She has been recognized by Sigma Theta Tau as a Distinguished Research Fellow and was the recipient of the Excellence in Nursing Award, as well as the first Presidential Award. She was awarded the Allied Signal Award for her groundbreaking research in aging. The Institute of Medicine presented her with the Gustav O. Lienhard Award in recognition of her contributions to the environment and healthier lifestyles. In addition, she has received the following military awards: Surgeon General's Medallion and Medal; two Distinguished Service Medals; Uniformed Services University of the Health Sciences Distinguished Service Medal; Meritorious Service Medal; the Secretary of Department of Health, Education and Welfare Distinguished Service Award; and two Founders Medals from the Association of Military Surgeons of the United States (McFadden, 2000).

PATIENT-CENTERED CARE   In 1955, a subcommittee of the National League for Nursing Committee on Records was charged with developing a meaningful clinical record for professional student nurses. Dr. Abdellah chaired this subcommittee, which soon identified three barriers to its task: the lack of a clear definition of nursing, the current philosophy of nursing education was cherished but not practiced, and nursing education curricula were not patient-centered. The old disease and procedure approach to nursing was deemed to be no longer adequate, and problem solving was identified as a means of meeting patient needs (Abdellah, Beland, Martin, & Matheney, 1960). Using a typology of nursing problems developed in 1953 (Abdellah & Levine, 1954), the original 58 problems were refined to 21 and validated with the assistance of faculty from 40 basic collegiate schools of nursing. This resulted in the publication of *Patient-Centered Approaches to Nursing* in 1960 after at least three research studies over a five-year period.

In this 1960 publication, nursing is described as serving individuals, families, and, thus, society. The basis of nursing is both an art and a science; these mold the "attitudes, intellectual competencies, and technical skills of the individual nurse into the desire and ability to help people, sick or well, cope with their health needs" (Abdellah et al., 1960, p. 34). Nursing may be carried out under general or specific medical direction. As a comprehensive service, nursing includes the following:

1. Recognizing the nursing problems of the patient;
2. Deciding the appropriate courses of action to take in terms of relevant nursing principles;
3. Providing continuous care of the individual's total health needs;
4. Providing continuous care to relieve pain and discomfort and providing immediate security for the individual;
5. Adjusting the total nursing care plan to meet the patient's individual needs;
6. Helping the individual to become more self-directing in attaining or maintaining a healthy state of mind and body;
7. Instructing nursing personnel and family to help the individual do for himself that which he can within his limitations;
8. Helping the individual to adjust to his limitations and emotional problems;
9. Working with allied health professions in planning for optimum health on local, state, national, and international levels; and
10. Carrying out continuous evaluation and research to improve nursing techniques and to develop new techniques to meet the health needs of people. (Abdellah et al., 1960, pp. 24–25)

In 1973, the third listed service, "providing continuous care of the individual's total health needs," was removed from the list (Abdellah, Beland, Martin, & Matheney, 1973).

The 21 Nursing Problems   The 21 nursing problems identified in 1960, after being validated through research, are the following:

Basic to all patients

1. To maintain good hygiene and physical comfort.
2. To promote optimal activity; exercise, rest, and sleep.
3. To promote safety through the prevention of accident, injury, or other trauma and through the prevention of the spread of infection.
4. To maintain good body mechanics and prevent and correct deformities.

Sustenal care needs

5. To facilitate the maintenance of a supply of oxygen to all body cells.
6. To facilitate the maintenance of nutrition of all body cells.
7. To facilitate the maintenance of elimination.
8. To facilitate the maintenance of fluid and electrolyte balance.
9. To recognize the physiological responses of the body to disease conditions—pathological, physiological, and compensatory.

Remedial care needs

10. To facilitate the maintenance of regulatory mechanisms and functions.
11. To facilitate the maintenance of sensory functions.
12. To identify and accept positive and negative expressions, feelings, and reactions.
13. To identify and accept the interrelatedness of emotions and organic illness.
14. To facilitate the maintenance of effective verbal and nonverbal communication.
15. To promote the development of productive interpersonal relationships.
16. To facilitate progress toward achievement of personal spiritual goals.
17. To create and/or maintain a therapeutic environment.
18. To facilitate awareness of self as an individual with varying physical, emotional, and developmental needs.

Restorative care needs

19. To accept the optimum possible goals in the light of limitations, physical and emotional.
20. To use community resources as an aid in resolving problems arising from illness.
21. To understand the role of social problems as influencing factors in the cause of illness. (Abdellah & Levine, 1965, pp. 78–79; Abdellah et al., 1960, pp. 16–17)

These 21 nursing problems focus on the biological, sociological, and psychological needs of the patient in an effort to provide a more meaningful basis for organization of nursing care than the categories of body systems. The most difficult problems were thought to be numbers 12, 14, 15, 17, 18, and 19 (Abdellah et al., 1973). It is of interest that all of these problems fall into the realm of socio-psychological needs and are likely to be covert in nature. The challenge of covert problems is supported in the discussion that such problems are often overlooked or misinterpreted. This discussion includes reference to Florence Nightingale's emphasis on the importance of accurate observations (Abdellah et al., 1960, p. 7).

The patient's health needs may be *overt*, obvious or apparent, or *covert*, hidden or concealed. Because covert problems can be emotional, sociological, and interpersonal in nature, they are often missed or perceived incorrectly. Yet, in many instances, solving the covert problems solves the overt problems as well (Abdellah et al., 1960). Abdellah's interest in dealing with covert problems is apparent in her 1955 dissertation, *Methods of Determining Covert Aspects of Nursing Problems as a Basis for Improved Clinical Teaching*.

It is important to note that there is a potential conflict of interpretation between the title of the book (*Patient-Centered Approaches*) and the developed typology (nursing problems). In an effort to differentiate nursing problems from medical problems, Abdellah says a nursing problem is a condition faced by the patient or patient's family that the nurse, through the performance of professional functions, can assist them to meet (Abdellah et al., 1960). It is possible to interpret Abdellah's use of the term *nursing problems* as more consistent with "nursing functions" or "nursing goals" than with patient-centered problems. This viewpoint could lead to an orientation that is more nursing centered than patient centered (Nicholls & Wessells, 1977). However, while the problems are labeled nursing problems, it is clear that the problems are those being experienced by the patient or family that the nurse can help meet. The problems identify where nursing can help. Note that Abdellah recognized the need to shift from nursing problems to patient outcomes (Abdellah & Levine, 1986). However, there has been no further development of the framework to provide guidance in doing this.

Problem Solving   Quality professional nursing care requires that nurses be able to identify and solve overt and covert nursing problems. These requirements can be met by the problem-solving approach that involves identifying the problem, selecting pertinent data, formulating hypotheses, testing hypotheses through the collection of data, and revising hypotheses when necessary on the basis of conclusions obtained from the data. The assumption underlying the selection of the problem-solving approach was that the correct identification of the patient's nursing problems influences the nurse's judgment in selecting the next steps in solving those problems (Abdellah & Levine, 1986). Problem solving is also consistent with such basic elements of nursing practice supported by Abdellah as observing, reporting, and interpreting the signs and symptoms that comprise the deviations from health and constitute nursing problems and with analyzing the nursing problems and selecting the necessary course of action (Abdellah et al., 1960). Note also that Abdellah advocated the use of the problem-solving process before the nursing process was developed and discussed nursing diagnosis as an independent function of the professional nurse during a time when diagnosis was considered the sole prerogative of the medical practitioner. She defined nursing diagnosis as "the determination of the nature and extent of nursing problems presented by individual patients or families receiving nursing care" (Abdellah et al., 1960, p. 9).

Essential to Abdellah's theory is the correct identification of nursing problems. Abdellah (1957) described the steps involved in this correct identification as learning to know the patient through use of available data, observation of and socialization with the patient, and discussion with other nurses and members of other disciplines; sorting out data that are significant and relevant; making generalizations (comparing the specific data about the patient with that of others with similar nursing problems); identifying the therapeutic plan; testing the generalizations with the patient (leads to further generalizations); validating the patient's conclusions about his problems with the conclusions of the nurse; continuing to observe and evaluate; exploring the patient and family reactions to the therapeutic plan while involving them in the plan; identifying how the nurse feels about the patient's problems; and, finally, discussing and developing an overall plan of nursing care. The nursing skills involved in this process include observation, communication, applying knowledge, teaching patients and families, planning and organizing work, using resource materials and personnel, problem solving to implement and evaluate the plan of care, directing the work of others, therapeutic use of self, and carrying out nursing procedures (Abdellah et al., 1960, pp. 17–19).

Within the practice of nursing, it was anticipated that these 21 problems as broad groupings would encourage generalization from specific patient data to principles to guide nursing care and promote development of the nurse's judgmental ability. Each of the broad nursing problems can be associated with numerous specific overt and covert problems. It was anticipated that the constant relating of the broad basic nursing problems to the specific problems of the individual patient and vice versa would encourage the development of an increased ability to use theory in clinical practice. Thus, a greater understanding of the relationship between theory and practice would strengthen the usefulness of the nursing problems (Abdellah et al., 1960).

Abdellah has suggested that the following criteria might be used to determine the effectiveness of patient-centered care:

1. The patient is able to provide for the satisfaction of his own needs.
2. The nursing care plan makes provision to meet four needs—sustenal care, remedial care, restorative care, and preventive care.
3. The care plan extends beyond the patient's hospitalization and makes provision for continuation of the care at home.
4. The levels of nursing skills provided vary with the individual patient care requirements.
5. The entire care plan is directed at having the patient help himself.
6. The care plan makes provision for involvement of members of the family throughout the hospitalization and after discharge. (Abdellah & Levine, 1965, pp. 77–78)

METAPARADIGM, RESEARCH, AND PRACTICE WITH PATIENT-CENTERED APPROACHES
While Abdellah did not specifically address the concepts in nursing's metaparadigm, some connection can be made to each. See Table 9-2.

This theory was developed through multiple research projects conducted over a five-year period. Testing of the theory in the clinical environment has not been undertaken, possibly because Abdellah's presentations of the nursing problems have focused on nursing education and hospital organization. Research questions and hypotheses generated from the theory would determine the research approach to be used. Abdellah used methodological research to identify the nursing problems of patients (Abdellah & Levine, 1965, p. 490). While Abdellah included discussion of the 21 nursing problems in her research texts written with Levine, she has not extended this particular area of her work. Her later publications focused on advanced practice (Abdellah, 1997), management (Abdellah, 1995), graduate education (Abdellah, 1993), and research (Abdellah 1991a, 1991b, 1991c, 1991d; Abdellah et al., 2005).

Abdellah has indicated that nursing research needs are to "focus on evidence based research . . . identify clinical practice guidelines that identify indicators that measure quality of care . . . and identify methods or instruments that monitor the extent to which actions of health care practitioners conform to practice guidelines, medical

TABLE 9-2   Abdellah's Patient-Centered Approach and Nursing's Metaparadigm

Metaparadigm Concept	Abdellah's Patient-Centered Approach
Human	Characteristics of humans are not identified; the 21 nursing problems cover biological, psychological, and social areas
Health	Not specifically defined, although total health needs and a healthy state of mind and body are included as part of comprehensive nursing service
Society/environment	The focus is on the individual and family; society is served through serving individuals
Nursing	Discussed as a comprehensive service, based on art and science, and aiming to help people cope with health needs

review criteria, or standards of quality, and then point out the policy implications of the research" (Abdellah, 1998, p. 216). These are compatible with investigations using the 21 nursing problems—what evidence is needed that the problems have been solved? What related guidelines indicate quality of care? She also says nursing research needs to be linked to "practice, cost, or policy" as well as to have interdisciplinary and collaborative aspects (Abdellah, 1998, p. 216).

At this time, Abdellah's theory is not in popular use as a field of study. Its uses may be seen more in the organization of teaching content within educational programs, the evaluation of a student's performance for providing total care in the clinical area, and the grouping of patients in clinical settings according to anticipated nursing needs. However, as indicated in her biographical sketch, Abdellah is known internationally for her contributions to nursing and to health policy.

A strength and a limitation are related to research. A major strength of Abdellah's work is that the 21 nursing problems were developed through extensive research—at least three separate research projects over a five-year period. A major limitation is the lack of continued research to link the effectiveness of use of the 21 nursing problems to successful outcomes of nursing care.

Another strength is the driving force behind the development of the 21 nursing problems. Abdellah wanted to move nursing care from a base in medical diagnosis and procedures to a patient-centered base. Interestingly, an approach taken to achieve this was to encourage the use of the 21 nursing problems in shaping the curricula of nursing education programs. In *Patient-Centered Approaches to Nursing*, Matheny discusses application in an associate degree program, Martin discusses application in a diploma program, and Beland discusses application in a bachelor of science program. Abdellah also discusses application in nursing service (Abdellah et al., 1960). While the use of the 21 nursing problems to structure nursing curricula has not been widely documented, the concept of patient-centered care and care of the total person has certainly evolved over the decades since the problems were initially identified.

Another strength can be seen in the emphasis placed on the importance of recognizing and correctly identifying both overt and covert problems. The link to Nightingale's emphasis on the value of careful observations only enhances the significance of this idea. Abdellah made a major contribution in reminding us to look below the surface—to seek out the covert problems since they are often the cause of the overt problems.

The label of "nursing problems" is a limitation. Labeling the list of 21 problems as nursing problems tends to lead the reader to the belief that Abdellah's work is nursing centered when she stated she was seeking to move nursing to being patient centered. It would have been helpful had she used other terminology or explained more clearly how this label relates to patient-centered care.

Also, especially in care settings where a nurse has very limited time to spend with each patient, the use of the 21 nursing problems could further fractionalize care. This could happen if the focus is placed only on a problem or a series of problems rather than on the total person. Abdellah's intention was for a total person approach. Having a list of discrete problems and using this list in time-constrained circumstances could easily lead to dealing with parts rather than the whole. Overall, the strengths of this work outweigh the limitations. This is particularly true when the limitations are taken into careful consideration; overcoming the limitations is within the capacity of the individual nurse.

PRESCRIPTIVE THEORY

Ernestine Wiedenbach

Ernestine Wiedenbach was born in Germany in August 1900 to an affluent family, the fourth of four daughters. Her family returned to the United States when she was around eight years old. She graduated from Wellesley College, Wellesley, Massachusetts, in 1922 with a liberal arts degree. Her interest in nursing had been stimulated by the care given her ailing grandmother and the stories told by a medical student friend of her sister. Much to the distress of her family, she enrolled in the Post Graduate Hospital School of Nursing, New York, New York (Nickel, Gesse, & MacLaren, 1992). She was expelled from this program after she served as the spokesperson for student grievances. Adelaide Nutting arranged for Wiedenbach to continue her nursing preparation at the Johns Hopkins School of Nursing, Baltimore, Maryland, but only after she agreed that she would neither organize nor encourage any student dissent. She received her nursing diploma from Johns Hopkins in 1925. Since she held a bachelor's degree she was offered supervisory positions after graduation and worked at Johns Hopkins and at Bellevue in New York City. She attended night classes and received her master's degree and a certificate in public health nursing from Teachers College, Columbia University, New York, New York, in 1934. For a time she worked with the Association for Improving Conditions of the Poor from the Henry Street Settlement, New York City. She then became a professional writer with the Nursing Information Bureau of the *American Journal of Nursing,* where she also worked to prepare nurses to enter World War II. She was unable to serve overseas because of a minor cardiac problem. Interested in returning to patient care, Wiedenbach obtained a certificate in nurse midwifery from the Maternity Center Association in New York in 1946. She practiced as a nurse midwife and a public health nurse and taught in a number of schools of nursing. She retired as Associate Professor Emeritus from Yale University School of Nursing, New Haven, Connecticut, where she had been director of the graduate program in maternal-newborn health nursing. She served as a visiting professor at California State University, Los Angeles, and at the College of Nursing, University of Florida, Gainesville. In 1978, she received the Hattie Hemschemeyer Award from the American College of Nurse Midwives for exceptional achievements in her professional life (Burst, 1979). Ernestine Wiedenbach died in March 1998 in Florida.

WIEDENBACH'S PRESCRIPTIVE THEORY   Ernestine Wiedenbach, a progressive nursing leader, first published *Family-Centered Maternity Nursing* in 1958. It is of interest that in this book she recommended that babies be in hospital rooms with their mothers rather than in a central nursery. This innovative concept was not widely implemented until 20 years later. In 1964 she wrote *Clinical Nursing—A Helping Art,* in which she described her ideas about nursing as a "concept and philosophy" derived from 40 years of nursing experience. She credited Patricia James, James Dickoff, and Ida Orlando Pelletier as great influences in her nursing writing and theory development. In collaboration with Dickoff and James, she presented the symposium and coauthored "Theory in a Practice Discipline" (1968a, 1968b). In 1970 Wiedenbach defined the essentials of her prescriptive theory in "Nurses' Wisdom in Nursing Theory."

According to Wiedenbach (1964), nursing is nurturing and caring for someone in a motherly fashion—that care is given in the immediate present and can be given by any caring person. Nursing wisdom is acquired through meaningful experience. Nursing is a helping service that is rendered with compassion, skill, and understanding to those in need of care, counsel, and confidence in the area of health (Wiedenbach, 1977). Sensitivity alerts the nurse to an awareness of inconsistencies in a situation that might signify a problem. It is a key factor in assisting the nurse to identify the patient's need for help. The nurse's beliefs and values regarding reverence for the gift of life, the worth of the individual, and the aspirations of each human being determine the quality of the nursing care. The nurse's purpose in nursing represents a professional commitment (Wiedenbach, 1970).

Wiedenbach (1964) states that the characteristics of a professional person that are essential for the professional nurse include the following (italics added):

1. *Clarity* of purpose.
2. *Mastery* of skills and knowledge essential for fulfilling the purpose.
3. *Ability* to establish and sustain purposeful working relationships with others, both professional and nonprofessional individuals.
4. *Interest* in advancing knowledge in the area of interest and in creating new knowledge.
5. *Dedication* to furthering the good of mankind rather than to self-aggrandizement. (p. 2)

The practice of nursing comprises a wide variety of services, each directed toward the attainment of one of its three components: (1) *identification* of the patient's need for help, (2) *ministration* of the help needed, and (3) *validation* that the help provided was indeed helpful to the patient (Wiedenbach, 1977). Within Wiedenbach's (1964) "identification of the patient's need for help," she presents three principles of helping: (1) the principle of inconsistency/consistency, (2) the principle of purposeful perseverance, and (3) the principle of self-extension. The *principle of inconsistency/ consistency* refers to the assessment of the patient to determine some action, word, or appearance that is different from that expected—that is, something out of the ordinary for this patient. It is important for the nurse to observe the patient astutely and then critically analyze her observations. The *principle of purposeful perseverance* is based on the nurse's sincere desire to help the patient. The nurse needs to strive to continue her efforts to identify and meet the patient's need for help in spite of difficulties she encounters while seeking to use her resources and capabilities effectively and with sensitivity. The *principle of self-extension* recognizes that each nurse has limitations that are both personal and situational. It is important that she recognize when these limitations are reached and that she seek help from others, including through prayer.

Prescriptive Theory   Theory may be described as a system of conceptualizations invented to serve some purpose. Prescriptive theory (a situation-producing theory) may be described as one that conceptualizes both a desired situation and the prescription by which it is to be brought about. Thus, a prescriptive theory directs action toward an explicit goal. As shown in Figure 9-2, Wiedenbach's (1969) prescriptive theory is made up of three factors, or concepts (italics added):

1. The *central purpose* that the practitioner recognizes as essential to the particular discipline.
2. The *prescription* for the fulfillment of the central purpose.
3. The *realities in the immediate situation* that influence the fulfillment of the central purpose. (p. 2)

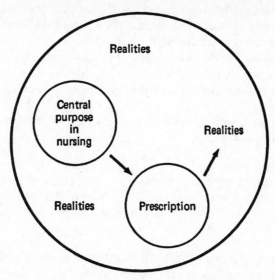

FIGURE 9-2   Wiedenbach's prescriptive theory. (*Adapted from Wiedenbach, E., (1969).* Meeting the realities in clinical teaching. *New York: Springer, p. x. Used with permission.*)

The Central Purpose: The nurse's central purpose in nursing defines the quality of health she desires to affect or sustain in her patient and specifies what she recognizes to be her special responsibility in caring for the patient (Wiedenbach, 1970). This central purpose (or commitment) is based on the individual nurse's philosophy. Wiedenbach (1964) states,

> Purpose and philosophy are, respectively, goal and guide of clinical nursing. . . . Purpose—that which the nurse wants to accomplish through what she does—is the overall goal toward which she is striving, and so is constant. It is her reason for being and doing. . . . Philosophy, an attitude toward life and reality that evolves from each nurse's beliefs and code of conduct, motivates the nurse to act, guides her thinking about what she is to do and influences her decisions. It stems from both her culture and subculture, and is an integral part of her. It is personal in character, unique to each nurse, and expressed in her *way* of nursing. Philosophy underlies purpose, and purpose reflects philosophy. (p. 13)

Wiedenbach (1970) identifies three essential components for a nursing philosophy: (1) a reverence for the gift of life; (2) a respect for the dignity, worth, autonomy, and individuality of each human being; and (3) a resolution to act dynamically in relation to one's beliefs. Any of these concepts might be further developed. However, Wiedenbach (1964, 1970) emphasizes the second in her work, formulating the following beliefs about the individual:

1. Human beings are endowed with unique potential to develop within themselves the resources that enable them to maintain and sustain themselves.

2. Human beings basically strive toward self-direction and relative independence and desire not only to make the best use of their capabilities and potentialities but also to fulfill their responsibilities.
3. Human beings need stimulation in order to make the best use of their capabilities and realize their self-worth.
4. Whatever individuals do represents their best judgment at the moment of doing it.
5. Self-awareness and self-acceptance are essential to the individual's sense of integrity and self-worth.

Thus, the central purpose is a concept the nurse has thought through—one she has put into words, believes in, and accepts as a standard against which to measure the value of her action to the patient. It is based on her philosophy and suggests the nurse's reason for being—the mission she believes is hers to accomplish (Wiedenbach, 1970).

The Prescription: Once the nurse has identified her own philosophy and recognizes that the patient has autonomy and individuality, she can work *with* the individual to develop a *prescription* or plan for his care. A *prescription* is a directive to activity (Wiedenbach, 1969). It "specifies both the *nature of the action* that will most likely lead to fulfillment of the nurse's central purpose and the *thinking process* that determines it" (Wiedenbach, 1970, p. 1059). A prescription may indicate the broad general action appropriate to implementation of the basic concepts as well as suggest the kind of behavior needed to carry out these actions in accordance with the central purpose. These actions may be voluntary or involuntary. Voluntary action is an intended response, whereas involuntary action is an unintended response.

A prescription is a directive to at least three kinds of voluntary action: (1) *mutually understood and agreed upon* action ("the practitioner has . . . evidence that the recipient understands the implications of the intended action and is psychologically, physically and/or physiologically receptive to it"), (2) *recipient-directed* action ("the recipient of the action essentially directs the way it is to be carried out"), and (3) *practitioner-directed* action ("the practitioner carries out the action . . .") (Wiedenbach, 1969, p. 3). Once the nurse has formulated a central purpose and has accepted it as a personal commitment, she not only has established the prescription for her nursing but also is ready to implement it (Wiedenbach, 1970).

The Realities: When the nurse has determined her central purpose and has developed the prescription, she must then consider the realities of the situation in which she is to provide nursing care. Realities consist of all factors—physical, physiological, psychological, emotional and spiritual—that are at play in a situation in which nursing actions occur at any given moment. Wiedenbach (1970) defines the five realities as (1) the agent, (2) the recipient, (2) the goal, (4) the means, and (5) the framework.

The *agent*, who is the practicing nurse or her delegate, is characterized by personal attributes, capacities, capabilities, and, most important, commitment and competence in nursing. As the agent, the nurse is the propelling force that moves her practice toward its goal. In the course of this goal-directed movement, she may engage in innumerable acts called forth by her encounter with actual or discrepant factors and situations within the realities of which she herself is a part (Wiedenbach, 1967). The agent or nurse has the following four basic responsibilities:

1. To reconcile her assumptions about the realities . . . with her central purpose.
2. To specify the objectives of her practice in terms of behavioral outcomes that are realistically attainable.
3. To practice nursing in accordance with her objectives.
4. To engage in related activities which contribute to her self-realization and to the improvement of nursing practice. (Wiedenbach, 1970, p. 1060)

The *recipient*, the patient, is characterized by personal attributes, problems, capacities, aspirations, and, most important, the ability to cope with the concerns or problems being experienced (Wiedenbach, 1967). The patient is the recipient of the nurse's actions or the one on whose behalf the action is taken. The patient is vulnerable, is dependent on others for help, and risks losing individuality, dignity, worth, and autonomy (Wiedenbach, 1970).

The *goal* is the desired outcome the nurse wishes to achieve. The goal is the end result to be attained by nursing action. The stipulation of an activity's goal gives focus to the nurse's action and implies her reason for taking it (Wiedenbach, 1970).

The *means* comprises the activities and devices through which the practitioner is enabled to attain her goal. The means includes skills, techniques, procedures, and devices that may be used to facilitate nursing practice. The nurse's way of giving treatments, of expressing concern, and of using the means available is individual and is determined by her central purpose and the prescription (Wiedenbach, 1970).

The *framework* consists of the human, environmental, professional, and organizational facilities that not only make up the context within which nursing is practiced but also constitute its currently existing limits (Wiedenbach, 1967). The framework is composed of all the extraneous factors and facilities in the situation that affect the nurse's ability to obtain the desired results. It is a conglomerate of "objects, existing or missing, such as policies, setting, atmosphere, time of day, humans, and happenings that may be current, past, or anticipated" (Wiedenbach, 1970, p. 1061).

The realities offer uniqueness to every situation. The success of professional nursing practice is dependent on them. Unless the realities are recognized and dealt with, they may prevent the achievement of the goal.

The concepts of central purpose, prescription, and realities are interdependent in Wiedenbach's theory of nursing. The nurse develops a prescription for care that is based on her central purpose, which is implemented in the realities of the situation.

Wiedenbach's Conceptualization of Nursing Practice   According to Wiedenbach (1967), nursing practice is an art in which the nursing action is based on the principles of helping. Nursing action may be thought of as consisting of the following four distinct kinds of actions:

- Reflex (spontaneous)
- Conditioned (automatic)
- Impulsive (impulsive)
- Deliberate (responsible)

Nursing as a practice discipline is goal directed. The nature of the nursing act is based on thought. The nurse thinks through the kind of results she wants, gears her actions to obtain those results, and then accepts responsibility for the acts and the outcome of those acts (Wiedenbach, 1970). Since nursing requires thought, it can be considered a deliberate responsible action.

Nursing practice has three components: (1) identification of the patient's need for help, (2) ministration of the help needed, and (3) validation that the action taken was helpful to the patient (Wiedenbach, 1977). Within the identification component, there are four distinct steps. First, the nurse observes the patient, looking for an inconsistency between the expected behavior of the patient and the apparent behavior. Second, she attempts to clarify what the inconsistency means. Third, she determines the cause of the inconsistency. Finally, she validates with the patient that her help is needed.

The second component is the ministration of the help needed. In ministering to her patient, the nurse may give advice or information, make a referral, apply a comfort measure, or carry out a therapeutic procedure. Should the patient become uncomfortable with what is being done, the nurse will need to identify the cause and, if necessary, make an adjustment in the plan of action.

The third component is validation. After help has been ministered, the nurse validates that the actions were indeed helpful. Evidence must come from the patient that the purpose of the nursing actions has been fulfilled (Wiedenbach, 1964).

Wiedenbach (1977) views the nursing process essentially as an internal personalized mechanism. As such, it is influenced by the nurse's culture, purpose in nursing, knowledge, wisdom, sensitivity, and concern. In Wiedenbach's (1977) nursing process (see Figure 9-3), she identifies seven levels of awareness: sensation, perception, assumption, realization, insight, design, and decision. Wiedenbach's nursing process begins with an activating situation. This situation exists among the realities and serves as a stimulus to arouse the nurse's consciousness. This consciousness arousal leads to a subjective interpretation of the first three levels, which are defined as *sensation* (experienced sensory impression), *perception* (the interpretation of a sensory impression), and *assumption* (the meaning the nurse attaches to the perception). These three levels of awareness are obtained through the focus of the nurse's attention on the stimulus; they are intuitive rather than cognitive and may initiate an involuntary response. For example, a nurse enters a patient's room and states, "My, it's hot in here!" She immediately goes to the thermostat and sets it to a lower temperature. The *sensation* is the room temperature. The *perception* is "It feels hot." The *assumption* is "If I am hot, then the patient must be hot." The involuntary response is to adjust the thermostat.

Progressing from intuition to cognition, the nurse's actions become voluntary rather than involuntary. The next four levels of awareness occur in the voluntary phase: *realization* (in which the nurse begins to validate the assumption previously made about the patient's behavior), *insight* (which includes joint planning and additional knowledge about the cause of the problem), *design* (the plan of action decided on by the nurse and confirmed by the patient), and *decision* (the nurse's performance of a responsible action) (Wiedenbach, 1977).

To continue with the previous example, the nurse asks, "Are you too warm?" and the patient replies, "No, I'm not. I have felt cold since I washed my hair." The nurse responds, "I will readjust the thermostat and get you a blanket." The patient agrees, "That would be wonderful!" The nurse readjusts the thermostat and gets a blanket for the patient.

The *realization* is the validation of the patient's perception of temperature comfort. The *insight* is the additional information that the patient had washed his or her hair. The *design* is the plan to readjust the thermostat and get a blanket as confirmed by the patient. The *decision* is the nurse readjusts the thermostat and gets a blanket for the patient.

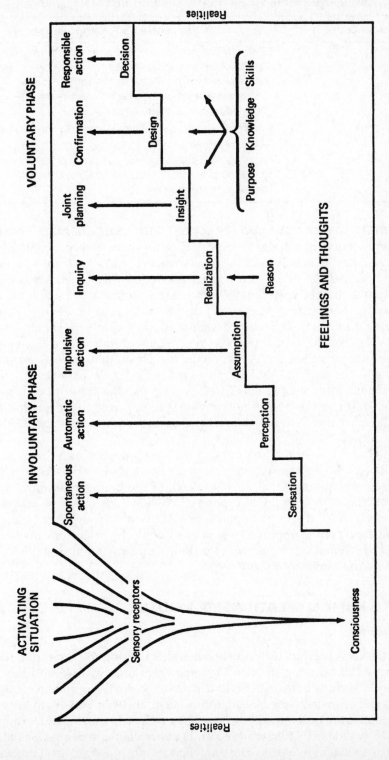

FIGURE 9-3 Conceptualization of the nursing process. *(Reproduced from Clausen, J. P. et al. (1977). Maternity nursing today. New York: McGraw-Hill, p. 43. Used with permission.)*

TABLE 9-3   Wiedenbach's Prescriptive Theory and Nursing's Metaparadigm

Metaparadigm Concept	Wiedenbach's Prescriptive Theory
Human	The individual possesses unique potential, strives toward self-direction, and needs stimulation; does what represents personal best judgment at the moment; needs self-awareness and self-acceptance for integrity and self-worth
Health	Does not define; accepts WHO definition
Society/environment	Incorporated into the realities—especially the framework
Nursing	A clinical discipline and a practice discipline designed to produce explicit desired results; a helping process designed to extend or restore the patient's ability to cope with the demands of the situation

METAPARADIGM, RESEARCH, AND PRACTICE WITH WIEDENBACH'S PRESCRIPTIVE THEORY   While Wiedenbach did not speak directly to the four concepts in nursing's metaparadigm, she did include all of the concepts in her work. See Table 9-3 for examples.

While little research has been reported, Wiedenbach's theory has been tested using qualitative methods. Trefz (1999) addressed nurses' satisfaction in relation to patient teaching. Gustafson (1988) used naturalistic inquiry to identify behaviors of women during the first stage of labor that signaled a need for help. Thompson (1998) incorporated Wiedenbach's central purpose in her study of staff nurses' lived experiences in relating to student nurses in clinical practice and found that the expectations (central purpose) of both the staff and student nurses influenced the experience.

A potential limitation of Wiedenbach's work is that the prescription is determined by the nurse. The theory itself does not provide specific direction for action in any given situation. The nurse must have developed enough self-knowledge to be able to identify her central purpose.

Although it is one of the first nursing theories proposed as a theory rather than being developed with another primary purpose, Wiedenbach's prescriptive theory has not been very contagious. An electronic search of the literature identified a limited number of articles with very limited recent discussion. One article by Carlson, Kotze, and Van Rooyen (2005) discusses application of Wiedenbach's work for theory generation. A major aspect of the importance of Wiedenbach's theory historically is that it was intentionally developed as a framework for clinical nursing practice—both for the practitioner and for the teacher of practitioners.

HUMAN-TO-HUMAN RELATIONSHIP MODEL

Joyce Travelbee

Joyce Travelbee was born in 1926. She obtained her nursing diploma from the Charity Hospital School of Nursing in New Orleans, Louisiana, in 1946 and her B.S.N. in education in 1956 from Louisiana State University, New Orleans. She completed her M.S.N. at Yale University, New Haven, Connecticut, in 1959. Initially in her career she worked in psychiatric nursing and then taught psychiatric nursing at DePaul Hospital Affiliate in New Orleans while working on her baccalaureate degree. She also taught psychiatric nursing at Charity Hospital School of Nursing; at Louisiana State

University, Baton Rouge; and at New York University, New York City, and was an associate professor at the University of Mississippi Medical Center's School of Nursing in Jackson. She served as the project director at Hotel Dieu School of Nursing in New Orleans and was the director of graduate education, School of Nursing, Louisiana State University Medical Center, New Orleans. Later, she worked as a nursing consultant at the Veterans Administration Hospital in Gulfport, Mississippi.

Travelbee was a progressive thinker. In 1949 she proposed that obstetrical care should include natural childbirth, prenatal instruction, the father's participation in birth, and rooming-in. In her 1966 text, Travelbee recognized that the prevention of illness or disease would need to become a priority area for health care and that the future would bring about "well-adult" clinics. She recognized that we in America must reduce admission rates to hospitals and increase our health teaching while implementing measures to conserve health and control symptoms of illness. She also emphasized that we must assist others to find meaning in illness as we support patients' acts of self-denial and sacrifice in order to preserve health. This concept has greatly supported the hospice movement. Another clear example of her forward thinking was demonstrated in her 1969 statement that there must be a "competency in nursing practice . . . [which] cannot be developed, much less improved without a continual appraisal of one's nursing intervention" (p. 44). Joyce Travelbee died in 1973, at the age of 47, as she was just beginning her doctoral studies.

HUMAN-TO-HUMAN RELATIONSHIP MODEL   Travelbee (1963a, 1963b, 1964) first published her concepts of sympathy, empathy, and rapport in the early 1960s, followed by *Interpersonal Aspects of Nursing* in 1966 and 1971. She also published *Intervention in Psychiatric Nursing: Process in the One-to-One Relationship* in 1969, with the second edition edited by Doona in 1979. Travelbee, like other early nursing theorists, focuses on nurse–patient relationships, patient perceptions, and nursing as a process. In her works, Travelbee acknowledges the influence of Viktor Frankl, Frieda Fromm-Reichmann, M. Eunice Lyle, and Catherine Norris as well as nursing theorists Ida Jean Orlando, Lydia Hall, Myra Levine, Faye Abdellah, Virginia Henderson, Dorothy Johnson, Hildegard Peplau, Martha Rogers, Ernestine Wiedenbach, and Florence Nightingale.

Purpose of Nursing   Travelbee (1971) defines nursing as "an interpersonal process whereby the professional nurse practitioner assists an individual, family, or community to prevent, or cope with the experience of illness and suffering and, if necessary, to find meaning in these experiences" (p. 7). She also discusses finding meaning in illness in 1972. The purpose of nursing is achieved through the establishment of a human-to-human relationship. The nursing needs of the individual, family, or community are met by a nurse who possesses and uses a disciplined intellectual approach to problems combined with the therapeutic use of self. The *purpose of nursing* represents a goal since many persons require continuous assistance in coping with the stress of illness and suffering. The need for assistance may be met temporarily, and another need may emerge. Therefore, the purpose of nursing is an unchanging overall objective and the terminus of all nursing endeavor. Professional nurses who work in any setting have the opportunity to perform two major functions of nursing that are inseparable:

1. To assist individuals and families and communities to prevent or cope with the stress of illness and suffering and
2. To assist individuals, families and communities to find meaning in illness and suffering if this be necessary. (p. 22)

These functions suggest appropriate nursing activities are carried out by the professional nurse practitioner who has the educational background and skill and understanding needed to perform the functions in an effective, competent, intelligent, tactful, and creative manner.

Disciplined Intellectual Approach   Professional nursing requires a *disciplined intellectual approach* that provides a logical method to approach nursing problems, which Travelbee (1971) believes should be learned in a collegiate school of nursing. To use a disciplined intellectual approach, the nurse must think logically, reflect, reason, deliberate, validate, analyze, and synthesize. Travelbee contends that nursing is composed of both cognitive and affective components. The nurse must know technical, scientific information from the natural, physical, biological, behavioral, nursing, and medical sciences as well as be able to apply information in a logical, caring manner. The nurse possesses a body of specialized knowledge and has the ability to use this knowledge for the purpose of assisting other human beings to prevent illness, regain health, or maintain the highest maximal degree of health. This requires a broad, general educational background in the humanities as well as in the sciences.

The professional nurse is an individual who has been irrevocably changed as a result of her specialized knowledge and education. She has learned a body of scientific knowledge and has the ability to use it. She has developed new strengths, but, more important, she has been confronted with the vulnerability of the human being. In practice the professional nurse uses a disciplined intellectual approach in combination with the therapeutic use of self. Both abilities are equally important.

Therapeutic Use of Self   The *therapeutic use of self* is the "ability to use one's personality consciously and in full awareness in an attempt to establish relatedness and to structure nursing intervention" (Travelbee, 1971, p. 19). This requires self-insight, self-understanding, and understanding of the dynamics of human behavior; an ability to interpret one's own behavior as well as the behavior of others; and the ability to intervene effectively in nursing situations. The therapeutic use of self involves consciously using one's personality and knowledge to effect change in the patient. Nursing is a service initiated for the purpose of effecting change. A nurse must be able to identify needed changes and be able to bring about change in a purposeful, thoughtful manner. To use oneself effectively as a change agent or to intervene effectively in the nurse–patient situation, it is essential to know how one's behavior affects others. Change is therapeutic when it alleviates the patient's distress.

Travelbee (1971) indicates the therapeutic use of self implies the use of reasoning and intellect; it is both an art and a science, and it requires discipline, self-insight, reasoning as well as empathy, and logic as well as compassion. Emotions and feelings must be guided by but not suppressed by intellect. The therapeutic use of self implies an educated heart and an educated mind and is not to be confused with kindly feelings. It must be synthesized with a disciplined intellectual approach over time, in the process of becoming, and is ultimately commitment and affirmation. It is the role of the professional school of nursing to help students think through ideas about inevitable situations, to assist students to understand the human condition, and to learn how to establish a helping nurse–patient relationship.

Human-to-Human Relationships   The purpose of nursing is achieved through the establishment of a *nurse–patient relationship*, an experience or a series of experiences between the nurse and patient. Travelbee (1971) identifies the patient as an individual in need of the services of the nurse. Every interaction between nurse and patient can be a step toward a relationship, but it is important to note that there is a difference between a nurse–patient interaction and a nurse–patient relationship. Travelbee emphasizes that as the nurse–patient relationship develops, there is a dynamic interchange that includes both verbal and nonverbal exchanges. As a process, it is a happening or a series of happenings between a nurse, an individual, or a group of individuals. This nursing situation is dynamic and fluid in character, with continuous movement, activity, and change, an experience in time and space, continually evolving and becoming. There is an ebb and flow of influence and counter influence from one to the other, the nurse influencing the patient and in turn being influenced by the patient. With each interaction there is growth, a change, and a progression in the relationship.

A nurse sustains, supports, and encourages the ill individual. By her words or behavior, she imparts confidence and the assurance that he will recover. Kindness and good intentions are important, but neither will compensate for a lack of knowledge or the ability to apply this knowledge. Travelbee (1971) asserts the nurse must communicate to the patient that he is not alone. As the nurse confronts illness, suffering, and death, she must first confront her own personal vulnerability. In this process, she absorbs certain beliefs and value systems and develops a nursing conscience—that is, the nurse experiences guilt if she has not fulfilled her responsibilities.

Travelbee also recognizes the importance of the family for the ill individual. She states, "If a nurse could remember that whenever she assists a family member, whenever she encourages or supports him, talks with him, is considerate of him and performs small acts of kindness, she is assisting the patient. If she could remember this, then perhaps relatives would be accorded the consideration which is due them" (1971, p. 188). Travelbee believed that nursing is in need of a humanistic revolution—a return to focus on the "caring" function of the nurse—in caring for and caring about—a reestablishment of the relatedness with the human beings called patients.

A relationship does not "just happen"; it is deliberately and consciously planned for by the nurse (Doona, 1979). According to Travelbee (1971), "The establishment of a nurse–patient relationship and the experience that is rapport, is the terminus of all nursing endeavor" (p. 150). In order for the nurse–patient relationship to develop and to move to the ultimate, the rapport phase, or Phase 5 (see Figure 9-4), the nurse and patient must move through four preceding phases:

1. The phase of the original encounter
2. The phase of emerging identities
3. The phase of empathy
4. The phase of sympathy

The phases leading to the establishment of a nurse–patient relationship are described by Travelbee (1971) as follows:

1. *Phase of the Original Encounter:*   In this phase, the patient and nurse usually view each other as "nurse" and "patient"—with little or no recognition of uniqueness. During this phase each observes and develops inferences and value judgments about the other. Feelings that are aroused in the interaction are a result of the inferences developed. The judgments and inferences are triggered by the perception of interpersonal cues and by the verbal and nonverbal communication. These first impressions tend to be determined by the background experiences of the individuals involved. Distortions may occur. In this phase, both the nurse and the patient are

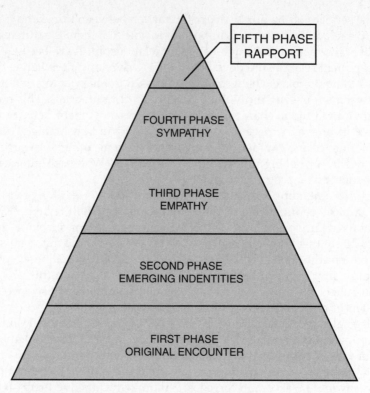

FIGURE 9-4   Phases of Travelbee's human-to-human relationship.

stereotyped and categorized. Travelbee (1969) recognizes that within the psychiatric nursing setting, the time for termination should be discussed with the patient during this phase. However, this limit setting may be helpful for patients in all settings to assist them to establish some boundaries of what to expect from their nurse.

2. *Phase of Emerging Identities:*   Both the nurse and the patient begin to establish a bond as they start to appreciate the uniqueness of another person. Similarities and dissimilarities are emerging and being recognized. The critical requirement in this phase is that the nurse must be able to transcend self to some extent. Inability to progress through this phase is exemplified in superficial types of nurse–patient interaction and by the semihelpful nurse–patient interaction. The nurse must become aware of how she is perceiving the other individual and assess similarities and differences between herself and the patient.

3. *Phase of Empathy:*   As the nurse and patient move into this phase, a conscious, almost instantaneous process occurs in which there is a sharper separation of identity, the uniqueness of each individual is more clearly perceived, the ability to transcend self is increased, and the likenesses and differences between nurse and patient become more apparent. Empathy is the ability to share in and to comprehend the momentary psychological state of another individual. It allows one individual to see through the outward behavior of another, to accurately sense that person's inner experience at a given point in time, and to comprehend the meaning and relevance of the thoughts and feelings of that individual.

Empathy is based on the similarity between two individuals and on the desire to comprehend or understand the other person. This comprehension is desirable because it helps us predict that individual's behavior and to perceive accurately his thinking and feeling. However, empathy is essentially a neutral process; it does not necessarily imply that a person takes action on the basis of the comprehension that has been gained (Travelbee, 1964).

4. *Phase of Sympathy:*   Travelbee (1971) describes sympathy as a basic urge, desire, or compulsion to alleviate another human's distress. Sympathy is warmth and kindness, a specific expression of compassion, a caring quality experienced on a feeling level and communicated by one human being to another. It is a predisposition, an attitude, a type of thinking and feeling characterized by deep personal interest and concern for one individual human being by an authentic human being. Sympathy is much more than being courteous and cannot be feigned. To sympathize is to give part of ourselves to others and, in the giving and sharing, to become vulnerable (Travelbee, 1964). Sympathy requires an act of courage because with feeling and the expression of sympathy may come pain—this is especially true if one is unable to relieve the distress of the other. The nurse then must take a risk—the risk that she, herself, may be hurt if the other human cannot get well or become cured or if his stress in the situation cannot be alleviated.

Sympathetic persons are authentic. They assist others not because it is assigned but because they are motivated by the compassion that underlies and is a fundamental element of sympathy. This transmission of caring may be nonverbal—by look or glance or gesture or in the manner by which a nurse performs her physical care. Sympathy may affect the physiological as well as the psychological well-being of another. When one experiences sympathy, another human being enters into and shares distress, thus relieving the individual's burden of carrying it alone. It is as though one is saying, "I will walk the walk with you." In and through that caring, this emotional support can sustain another human being in his time of crisis.

5. *Phase of Rapport:*   Rapport is that which is experienced when the nurse and patient have progressed through the four preceding phases and the establishment of a nurse–patient relationship. Rapport is a dynamic, fluctuating and ever-changing process. As such, it does not just happen; it grows. Rapport is a happening, an experience or a series of experiences undergone simultaneously between two persons (the nurse and the patient) relating as human being to human being. Rapport is the ability to truly care for and about others—to translate the quality of caring into action in nursing situations.

Rapport is composed of a cluster of interrelated thoughts, feelings, and attitudes and interest in and concern for others being transmitted or communicated by one human being to another through intelligent and creative actions. In order to achieve rapport it is necessary that the actions initiated by the nurse are consistent to alleviate the patient's distress. Rapport is bound and enmeshed into the nurse's philosophy of life; it is a part of her value system. Rapport is not only something a nurse has but also something she is. A nurse is able to establish rapport because she possesses the necessary knowledge and skills required to assist people and because she is able to perceive, to respond to, and to appreciate the uniqueness of the human being who is the patient. An outcome of rapport is that both the nurse and the patient grow as human beings as a result of this experience.

The purpose of all these activities is to assist the individual or family to prevent or cope with the experience of illness and suffering, to regain health, or to maintain the highest optimal level of health possible.

Communication Process   Communication with ill persons is one of the primary methods by which nurses accomplish the goals of nursing intervention. The skillful use of communication is essential if the goals of nursing interventions are to be accomplished (Travelbee, 1969). Every interaction between nurse and patient can be a step toward a relationship, but it is important to remember that there is a difference between a nurse–patient interaction and a nurse–patient relationship. "Everything the nurse says and does for and with patients helps to fulfill the purpose of nursing" (Travelbee, 1971, p. 119). The skills of communication are learned as the nurse learns the disciplined approach and the therapeutic use of self.

Communication is a process that enables the nurse to establish a nurse–patient relationship. Travelbee (1971) defines communication as the sending and receiving of messages by means of symbols, words (spoken or written), signs, gestures, and other nonverbal means. For communication to take place, the message must be sent, received, and understood by both sender and receiver (Travelbee, 1969). Nurses must know if communication is taking place in nursing situations—if messages have been understood by all concerned.

Communication abilities are interdependent. These communication skills may be divided into general abilities, or those needed by all educated individuals, and specific abilities, or those having implications for nursing situations. General abilities would include (1) the ability to read, comprehend, and interpret what was read and then to apply the knowledge gained through reading; (2) the ability to express oneself in writing, using correct spelling and grammar; (3) the ability to express oneself in speaking, to speak clearly and concisely with and not at or to others and to use appropriate vocabulary and to speak with others at their level of understanding; and (4) the ability to listen, hear, and interpret accurately both the verbal and the nonverbal communication of others. Specific abilities required by nurses would include (1) the ability to observe and interpret observations—to generalize, to develop valid inferences, to validate inferences, to plan nursing interventions; (2) the ability to direct or guide the nurse–patient interaction to accomplish goals and objectives; (3) the ability to ascertain if communication is occurring in the interpersonal process; (4) the ability to know when to speak and when to be silent; (5) the ability to proceed at the patient's pace; and (6) the ability to evaluate the nurse–patient interaction to determine if goals were achieved and to plan further interventions if needed (Travelbee, 1971).

Communication techniques refer to various devices or methods, used consciously and intentionally in interactions. Travelbee (1971) encourages the nurse to use any communication technique that she may need to explore and understand the meaning of the patient's communication. She identifies these techniques as those that include open-ended comments or questions, reflection, the sharing of perceptions, and the deliberate use of clichés. Factors that influence the communication process include (1) the perceptions, thoughts, and feelings of the sender/receiver immediately prior to the message transmission; (2) the relationship between sender/receiver; (3) the intention (s) of the sender; (4) the content of the message; (5) the context in which the communication takes place; (6) the manner of the transmission; and (7) the effect of the message on the receiver (Travelbee, 1969). She recognizes that breakdowns in nurse–patient communication may occur and that the major causes include failure to perceive the patient as a human being, failure to recognize levels of meaning, failure to listen, use of value statements without reflection, use of automatic responses, failure to interpret a message correctly, failure to focus on the ill person's problems, the nurse talking too much or too little, failure to interrupt when it is indicated, ineffective reassurance, and failure to adapt communication techniques to the situation.

Assisting Patients to Find Meaning in Illness and Suffering   Nursing has an advantage over other health professions in that a nurse has unlimited access to patients and is present when patients are undergoing the stress of illness. Travelbee (1971) asserts that the nurse cannot know how the patient perceives his illness until she helps him clarify the meanings he attaches to his condition. Any nursing action designed to assist the patient to arrive at meaning will be effective only to the extent that the nurse truly believes that meaning can be found. The quality of nursing care given any patient is determined by the nurse's beliefs about illness, suffering, and death. The spiritual values of the nurse or her philosophical beliefs about illness and suffering will determine the extent to which she will be able to help patients find meaning (or no meaning) in these situations. A major task of professionals is to assist patients to find some meaning in the acts of self-denial and sacrifices they are asked to make. It is the role of the professional nurse to intervene before the individual progresses to not caring. Nursing is an act of courage because in caring for another, she exposes herself to the chance of being hurt by him.

Achieving a sense of one's identity as a person and as a unique human being precedes the developmental task of finding a meaning or purpose to life. Human beings need a sense of direction and a purpose for living—not to merely exist. Travelbee (1971) contends that human experiences have no meaning in and of themselves and that only the person experiencing the illness or event can determine its value and meaning. A philosophy of life should include the finding of meaning and purpose in living. It is in times of great stress, suffering, pain, illness, and loneliness that one's purpose or meaning is most tested (Travelbee, 1969). The human being is motivated by a search for meaning in life experiences, and that meaning can be found in the experiences of illness, suffering, and pain. For Travelbee, suffering is a part of illness and comes about as the human being is subjected to physical or mental pain and/or in a loss that causes distress.

The professional nurse has the difficult responsibility to assist the patient to find meaning in the experience of illness, suffering, and pain (Travelbee, 1971). The human being must be assisted also to find meaning in the very measures he must take to conserve his health and control his illness—this may include finding meaning in the acts of self-denial and sacrifice he may be asked to make. An example of this would be supporting the diabetic patient who must check his blood sugar, eat the appropriate foods, take insulin as needed, and at times deny himself the food or beverages that he desires because to do otherwise might jeopardize his health and possibly his life.

As a patient suffers, his feelings of displeasure may vary and range on a continuum from a simple transitory mental, physical, or spiritual discomfort, to a level of extreme anguish, to the malignant phase of despairful "not caring," and finally to the terminal phase of apathetic indifference (Travelbee, 1971). Patients may develop specific reactions to illness. These can include reactions of nonacceptance, being unjustly afflicted, being punished, self-pity, being full of despair and not caring, indifference, complete apathy, or complete acceptance. The nurse's task is to assist the patient to arrive at a meaning for illness without imposing her own meaning on the patient or family. This is possible only if she is able to establish and maintain a nurse–patient relationship.

TABLE 9-4	Travelbee's Human-to-Human Relationship Model and Nursing's Metaparadigm
Metaparadigm Concept	**Travelbee's Human-to-Human Relationship Model**
Human	A major focus—biological organisms with basic needs; unique, irreplaceable individuals, thinking organisms, capable of maturity with a core of immaturity, both time bound and time free, always becoming and evolving
Health	Acknowledged WHO definition; described health as a value judgment
Society/environment	Discussed only briefly; acknowledges influence of culture on individual values
Nursing	An interpersonal process—the professional nurse assists the patient (family, community) to prevent or cope with illness and to find meaning in the experience

METAPARADIGM, RESEARCH, AND PRACTICE WITH THE HUMAN-TO-HUMAN RELATIONSHIP MODEL   Travelbee did not emphasize all four of the major concepts in nursing's metaparadigm. She discussed human beings and nursing in depth with some recognition of health and society. See Table 9-4 for examples.

This theory seems to be more applicable for qualitative research than for quantitative studies since much of the theory is in the affective realm. Travelbee's theory has been tested in the real world, but only to a limited extent. Examples include the following: Bennett (1993) tested Travelbee's concept of nursing empathy in relation to homophobia with patients with AIDS, and Betta (1993) tested the concept of empathy in situations in which the nurse and patient experienced mutual crying. Wadensten and Carlsson (2003) used Travelbee's theory in their work looking at "meaning in illness" as the patient ages. Baier (1995) investigated the search for meaning and the transcendence of illness in a qualitative study with persons diagnosed with schizophrenia. Lange (1999) considered patient satisfaction in the quality of the nurse–patient relationship and the ability of the patient to identify a licensed professional based on that relationship. In Sweden, Jormin, Augustsson, and Forsberg (2003) studied Travelbee's theory as it related to nurse–patient relationships that fostered a sense of hope and promoted adherence to treatment plans for patients with both psychiatric disorders and a history of substance abuse. In Brazil, studies have investigated the application of Travelbee's theory in the areas of neonatal intensive care (Olivera, DeAlmeida, deAraújo, & Galvão, 2005), an adult intensive care unit (daSilveira, Lunardi, Filho, & deOliveira, 2005), and with patients with cancer (Bobroff, Furegato, & Scatena, 2003) and patients with psychiatric/mental conditions (Foschiera & Durman, 2004; Waidman, Elsen, & Marcon, 2006).

Travelbee focuses on nursing at the bedside and the importance of the establishment of a relationship with the patient as human being to human being. She stresses that even if the individual is suffering from a condition that cannot be cured, the nurse can still assist the patient to find meaning in his situation.

Even though it was one of the early models proposed in the development of nursing theory, Travelbee's human-to-human relationship model has not been very contagious. An electronic search of the literature identified very limited use of this model for research. This may in part be true because of the multiple variables within a human-to-human interaction that would be difficult to quantify and test objectively in the research arena.

Travelbee's model has much utility for the nurse at the bedside to develop a relationship with patients in order to provide the highest quality of care as rapport develops. Travelbee emphasizes that every nurse is a human being and can provide excellent care, even though in some situations the nurse cannot establish the ultimate: rapport. Her work would seem to have the highest utility for the patient in a psychiatric setting or for the nurse working with terminally ill persons or in the hospice setting, when the nurse can help one find meaning in his illness or inevitable outcome. There would be less application in a clinical situation when the patient has great physical needs but is unable to communicate verbally.

Travelbee's model is a focus on the caring aspect of nursing. She identifies a personal approach to nursing care in which the nurse must develop a relationship with the individual and family. Each interaction between the nurse and the patient affects the growth of the dyad. She recognizes that both the nurse and the patient are humans and as such have definite characteristics and limitations. Their relationship is affected by the spiritual values of each. Whenever there is a relationship, both must give of themselves and in so doing take a risk of being hurt, but also if the relationship progresses to the establishment of rapport, the gamble may produce immeasurable rewards—the terminus of all nursing endeavors.

This theory applies to all nurses as the nurse–patient relationship develops but seems to apply more specifically when there are multiple dynamic interchanges over time between the nurse and patient. However, the theory can be applied to other relationships involved in the provision of health care (e.g., the therapeutic use of self when communicating with physicians and other professionals in the work environment). Group process and trust would be enhanced if all professionals communicated at the rapport level, knowing each other so well that initial interactions and superficialities have been progressed through and a deep trusting relationship has developed in the work environment. Each person would know and accept all other team members, valuing their abilities, strengths, weaknesses, and humanness. At this level communication would be from one authentic human being to another.

PEARSON
EXPLORE mynursingkit™

MyNursingKit is your one stop for online chapter review materials and resources. Prepare for success with additional NCLEX®-style practice questions, interactive assignments and activities, web links, animations and videos, and more!

Register your access code from the front of your book at
www.mynursingkit.com.

References for Hall

Bowar-Ferres, S. (1975). Loeb Center and its philosophy of nursing. *American Journal of Nursing, 75,* 810–815.

Brown, E. L. (1970). *Nursing reconsidered: A study of change, part 1: The professional role in institutional nursing.* Philadelphia: Lippincott.

Griffiths, P. (1997). In search of the pioneers of nurse led care. . . . The Loeb Centre. *Nursing Times, 93*(21), 46–48.

Griffiths, P., & Willis-Barnett, J. (1998). The effectiveness of "nursing beds": A review of the literature. *Journal of Advanced Nursing, 27,* 1184–1192.

Hall, L. (1955). Quality of nursing care. *Public Health News, New Jersey State Department of Health, 36,* 212–215.

Hall, L. (1959). *Nursing—What is it?* Publication of the Virginia State Nurses Association.

Hall, L. (1965). *Another view of nursing care and quality.* Address given at Catholic University Workshop, Washington, DC.

Hall, L. (1969). The Loeb Center for Nursing and Rehabilitation at Montefiore Hospital and Medical Center. *International Journal of Nursing Studies, 6,* 81–95.

Loeb Center for Nursing and Rehabilitation Project Report. (1963, May–June). *Congressional Record,* 1515–1562.

Loose, V. (1994). Lydia E. Hall: Rehabilitation nursing pioneer in the ANA Hall of Fame. *Rehabilitation of Nursing, 19,* 174–176.

Bibliography for Hall

Alfano, G. (1969). Loeb Center. *Nursing Clinics of North America, 4,* 3.

Alfano, G. (1984). Administration means working with nurses. *American Journal of Nursing, 64,* 83–85.

Bernardin, E. (1964). Loeb Center—as the staff nurse sees it. *American Journal of Nursing, 64,* 85–86.

Hall, L. (1963). A center for nursing. *Nursing Outlook, 2,* 805–806.

Hall, L. (1964). Can nursing care hasten recovery? *American Journal of Nursing, 64,* 6.

Isler, C. (1964). New concepts in nursing therapy: More care as the patient improves. *RN, 27,* 58–70.

References for Abdellah

Abdellah, F. G. (1955). *Methods of determining covert aspects of nursing problems as a basis for improved clinical teaching.* Unpublished doctoral dissertation, Teachers College, Columbia University, New York, NY.

Abdellah, F. G. (1957, June). Methods of identifying covert aspects of nursing problems. *Nursing Research, 6,* 4.

Abdellah, F. G. (1991a). The funding crisis in biomedical research, part I—Addressing the issue. *Journal of Professional Nursing, 7,* 7.

Abdellah, F. G. (1991b). The funding crisis in biomedical research, part II—Options for action. *Journal of Professional Nursing, 7,* 75.

Abdellah, F. G. (1991c). The human genome initiative—Implications for nurse researchers. *Journal of Professional Nursing, 7,* 332.

Abdellah, F. G. (1991d). Summary statements of the NIH Nursing Research Grant Applications. *Nursing Research, 40,* 346–351.

Abdellah, F. G. (1993). Doctoral preparation and research productivity. *Journal of Professional Nursing, 9,* 71.

Abdellah, F. G. (1995). Management perspectives. I'm the aspiring vice president of nursing at a university hospital and I'm wondering how to avoid hitting the "glass ceiling." *Nursing Spectrum, 5*(9), 7.

Abdellah, F. G. (1997). Managing the challenges of role diversification in an interdisciplinary environment. *Military Medicine, 162,* 453–458.

Abdellah, F. G. (1998). An interview with Faye G. Abdellah on nursing research and health policy. *Image: Journal of Nursing Scholarship, 301,* 215–219.

Abdellah, F. G., Beland, I. L., Martin, A., & Matheney, R. V. (1960). *Patient-centered approaches to nursing.* New York: Macmillan. [out of print]

Abdellah, F. G., Beland, I. L., Martin, A., & Matheney, R. V. (1973). *New directions in patient-centered nursing.* New York: Macmillan.

Abdellah, F. G., & Levine, E. (1954). *Appraising the clinical resources in small hospitals* (Public Health Service Monographs No. 24). Washington, DC: Department of Health, Education, and Welfare.

Abdellah, F. G., & Levine, E. (1965). *Better patient care through nursing research.* New York: Macmillan.

Abdellah, F. G., & Levine, E. (1986). *Better patient care through nursing research* (3rd ed.). New York: Macmillan.

Abdellah, F. G., Levine, E., Sylvia, B., Kelley, P. W., Saba, V., & Tenebaum, S. (2005). Military nursing research by students at the Graduate School of Nursing, Uniformed Services University of Health Sciences. *Military Medicine, 170,* 188–192.

McFadden, W. (2000). Message from the Dean Graduate School of Nursing. Available online at http://www.usuhs.mil/gsn/msgdean.html.

Nicholls, M. E., & Wessells, V. G. (Eds.). (1977). *Nursing standards and nursing process.* Wakefield, MA: Contemporary Publishing.

References for Wiedenbach

Burst, H. V. (1979). Presentation of the Hattie Hemschemeyer Award. *Journal of Nurse-Midwifery, 24*(5), 35–36.

Carlson, S., Kotze, W. J., & Van Rooyen, D. (2005). A self-management model toward professional maturity for the practice of nursing. *Curationis, 28*(5), 44–52

Dickoff, J., James, P., & Wiedenbach, E. (1968a). Theory in a practice discipline I: Practice-orientated research. *Nursing Research, 17,* 415–435.

Dickoff, J., James, P., & Wiedenbach, E. (1968b). Theory in a practice discipline II: Practice-orientated research. *Nursing Research, 17,* 545–554.

Gustafson, D. C. (1988). Signaling behavior in stage I labor to elicit care: A clinical referent for Wiedenbach's need-for-help. *Dissertation Abstracts International, 49*(10B), 4230. Abstract retrieved November 5, 2007, from Dissertation Abstracts Online.

Nickel, S., Gesse, T., & MacLaren, A. (1992). Ernestine Wiedenbach: Her professional legacy. *Journal of Nurse-Midwifery, 37*(3), 161–167.

'Trefz, L. M. (1999). *Nursing staff perceptions about breastfeeding: An education task force survey.* Unpublished master's thesis, University of Cincinnati, Ohio.

Wiedenbach, E. (1958). *Family-centered maternity nursing.* New York: G. P. Putnam's.

Wiedenbach, E. (1964). *Clinical nursing—A helping art.* New York: Springer.

Wiedenbach, E. (1967). *Family-centered maternity nursing* (2nd ed.). New York: G. P. Putnam's.

Wiedenbach, E. (1969). *Meeting the realities in clinical teaching.* New York: Springer.

Wiedenbach. E. (1970). Nurse's wisdom in nursing theory. *American Journal of Nursing, 70,* 1057–1062.

Wiedenbach, E. (1977). The nursing process in maternity nursing. In J. P. Clausen, M. H. Flook, & B. Ford (Eds.), *Maternity nursing today* (2nd ed., pp. 39–51). New York: McGraw-Hill.

Bibliography for Wiedenbach

Dickoff, J. J. (1968). Symposium in theory development in nursing: Researching research's role in theory development. *Nursing Research, 17,* 204–206.

Dickoff, J. J., & James, P. A. (1968). Symposium of theory development in nursing: A theory of theories: A position paper. *Nursing Research, 17,* 197–203.

Holland, M. A. (1989). *An examination of the propositions of James Dickoff, Patricia James: Implications for nursing research.* Unpublished doctoral dissertation, Temple University.

Wiedenbach, E. (1949). Childbirth as mothers say they like it. *Public Health Nursing, 51,* 417–421.

Wiedenbach, E. (1960). Nurse-midwifery, purpose, practice and opportunity. *Nursing Outlook, 8,* 256.

Wiedenbach, E. (1963). The helping art of nursing. *American Journal of Nursing, 63,* 54–57.

Wiedenbach, E. (1965). Family nurse practitioner for maternal and child care. *Nursing Outlook, 13,* 50.

Wiedenbach, E. (1968a). Genetics and the nurse. *Bulletin of the American College of Nurse Midwifery, 13,* 8–13.

Wiedenbach, E. (1968b). The nurse's role in family planning—A conceptual base for practice. *Nursing Clinics of North America, 3,* 355–365.

Wiedenbach, E. (1970). Comment on beliefs and values: Basis for curriculum design. *Nursing Research, 19,* 427.

Wiedenbach, E., & Falls, C. (1978). *Communication: Key to effective nursing.* New York: Tiresias Press.

References for Travelbee

Baier, M. (1995). The process of developing insight and finding meaning within persons with schizophrenia. *Dissertation Abstracts International*, 57(02B), 986. Abstract retrieved October 30, 2007, from Dissertation Abstracts Online.

Bennett, J. A. (1993). The effects of empathy, knowledge and attitudes about sex, and homophobia on nurses' attitudes about AIDS care: An exploration of Orem's concept of nursing agency using propositions from Travelbee's theory of interpersonal relations in nursing. *Dissertation Abstracts International*, 54(04B), 4598. Abstract retrieved October 30, 2007, from Dissertation Abstracts Online.

Betta, P. A. (1993). Mutual crying: Experiences of adult female patients who have had nurses cry with them. *Dissertation Abstracts International*, 53(12B), 6217. Abstract retrieved October 30, 2007, from Dissertation Abstracts Online.

Bobroff, M. S., Furegato, A. R. F., & Scatena, M. C. M. (2003). Nurses in the help relationship with cancer patients [Portuguese]. *Revista Paulista DeEnfermagem*, 22(2), 158–65. Abstract in English retrieved October 30, 2007, from EBSCOhost.

daSilveira, R. S., Lunardi, V. L., Filho, W. D. L., & deOliveira, A. M. N. (2005). An attempt to humanize the relationship of the nursing staff with the family of patients in the unit of intensive therapy [Portuguese]. *Texto & Contexto Enfermagem*, 14(4), 125–130. Abstract in English retrieved October 30, 2007, from EBSCOhost.

Doona, M. E. (1979). *Travelbee's intervention in psychiatric nursing* (2nd ed.). Philadelphia: F. A. Davis.

Foschiera, F., & Durman, S. (2004). Caring the therapeutic relationship help with a female patient with a psyche suffering [Portuguese]. *Revista Electronica de Enfermagem*, 6(1), 98–104. Abstract in English retrieved October 30, 2007, from EBSCOhost.

Jormin, R., Augustsson, B., & Forsberg, A. (2003). Patients with dual diagnosis—A caring perspective based on Travelbee's theory of nursing [Swedish]. *Theoria Journal of Nursing Theory*, 12(4), 3–14. Abstract in English retrieved October 30, 2007, from EBSCOhost.

Lange, J. C. W. (1999). Hospitalized patient's ability to identify licensed nurse versus unlicensed assistive personnel and prediction of patient satisfaction. *Dissertation Abstracts International*, 60(04B), 1532. Abstract retrieved October 30, 2007, from Dissertation Abstracts Online.

Olivera, M. M. S., deAlmeida, C. B., deAraújo, T. L., & Galvão, M. T. G. (2005). Use of Travelbee's interpersonal relation process with mothers of newborns in a neonatal unit [Portuguese]. *Revista da Escola de Enfermagem da USP, 39*, 430–436. Abstract in English retrieved October 30, 2007, from EBSCOhost.

Travelbee, J. (1963a). Humor survives the test of time. *Nursing Outlook, 11*, 128.

Travelbee, J. (1963b). What do we mean by rapport? *American Journal of Nursing, 63*, 70.

Travelbee, J. (1964). What's wrong with sympathy? *American Journal of Nursing, 64*, 68–70.

Travelbee, J. (1966). *Interpersonal aspects of nursing*. Philadelphia: F. A. Davis.

Travelbee, J. (1969). *Intervention in psychiatric nursing: Process in the one-to-one relationship*. Philadelphia: F. A. Davis.

Travelbee, J. (1971). *Interpersonal aspects of nursing* (2nd ed.). Philadelphia: F. A. Davis.

Travelbee, J. (1972). To find meaning in illness. *Nursing '72, 2*(12), 6–7.

Wadensten, G., & Carlsson, M. (2003). Nursing theory views on how to support the process of ageing. *Journal of Advanced Nursing, 42*, 118–124.

Waidman, M. A. P., Elsen, I., & Marcon, S. S. (2006). Possibilities and limits of Joyce Travelbee's theory for the construction of a family care methodology [Portuguese]. *Revista Electronica de Enfermagem, 8*, 282–291. Abstract in English retrieved October 30, 2007, from EBSCOhost.

CHAPTER 10

The Conservation Principles: A Model for Health

Myra Estrin Levine

Julia B. George

Myra E. Levine (1920–1996) was born in Chicago, Illinois, the first child in a family of three siblings. Her experiences during her father's frequent illnesses contributed to her interest in and dedication to nursing. She received a diploma from Cook County School of Nursing, Chicago, in 1944; a B.S. from the University of Chicago in 1949; and an M.S. in nursing from Wayne State University, Detroit, Michigan, in 1962. Her career in nursing was varied. Clinically, she held positions as a private-duty nurse, a civilian nurse for the U.S. Army, surgical supervisor, and director of nursing. She held faculty positions at Bryan Memorial Hospital, Lincoln, Nebraska, and Cook County School of Nursing, Loyola University, Rush University, and the University of Illinois, Chicago. She was Professor Emerita, medical-surgical nursing, University of Illinois, Chicago. Levine filled visiting professorships at Tel-Aviv University and the Department of Nursing, Recanati School for Community Health Professions, Ben Gurion University of the Negev, both in Israel.

Levine was a charter fellow in the American Academy of Nursing and was honored by the Illinois Nurses Association. She was the first recipient of Sigma Theta Tau's Elizabeth Russell Belford Award for teaching excellence. She was granted an honorary doctorate by Loyola University, Chicago, in 1992.

Levine has been described as "a daughter, sister, wife, mother, friend, educator, administrator, student of humanities, scholar, enabler, and confidante . . . amazingly intelligent, opinionated, quick to respond, loving, caring , trustworthy, and global in her vision of nursing" (Schaefer, 2006, p. 94), or, in other words, a very human being who is more than deserving of our respect and attention.

Myra Levine said she had no intention of developing a theory when she first began putting her ideas about nursing into writing (Trench, Wallace, & Coberg, 1987). In fact, nearly two decades after the initial publication of *Introduction to Clinical Nursing* (Levine, 1969, 1973), she referred to her work as a theory but preferred to identify it as a conceptual model. She stated she was looking for a way to teach all the major concepts in medical-surgical nursing in three quarters and for a way to generalize the content, to move away from a procedurally oriented educational process. She was interested in helping nurses realize that every nurse–patient contact leads to a puzzle in relation to nursing care that needs to be solved in an individualized manner. Her work evolved over the years, with the most recent comprehensive update of the theory published in 1989 and additional discussions in 1990, 1991, and 1996.

Levine (1990) believed that entry into the health care system is associated with giving up some measure of personal independence. To designate the person who has entered the health care system a client reinforces the state of dependency, for a client is a follower. She supported the term *patient* because patient means sufferer, and dependency is associated with suffering.

> It is the condition of suffering that makes it possible to set independence aside and accept the services of another person. It is the challenge of the nurse to provide the individual with appropriate care without losing sight of the individual's integrity, to honor the trust that the patient has placed in the nurse, and to encourage the participation of the individual in his or her own welfare. The patient comes in trust and dependence only for as long as the services of the nurse are needed. The nurse's goal is always to impart knowledge and strength so that the individual can . . . walk away . . . as an independent individual. (p. 199)

It was Levine's intent that such dependency be a very temporary state of affairs (Trench et al., 1987). In accord with Levine's belief, the term *patient* is used throughout this chapter.

Levine (1989, 1990, 1991, 1996) was careful to credit the scientists' works upon which she built. She spoke to the importance of recognizing and building on these vital adjuncts to knowledge. This knowledge is not borrowed but, rather, is shared. In discussing physiological mechanisms, she drew on Cannon's (1939) description of the flight-or-fight response. Selye's (1956) stress theories provided further information about protection from the hazards of living. Gibson's (1966) perceptual systems about how people are actively involved in gathering information from their environments to aid them in moving safely through those environments were drawn on. Erikson's (1969, 1975) discussions of the influence of environment on development further expanded Levine's information about the person–environment interaction. Bates's (1967) description of three types of environment was also important. The works of Dubos (1965), Cohen (1968), and Goldstein (1963) contributed to Levine's concept of adaptation.

LEVINE'S THEORY

Levine discussed adaptation, conservation, and integrity. *Adaptation* is the process by which *conservation* is achieved, and the purpose for conservation is *integrity*. The core of Levine's theory is her four principles of conservation.

Adaptation

Adaptation is the life process by which, over time, people maintain their wholeness or integrity as they respond to environmental challenges; it is the consequence of interaction between the person and the environment (Levine, 1989; Trench et al., 1987).

Successful engagement with the environment depends on an adequate store of adaptations (Levine, 1990).

Both physiological and behavioral responses are different under different conditions—for example, responses to intensely quiet or extremely noisy environments will vary. It is possible to anticipate certain kinds of reactions, but the individuality of responses prevents accurate prediction. Adaptation is explanatory rather than predictive.

Adaptation includes the concepts of *historicity, specificity,* and *redundancy.* Adaptation is a historical process; responses are based on past experiences, both personal and genetic. Each individual's genetic pattern is unique. This uniqueness is further developed by the individual's experiences.

Adaptation is also specific. Each system has very specific responses. The physiological responses that "defend oxygen supply to the brain are distinct from those that maintain the appropriate blood glucose levels" (Levine, 1989, p. 328). Particular responses are called into action by a particular challenge; responses are task specific. They are also synchronized. Although the changes that occur are sequential, they should not be viewed as linear. Rather, Levine (1989) describes them as occurring in "cascades" in which there is an interacting and evolving effect in which one sequence is not yet completed when the next begins.

"One of the most remarkable things about living species is the number of levels of response which permit them to confront the reality of their environment in ways that somehow maintain their well being" (Trench et al., 1987). These redundant systems are both protective and adaptive. If one system does not adapt, another can take over. Levine (1989) indicated that redundant systems may function in a time frame; some are corrective, whereas others permit a previously failed response to be reestablished. Redundancy results in the most parsimonious use of energy (Levine, 1996).

Levine described adaptation as the best "fit of the person with his or her predicament of time and space" (Trench et al., 1987). She differentiated between fit and congruence by using an example of shoes. Most of us have many pairs of shoes that are congruent with our feet. We also have certain pairs that we prefer to wear because they are the most comfortable—they are the best fit.

Conservation

The product of adaptation is conservation. Conservation is a universal concept, a natural law, that deals with defense of wholeness and system integrity (Levine, 1990, 1991, 1996). "Conservation defends the wholeness of living systems by ensuring their ability to confront change appropriately and retain their unique identity" (Levine, 1990, p. 192). Conservation describes how complex systems continue to function in the face of severe challenges; it provides not only for current survival but also for future vitality through facing challenges in the most economical way possible. An example Levine used to illustrate conservation is that of the thermostat. The thermostat is set at a selected temperature. As long as the temperature in the room is the same as the set temperature, nothing occurs. When the room temperature falls below the selected temperature, the thermostat activates the heating system—but only until the room temperature again reaches the thermostat setting. When the setting is reached, the thermostat turns the heating system off. Levine (1990) describes this as conserving energy—using it in "the most frugal, economic, and energy-sparing fashion" (p. 192). The essence of conservation is the successful use of responses that cost the least (Levine, 1989). "Conservation is clearly the consequence of the multiple, interacting, and synchronized negative feedback systems that provide for the stability of the living organism" (Levine, 1989, p. 329). As long as systems are physiologically stable, or in balance, negative feedback systems can function at minimal cost. Energy resources are conserved for use when needed to restore balance. Homeostasis is a state of conservation, a state of synchronized sparing of energy.

Levine (1989) stated that physiological and behavioral responses are essential components of the same activity. They are not parallel or simultaneous but part of the same whole. She also recognized that it is difficult to break down a body of knowledge and that often information must be gathered piece by piece (Trench et al., 1987). Thus, physiological and behavioral responses are often identified and described as separate things. Since they represent the same whole, it is important to put the pieces together to represent that whole.

Levine (1989) described four levels of behavior. The first is Cannon's (1939) "fight-or-flight" response, the adrenocortical-sympathetic reactions that provide both physiological and behavioral readiness in the face of sudden and unexplained challenges in the environment. The second is the inflammatory-immune response, which we rely on for restoration of physical wholeness and healing. The third is Selye's (1956) stress response, described as an integrated defense that occurs over time and is "influenced by the accumulated experience of the individual" (p. 330). The fourth is Gibson's (1966) perceptual systems, in which the senses not only provide access to environmental energy sources but also convert these sources into meaningful experiences; people not only see, they *look*; they not only hear, they *listen*. These levels of behavior support the individual as an active participant with the environment, not merely as a reactive being. The levels of responses are not sequential but rather redundant and integrated within the individual.

Nursing's role in conservation is to help the person with the process of "keeping together" the total person through the least expense of effort. Levine (1989) proposed the following four principles of conservation:

1. The conservation of energy of the individual
2. The conservation of the structural integrity of the individual
3. The conservation of the personal integrity of the individual
4. The conservation of the social integrity of the individual (p. 331)

The conservation of *energy* is basic to the natural, universal law of conservation. Levine (1989) stated that energy is not hidden; "it is eminently identifiable, measurable, and manageable" (p. 331). Within nursing practice, the measurement of vital signs is a daily measurement of energy parameters. For example, body temperature is an indication of the heat (energy) generated by living cells as they accomplish their work. Energy conservation is encouraged through the limitation of activities for coronary patients or the planned gradual resumption of activities postoperatively. It is important that, even at rest, energy costs are incurred through the activities necessary to support living. Levine (1989) identified these as those activities involved in growth, transport, and biochemical and bioelectrical change. She stated, "The conservation of energy is clearly evident in the very sick, whose lethargy, withdrawal, and self-concern are manifested while, in its wisdom, the body is spending its energy resources on the processes of healing" (p. 332). Levine (1996) also discussed conservation of energy as universal and increasingly justified through scientific data.

The second, third, and fourth principles continue the theme of conservation and include integrity—structural integrity, personal integrity, and social integrity. Levine (1990) also described the conservation of energy as protecting functional integrity. Levine presented the idea that "health" and "whole" are derived from the same root word and that another synonym for "whole" is "integrity." "Integrity means being in control of one's life . . . having the freedom to choose: to move without constraint . . . to exercise decisions on all matters . . . without apology, indebtedness, or guilt" (Levine, 1990, p. 193). We are concerned with the integrity of the whole person; the essence of wholeness is integrity.

Conservation of *structural integrity* focuses on the healing process (Levine, 1989). Through multiple experiences with scraped knees and such that heal with no scarring, humans develop a mind-set that expects perfect restoration of structural integrity throughout life. "Healing is the defense of wholeness" (p. 333). Nurses support structural integrity through efforts to limit injury and thus limit scarring through proper positioning and range of motion to prevent skeletal deformity, pressure areas, or loss of muscle tone. To Levine the phantom limb phenomenon (Sacks, 1985) supports the idea that a sense of structural integrity is more than a physiological need.

Conservation of *personal integrity* focuses on a sense of self—"that intensely private, always unique and secret knowledge that we use to define ourselves" (Levine, 1996, p. 40). Levine described Goldstein's (1963) identification of self-actualization as observed in efforts of severely brain-injured persons to retain their personal identity. She pointed out that both Maslow (1968) and Rogers (1961) discussed self-actualization as a reaching beyond. Goldstein's concept, the one supported by Levine, is a reaching into the person rather than a reaching beyond. Humans have both a public and a very private self. At least some portion of the private self is not known even to those who are closest to the person. The self "is defined, defended, and described only by the soul that owns it. That private self is unique and whole. A person can share mere fragments of it with others" (Levine, 1990, p. 194). In this way a separation between self and other is maintained. Levine (1989) stated that efforts at collecting a complete psychosocial database may well violate this need to maintain separation, and therefore these efforts violate personal integrity. She stated, "The most generous psycho–social approach would be to limit the recording of confidences to only those generalizations that actually make a difference in the choice of treatment plans" (p. 334). She likened the awareness of self to independence.

Conservation of *social integrity* involves a definition of self that goes beyond the individual and includes the holiness of each person (Levine, 1989, 1996). Individuals use their relationships to define themselves. One's identity is connected to family, friends, community, workplace, school, culture, ethnicity, religion, vocation, education, and socioeconomic status. To function successfully in this wide variety of social environments requires a broad behavioral repertoire. The ultimate direction for social integrity is derived from the ethical values of the social system. "The health care system is a vast social order with its own rules, but it is an instrument of society and must guarantee privacy, personhood, and respect as moral imperatives" (Levine, 1989, p. 336). Levine (1990) pointed out that disease prevention is an issue of social integrity and discusses the need both to discuss and to fund studies and programs to deal with overwhelming health problems such as smoking, drug abuse, HIV, and cancer. She also stated, "It is difficult to foresee a time when conservation of social integrity is realistically possible" (Levine, 1996, p. 41).

The conservation principles do not, of course, operate singly and in isolation from each other. They are joined within the individual as a cascade of life events, churning and changing as the environmental challenge is confronted and resolved in each individual's unique way. The nurse as caregiver becomes part of that environment, bringing to every nursing opportunity his or her own cascading repertoire of skill, knowledge, and compassion. It is a shared enterprise and each participant is rewarded. (Levine, 1989, p. 336)

LEVINE'S THEORY AND NURSING'S METAPARADIGM

Levine skillfully wove her beliefs about human beings, environment, health, and nursing throughout her discussions of conservation and adaptation. They are fundamental to her work.

In relation to *human beings*, Levine (1990) stated that when a person is being studied, the focus should be on wholeness. She also maintained that a person cannot be understood outside the context of the place and time in which he or she is functioning or separated from the influence of everything that is happening around him or her. Not only are human beings influenced by their current circumstances, they also are "burdened by a lifetime of experience," which has been recorded on the tissues of the body as well as on the mind and spirit (p. 197). Human beings are continually adapting in their interactions with their environment. The process of adaptation results in conservation. Human beings have need for nursing when they are suffering and can set aside independence and accept the services of another.

Levine (1984) indicated that *health* and disease are patterns of adaptive change. Some adaptations are more successful than others; all adaptations are seeking the best fit with the environment. The most successful adaptations are the ones that achieve the best fit in the most conserving manner. Health is the goal of conservation (Levine, 1990). She also discusses the words *health, whole,* and *integrity* as all being derived from the same root word and that even with a multiplicity of definitions of health, each individual still defines health for him- or herself (Levine, 1991).

In defining *environment* Levine (1990) drew upon Bates's (1967) classifications of three aspects of environment. The *operational environment* consists of those undetected natural forces that impinge on the individual. The *perceptual environment* consists of information that is recorded by the sensory organs. The *conceptual environment* is influenced by language, culture, ideas, and cognition. Levine also said that even with definition, the environment is difficult to measure. However, because adaptation and conservation are based on the human being's interaction with the environment, efforts to understand the environment and the role it plays in an individual's predicament are vital. The *social context* is also important to consideration of the wholeness of an individual. Levine (1991) included the individual's "ethnic and cultural heritage, economic niche, the opportunities ignored or seized" in social context (p. 9). She said, "It is the social system that, in every place and in every generation, establishes the values that direct it and sets the rules by which its members are judged. The social integrity of the individual mirrors the community to which he or she belongs" (p. 9).

For Levine (1989) the purpose of *nursing* is to take care of others when they need to be taken care of. The dependency created by this need is a very temporary state. Nursing takes place wherever there is an individual who needs care to some degree. Levine discussed the fact that the person who provides nursing care has special burdens of concern since the "permission to enter into the life goals of another human being bears onerous debts of responsibility and choice" (p. 336). The nurse–patient relationship is based on the willful participation of both parties, and in such a relationship there cannot be "a substitute for honesty, fairness, and mutual respect" (p. 336). Nursing theory "is tested finally in the pragmatic, humble daily exchanges between nurse and patient . . . [its] success [is demonstrated in its ability to] equip individuals with renewed strength to pursue their lives in independence, fulfillment, hope, and promise" (pp. 336–337).

LEVINE'S THEORY AND THE NURSING PROCESS

Levine's concepts of adaptation, conservation, and integrity can be used to guide patient care within the nursing process.

In *assessment,* an understanding of the wholeness of the patient needs to be the end result. However, because we lack the mechanisms for assessing the whole as such, the principles of conservation can be used as a guide to structure the assessment. The assessment would not be initiated unless the person is suffering and willing to become to some degree dependent on the nurse. The overarching question could be, "What adaptation is needed, or has not been successful?" The history, specificity, and potential for redundancy in this area of adaptation need to be investigated. For example, with the cardiac patient it is important to gather information about the signs and symptoms that brought the person into the health care system. Is there a family or personal history of cardiac problems or of being at risk for such problems? Can the incident that initiated this problem be identified (e.g., response to sudden change in temperature would indicate a different specific response than to overexertion)? Have compensating efforts been made?

Under the first principle, conservation of energy, assessment data would relate to energy sources and expenditure. Data would include vital signs, laboratory values related to uptake and use of oxygen and nutrients, activities of daily living, nutrition, exercise, elimination, menstrual cycles—any aspect of living that requires energy. The primary focus would be on identifying the areas of energy expenditure that are related to the suffering that brought the patient into contact with the nurse. Information about the balance between energy input and output is also important.

Assessment data in relation to conservation of structural integrity would relate to information about injury and disease processes. Data would include laboratory values that reflect the immune/inflammatory response, direct observations of wounds, any visible indications of disease (e.g., the "pox" in chicken pox), and information from the patient about symptoms that are not observable (e.g., nausea, pain).

Assessment data related to conservation of personal integrity need to be collected very carefully. Levine (1989) warns about the threat to the self of the patient that can be created if the nurse seeks a too thorough investigation of the self of that patient. Her guideline to use "only those generalizations that actually make a difference in the choice of treatment plans" is helpful (p. 334). For example, knowing that the person prefers to learn from reading material and receiving instruction individually rather than in a group setting would influence the choice of treatment plans. The patient will be comfortable in sharing his public self but reluctant to share the private self. To assist in maintaining independence, assessment needs to be limited to those portions of the self that the person is willing to share and is capable of sharing.

Assessment data related to the conservation of social integrity include information about others who have influenced the person's identification of self. Again, the kind and amount of data collected in this area need to be constructed carefully, with due sensitivity to the needs of the person to maintain privacy. Information may be obtained about family, the community in which the person lives and works, religious preferences, cultural and ethnic influences, and any other social information that the person deems important to share and that could influence the plan of care.

Assessment of the patient's nursing requirements leads to the development of *trophicognosis*. Trophicognosis is a nursing care judgment that is arrived at through the use of the scientific method (Trench et al., 1987). Levine proposed the use of the term *trophicognosis* as an alternative to *nursing diagnosis* in 1966. In her more recent writings (1989, 1990) she does not include trophicognosis. She does state, "No diagnosis should be made that does not include the other persons whose lives are entwined with that of the individual" (1989, p. 336). The *nursing diagnosis* focuses on the cause of the patient's suffering—what has put him in the predicament of need—and on the areas in which adaptation needs to be supported in order to achieve conservation and integrity.

Outcomes would center on Levine's goal of returning the patient to independence. In Levine's terms, an outcome might be that the patient can walk away from the nurse.

Planning focuses on what the nurse needs to do to aid the patient in again becoming independent. The goals that are set will reflect the patient's behavior and the planned activities will include both willing participants—the nurse and the patient. Levine has made no effort to be prescriptive about the kinds of actions that would be planned. She is very clear, however, that the intent is to return the patient to a state of independence as quickly and fully as possible.

Implementation is structured according to the four conservation principles. For conservation of energy, actions will seek to balance energy input with energy output. The actions may focus on increasing energy input through improved nutrition or in decreasing energy output through changes in activity. The classic example of decreasing energy output is full bed rest. However, it is important to remember, as Levine (1989) pointed out, even at purportedly complete rest, the body is still using energy. Levine reported that Winslow's research demonstrates that energy conservation can be *predicted* (personal communication, 1994). For structural integrity, nursing actions will be "based on limiting the amount of tissue involvement in infections and disease" (Trench et al., 1987). Such actions could include appropriate positioning to prevent the formation of decubiti, dressing changes, and administration of antibiotics. For personal integrity, efforts will be "based on helping the person to preserve his or her identity and selfhood" (Trench et al., 1987). These actions may begin in deciding to protect the private self by *not* collecting complete psychosocial data and continue through the design of treatment plans that take individual characteristics into account. Levine indicated it is important to observe a strict moral approach. For social integrity, nursing actions are "based on helping the patient to preserve his or her place in a family, community, and society" (Trench et al., 1987). Such nursing actions may include teaching the family about the patient's care needs or teaching persons with new colostomies how to handle food and fluid intake and how to change the ostomy bag in a manner that helps to minimize its being evident to those they meet.

Evaluation is not specifically discussed by Levine but outcomes were discussed by Taylor (1974) for neurological patients. However, Levine's emphasis on the importance of assisting the person to return to independence as soon as possible supports the need for evaluation. It is important to know that the person's suffering has been relieved and that he or she is willing and capable of no longer being dependent. The evaluation data focus on the effectiveness of adaptation in achieving conservation and integrity in the four areas of energy, structural integrity, personal integrity, and social integrity. See Table 10-1 for an example of an application to clinical practice.

TABLE 10-1   Application of Conservation Principles to Clinical Practice

Patient: Lester Douglas, admitted with medical diagnoses of hypertension and peripheral vascular disease.

Assessment:

Conservation of Energy:

> Mr. Douglas reports he cannot walk more than 1/2 block without resting because of pain in his legs. He must climb three steps to enter his house and can usually do so without difficulty. He lives in a two-story house but has a bedroom on the first floor.

> Vital signs are within normal limits—Mr. Douglas says that as long as he takes his antihypertension medicine and limits the salt in his diet, his high blood pressure is controlled.

> Chest X-ray clear

> Lab values: Only abnormal level is cholesterol at 260

> Mr. Douglas reports he takes care of himself and hires someone to come in to clean his house and do his laundry once a week. He states he eats two meals a day and he cooks for himself.

> He has to get up at least once a night to void. His bowels are usually regular—sometimes he is constipated.

Conservation of Structural Integrity:

> Medical diagnosis of peripheral vascular disease is consistent with Mr. Douglas's description of difficulty walking and indicates impairment of his vascular system.

> Mr. Douglas reports that his left leg either hurts or "feels strange" most of the time. Pedal pulses on the left are diminished.

> History of smoking 1/2 pack per day for 40 years—stopped smoking 10 years ago and reports his breathing is better since then.

> Reports arthritis in both hands; physical examination indicates arthritic nodules distal joints of index fingers. Mr. Douglas reports pain in the proximal joints of both thumbs and that this has weakened his grip strength. He can fully close each hand.

Conservation of Personal Integrity:

> 89-year-old male

Conservation of Social Integrity:

> Widower, lives alone

> Believes in God but doesn't "get out to church much anymore. It's just too much effort."

> Has three living children—all are in their 60s and live out of state. Mr. Douglas states they call and write regularly and each visits once or twice a year.

> He has neighbors on either side of him who "keep an eye out." One of these neighbors likes to cook and regularly brings food over—"he can't seem to make a recipe small enough for just him so he shares with me. He's a pretty good cook, too!"

Nursing Diagnoses:

> Pain related to arthritis in hands and peripheral vascular disease in legs.

> Limited mobility associated with pain and peripheral vascular disease.

Desired Outcome: Able to continue to care for self and live in own home.

(continued)

TABLE 10-1   (Continued)

Planning:

Pain control using prescribed medication and possible physical therapy to support continued function.

Support for medical work-up that could result in the recommendation of vascular surgery—provide appropriate education and opportunity for questions and discussion. Explain all tests in the level of detail he desires. Be sensitive to how much detail he really wants.

Implementation:

Conservation of Energy:

Increase the servings of fruits and vegetables to at least five daily to help assure regularity of his bowels.

Arrange his bath and other care activities to allow rest before and after his physical therapy.

Conservation of Structural Integrity:

Work with physician and patient to establish an effective plan of analgesia to decrease his pain—help him accept that the pain will not totally disappear.

Conservation of Personal and Social Integrity:

Encourage him to keep up the good work!

Evaluation:

Can he walk with more comfort?

Can he use his hands for activities of daily living and desired recreation?

Is he ready to resume independence?

CRITIQUE OF LEVINE'S CONSERVATION PRINCIPLES

1. *What is the historical context of the theory?*   Levine developed her work to teach nursing students the practice of medical-surgical nursing. She had a practice-oriented focus in doing so and began to discuss the work in terms of a theory only about two decades after the initial publication. She was attuned to the origin of words and took care in her use of words and how they relate to one another.

   Levine clearly identified those ideas from adjunctive disciplines that she used in her work. These include Cannon's (1939) flight-or-fight response, Selye's (1956) stress theories, Gibson's (1966) perceptual systems, Erikson's (1969, 1975) discussions of the influence of environment on development, Bates's (1967) three types of environment, and the works of Dubos (1965), Cohen (1968), and Goldstein (1963) in relation to adaptation. She clearly and carefully includes information about how she used these ideas. Her work is consistent with these works but builds on them in a way that creates questions to be answered. Such questions could include the following: Does change in one type of environment have a greater effect on adaptation than changes in the other two types? Why are some people more (or less) effective than others in adapting, conserving, and thus maintaining integrity? What are the most effective ways of conserving social integrity through disease prevention activities?

   Levine's work is most consistent with the totality paradigm. She supported holism and stressed the importance of the whole person. However, she indicated that we must look at the parts to understand the whole.

2. *What are the basic concepts and relationships presented by the theory?*   The basic concepts are adaptation, conservation, and integrity. The relationships are presented in the theory statement; *adaptation* is the process by which *conservation* is achieved, and the purpose for conservation is *integrity*. The conservation concepts include *energy, structural integrity, personal integrity,* and *social integrity.*

3. *What major phenomena of concern to nursing are presented? (These phenomena may include* **but are not limited to** *human beings, environment, health, interpersonal relations, caring, goal attainment, adaptation, and energy fields.)*   The major phenomena begin with the basic concepts of adaptation, conservation, and integrity. In addition, the conservation principles include the phenomena of energy, structural integrity, personal integrity, and social integrity. The human being who needs nursing is seen as a person who is in a predicament of illness, who is willing to enter a dependent state, and who needs to return to independence as soon as possible. Levine emphasized that the person who is receiving nursing should be identified as a patient.

4. *To whom does this theory apply? In what situations? In what ways?*   Because Levine's three major concepts apply to all living human beings and, according to Levine, nursing is not setting specific, the theory is widely generalizable. It can be used in any setting with any human being who is suffering and willing to seek assistance from a nurse.

   Critical thinking is required for effective use of the principles of conservation. Critical thinking is particularly important in the conservation of personal integrity since the nurse must be sensitive to what data are imperative to identifying appropriate therapeutic measures and which are best left to the person rather than filling in the blanks in a standardized assessment form.

5. *By what method or methods can this theory be tested?*   Both qualitative and quantitative studies have been conducted in relation to Levine's theory. The results of these research studies have contributed to the general body of knowledge in nursing. Levine (1989) discusses the studies conducted by Wong (1968) and Winslow, Lane, and Gaffney (1985) that support the importance of energy conservation for patients with myocardial infarctions. Research has also been conducted in using Levine's theory with confused patients over age 60 and caring for neonates and for women in labor (Foreman, 1989; 1991; Newport, 1984; Yeates & Roberts, 1984). Pappas (1990) investigated the relationship between nursing care and anxiety in patients with sexually transmitted diseases and found significant relationships between constructs of nursing and components of anxiety. MacLean (1987) used the principles of conservation of energy and conservation of structural integrity in identifying cues that nurses use to diagnose activity intolerance. Foreman (1987) found that variables that represented the four conservation principles were more important in combination than separately when used to diagnose confusion in hospitalized elderly patients. Nagley (1984) did not find significant differences in groups of hospitalized elderly in relation to confusion between those treated with nursing measures derived from the four principles of conservation and those who did not receive such treatment. However, she questioned the accuracy of the initial diagnosis of confusion for these patients.

   These and other studies are listed in Table 10-2. A number of these are included in Schaefer and Pond (1991). Others are unpublished master's theses or doctoral dissertations and thus are less accessible than published materials,

TABLE 10-2   Research Involving the Conservation Principles

Author/Year	Area of Research	Type of Research
	DESCRIPTIVE RESEARCH	
*Cresci, 1997	Hip surgery recovery, women 65 and over	Cross-sectional, exploratory
*Delmore, 2003, 2006	Weaning long-term ventilated adults	Longitudinal, descriptive
*Fleming, 1987	Childbirth, perineal status	Descriptive
*Foreman, 1987, 1989, 1991	Hospitalized elderly, cognitive integrity	Descriptive correlational
Gagner-Tjellesen, Yurkovich, & Gragert, 2001	Acute care, use of independent therapeutic nursing interventions	Descriptive
Hanna, Avila, Meteer, Nicholas, & Kaminsky, 2008	Exercise, patients with cancer	Descriptive
Hanson et al., 1991	Hospice, pressure ulcers	Descriptive
*Higgins, 1996, 1998	Long-term mechanical ventilation, fatigue	Descriptive, correlational
Lowe & Miller, 1998	School nursing services	Descriptive
Ludington, 1990	Premature infants and their mothers	Pilot study; correlational
MacLean, 1987	Activity intolerance, cues used by nurses	Survey—Delphi technique
Melancon & Miller, 2005	Low back pain, massage versus traditional therapy	Factorial, comparative
Mock et al., 2007	Fatigue in cancer patients	Descriptive, use of conceptual model
*Pappas, 1990	Satisfaction with nursing care, anxiety level	Correlational
Basso & Piccoli, 2004; Flório & Galvão, 2003; Piccoli & Galvão, 2001, 2005	Perioperative	Descriptive
Schaefer & Potylycki, 1993	Congestive heart failure, fatigue	Descriptive
Zalon, 2004	Major abdominal surgery, recovery patterns	Correlational
	EVALUATIVE RESEARCH	
*Blasage, 1987	Theory and nursing practice	Critical analysis
Burd et al., 1994	Skilled nursing home skin care	Formative evaluation
	EXPERIMENTAL/QUASI-EXPERIMENTAL RESEARCH	
Clark, Fraaza, Schroeder, & Maddens, 1996	Dayroom program	Experimental

(*continued*)

TABLE 10-2   (Continued)

Author/Year	Area of Research	Type of Research
Deiriggi & Miles, 1995	Preterm infants, waterbeds and heart rate	Experimental
Lane & Winslow, 1987	Healthy adults, exertion	Quasi-experimental
Mock et al., 2007	Men with prostate cancer, exercise	Experimental
*Nagley, 1984	Hospitalized elderly, confusion prevention	Quasi-experimental
Newport, 1984	Newborn, conserving thermal energy and social integrity	Experimental
Roberts, Brittin, Cook, & deClifford, 1994	Respiratory capacity, boomerang pillows	Experimental
Winslow, Lane, & Gaffney, 1985	Oxygen consumption and cardiovascular response	Experimental
*Yeates, 1982; Yeates & Roberts, 1984	Bearing-down techniques, perineal integrity	Experimental
QUALITATIVE RESEARCH		
Ballard, Robley, Barrett, Fraser, & Mendoza, 2006	Intensive care unit, therapeutic paralysis	Phenomenology

*Master's thesis or doctoral dissertation.

especially when they are not included in either *Masters Abstracts International* or *Dissertation Abstracts International.*

6. ***Does this theory direct nursing actions that lead to favorable outcomes?*** For Levine, the desired outcome of nursing interventions is to return a person who has become dependent because of the predicament of an illness to a state of independence as quickly as possible. Thus, she defined the outcomes that would be favorable when using her theory. Areas of nursing practice that have been reported in the literature as using Levine's work are reflected in Table 10-3. Levine's work has also been used in both undergraduate and graduate education (Grindley & Paradowski, 1991; Schaefer, 1991b).

7. ***How contagious is this theory?*** Unfortunately, a search of the literature does not clearly reflect the full use of Levine's work. The literature does support its use in a variety of clinical settings, and some research has been conducted using the theory as a framework for the study or as a guide in assessing the data. There is also documentation of its use in Brazil (Basso & Piccoli, 2004; Fagundes, 1983; Flório & Galvão, 2003; Piccoli & Galvão, 2001, 2005), Great Britain (Webb, 1993), and Australia (Leach, 2006; Roberts et al., 1994).

TABLE 10-3   Applications of the Conservation Principles in Clinical Practice

Author/Year	Area of Clinical Practice
Bayley, 1991	Burn patients
Brunner, 1985; Fawcett et al., 1987; Lynn-McHale & Smith, 1991	Critical care
Cooper, 1990; Leach, 2006	Wound healing
Cox, 1991	Long-term care
Crawford-Gamble, 1986	Perioperative
Dever, 1991; Savage & Culbert, 1989	Care of children
Dow & Mest, 1997	Psychosocial interventions, persons with chronic obstructive pulmonary disease
Erwin & Biordi, 1991	Smoking cessation
Fagundes, 1983	Community health
Jost, 2000	Nursing administration
Langer, 1990; Mefford, 2004	Neonatal intensive care nursery, preterm infants
McCall, 1991; Taylor, 1974	Neurological care/monitoring
Neswick, 1997; Webb, 1993	Enterostomal therapy
O'Laughlin, 1986	Oncology, bladder function post-radical hysterectomy
Pasco & Halupa, 1991	Chronic pain
Pond, 1991	Ambulatory care, homeless
Pond & Taney, 1991	Emergency care
Schaefer, 1991a; Schaefer & Pond, 1994	Adult with congestive heart failure

Strengths and limitations

A major strength of Levine's work is its universality. Her concepts apply to all human beings wherever they may be. She also indicates when nursing is needed—it is needed by the person in a predicament of illness who is willing to become dependent in relation to that predicament. Thus, the use of this work is not limited to any given setting but may be used wherever there is a nurse and a patient.

Levine's careful use of words is also a strength. Her careful selection of terminology provides clarity to the reader. She provides clear connections to the works of others (the adjunctive disciplines) and certainly helps the reader understand how these works can be used in a way that is specific to nursing.

Her stress on the wholeness of the person, the importance of integrity, is very useful. Also, her statement that adaptation is a process, not a value, helps us understand that adaptation is what is rather than a positive or negative state. She describes adaptation as a bridge between environments (Levine, 1996).

A limitation could be considered to be the need for each nurse to create her own assessment tool to use Levine's conservation principles. This could also be viewed as providing flexibility and allowing each nurse to create a personal fit with the principles.

Summary

Myra Levine's theory has evolved from a publication whose initial intention was the organization of medical-surgical nursing content to facilitate student learning. Her theory interrelates the concepts of adaptation, conservation, and integrity. Adaptation is the process by which conservation occurs. Human beings are constantly in interaction with their environments. It is this interaction that creates the need for adaptation. As the environment changes, the human must adapt. Successful adaptation will achieve the best fit with the environment and will do so in a manner that conserves energy, structural integrity, personal integrity, and social integrity. The purpose of conservation is health, or integrity—the wholeness of the individual. This theory has been tested through research, and its usefulness has been demonstrated in clinical practice and education.

Thought Questions

1. For each of the conservation principles, identify at least two ways to promote conservation.
2. How does Levine's definition of adaptation agree with or differ from how you think about adaptation?
3. Give an example of historicity, specificity, and redundancy.
4. Is Levine's theory confined to individuals, or could it be utilized with groups or families? Justify your response.
5. Create an assessment tool using Levine's theory as a guide. Will you be able to gather all the information you need to provide appropriate care? Why or why not?

PEARSON

EXPLORE mynursingkit™

MyNursingKit is your one stop for online chapter review materials and resources. Prepare for success with additional NCLEX®-style practice questions, interactive assignments and activities, web links, animations and videos, and more!

Register your access code from the front of your book at
www.mynursingkit.com.

References

Ballard, N., Robley, L., Barrett, D., Fraser, D., & Mendoza, I. (2006). Patients' recollections of therapeutic paralysis in the intensive care unit. *American Journal of Critical Care, 15*(1), 86–94.

Basso, R. S., & Piccoli, M. (2004). Post-anesthetic [sic] recuperation unit: Nursing diagnosis based in Levine conceptual framework [Portuguese]. *Revista Electronica de Enfermagem, 6*(3), 309–323. Abstract in English retrieved May 29, 2007, from CINAHL Plus with Full Text database.

Bates, M. (1967). A naturalist at large. *Natural History, 76*(6), 8–16.

Bayley, E. W. (1991). Care of the burn patient. In K. M. Schaefer & J. B. Pond (Eds.), *Levine's conservation model: A framework for nursing practice* (pp. 91–99). Philadelphia: F. A. Davis.

Blasage, M. C. (1987). Toward a general understanding of nursing education: A critical analysis of the work of Myra Estrin Levine (Doctoral dissertation, Loyola University of Chicago, 1987). *Dissertation Abstracts International, No. 8704833.*

Brunner, M. (1985). A conceptual approach to critical care nursing using Levine's model. *Focus on Critical Care, 12*(2), 39–44.

Burd, C., Olson, B., Langemo, D., Hunter, S., Hanson, D., Osowski, K. F., et al. (1994). Skin care strategies in a skilled nursing home. *Journal of Gerontological Nursing, 20*(11), 28–34.

Cannon, W. B. (1939). *The wisdom of the body*. New York: Norton.

Clark, L. R., Fraaza, V., Schroeder, S., & Maddens, M. E. (1995). Alternative nursing environments: Do they affect hospital outcomes? *Journal of Gerontological Nursing, 21*(11), 32–38.

Cohen, Y. (1968). *Man in adaptation: The biosocial background*. Chicago: Aldine.

Cooper, D. M. (1990). Optimizing wound healing: A practice within nursing's domain. *Nursing Clinics of North America, 25*(1), 165–180.

Cox, R. A., Sr.(1991). A tradition of caring: Use of Levine's model in long-term care. In K. M. Schaefer & J. B. Pond (Eds.), *Levine's conservation model: A framework for nursing practice* (pp. 179–197). Philadelphia: F. A. Davis.

Crawford-Gamble, P. E. (1986). An application of Levine's conceptual model. *Perioperative Nursing Quarterly, 2*(1), 64–70.

Cresci, M. K. (1997). Social integrity and level of health in women 65 years of age and older recovering from hip surgery (Doctoral dissertation, Wayne State University, 1997). *Dissertation Abstracts International, No. 98152388.*

Deiriggi, P. M., & Miles, K. E. (1995). The effects of waterbeds on heart rate in preterm infants. *Scholarly Inquiry for Nursing Practice, 9*, 245–262.

Delmore, B. A. (2003). Fatigue and prealbumin levels during the weaning process in long-term ventilated patients (Doctoral dissertation, New York University, 2003). *Dissertation Abstracts International, No. 2005066090.*

Delmore, B. A. (2006). Levine's framework in long-term ventilated patients during the weaning course. *Nursing Science Quarterly, 19*, 247–258.

Dever, M. (1991). Care of children. In K. M. Schaefer & J. B. Pond (Eds.), *Levine's conservation model: A framework for nursing practice* (pp. 71–82). Philadelphia: F. A. Davis.

Dow, J. S., & Mest, C. G. (1997). Psychosocial interventions for patients with chronic obstructive pulmonary disease. *Home Healthcare Nurse, 15*, 414–420.

Dubos, R. (1965). *Man adapting*. New Haven, CT: Yale University Press.

Erikson, E. (1969). *Ghandi's truth*. New York: Norton.

Erikson, E. (1975). *Life history and the historical moment*. New York: Norton.

Erwin, S., & Biordi, D. (1991). A smoke-free environment: Psychiatric nurses respond. *Journal of Psychosocial Nursing and Mental Health Services, 29*(5), 12–18.

Fagundes, N. C. (1983). O processo de enfermagem em saude comunitaria a partir de teoria de Myra Levine (The nursing process in community health as derived from Myra Levine's theory). *Revista Brasileira de Enfermagem, 38*, 265–273.

Fawcett, J., Cariello, F. P., Davis, D. A., Farley, J., Zimmaro, D. M., & Watts, R. J. (1987). Conceptual models of nursing: Application to critical care nursing practice. *Dimensions of Critical Care Nursing, 6*, 202–213.

Fleming, N. (1987). Comparison of women with different perineal conditions after childbirth (Doctoral dissertation, University of Illinois at Chicago, Health Sciences Center, 1987). *Dissertation Abstracts International, No. 8728762.*

Flório, M. C. S., & Galvão, C. M. (2003). Surgery in out patient units: Identification of nursing diagnoses in the perioperative period [Portuguese]. *Revista Latino-Americana de Enfermagem, 11*, 630–637. Abstract in English retrieved May 29, 2007, from CINAHL Plus with Full Text database.

Foreman, M. D. (1987). The development of confusion in the hospitalized elderly. *Dissertation Abstracts International, 48-08B*, 2261.

Foreman, M. D. (1989). Confusion in the hospitalized elderly: Incidence, onset, and associated factors. *Research in Nursing and Health, 12*, 21–29.

Foreman, M. D. (1991). Conserving cognitive integrity of the hospitalized elderly. In K. M. Schaefer & J. B. Pond (Eds.), *Levine's conservation model: A framework for nursing practice* (pp. 133–149). Philadelphia: F. A. Davis.

Gagner-Tjellesen, D., Yurkovich, E. E., & Gragert, M. (2001). Use of music therapy and other ITNIs in acute care. *Journal of Psychosocial Nursing and Mental Health Services, 39*(10), 26–37, 52–53.

Gibson, J. E. (1966). *The senses considered as perceptual systems*. Boston: Houghton Mifflin.

Goldstein, K. (1963). *Human nature*. New York: Schocken.

Grindley, J., & Paradowski, M. (1991). Developing an undergraduate program using Levine's model. In K. M. Schaefer & J. B. Pond (Eds.), *Levine's conservation model: A framework for nursing practice* (pp. 199–208). Philadelphia: F. A. Davis.

Hanna, L. R., Avila, P. F., Meteer, J. D., Nicholas, D. R., & Kaminsky, L. A. (2008). The effects of a comprehensive exercise program on physical function, fatigue, and mood in patients with various types of cancer. *Oncology Nursing Forum, 35*, 461-469.

Hanson, D., Langemo, D. K., Olson, B., Hunter, S., Sauvage, T. R., Burd, C., et al. (1991). *American Journal of Hospice and Palliative Care, 8*(5), 18–22.

Higgins, P. A. (1996). Fatigue in the long-term ventilator patient: Incidence and associated factors (Doctoral dissertation, Case Western University, 1996). *Dissertation Abstracts International, No. 1999084251.*

Higgins, P. A. (1998). Patient perception of fatigue while undergoing long-term mechanical ventilation: Incidence and associated factors. *Heart and Lung, 27*(3), 177–183.

Jost, S. G. (2000). An assessment and intervention strategy for managing staff needs during change. *Journal of Nursing Administration, 30*(1), 34–40.

Lane, L. D., & Winslow, E. H. (1987). Oxygen consumption, cardiovascular response, and perceived exertion in health adults during rest, occupied bedmaking, and unoccupied bedmaking activity. *Cardiovascular Nursing, 23*(6), 31–36.

Langer, V. S. (1990). Minimal handling protocol for the intensive care nursery. *Neonatal Network, 9*(3), 23–27.

Leach, M. J. (2006). Wound management: Using Levine's conservation model to guide practice. *Ostomy Wound Management, 52*(8), 74–76, 78–80.

Levine, M. E. (1966). Trophicognosis: An alternative to nursing diagnosis. In *American Nurses Association Regional Clinical Conference Vol. 23* (pp. 55–70). New York: American Nurses Association.

Levine, M. E. (1969). *Introduction to clinical nursing.* Philadelphia: F. A. Davis. [out of print]

Levine, M. E. (1973). *Introduction to clinical nursing* (2nd ed.). Philadelphia: F. A. Davis. [out of print]

Levine, M. E. (1989). The conservation principles of nursing: Twenty years later. In J. Riehl-Sisca (Ed.), *Conceptual models for nursing practice* (3rd ed., pp. 325–337). Norwalk, CT: Appleton & Lange.

Levine, M. E. (1990). Conservation and integrity. In M. E. Parker (Ed.), *Nursing theories in practice* (pp. 189–201) (Pub. No. 15-2350). New York: National League for Nursing.

Levine, M. E. (1991). The conservation principles: A model for health. In K. M. Schaefer & J. B. Pond (Eds.), *Levine's conservation model: A framework for nursing practice* (pp. 1–11). Philadelphia: F. A. Davis.

Levine, M. E. (1996). The conservation principles: A retrospective. *Nursing Science Quarterly, 9*, 38–41.

Lowe, J., & Miller, W. (1998). Health services provided by school nurses for students with chronic health problems: A 1996 NASN research award winner. *Journal of School Nursing, 14*(5), 4–10, 12–16.

Ludington, S. M. (1990). Energy conservation during skin-to-skin contact between premature infants and their mothers. *Heart and Lung, 19*, 445–451.

Lynn-McHale, D. J., & Smith, A. (1991). Comprehensive assessment of families of the critically ill. *AACN Clinical Issues in Critical Care Nursing, 2*, 195–209.

MacLean, S. L. (1987). Description of cues nurses use for diagnosing activity intolerance. *Dissertation Abstracts International, 48–08B,* 2264.

Maslow, A. (1968). *Toward a psychology of being* (2nd ed.). Princeton, NJ: VanNostrand.

McCall, B. H. (1991). Neurological intensive monitoring system: Unit assessment tool. In K. M. Schaefer & J. B. Pond (Eds.), *Levine's conservation model: A framework for nursing practice* (pp. 83–90). Philadelphia: F. A. Davis.

Mefford, L. C. (2004). A theory of health promotion for preterm infants based on Levine's Conservation Model of Nursing. *Nursing Science Quarterly, 17*, 260–272.

Melancon, B., & Miller, L. H. (2005). Massage therapy versus traditional therapy for low back pain relief. *Holistic Nursing Practice, 19*(3), 116–121.

Mock, V., Krumm, S., Belcher, A., Stewart, K., De Weese, T., Shang, J, et al. (2007). Exercise during prostate cancer treatment: Effects on functional status and symptoms. *Oncology Nursing Forum, 34*(1), 189–190.

Mock, V., St. Ours, C., Hall, S., Bositis, A., Tillery, M., Belcher, A., et al., (2007). Using a conceptual model in nursing research—Mitigating fatigue in cancer patients. *Journal of Advanced Nursing, 58*, 503-512.

Nagley, S. J. (1984). Prevention of confusion in hospitalized elderly persons. *Dissertation Abstracts International, 45–06B,* 1732.

Neswick, R. S. (1997). Myra E. Levine: A theoretic basis for ET nursing. *Journal of WOCN, 21*(1), 6–9.

Newport, M. A. (1984). Conserving thermal energy and social integrity in the newborn. *Western Journal of Nursing Research, 6*, 176–197.

O'Laughlin, K. M. (1986). Changes in bladder function in the woman undergoing radical hysterectomy for cervical cancer. *JOGNN:*

Journal of Obstetric, Gynecologic, and Neonatal Nursing, 15, 380–385.

Pappas, W. S. (1990). The sexually transmitted disease patient's satisfaction with nursing care and impact on anxiety level. *Masters Abstracts International, 29–01*, 97.

Pasco, A., & Halupa, D. (1991). Chronic pain management. In K. M. Schafer & J. P. Pond (Eds.), *Levine's conservation model: A framework for nursing practice* (pp. 101–117). Philadelphia: F. A. Davis.

Piccoli, M., & Galvão, C. M. (2001). Perioperative nursing: Identification of the nursing diagnosis infection risk based on Levine's conceptual model [Portuguese]. *Revista Lation-Americana de Enfermagem, 9*(4), 37–43. Abstract in English retrieved May 29, 2007, from CINAHL Plus with Full Text database.

Piccoli, M., & Galvão, C. M. (2005). Pre-operative nursing visit: A methodological proposal based on Levine's Conceptual Model [Portuguese]. *Revista Electronica de Enfermagem, 7*, 365–371. Abstract in English retrieved May 29, 2007, from CINAHL Plus with Full Text database.

Pond, J. B. (1991). Ambulatory care of the homeless. In K. M. Schaefer & J. B. Pond (Eds.), *Levine's conservation model: A framework for nursing practice* (pp. 167–178). Philadelphia: F. A. Davis.

Pond, J. B., & Taney, S. G. (1991). Emergency care in a large university emergency department. In K. M. Schaefer & J. B. Pond (Eds.), *Levine's conservation model: A framework for nursing practice* (pp. 151–166). Philadelphia: F. A. Davis.

Roberts, K. L., Brittin, M., Cook, M., & deClifford, J. (1994). Boomerang pillows and respiratory capacity. *Clinical Nursing Research, 3*(2), 157–165.

Rogers, C. R. (1961). *On becoming a person*. Boston: Houghton Mifflin.

Sacks, O. (1985). *The man who mistook his wife for a hat*. New York: Summit.

Savage, T. A., & Culbert, C. (1989). Early intervention: The unique role of nursing. *Journal of Pediatric Nursing, 4*, 339–345.

Schaefer, K. M. (1991a). Care of the patient with congestive heart failure. In K. M. Schaefer & J. B. Pond (Eds.), *Levine's conservation model: A framework for nursing practice* (pp. 119–132). Philadelphia: F. A. Davis.

Schaefer, K. M. (1991b). Developing a graduate program in nursing: Integrating Levine's philosophy. In K. M. Schaefer & J. B. Pond (Eds.), *Levine's*

conservation model: A framework for nursing practice (pp. 209–217). Philadelphia: F. A. Davis.

Schaefer, K. M. (2006). Myra Levine's Conservation Model and its applications. In M. E. Parker, *Nursing theories and nursing practice* (pp. 94–112). Philadelphia: F. A. Davis.

Schaefer, K. M., & Pond, J. B. (Eds.). (1991). *Levine's conservation model: A framework for nursing practice*. Philadelphia: F. A. Davis.

Schaefer, K. M., & Pond, J. B. (1994). Levine's conservation model as a guide to nursing practice. *Nursing Science Quarterly, 7*, 53–54.

Schaefer, K. M., & Potylycki, M. J. S. (1993). Fatigue associated with congestive heart failure: Use of Levine's Conservation Model. *Journal of Advanced Nursing, 18*(2), 260–268.

Selye, H. (1956). *The stress of life*. New York: McGraw-Hill.

Taylor, J. W. (1974). Measuring the outcomes of nursing care. *Nursing Clinics of North America, 9*, 337–349.

Trench, A. S. (Executive producer), Wallace, D. (Producer), & Coberg, T. (Director). (1987). *Myra E. Levine—The nurse theorists: Portraits of excellence* [Videotape]. Oakland, CA: Studio Three Production, Samuel Merritt College of Nursing.

Webb, H. (1993). Holistic care following a palliative Hartmann's procedure. *British Journal of Nursing, 2*(2), 128–132.

Winslow, E., Lane, L. D., & Gaffney, F. A. (1985). Oxygen consumption and cardiovascular response in control adults and acute myocardial infarction patients during bathing. *Nursing Research, 34*, 164–169.

Wong, S. (1968). *Rehabilitation of a patient following myocardial in/out*. Unpublished master's thesis, Loyola University of Chicago School of Nursing.

Yeates, D. (1982). *A comparison of two bearing-down techniques during the second stage of labor*. Master's thesis, University of Illinois at the Medical Center, Graduate College, Department of Nursing Sciences, Chicago.

Yeates, D. A., & Roberts, J. E. (1984). A comparison of two bearing-down techniques during the second stage of labor. *Journal of Nurse-Midwifery, 29*, 3–11.

Zalon, M. L. (2004). Correlates of recovery among older adults after major abdominal surgery. *Nursing Research, 53*(2), 99–106.

Bibliography

Levine, M. E. (1967). The four conservation principles of nursing. *Nursing Forum, 6*, 45–59.

Levine, M. E. (1969). The pursuit of wholeness. *American Journal of Nursing, 69*, 93–98.

Levine, M. E. (1970). The intransigent patient. *American Journal of Nursing, 70*, 2106–2111.

Levine, M. E. (1971). Holistic nursing. *Nursing Clinics of North America, 6*, 253–264.

Levine, M. E. (1988). Antecedents from adjunctive disciplines: Creation of nursing theory. *Nursing Science Quarterly, 1*, 16–21.

Levine, M. E. (1989). The ethics of nursing rhetoric. *Image: Journal of Nursing Scholarship, 21*, 4–6.

Annotated Bibliography

Blasage, M. C. (1987). Toward a general understanding of nursing education: A critical analysis of the work of Myra Estrin Levine. *Dissertation Abstracts International, 47-11B*, 4467.

The purpose of this research was to review and identify trends in the writings of Myra Estrin Levine. In addition, the study compared and contrasted Levine's model with those of Imogene King and Dorothea Orem. Levine's model was identified as one of her greatest contributions to nursing. Four trends were identified in her writings. These trends were holistic patient care, communication, nursing education, and ethics in nursing practice.

Mefford, L. C. (2004). A theory of health promotion for preterm infants based on Levine's Conservation Model of Nursing. *Nursing Science Quarterly, 17*, 260–272.

Mefford developed a new middle range theory of health promotion for preterm infants, using Levine's conservation principles, to guide neonatal nursing. She identifies threats to the balance of energy, structural integrity, personal integrity, and social integrity. In this article, she also discusses nursing care needed to help the preterm infant achieve conservation of wholeness, as represented by being discharged from the neonatal intensive care unit into the care of the family on or before the expected date of term gestation.

Mock, V., Krumm, S., Belcher, A., Stewart, K., De Weese, T., Shang, J., et al. (2007). Exercise during prostate cancer treatment: Effects on functional status and symptoms. *Oncology Nursing Forum, 34*(1), 189–190.

This interdisciplinary study investigated effects of a walking exercise program on maintenance of physical functioning and management of symptoms in patients undergoing radiation therapy to treat prostate cancer. The exercise program was nurse directed and based on the framework that by increasing functional capacity, conservation of energy and structural integrity would be supported. Overall results supported that a nurse-directed exercise program improved functional capacity during radiation therapy for prostate cancer.

CHAPTER **11**

Conceptual System and Theory of Goal Attainment

Imogene M. King

Julia B. George

Imogene M. King was born in 1923, the youngest of three children. She received her basic nursing education from St. John's Hospital School of Nursing in St. Louis, Missouri, graduating in 1945. Her B.S. in nursing and education with minors in philosophy and chemistry (1948) and M.S. in nursing (1957) were from St. Louis University, and her Ed.D. (1961) was from Teachers College, Columbia University, New York. She also did postdoctoral study in research design, statistics, and computers (King, 1986b).

King had experience in nursing as an administrator, an educator, and a practitioner. Her area of clinical practice was adult medical-surgical nursing. She served as a faculty member at St. John's Hospital School of Nursing, St. Louis; Loyola University, Chicago, Illinois; and the University of South Florida, Tampa. She also was director of the School of Nursing at Ohio State University, Columbus. She was an assistant chief of the Research Grants Branch, Division of Nursing, Department of Health, Education, and Welfare, in the mid-1960s and on the Defense Advisory Committee on Women in the Services for the Department of Defense in the early 1970s. King received many honors, including induction into the American Academy of Nursing in 1994, receiving the American Nurses Association Jessie M. Scott Leadership Award in 1996, being granted lifetime membership in the Florida Nurses Association, and having the University of Tampa annual research award named for her.

She was Professor Emeritus from the University of South Florida and continued to consult and work on the further application of her theory during her so-called retirement years. She was actively involved in the establishment of the King International Nursing Group, which was headquartered at Oakland University's School of Nursing, Rochester, Michigan. King died in Florida on December 24, 2007 (Kennedy, 2008; Stevens & Messmer, 2008).

During the 20th century, the rapidity of knowledge development in many arenas had as great an impact on the profession of nursing as on the rest of society. In the 1960s, as emerging professionals, nurses were identifying the knowledge base specific to nursing practice and to an expanding role for nurses. In 1964, Imogene M. King published a paper discussing problems and prospects for the development of nursing knowledge. In 1968, she first identified several concepts she later used in her conceptual system and continued to discuss the need for a nursing knowledge base. In this environment, King (1971) sought to answer several questions:

1. What are some of the social and educational changes in the United States that have influenced changes in nursing?
2. What basic elements are continuous throughout these changes in nursing?
3. What is the scope of the practice of nursing, and in what kind of settings do nurses perform their functions?
4. Are the current goals of nursing similar to those of the past half century?
5. What are the dimensions of practice that have given the field of nursing unifying focus over time? (p. 19)

In exploring the literature on systems analysis and general system theory, King (1971) developed additional questions:

1. What kind of decisions are nurses required to make in the course of their roles and responsibilities?
2. What kind of information is essential for them to make decisions?
3. What are the alternatives in nursing situations?
4. What alternative courses of action do nurses have in making critical decisions about another individual's care, recovery, and health?
5. What skills do nurses now perform and what knowledge is essential for nurses to make decisions about alternatives? (pp. 19–20)

Even though these questions were posed several decades ago, they still provide food for thought. Their continued importance and the importance of their answers demonstrate the timelessness of King's thinking and scholarship about nursing knowledge.

King's *Toward a Theory for Nursing: General Concepts of Human Behavior* was published in 1971 and *A Theory for Nursing: Systems, Concepts, Process* in 1981 (reprinted in 1990). These publications grew from King's thoughts about the vast amount of knowledge available to nurses and the difficulty this presents to the individual nurse in choosing the facts and concepts relevant to a given situation. In the preface to *Toward a Theory for Nursing* (1971), King clearly states she was proposing a conceptual framework for nursing and not a nursing theory. As she denoted in the title, her purpose was to help move *toward* a theory for nursing. In contrast, in the preface to *A Theory for Nursing* (1981/1990a), she indicates that she has expanded and built on the original framework. In this second publication, she again presents her system-based conceptual framework and discusses the relationship of the concepts she identifies as fundamental to comprehending nursing as a system in the health care systems. In this text she also discusses concept development and knowledge application in nursing and, through explication of her Theory of Goal Attainment, derived from the open systems framework, shows one way of constructing a theory.

King (1997, 2001, 2006a) now identifies her framework as a conceptual system. The function of a conceptual system is to give support for arranging ideas or concepts into a grouping that provides meaning. As her extensive documentation indicates (see King, 1971, 1981/1990a), she has drawn from a wide variety of sources in developing the conceptual system and deriving the theory from that conceptual system. Because the Theory of Goal Attainment is derived from the conceptual system, the conceptual system and its assumptions and concepts are presented first, and then the goal attainment theory is discussed.

KING'S CONCEPTUAL SYSTEM

The purposes of the conceptual system are to (1) name concepts necessary to nursing as a discipline, (2) provide for the derivation of theories that are tested through research as part of the development of the scientific base for nursing knowledge, (3) provide an organizing structure for nursing curricula, and (4) lead to nursing practice, based in theory, that supports quality care in all settings in which nursing occurs (King, 1990c, 1997). Concepts and knowledge may be similar across disciplines, but the way each profession uses them will differ (King, 1989). The conceptual system includes goal, structure, functions, resources, and decision making, which King (1990c, 1997) says are essential elements. The conceptual system has health as the *goal* for nursing. *Structure* is represented by three open systems. *Functions* are demonstrated in reciprocal relations of individuals in interaction and transactions. *Resources* include both people (health professionals and their clients) and money, goods, and services for items needed to carry out specific activities. *Decision making* occurs when choices are made in resource allocation to support attaining system goals.

King (1989) presents several assumptions that are basic to her conceptual system. These include the assumptions that human beings are open systems in constant interaction with their environment, that nursing's focus is human beings interacting with their environment, and that nursing's goal is to help individuals and groups maintain health.

The conceptual system is composed of three interacting systems: the personal systems, the interpersonal systems, and the social systems. Figure 11-1 presents a schematic diagram of these interacting systems. King (1995a) summarizes the conceptual system as focusing on human behavior. Each personal system represents an individual. When individuals interact with others, they form interpersonal systems that may range in size from two people to a large group. Groups interact with one another and form social systems that in turn are part of a community; communities reside in societies.

The unit of analysis for the conceptual system is the behavior of humans in various social environments (King, 1995a). King identifies several concepts as relevant for each of these systems. However, she also states that the placement of concepts with each system is arbitrary because all the concepts are interrelated in the human–environment interaction, and knowledge of all the concepts is used by the nurse in most situations. King (1981/1990a) has defined most of these concepts and refers back to these definitions in her later publications. Over time, concepts have been added or apparently deleted. See Table 11-1 for the conceptual system concepts as they have been discussed in various publications (King, 1971, 1981/1990a, 1989, 1990c, 1992, 1995a, 2001, 2006a).

Personal Systems

Each individual is a personal system. For a personal system the most current concepts are perception, self, growth and development, and body image (King, 2001, 2006a). *Perception* is presented as the major concept of a personal system, the concept that influences all

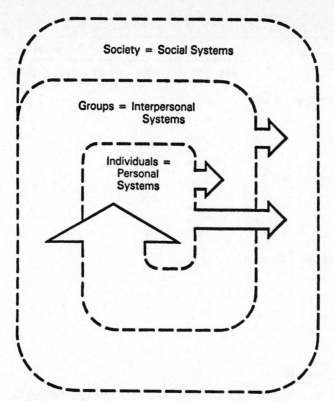

FIGURE 11-1 Dynamic interacting systems. (*Adapted from King, I. M. (1971). Toward a theory for nursing. New York: Wiley, p. 20. Copyright © 1971, by John Wiley & Sons, Inc. Used with permission.)*

behaviors or to which all other concepts are related. The characteristics of perception are that it is universal, or experienced by all; subjective or personal; and selective for each person, meaning that any given situation will be experienced in a unique manner by each individual involved. Perception is focused on activity in the present that is based on the available information. Also, perception is transactions; that is, individuals are active participants in situations, and their identities are affected by their participation (King, 1981/1990a). King further discusses perception as a process in which data obtained through the senses and from memory are organized, interpreted, and transformed. This process of human interaction with the environment influences behavior, provides meaning to experience, represents the individual's image of reality, and includes learning.

The characteristics of *self* are the dynamic person who is an open system and whose actions are oriented toward achieving goals. King (1981/1990a) accepts Jersild's (1952) definition of self that includes self as made up of those thoughts and feelings related to one's awareness of being a person separate from others and influencing one's view of who and what he or she is. Included are attitudes, ideas, values, and commitments. Also, self differentiates one's inner world from the outer world in which other people and objects exist.

TABLE 11-1   Concepts Included in King's Conceptual System

Concept	Year of Publication							
	1971	1981	1989	1990c	1992	1995a	2001	2006a
Personal Systems (Individuals)								
Perception	•	•	•	•	•	•	•	•
Information	•							
Energy	•							
Self		•	•	•	•	•	•	•
Growth and development		•	•	•	•	•	•	•
Body image		•	•	•	•	•	•	•
Space		•	•		*	•		
Time		•	•		•	•		
Learning			•		•	•		
Interpersonal Systems (Groups)								
Interpersonal relations	•				•			
Communication	•	•	•	•	•	**	•	•
Interaction		•	•	•	•	•	•	•
Transactions		•	•	•	•	•	•	•
Role		•	•	•	•	•	•	•
Stress		•	•		•	•		
Social Systems (Society)								
Social organization	•	•	***	•	•	•	•	•
Role	•							
Status		•	•		•	•		
Authority			•	•	•	•	•	•
Power			•	•	•	•	•	•
Decision making			•	•	•	•	•	•
Control			•					

* Listed as personal space beginning in 1992.
**Described as verbal and nonverbal communication beginning in 1995.
***Became organization in 1989.

The characteristics of *growth and development* include changes in behavior at the cellular and molecular levels in individuals. These changes usually occur in an orderly manner, one that is predictable but has individual variations. They are influenced by genetic makeup; by life experiences, especially those that have meaning and lead to satisfaction; and by an environment that supports movement toward maturity (King, 1981/1990a). Growth and development can be defined as the processes in people's lives through which they move from a potential for achievement to actualization of self. Theorists mentioned are Freud (1966), Erikson (1950), Piaget (Inhelder & Piaget, 1964), Gesell (1952), and Havinghurst (1953), but no particular model, theory, or framework of growth and development is specifically selected.

Body image is characterized as very personal and subjective, acquired or learned, dynamic and changing as the person redefines self. Body image is part of each stage of growth and development. King (1981/1990a) indicates that body image includes both the way one perceives one's body and others' reactions to one's appearance.

In earlier publications, King (1981/1990a, 1989, 1992, 1995a) included space and time as concepts in the personal system and has defined them. *Space* is characterized as universal because everyone has some concept of it. It may be personal and subjective; situational and dependent on the relationships in the situation; dimensional as a function of volume, area, distance, and time; and transactional or based on the individual's perception of the situation. King (1981/1990a) states that space occurs in every direction, is universally the same, and is defined by the physical area known as territory and by the behaviors of those who occupy it. Individual definitions of space are influenced by culture.

Time is characterized as universal and inherent in life processes, relational or dependent on distance and the amount of information occurring, unidirectional or irreversible as it moves from past to future with a continuous flow of events, measurable, and subjective because it is based on perception. King (1981/1990a) defines time as an interval between the two events that is experienced differently by each person.

In 1986, King (1986a) added *learning* as a concept in the personal system. She did not further define learning as a concept. Learning is included in 1995 but is not discussed as a separate concept in later publications. In 2001, King states that coping was added to the personal system but does not discuss this concept in any more detail. In 1992, she discussed coping in relation to stress and stressors in the interpersonal system.

Perception, self, growth and development, and body image are the current concepts of the personal system. The focus of nursing in the personal system is the person (King, 1986a). When personal systems come in contact with one another, they form interpersonal systems.

Interpersonal Systems

Interpersonal systems are formed by human beings interacting. Two interacting individuals form a dyad, three form a triad, and four or more form small or large groups. The complexity of the interactions increases as the number of people interacting increases. The most current concepts for interpersonal systems are interaction, communication, transaction, and role (King, 2001, 2006a). The concepts from the personal system are also used in understanding interactions (King, 1989). In 1992, King included interpersonal relations as a concept of interpersonal systems. She did not define this concept, and it has not been included in later works.

Interaction is characterized by values, mechanisms for establishing human relationships, being universally experienced, being influenced by perceptions, reciprocity, being mutual or interdependent, containing verbal and nonverbal communication, learning occurring when communication is effective, unidirectionality, irreversibility, dynamism, and existing in time and space (King, 1981/1990a). Interactions are defined as the observable behaviors of two or more persons in mutual presence.

Characteristics of *communication* are that it is verbal and nonverbal; situational; perceptual; transactional; irreversible, or moving forward in time; personal; and dynamic (King, 1981/1990a). Symbols for verbal communications are provided by language, for such communication includes the spoken and written language that conveys ideas from one person or group to another. An important aspect of nonverbal behavior is touch. Other aspects of nonverbal behavior are distance, posture, facial expression, physical appearance, and body movements. Communication involves the exchange of information between persons. This may occur face-to-face, through electronic media, and through the written word. Communication as a fundamental social process develops and maintains human relations and facilitates the ordered functioning of human groups and societies. As the information component of human interactions, communication occurs in all behaviors. King also discusses communication as intrapersonal or occurring within the person. She includes genetics, metabolic changes, hormonal fluctuations, neurological signals, as well as psychological processes and indicates that intrapersonal communication can affect the person's social exchanges.

Transactions, for this conceptual system, are derived from cognition and perceptions and not from transactional analysis. The characteristics of transactions are that they are unique because each person has a distinctive view of the world based on that person's perceptions, they occur in space and time, and they are experience—a series of events in time. King (1981/1990a) defines transactions as a series of exchanges between human beings and the environment that include observable behaviors that seek to reach goals of worth to the participants.

The characteristics of *role* include reciprocity in that a person may be a giver at one time and a taker at another time, with a relationship between two or more individuals who are functioning in two or more roles that are learned, social, complex, and situational (King, 1981/1990a). There are three major elements of role. The first is that role consists of a set of expected behaviors of those who occupy an identified position in a social system. The second is a set of procedures or rules that define the obligations and rights associated with a position in an organization. The third is a relationship of two or more persons who are interacting for a purpose in a particular situation. The nurse's role can be defined as interacting with one or more others in a nursing situation in which the nurse as a professional uses the skills, knowledge, and values identified as belonging to nursing to identify goals with others and help them achieve the goals.

Stress and coping with stress were included and defined by King in earlier publications (1981/1990a, 1989, 1992, 1995a). The characteristics of *stress* are that it is a universal dynamic as a result of open systems being in continuous exchange with the environment; the intensity varies; there is a temporal-spatial dimension that is influenced by past experiences; and it is individual, personal, and subjective—a response to life events that is uniquely personal. King (1981/1990a) defines stress as an ever-changing condition in which an individual, through environmental interaction, seeks to keep equilibrium to support growth and development and activity. This environmental interaction is based on an open system process of exchange of information and energy with the purpose of regulating and controlling stressors. In addition, stress involves objects, persons, and events as stressors that evoke an energy response from the person. Stress may be positive or negative and may simultaneously help an individual to a peak of achievement and wear the individual down.

The defined concepts of interpersonal systems are interaction, communication, transaction, role, and stress. Those currently used in the conceptual system are interaction, communication, transaction, and role. The focus of nursing in the interpersonal system is the environment (King, 1986a). Interpersonal systems join together to form larger systems known as social systems.

Social Systems

A social system is a structured large group in a system that includes the roles, behaviors, and practices defined by the system for the purposes of sustaining desirable attributes and for creating methods to maintain the practices and rules of the system

(King, 1981/1990a). Examples of social systems include peers, families, community groups, religious groups, educational organizations, governments, and work systems. The most current concepts relevant to social systems are organization, authority, power, and decision making, plus all the concepts from the personal and interpersonal systems (King, 1989, 2001, 2006a).

King (1981/1990a) proposes four parameters for *organization*. The first is those values held by human beings as well as the patterns of behavior and the expectations, needs, and desired outcomes of the individuals in the system. The second is the environment in which the system exists and that influences the availability of resources, both material and human. The third is the humans in the system—family members, administration and staff, officers and members. The fourth involves the technology used to reach the goals of the organization.

An *organization* is characterized by a structure that orders positions and activities and includes formal and informal arrangements of people to gain both personal and organizational goals, has functions that describe the roles and positions of people as well as the activities to be performed, has goals or outcomes to be achieved, and has resources. King (1981/1990a) defines an organization as being made up of individuals who have prescribed roles and positions and who make use of resources to meet goals—both personal and organizational.

The characteristics of *authority* include that it is observable through the regularity, direction, and responsibility for actions it provides; universal; necessary to formal organizations; reciprocal because it requires cooperation; resides in a holder who must be perceived as legitimate; situational; essential to goal achievement; and associated with power (King, 1981/1990a). Assumptions about authority include that it can be discerned by human beings and seen as legitimate, it can be associated with a position in which the position holder distributes rewards and sanctions, it can be held by professionals through their competence in using special knowledge and skills, and it can be exercised through group leadership by those with human relations skills. King defines authority as an active, reciprocal process of transaction in which the actors' experience, understanding, and values influence the meaning, legitimacy, and acceptance of those in organizational positions associated with authority.

Power is characterized as universal, situational (i.e., not a personal attribute but existing in the situation), necessary in the organization, influenced by resources in a situation, dynamic, and goal directed (King, 1981/1990a). Premises about power are that it is energy that is potential rather than actual, is necessary to avoid chaos in society, increases group integration, is related to organizational position, has a direct association with authority, is a function of the communication of human beings, and is associated with decision making. King defines power in a variety of ways, including organizational capacity to use resources to meet goals, one person influencing others, capability to attain goals, existing in every area of life with all having potential for power, and a social force.

Decision making is characterized as necessary to provide order in an individual's or group's living and working, universal, individual, personal, subjective, situational, a continuous process, and goal directed. Decision making in organizations is defined as a changing and orderly process through which choices related to goals are made among identified possible activities and individual or group actions are taken to move toward the goal (King, 1981/1990a).

In her earlier publications, King includes and defines status as a concept in social systems. Status is characterized as situational, position dependent, and reversible. King

(1981/1990a) defines status as the relationship of one's place in a group to others in the group or of a group to other groups. She also identifies that status is accompanied by advantages, accountabilities, and requirements. In 1989 control was included as a concept of social systems but was not defined.

The major theses of King's (1981/1990a) conceptual system are that every individual views the world as a whole as goals are identified and sought with other people and with objects in the environment. Also, the establishment of and movement toward goals occur in life situations characterized by the interaction of the perceiver and the perceived (person or object), with each person being an active participant and each participant changed by the activities and exchanges that occur.

Theories may be derived from conceptual frameworks. King has derived a Theory of Goal Attainment from the concepts and systems of her conceptual system.

KING'S THEORY OF GOAL ATTAINMENT

The major elements of King's middle-range Theory of Goal Attainment are seen "in the interpersonal systems in which two people, who are usually strangers, come together in a health care organization to help and be helped to maintain a state of health that permits functioning in roles" (King, 1981/1990a, p. 142). The theory's focus on interpersonal systems reflects King's belief that the practice of nursing is differentiated from that of other health professions by what nurses do with and for individuals. The original concepts of the theory are interaction, perception, communication, transaction, self, role, stress, growth and development, time, and personal space (King, 1981/1990a, 1986b, 1987b, 1989, 1990c, 1992, 1995b, 1997, 1999). In her 2001 overview, King added decision making and omitted growth and development, stress, time, and space, without discussion of a rationale for change. Table 11-2 identifies the concepts included/excluded from the theory over time. The most current concepts will be used in the following discussion.

The concepts of the theory are interrelated in every nursing situation (King, 1989, 1995b). Although these terms have already been defined in the conceptual system discussion, they are defined again here as part of the Theory of Goal Attainment. King states that although all concepts have been conceptually defined, only transaction has been operationally defined. However, the operational definition given for transaction is also used for interaction in another publication (King, 1990c).

Interaction is the observable verbal and nonverbal goal-directed behaviors of two or more people in mutual presence and includes perception and communication (King, 1981/1990a). King diagrams interaction as shown in Figure 11-2. This is also known as the transaction process model. Each of the individuals involved in an interaction brings different ideas, attitudes, and perceptions to the exchange. The individuals come together for a purpose and perceive each other; each makes a judgment and takes mental action or decides to act. Then each reacts to the other and the situation (perception, judgment, action, reaction). King indicates that only the interaction and transaction are directly observable. Her law of nurse–patient interaction is that "nurses and patients in mutual presence, interacting purposefully, make transactions in nursing situations based on each individual's perceptions, purposeful communication and valued goals" (King, 1997, p. 184).

Perception is reality as seen by each individual (King, 1981/1990a). The elements of perception are the importing of energy from the environment and organizing it by information, transforming energy, processing information, storing information, and exporting information in the form of observable behaviors.

TABLE 11-2   Concepts in the Theory of Goal Attainment

Concept	Year of Publication										
	1981	1986b	1987b	1989	1990c	1992	1995b	1997	1999	2001	2006a
Interaction	•	•	•	•	•	•	•	•	•	•	•
Perception	•	•	•	•	•	•	•	•	•	•	•
Communication			•	•	•	•	•	•	•	•	•
Transaction	•	•	•	•	•	•	•	•	•	•	•
Self	•	•	•	•	•	•	•	•	•	•	•
Role	•	•	•	•	•	•	•	•	•		
Stress	•	•	•	•	•	**	•	•***	•		
Growth and development	•	•	•	•	•	•	•	•	•		
Time	•	•	•		•	•	•	•	•		
Space	•	•	•	•	*	•	•	•	•		
Coping								•			
Decision making****										•	•

*Became personal space beginning in 1990.

**Identified as coping with stress in 1992.

***Identified as stress-stressors in 1997; coping listed as a separate concept.

****Decision making was discussed as an essential characteristic of an open system in earlier writings.

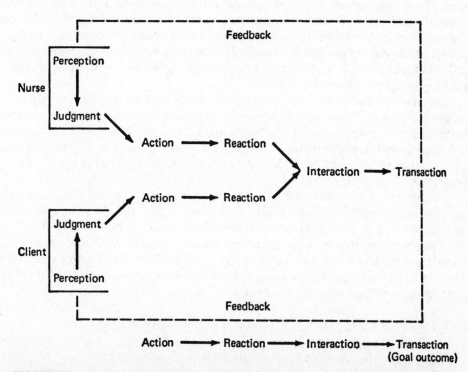

FIGURE 11-2   Interaction. *(Adapted from King, .I M. (1971). Toward a theory for nursing. New York: Wiley, pp. 26, 92. Copyright ©1971, by John Wiley & Sons, Inc. Used with permission.)*

Communication is the exchange of information between people that may occur during a face-to-face meeting, through electronic media, and through the written word (King, 1981/1990a). Communication represents and is part of the information aspect of interaction and may occur within a person as well as between people.

Transaction is a series of exchanges between human beings and their environment that includes observable behaviors that seek to reach goals of worth to the participants (King, 1981/1990a). Transactions represent the aspect of human interactions in which values are apparent and involve compromising, conferring, and social exchange. When transactions occur between nurses and clients, goals are attained.

Role is defined as a set of expected behaviors (King, 1981/1990a). Related to role is the position held by the person, the rights and responsibilities associated with that position, and the relationship between the interacting individuals. It is important that roles be understood and interpreted clearly by all persons involved in defining the expected behaviors to avoid conflict and confusion.

Decision making is defined as the process of making choices from the many available, based upon facts and values, implementing the choice made, and then evaluating the results in relation to the goals achieved (King 1981/1990a). Decision making permeates the lives of individuals and organizations.

Health is not stated as a concept in the theory but is identified as the goal for nursing (King, 1990b). King (1986b) indicates the outcome is an individual's state of health or ability to function in social roles.

King's (1981/1990a, 1989, 1990c) operational definition of transaction has been used to identify the elements in interactions, at other times called a model of transactions. These elements are *action, reaction, disturbance (problem), mutual goal setting, exploration of means to achieve the goal, agreement on means to achieve the goal, transaction,* and *goal attainment.* The model initially described an interpersonal dyad (nurse and client) in interactions, using mutual goal setting or decision making as a process that leads to goal attainment. However, the model may also be applied to a nurse interacting with a family, group, or community as client.

From the Theory of Goal Attainment, King (1990c) has developed predictive propositions that (1) perceptual accuracy, role congruence, and communication in a nurse–client interaction lead to transactions; (2) transactions lead to goal attainment and growth and development; and (3) goal attainment leads to satisfaction and to effective nursing care (pp. 80–81). She suggests that additional propositions may be generated.

Originally, King (1981/1990a) specified internal and external boundary determining criteria. Internal boundary criteria were derived from the characteristics of the concepts of the theory and spoke to the theory itself. External boundary criteria spoke to the domain of the theory. King (personal communication, 2001) no longer supports boundary criteria, as she states that open systems do not have boundaries. However, these former boundary criteria do point out some important aspects of the Theory of Goal Attainment that are still pertinent:

- The nurse is a licensed practitioner of professional nursing.
- The client has a need for services provided by nursing.
- Generally, the nurse and client initially meet as strangers.
- The nurse and client meet in mutual presence and interact with the purpose of meeting goals.

- The nurse–client relationship is one of reciprocity:
  - The nurse brings specialized knowledge and skills and can communicate information that is helpful in setting goals.
  - The client has information and knowledge about self and can communicate concerns and viewpoints to help in mutual goal setting.
- Interactions occur in a dyad (this is the original statement; more recently King has spoken to working with families, groups, and communities and identified the work of others in relation to interactions beyond the dyad).
- Interactions occur between the professional nurse and the client in need of nursing.
- The environment for interactions is a natural one.

King (1995b) includes these ideas in her discussion of the transaction process model and adds that nurses may interact with family members when the client is not verbal. King (1987a) discusses the idea of client locus of control and stated that it is difficult to achieve mutual goal setting with a client who has an external locus of control.

Thus, King is saying that, with individuals, a professional nurse, with special knowledge and skills, and a client in need of nursing, with knowledge of self and perceptions of personal problems, meet as strangers in a natural environment. They interact mutually to identify problems and to establish and achieve goals. The personal system of the nurse and the personal system of the client meet in interaction with the interpersonal system of their dyad. Their interpersonal system is influenced by the social systems that surround them as well as by each of their personal systems. A similar process may occur with families or groups as clients.

KING'S THEORY AND NURSING'S METAPARADIGM

In discussing her conceptual system as an introduction to the presentation of her Theory of Goal Attainment, King (1981/1990a) indicates that the abstract concepts of the conceptual system are human beings, health, environment, and society. Because the theory is presented as a theory for nursing, King also defines nursing. Thus, the four major concepts of human beings, health, environment/society, and nursing are discussed by King.

King (1981/1990a) identifies several assumptions about *human beings*. She describes human beings as social, sentient, rational, reacting, perceiving, controlling, purposeful, action oriented, and time oriented. In 2001, she indicates that human beings are also spiritual and that this term was originally in her 1971 manuscript and was accidentally omitted during publication. From these beliefs about human beings, she has derived the following assumptions that are specific to nurse–client interaction:

- Perceptions of nurse and of client influence the interaction process.
- Goals, needs, and values of nurse and client influence the interaction process.
- Individuals have a right to knowledge about themselves.
- Individuals have a right to participate in decisions that influence their life, their health, and community services.
- Health professionals have a responsibility to share information that helps individuals make informed decisions about their health care.
- Individuals have a right to accept or to reject health care.
- Goals of health professionals and goals of recipients of health care may be incongruent. (1981/1990a, pp. 143–144)

King (1981/1990a) further states that a concern for nursing is helping people interact with their environment in a manner that will support health maintenance and growth toward self-fulfillment. Human beings have three fundamental health needs: (1) the need for health information that is usable at the time when it is needed and can be used, (2) the need for care that seeks to prevent illness, and (3) the need for care when human beings are unable to help themselves. King indicates that nurses have the opportunity to find out what health information the client has, how the client views his own health, and what actions the client takes for health maintenance.

King defines *health* as "dynamic life experiences of a human being, which implies continuous adjustment to stressors in the internal and external environment through optimum use of one's resources to achieve maximum potential for daily living" (King, 1989, p. 152) and as "a dynamic state of an individual in which change is constant and ongoing and may be viewed as the individual's ability to function in his or her usual roles" (King, 1990b, p. 76). King (1990b) affirms that health is not a continuum but a holistic state and identifies the characteristics of health as "genetic, subjective, relative, dynamic, environmental, functional, cultural, and perceptual" (p. 124). She discusses health as a functional state and illness as an interference with that functional state. She defines illness as a deviation from or imbalance in the person's normal functioning. This deviation may be related to biological structure, psychological makeup, or social relationships (King, 1981/1990a).

Environment and *society* are indicated as major concepts in King's conceptual system but are not specifically defined in her work. Society may be viewed as the social systems portion of her conceptual system. In 1983, King extended the ability to interact in goal setting and selection of means to achieve the goal to include mutual goal setting with family members in relation to clients and families. Although her definition of health mentions both internal and external environment and she has stated that "environment is a function of balance between internal and external interactions" (1990b, p. 127), the usual implication of the use of environment in *A Theory for Nursing* is that of external environment. Because she presents her material as based on open systems, it is assumed that a definition of external environment may be drawn from general system theory. Systems are considered to have semipermeable boundaries that help differentiate their internal components from the rest of the world. The external environment for a system is the portion of the world that exists outside of the system. Of particular interest as a system's external environment is the part of the world that is in direct exchange of energy and information with the system. King (1981/1990a) does say that the three systems form the environments that influence individuals.

Nursing is defined as the nurse and client using action, reaction, and interaction in a health care situation to share information about their perception of each other and the situation; this communication enables them to set goals and choose the methods for meeting the goals (King, 1981/1990a). *Action* is defined as a sequence of behaviors involving mental and physical activity. The sequence begins with mental action to recognize the presenting conditions, then physical action to initiate activities related to those conditions, and finally mental action in an effort to exert control over the situation, combined with physical action seeking to achieve goals. *Reaction* is not specifically defined but might be considered to be included in the sequence of behaviors described in action. *Interaction* has been discussed previously. Although King has altered her definition of nursing from that published in 1971, she has continued to refer to nursing as that which is done by nurses. "Lawyer" and "legal situation," "physical therapist" and "therapy situation," or any other practitioner who interacts with clientele could be substituted for "nurse" and "health care situation" in her definitions of nursing. Such substitution would create definitions that could be applied to these other practices. This weakens her definition.

In addition to the foregoing definition of nursing, King (1981/1990a) discusses the goal, domain, and function of the professional nurse. The goal of the nurse is "to help individuals maintain health or regain health" (King, 1990b, pp. 3–4). Nursing's domain includes promoting, maintaining, and restoring health and caring for the sick, injured, and dying. The function of the professional nurse is to interpret information in what is known as the nursing process to plan, implement, and evaluate nursing care for individuals, families, groups, and communities.

THEORY OF GOAL ATTAINMENT AND THE NURSING PROCESS

The basic assumption of the Theory of Goal Attainment—that nurses and clients communicate information, set goals mutually, and then act to attain those goals—is also the basic assumption of the nursing process. King (1990c, 1997) describes the steps of the nursing process as a system of interrelated actions and identifies concepts from her work that provide the theoretical basis for the nursing process as method.

According to King (1981/1990a, 1997), *assessment* occurs during the interaction of the nurse and client, who are likely to meet as strangers. Assessment may be viewed as paralleling action and reaction. The concepts King identifies are the perception, communication, and interaction of nurse and client. The nurse brings to this meeting special knowledge and skills, whereas the client brings knowledge of self and perceptions of the problems that are of concern. Assessment, interviewing, and communication skills are needed by the nurse, as is the ability to integrate knowledge of natural and behavioral sciences for application to a concrete situation.

All concepts of the theory apply to assessment. Growth and development, knowledge of self and role, and the amount of stress influence perception and in turn influence communication, interaction, and transaction. In assessment, the nurse needs to collect data about the client's level of growth and development, view of self, perception of current health status, communication patterns, and role socialization, among other things. Factors influencing the client's perception include the functioning of the client's sensory system, age, development, sex, education, drug and diet history, and understanding of why contact with the health care system is occurring. The perceptions of the nurse are influenced by the cultural and socioeconomic background and age of the nurse and the diagnosis of the client (King, 1981/1990a). Perception is the basis for gathering and interpreting data and thus the basis for assessment. Communication is necessary to verify the accuracy of perceptions. Without communication, interaction and transaction cannot occur.

For example, the nurse is meeting for the first time with Kelly Jenkins and gathers the following assessment data. She perceives Mrs. Jenkins as a well-groomed pregnant female who appears to be comfortable in the examination room and who makes eye contact with the nurse. As they interact, the nurse finds out that Kelly is 25 years old, married, and about six months pregnant and has gained 12 pounds so far during the pregnancy (growth and development); Kelly views herself as essentially healthy (self); she has a B.S. in English and taught high school English before the family's recent move to the area; she plans to look for a teaching position after the baby is born (role); and the family's recent move has been a bit stressful since they must change health care providers in the middle of her first pregnancy but also exciting because they have moved into their first house. Kelly indicates she is using e-mail and Facebook more than she ever did before because it helps her keep in touch with friends and family "back home." She asks questions about Lamaze classes and how she might locate a good dentist and pediatrician. She also reports she is very glad the nausea and vomiting she experienced during the first three months of her pregnancy are no longer bothering her. Her pregnancy appears to be progressing normally and without complications.

The information shared during assessment is used to derive a *nursing diagnosis*, defined by King (1981/1990a) as a statement that recognizes the distresses, difficulties, or worries identified by the client and for which help is sought. The implication is that the nurse makes the nursing diagnosis as a result of the mutual sharing with the client during assessment. Stress may be a particularly important concept in relation to nursing diagnosis because stress, distress, difficulty, and worry may be closely connected.

The nursing diagnoses for Kelly Jenkins would include "healthy primipara progressing normally through pregnancy" and "knowledge deficit about local resources for health care and childbirth related to recent move to the area." These are derived from the interactions that occurred during assessment.

After the nursing diagnosis is made, *outcomes* are identified and *planning* occurs. King (1997, 2001) indicates that goal attainment equates to outcomes. King (1997) says that the concepts involved are *decision making* about goals and *agreeing to means* to attain goals. King describes planning as setting goals and making decisions about how to achieve these goals. This is part of transaction and again involves mutual exchange with the client. She specifies that clients are requested to participate in decision making about how the goals are to be met. Although King assumes that in nurse–client interactions clients have the right to participate in decisions about their care, she does not say they have the responsibility. Thus, clients are requested to participate, not expected to do so. Carter and Dufour (1994) discuss that this ability of the client to decide not to decide enhances the cultural flexibility of King's work.

Implementation occurs in the activities that seek to meet the goals. Implementation is a continuation of transaction in King's theory. She states that the concept involved is the making of *transactions*.

With Kelly Jenkins, the mutually established desired outcome (or goal, in King's terminology) would be a healthy mother, father, and baby. The transactions would involve establishing and keeping a schedule of regular prenatal visits, the nurse providing referrals and information about community resources for the family to identify appropriate health care providers and childbirth education, as well as Kelly maintaining healthy personal habits such as regular exercise and good nutrition.

Evaluation involves descriptions of how the outcomes identified as goals are attained. In King's (1981/1990a) description, evaluation speaks not only to the attainment of the client's goals but also to the effectiveness of nursing care. She also indicates that the involved concept is goal attainment or, if not, why not (King, 1997).

Evaluation data would include the uncomplicated vaginal delivery of a nine-pound, two-ounce boy. Father is beaming and making plans for baseball and football games. The pediatrician selected by the family has seen the baby and pronounced him healthy. Mother and baby have had a successful initial experience with breastfeeding, with support of the nursing staff. The goal of a healthy mother, father, and baby has been attained.

Although all of the theory concepts apply throughout the nursing process, communication with perception, interaction, and transaction are vital for goal attainment and need to be apparent in each phase. King emphasizes the importance of mutual participation in interaction that focuses on the needs and welfare of the client and of verifying perceptions while planning and activities to achieve goals are carried out together. Although King emphasizes mutuality, she does not limit it to verbal communication, nor does she require the client's active physical participation in actions to achieve goal attainment. In situations where the nurse cannot interact directly with the client, Carter and Dufour (1994) and King (1983) support interaction with the family or other members of the client's interpersonal and social systems.

King (2001) has developed a documentation system, known as the goal-oriented nursing record, to facilitate the implementation of the transaction process model and the attainment of goals. She has also developed the Goal Attainment Scale for use in measuring goal attainment.

CRITIQUE OF KING'S THEORY OF GOAL ATTAINMENT

1. *What is the historical context of the theory?*   King began her study of the literature to answer her questions about the influence of changes on nursing as the rapid expansion of knowledge was being recognized. She supported her ideas from the literature and applied that information to the practice of nursing. She identifies an overall assumption for the Theory of Goal Attainment as including "that the focus of nursing is human beings interacting with their environment, leading to health for individuals, which is the ability to function in social roles" (King, 1992, p. 21). Assumptions about nurse–client interactions include that

   perceptions of nurse and client influence the interaction process. Individuals and families have a right to knowledge about their health. They have a right to accept or reject health care. They have a right to participate in decisions that influence their life, their health and community services. Health professionals have a responsibility to share information that helps individuals make informed decisions about their health. Health professionals have a responsibility to gather relevant information about the perceptions of the client so that their goals and the goals of the client are congruent. (p. 21)

   These latter assumptions were first presented for individuals in King's 1981 publication and include families in 1992. These assumptions are easily understood. King derived a Theory of Goal Attainment from her conceptual system of personal, interpersonal, and social systems. This middle-range theory was developed in the midst of the surge of nursing theory development in the latter part of the 20th century. With the emphasis on holistic systems and perceptions, this theory fits best with the simultaneity paradigm.

2. *What are the basic concepts and relationships presented by the theory?*   At various times, King uses the concepts of interaction, perception, communication, transaction, self, role, stress, growth and development, time, space, and decision making for the Theory of Goal Attainment. Her theory deals with a nurse–client dyad, a relationship to which each brings perceptions of self, role, and levels of growth and development. The nurse and client communicate, first in interaction

and then in transaction, to attain mutually set goals. The relationship takes place in space identified by their behaviors and occurs in forward-moving time as they make decisions and take action on those decisions. The specification of transaction as dealing with mutual goal attainment is a unique way of looking at the phenomenon of nurse–client relationships.

3. *What major phenomena of concern to nursing are presented? (These phenomena may include* **but are not limited to** *human beings, environment, health, interpersonal relations, caring, goal attainment, adaptation, and energy fields.)*   In addition to the four major concepts of human being, environment, health, and nursing, King has included the personal, interpersonal, and social systems. She also emphasizes the importance of interaction for transaction and of transaction for goal attainment. Health is identified as a goal.

4. *To whom does it apply? In what situations? In what ways?*   Even though King indicates that many of her concepts are situation dependent, they are not situation specific; that is, they are influenced by the situation but may occur in many different situations. The Theory of Goal Attainment is limited in setting only in regard to "natural environments" and, with growth and development as a concept, is certainly not limited in age. The Theory of Goal Attainment is generalizable to any nursing situation, with a possible limitation relating to difficulties associated with seeking mutual goal setting with a client who has an external locus of control. The emphasis on mutuality would initially appear to limit the theory to dealing with those clients who can verbally interact with the nurse and physically participate in implementations to meet goals. However, King points to observable behaviors and to both verbal and nonverbal communication. Indeed, even the comatose individual has observable behaviors in the form of vital signs and does communicate nonverbally. Also, family members may be involved in transactions for the nonverbal individual. King predicts that with transactions and mutual goal setting, the goals will be attained. King (2006b) has described the use of her systems approach in nursing administration, and Husting (1997) supports that King's theory is applicable in culturally diverse situations and useful in transcultural nursing care. King (1994) also states that her conceptual system is not culture bound.

5. *By what method or methods can this theory be tested?*   The research related to King's theory and conceptual system that has been reported in the literature has used primarily qualitative or descriptive methods. Some experimental and quasi-experimental research has been documented. Perhaps of even greater interest are the reports of testing of middle-range theories derived from King's work and of related measurement tools (Brooks, 1995; Brooks & Thomas, 1997; Davis, 1992; Doornbos, 1995; du Mont, 1998; Frey 1987, 1989, 1995; Killeen, 1996; Meighan, 1998; Rawlins, Rawlins, & Horner, 1990; Sieloff, 1996, 2003). See Table 11-3 for an overview of published research. Those studies that have investigated transactions or goal attainment have supported that mutual goal setting and transactions increase goal attainment or that, conversely, the lack of transactions is associated with lower levels of goal attainment (Binder, 1992; Bowman, 2004; Campbell-Begg, 1998; Ford, 1992; Froman, 1995; Hanna, 1993; Hanucharurnkui & Vinya-nguag, 1991; Kameoka, 1995; Lincoln, 1997; McKay, 1999; Quirk, 1995; Scott, 1998). A large number of studies have indicated the use of King as a guide or framework for studies involving perceptions (Bagby, 1994; Bowman, 2004; Bryant-Lukosius, 1993; Dispenza, 1989; Federowicz, 2002; Froman, 1995; Gellatly-Frey, 1997;

TABLE 11-3   Research with King's Conceptual System and Theory of Goal Attainment

Author/Date	Subjects	Topic
Content Analysis		
Bryant-Lukosius/1993	Patients with non-Hodgkin's lymphoma	Patient and nurse *perceptions* of patient needs
Correlational		
Allan/1995	36 frail elderly	*Goal attainment* and life satisfaction
Batchelor/1994	55 staff nurses	Budgetary knowledge and attitudes toward cost-effectiveness
Church/1997	250 low-income women	Relationship of *interaction* and duration of breastfeeding
Duffy/1990	86 adult med-surg patients	Relationship of nurse caring behaviors and outcomes of care
Froman/1995	40 nurse–client (adult med-surg) pairs	*Perception, transaction* (factor relating)
Gerstle/2001	Nurses	Moral judgment as part *growth and development, perception,* and judgment of pain
Glasgow/1998	30 African Canadian women and their partners	Preconceptual health and pregnancy outcomes
Hobdell/1995	68 mothers, 64 fathers, 69 children with neural tube defects	*Perception, self, growth and development*—relationship of chronic sorrow to parental perception of child's cognitive development
Krassa/1994	354 nurses	Factors influencing political participation
McKay/1999	Case management nurses and their patients	*Transactions, role,* including role strain and patient satisfaction
Monna/1989	Community health nurses	*Perception* of job satisfaction as related to educational preparation
Oates/1994	65 professional and practical nurses	*Perceptions* of participation in shaping the workplace
O'Shall/1988	Head nurses and staff nurses	Congruence of role conception with job satisfaction
Phillips/1995	102 diploma nursing students	*Perceptions* toward poverty and year in program
Rhodes/1995	African American adults	*Perceptions* of health and utilization of health services
Sharts-Hopko/1995	249 females	*Development, environmental change, health, perceptions* during menopause
Ventresca/1994	62 community health nurses	*Goal attainment* and job satisfaction
Wicks/1992	139 families	Relationship of family health and chronic illness
Winker/1996	A hospital	*Interaction* disturbance and organizational health

(continued)

TABLE 11-3 Continued		

Descriptive

Bagby/1994	Adults, ages 25–70	*Perceptions* of nurse caring behaviors
Binder/1992	50 adolescents	*Transactions* in *interactions* with health care providers
Bowman/2004	Parents of children in a hospital setting	Parent *perceptions* and *interactions* between nurses and families
Campbell-Begg/1998	Persons recovering from chemical addiction	*Transactions* during animal-assisted group therapy
Harrity/1992	17 military retirees who volunteered for a support program	Describes characteristics of the volunteers
Johnson/2005	116 public health nurses	*Perceptions* of job satisfaction, recruitment, and retention in the workplace
Keyworth/1998	63 visiting nurses	Responses to sexual harassment and hardiness
Kirkpatrick/1992	8 12th-grade females	*Perceptions* of death and dying
Lincoln/1997	33 nurses, 62 postpartum clients	*Perceptions* of information needs
Lockhart/1992, 2000	Female nurses	*Perceptions* of facial disfigurement
Lott/1996	Professional Black nurses, ages 30–60	*Perceptions* of acceptance and recognition
Mann/1997	57 home care nurses	*Perceptions* of continuing their education
Marasco/1990	5 postpartum couples	*Perceptions* of early discharge and family adjustment
McGeein/1992	Community health nurses	*Perceptions* of elder mistreatment
Monti/1992	40 mental health clients	*Perceptions* of *transactions* in a psychosocial club
Morris/1996	124 home care clients	*Perceptions* of nursing care
Olsson & Forsdahl/1996	62 newly employed nurses	*Perceptions* of competency
Omar/1989	40 stepfamily couples and 40 biological family couples	*Coping* and *interaction* related to life satisfaction
Parsons & Ricker/1993	140 nurse practitioners in Massachusetts	Practices used to promote breastfeeding
Petrich/2000	Medical and nursing students	*Perceptions* of obesity
Quirk/1995	30 registered nurses	Self-directed teams and job satisfaction
Richard-Hughes/1997	African American adults	Attitudes and beliefs about organ donation
Scott/1998	21 caregivers of critically ill children and 17 pediatric critical care nurses	*Perceptions* of the needs of parents/primary caregivers of critically ill children
Theobald/1992	Nursing faculty	Clinical teaching characteristics
Zurakowski/1990	91 nursing home residents	*Person–environment interaction*

TABLE 11-3	Continued	

Experimental

Hanna/1990,1993	51 adolescent females	*Transactions* and oral contraceptive use
Hanucharurnkui & Vinya-nguag/1991	40 adult surgical patients	*Interaction, mutual goal setting,* and self-care to achieve *goals* (used in conjunction with Orem)
Lockhart & Goodfellow, 2009	37 junior-level nursing students	*Patterns of perception*

Grounded Theory

| Desruisseaux/1991 | 5 post-ostomy surgery females | *Goal attainment* as a factor of learning |
| Kameoka/1995 | 19 process recordings from two orthopedic wards in Japan | *Transactions* |

Qualitative

Dispenza/1989	5 couples—husbands had recent myocardial infarction	*Perceptions* of *coping* responses
Federowicz/2002	8 home care clients	*Perception* of quality nursing care (used with modeling and role modeling by Erickson, Tomlin, and Swain)
Gellatly-Frey/1997	6 women who maintained weight loss	*Perceptions* about maintaining weight loss; use of *transactions* to facilitate such maintenance
Gunther/2001		Used Gadamer's philosophical hermeneutics with King's *A Theory of Nursing* to identify the characteristics of high-quality nursing care
Skariah/1999	60 third, fourth, and fifth graders	*Perceptions* of health
Talosi/1993	School-age children with asthma	*Goal attainment*
Villanueva-Noble/1998	203 drawings of fifth graders	*Perceptions* of health

Quasi-Experimental

Cox/1995	133 college students	*Goal attainment* in exercise adherence
Fredenburgh/1993	30 adult community mental health clients	*Mutual goal setting* and stress reduction
Glenn/1989	48 diploma nursing graduates	*Growth and development* (development of *self*) and autonomy
Harman/1998	Certified nurse assistants	Effects of preceptor program
Kaminski/1999	Home care nurses	Nurses *perceptions* as facilitators
Khowaja/2006	Patients undergoing transurethral resection of the prostate; health care providers	*Goal attainment* as improved outcomes
Sink/2001	89 expectant mothers	*Perceptions*, informational needs, and feelings of competency

(continued)

TABLE 11-3 Continued		
Secondary Analysis		
Dawson/1996		Social support, social network, prenatal care
Rexford/2001	Patients receiving home care for heart failure	Nursing approaches and quality of life
Tawil/1993	Spouse caregivers	Gender and *perception* of level of need for assistance
White-Linn/1994	117 adults	*Perceptions* of quality of life
Survey		
Casey/2002	75 unit managers and 269 staff nurses	Policies and practices on perinatal units and nurse attitudes toward breastfeeding
Konkle-Parker/1996	59 nurse practitioners	Health counseling strategies
McGirr, Rukholm, Salmoni, O'Sullivan, & Koren/1990	65 adults referred for cardiac rehabilitation	*Perceptions* of mood and exercise behaviors
Theory Testing		
Brooks/1995, Brooks & Thomas/1997	18 senior baccalaureate students	Theory of *intrapersonal perceptual* awareness
Doornbos/1995	84 families with a chronically mentally ill young adult	Theory of family health in the families of the young chronically mentally ill
du Mont/1998	327 female middle school students	Theory of asynchronous development (early menarche, health risk behaviors, and depressive symptoms)
Frey/1987 1989,1995	Families of children with diabetes or asthma	Theory of families, children, and chronic illness
May/2000	380 baccaluareate pre-nursing students	Theory of basic empathy, self-awareness, and learning styles (from the *personal system*)
Meighan/1998	46 families	Theory of *interaction* enhancement
Tool Development		
Davis/1992		Patient Outcome Documentation—a *goal-oriented* system
Killeen/1996		Killeen–King Patient Satisfaction with Nursing Care (patient–consumer *perceptions)*
Rawlins et al./1990		Family Needs Assessment Tool
Sieloff/1996	460 chief nurse executives	Sieloff–King Assessment of Department *Power*
Sieloff/2003	357 chief nurse executives	Sieloff–King Assessment of Group *Power* Within Organizations
Time-Series Analysis		
Ford/1992	Patient records	Patient-centered care and productivity and quality

Gerstle, 2001; Harrity, 1992; Hobdell, 1995; Johnson, 2005; Kaminiski, 1999; Kirkpatrick, 1992; Lincoln, 1997; Lockhart, 1992, 2000; Lott, 1996; Mann, 1997; Marasco, 1990; McGeein, 1992; McGirr et al., 1990; Monna, 1989; Monti, 1992; Morris, 1996; Oates, 1994; Olsson & Forsdahl, 1996; Petrich, 2000; Phillips, 1995; Rhodes, 1995; Scott, 1998; Sharts-Hopko, 1995; Sink, 2001; Skariah, 1999; Tawil, 1993; Theobald, 1992; Villaneuva-Noble, 1998; White-Linn, 1994). Some of these studies are clearly linked to King's conceptual system and Theory of Goal Attainment. However, in other of these studies the purpose of the study was to describe the perceptions of a group of people, such as nurses in a particular setting, rather than to investigate the effect of the nurse's perceptions and the client's perceptions on the ability of the nurse and client to interact and transact. It is questionable that these studies are testing relationships within the theory. Such testing needs to continue and be reported in the literature.

6. *Does this theory direct nursing actions that lead to favorable outcomes?* The focus of the theory is the attainment of goals. The nurse–client relationship of interaction and transaction occurs because the client's interactions with the environment in some way require support, information, or intervention. King indicates that the nurse and client bring knowledge and information to the relationship that will support the identification and development of interventions to attain mutually set goals. King (1981/1990a) has developed the goal-oriented nursing record in an effort to document the implementation of the transaction process model and goal attainment. She has also developed a criterion-referenced tool for measuring attainment of health goals (King, 1988, 2001). The theory predicts that the use of mutually set goals will lead to favorable outcomes.

7. *How contagious is this theory?* King's conceptual system and Theory of Goal Attainment are widely used, as evidenced by a growing body of literature about the conceptual system and theory. Studies reported in the literature include using King's conceptual system and/or Theory of Goal Attainment to investigate nurses' attitudes/characteristics/perceptions/knowledge (Batchelor, 1994; Gerstle, 2001; Glenn, 1989; Johnson, 2005; Kaminiski, 1999; Keyworth, 1998; Krassa, 1994; Lockhart, 1992, 2000; Lott, 1996; Mann, 1997; McGeein, 1992; Monna, 1989; Oates, 1994; Olsson & Forsdahl, 1996; O'Shall, 1988; Petrich, 2000; Phillips, 1995; Quirk, 1995; Ventresca, 1994), the effects of nursing actions (Church, 1997; Duffy, 1990; Rosendahl & Ross, 1982), client's perceptions and/or goal attainment (Allan, 1995; Bagby, 1994; Cox, 1995; Desruisseaux, 1991; Dispenza, 1989; Federowicz, 2002; Fredenburgh, 1993; Gellatly-Frey, 1997; Glasgow, 1998; Harrity, 1992; Hobdell, 1995; Kameoka, 1995; Kirkpatrick, 1992; Marasco, 1990; Monti, 1992; Morris, 1996; Rhodes, 1995; Richard-Hughes, 1997; Rooke, 1995a; Sharts-Hopko, 1995; Sink, 2001; Skariah, 1999; Talosi, 1993; Tawil, 1993; Villanueva-Noble, 1998; White-Linn, 1994), organizational structure and function (Batchelor, 1994; Casey, 2002; Dawson, 1996; Ford, 1992; Johnson, 2005; McKay, 1999; Monna, 1989; Oates, 1994; O'Shall, 1988; Ventresca, 1994; Winker, 1996), and care in a variety of clinical areas or topics, including children and adolescents, cardiac rehabilitation, chemical addiction, chronic illness, clinical pathways, community mental health, diabetic care, the elderly, families, health behavior change, high-quality care, home care, hospitalized adults, low-income/poverty, menopause, menarche, oncology, parenting, pregnancy,

postpartum and newborn care, and self-care (Binder, 1992; Bowman, 2004; Bryant-Lukosius, 1993; Campbell-Begg, 1998; Church, 1997; Dawson, 1996; Doornbos, 1995; Duffy, 1990; duMont, 1998; Fredenburgh, 1993; Frey, 1987, 1989, 1995; Froman, 1995; Funghetto, Terra, & Wolff, 2003; Glasgow, 1998; Gunther, 2001; Hanna, 1990, 1993; Hanucharunkui & Vinya-nguag, 1991; Hobdell, 1995; Khowaja, 2006; Kirkpatrick, 1992; Konkle-Parker, 1996; Laben, Dodd, & Sneed, 1991; Laben, Sneed, & Seidel, 1995; Lincoln, 1997; Machado & Vieira, 2004; Marasco, 1990; McGirr et al., 1990; Meighan, 1998; Norris & Hoyer, 1993; Omar, 1989; Parsons & Ricker, 1993; Phillips, 1995; Rexford, 2001; Scott, 1998; Sharts-Engel, 1984; Sharts-Hopko, 1995; Skariah, 1999; Talosi, 1993; Villaneuva-Noble, 1998; White-Linn, 1994; Wicks, 1992; Zurakowski, 1990).

Articles relating to the use of King's conceptual system or Theory of Goal Attainment in practice include such clinical areas and topics as carpal tunnel syndrome, case management, cultural diversity, diabetic care, discharge planning, documentation, the elderly, emergency care, genetics, health promotion, HIV, managed care, neonates, oncology, orthopedics, organizational structure, parenting, practice framework, pregnancy, psychotherapy, rural nursing, tertiary care, and quality care (Alligood, 1995; Bauer, 1998, 1999; Benedict & Frey, 1995; Byrne & Schreiber, 1989; Calladine, 1996; Coker et al., 1995; David, 2000; DeHowitt, 1992; Fawcett, Vaillancourt, & Watson, 1995; Gill et al., 1995; Hampton, 1994; Husband, 1988; Husting, 1997; Jolly & Winker, 1995; Jonas, 1987; Jones, Clark, Merker, & Palau, 1995; Kemppainen, 1990; Laben et al., 1995; Messmer, 1995; Messner & Smith, 1986; Norgan, Ettipio, & Lasome, 1995; Norris & Hoyer, 1993; Omar, 1989; Porter, 1991; Rooda, 1992; Shea et al., 1989; Smith, 1988; Sowell & Lowenstein, 1994; Temple & Fawdry, 1992; Tritsch, 1998; West, 1991; Williams, 2001; Woods, 1994). Publications in relation to education have included preparation of certified nursing assistants, curriculum development, teaching methods, and student perceptions and characteristics (Bello, 2000; Brooks, 1995; Brooks & Thomas, 1997; Brown, 1999; Daubenmire, 1989; Dougal & Gonterman, 1999; Gold, Haas, & King, 2000; Gulitz & King, 1988; Harman, 1998; May, 2000; Rooke, 1995b).

Internationally, King's work has been used in relation to practice in Canada and Germany (Bauer, 1998, 1999; Fawcett et al., 1995; Gill et al., 1995; Glasgow, 1998; Petrich, 2000; Porter, 1991; Shea et al., 1989; West, 1991; Woods, 1994). In addition, it has been extended and tested in Sweden and Japan as well as used for education in Sweden (Frey et al., 1995; Kameoka, 1995; Rooke, 1995b). It has been used as a basis for research in Pakistan and Norway (Khowaja, 2006; Olsson & Forsdahl, 1996) and for clinical practice, education, and research in Brazil (Bello, 2000; David, 2000; Franca & Pagliuca, 2002; Funghetto, Terra, & Wolff, 2003; Machado & Vieira, 2004; Moreira & Araújo, 2002a, 2002b). Killeen (2007) recommends the use of King's conceptual system and theory, along with nursing informatics, to frame global communication.

King's conceptual system and theory have demonstrated contagiousness. Further research is needed to establish the relationships among the concepts in the theory, and evaluation reports of use in nursing practice are needed. Lane-Tillerson (2007) predicts King's interpersonal system will have continued utility for practice through 2050 as the interaction between nurse and client will continue to be an essential part of health care. While Lane-Tillerson specifies only the interpersonal system, it is apparent that the personal systems of the nurse and the client as well as the social system of health care will also be pertinent, as the systems are interactive. Thus, the conceptual system, as well as the theory, will continue to provide guidance for nursing practice, education, and research.

STRENGTHS AND LIMITATIONS

It is obvious from the use of the conceptual system and theory across multiple cultures that King's work is not limited to use in the United States. This is a major strength in a time when communication can be instantaneous and multicultural situations are becoming the norm. Husting (1997) speaks to the importance of the cultural facets in each of the interacting systems in the conceptual system.

Although the presentation appears to be complex, King's Theory of Goal Attainment is relatively simple. Of the 12 concepts associated at some time with the theory, 10 are identified and defined and their relationships considered; two concepts are identified only. Six of these concepts are used in King's most current publications (2001, 2006a). King's Theory of Goal Attainment describes a logical sequence of events, and, for the most part, concepts are clearly defined. However, a major inconsistency within her writing is the lack of a clear definition of environment, which is identified as a basic concept for the conceptual system from which she derives her theory. In addition, she indicates that nurses are concerned about the health care of groups and communities but initially concentrated her discussion on nursing as occurring in a dyadic relationship. Thus, the theory essentially draws on only two of the three systems described in the conceptual system. The social systems portion of the conceptual system is less clearly connected to the Theory of Goal Attainment than are the personal and interpersonal systems. This may help explain Carter and Dufour's (1994) concern that critiques of King's work have not always differentiated between the conceptual system and the theory.

The definition of stress indicates that it is both negative and positive, but discussions of stress always imply that it is negative. Finally, King says that the nurse and client are strangers, yet she speaks of their working together for goal attainment and of the importance of health maintenance. Attainment of long-term goals, such as those concerning health maintenance, is not consistent with not knowing each other.

A limitation is the effort required of the reader to sift through the presentation of a conceptual system and a theory with repeated definitions to find the basic concepts. Another limitation relates to the lack of development of application of the theory in providing nursing care to groups, families, or communities. Fortunately, although the original presentations of the theory related to caring for individuals, more recent publications, by King and others, describe the utility of the theory in working with larger units such as groups or families. King (Fawcett, 2001; King, 2006b) also supports the use of her work in the practice of nursing administration.

Another limitation is the need for more public reporting of King-based research and nursing practice. The majority of research to date is found in master's theses and doctoral dissertations, few of which have been published in the nursing literature. Those who have published their studies are to be commended. Frey and Sieloff (1995) provided an excellent start on improving this situation. Others need to follow their example.

Summary

Imogene King has presented a conceptual system from which she derived a Theory of Goal Attainment. The conceptual system consists of three systems—personal, interpersonal, and social—all of which are in continuous exchange with their environments. The current concepts of the personal systems are perception, self, body image, and growth and development. The current concepts of the interpersonal systems are role, interaction, communication, and transaction. Social systems concepts are organization, power, authority, and decision making. Earlier concepts from the conceptual system that may be found in reports of applications related to the conceptual system are space, time, learning, stress, and status.

From these systems and their abstract concepts of human beings, health, environment, and society, King derives a Theory of Goal Attainment. The major concepts of the Theory of Goal Attainment are interaction, perception, communication, transaction, self, and decision making. Each of these is defined, and overall propositions and criteria for determining internal and external boundaries of the theory are presented. Earlier concepts included in the Theory of Goal Attainment are role, stress, growth and development, time, space, and coping.

Imogene King has developed a Theory of Goal Attainment that is based on a philosophy of human beings and a conceptual system. She presents the results of some of the research conducted to test the theory and proposes a goal-oriented nursing record to document, and a Goal Attainment Scale to measure, goal attainment. This chapter also provides an overview of the use of the conceptual system and Theory of Goal Attainment in nursing research, education, and practice.

The theory is useful, testable, and applicable to nursing practice. Although it is not the "perfect theory," it is widely generalizable and not situation specific. Dr. King's work is solidly based in the literature and provides the reader with a rich set of resources for further study. Her work provides nursing with an excellent example of scholarship.

Thought Questions

1. Select one of King's questions listed in the first portion of this chapter. How would you answer this question today?
2. Analyze a nursing situation in which you participated in order to describe how you and your client did or did not achieve transactions.
3. Describe how perceptions influence the other concepts in personal systems.
4. Discuss how the perceptions of each of the participants affects the transaction process.
5. According to King, what is necessary for goal attainment to occur? How do you know a goal has been attained?

References

Allan, N. J. (1995). Goal attainment and life satisfaction among frail elderly. *Masters Abstracts International, 33*(05), 1486.

Alligood, M. R. (1995). Theory of Goal Attainment: Application to adult orthopedic nursing. In M. A. Frey & C. L. Sieloff (Eds.), *Advancing King's systems framework and theory of nursing* (pp. 209–222). Thousand Oaks, CA: Sage.

Bagby, A. M. (1994). Nurse caring behaviors: The perceptions of potential health care consumers in a community setting. *Masters Abstracts International, 33*(03), 864.

Batchelor, S. G. (1994). Relationship of budgetary knowledge and staff nurses' attitudes toward cost-effectiveness. *Masters Abstracts International, 32*(05), 1365.

Bauer, R. (1998). A dialectical study of the psychotherapeutic effectives of nursing interventions [German]. *Pflege, 11*, 305–311.

Bauer, R. (1999). A dialectical perspective of the psychotherapeutic effectiveness of nursing therapeutics [German]. *Pflege, 12*, 5–10.

Bello, I. T. R. (2000). Imogene King's theory as the foundation for the set of a teaching-learning process with undergraduation [*sic*] students [Portuguese]. *Testo & Contexto Enfermagem, 9*, 646–657. Abstract in English retrieved May 18, 2007, from CINAHL Plus with Full Text database.

Benedict, M., & Frey, M. A. (1995). Theory-based practice in the emergency department. In M. A. Frey & C. L. Sieloff (Eds.), *Advancing King's systems framework and theory of nursing* (pp. 317–324). Thousand Oaks, CA: Sage.

Binder, B. K. (1992). King's transaction elements indentified in adolescents' interactions with health care providers. *Dissertation Abstracts International, 54*(01B), 163.

Bowman, A. M. (2004). Parents' perceptions of quality family-centered nursing care in pediatrics. *Masters Abstracts International, 42*(06), 1679.

Brooks, E. M. (1995). Exploring the perception and judgment of senior baccalaureate student nurses from a nursing theoretical perspective. *Dissertation Abstracts International, 56*(12B), 6667.

Brooks, E. M., & Thomas, S. (1997). The perception and judgment of senior baccalaureate student nurses in clinical decision making. *Advances in Nursing Science, 19*(3), 50–69.

Brown, S. J. (1999). Student nurses' perceptions of elderly care. *Journal of National Black Nurses' Assocation, 10*(2), 29–36.

Bryant-Lukosius, D. E. (1993). Patient and nurse perceptions of the needs of patients with non-Hodgkin's lymphoma: A qualitative study. *Masters Abstracts International, 31*(04), 1730.

Byrne, E., & Schreiber, R. (1989). Concept of the month: Implementing King's conceptual framework at the bedside. *Journal of Nursing Administration, 19*(2), 28–32.

Calladine, M. L. (1996). Nursing process for health promotion using King's theory. *Journal of Community Health Nursing, 13*(1), 51–57.

Campbell-Begg, T. (1998). Promotion of transactions during animal-assisted, group therapy with individuals who are recovering from chemical addictions. *Masters Abstracts International, 37*(04), 1175.

Carter, K. F., & Dufour, L. T. (1994). King's theory: A critique of the critiques. *Nursing Science Quarterly, 7*(3), 128–133.

Casey, E. H. (2002). *Breastfeeding support on perinatal units in Florida hospitals.* Unpublished master's thesis, Florida State University, Tallahassee. Abstract retrieved May 18, 2007, from http://etd.lib.fsu.edu/theses/available/etd-04122004-085346.

Church, C. J. (1997). The relationship of interaction between peer counselors and low-income women and duration of breastfeeding. *Masters Abstracts International, 36*(04), 1061.

Coker, E., Fradley, T., Harris, J., Tomarchio, D., Chan, V., & Caron, C. (1995). Implementing nursing diagnosis within the context of King's conceptual framework. In M. A. Frey & C. L. Sieloff (Eds.), *Advancing King's systems framework and theory of nursing* (pp. 161–175). Thousand Oaks, CA: Sage.

Cox, M. A. C. (1995). Exercise adherence: Testing a goal attainment intervention program. *Dissertation Abstracts International, 56*(09B), 4813.

Daubenmire, M. J. (1989). A baccalaureate nursing curriculum based on King's conceptual framework. In J. Riehl-Sisca (Ed.), *Conceptual models for nursing practice* (3rd ed., pp. 167–178). Norwalk, CT: Appleton & Lange.

David, G. L. B. (2000). Ethics in the relationship between nursing and AIDS-afflicted families (Portuguese). *Texto & Contexto Enfermagem, 9*,

590–599. Abstract in English retrieved May 18, 2007, from CINAHL Plus with Full Text database.

Davis, S. M. (1992). Patient Outcome Documentation: Development and implementation. *Masters Abstracts International, 30*(04), 1288.

Dawson, B. W. (1996). The relationship between functional social support, social network and the adequacy of prenatal care. *Masters Abstracts International, 35*(01), 361.

DeHowitt, M. C. (1992). King's conceptual model and individual psychotherapy. *Perspectives in Psychiatric Care, 28*(4), 11–14.

Desruisseaux, B. (1991). A qualitative study: Goal attainment is the path to mastery—A factor contributing to patients' learning following ostomy surgery. *Masters Abstracts International, 30*(02), 296.

Dispenza, J. M. (1989). Relationships of husband and wife perceptions of the coping responses of the female spouse of males in high level stress. *Masters Abstracts International, 28*(03), 407.

Doornbos, M. M. (1995). Using King's systems framework to explore family health in the families of the young chronically mentally ill. In M. A. Frey & C. L. Sieloff (Eds.), *Advancing King's systems framework and theory of nursing* (pp. 192–205). Thousand Oaks, CA: Sage.

Dougal, J., & Gonterman, R. (1999). A comparison of three teaching methods on learning and retention. *Journal for Nurses in Staff Development, 15*, 205–209.

Duffy, J. R. (1990). An analysis of the relationships among nurse caring behaviors and selected outcomes of care in hospitalized medical and/or surgical patients. *Dissertation Abstracts International, 51*(08B), 3777.

Du Mont, P. M. (1998). The effects of early menarche on health risk behaviors. *Dissertation Abstracts International, 60*(07B), 3200.

Erikson, E. (1950). *Childhood and society.* New York: Norton. [out of print]

Fawcett, J. (2001). The nurse theorists: 21st century updates—Imogene M. King. *Nursing Science Quarterly, 14*, 310–315.

Fawcett, J. M., Vaillancourt, V. M., & Watson, C. A. (1995). Integration of King's framework into nursing practice. In M. A. Frey & C. L. Sieloff (Eds.), *Advancing King's systems framework and theory of nursing* (pp. 176–191). Thousand Oaks, CA: Sage.

Federowicz, M. L. (2002). An investigation of clients' perceptions of what constitutes quality nursing care: A phenomenological approach. *Masters Abstracts International, 40*(06), 1501.

Ford, W. A. (1992). A study of productivity and quality on a pilot unit for patient centered care. *Masters Abstracts International, 30*(04), 1290.

Franca, I. S. X., & Pagliuca, L. M. F. (2002). Usefulness and the social significance of the Theory of Goal Attainment by King. *Revista Brasileira de Enfermagem, 55*, 44–51. Abstract retrieved July 11, 2007, from CINAHL Plus with Full Text database.

Fredenburgh, L. (1993). The effect of mutual goal setting on stress reduction in the community mental health client. *Masters Abstracts International, 32*(03), 934.

Freud, S. (1966). *Introductory lectures on psychoanalysis* (J. Strachey, Trans.). New York: Norton. [out of print]

Frey, M. A. (1987). Health and social support in families with children with diabetes mellitus. *Dissertation Abstracts International, 48*(04A), 841.

Frey, M. A. (1989). Social support and health: A theoretical formulation derived from King's conceptual framework. *Nursing Science Quarterly, 2*, 138–148.

Frey, M. A. (1995). Toward a theory of families, children, and chronic illness. In M. A. Frey & C. L. Sieloff (Eds.), *Advancing King's systems framework and theory of nursing* (pp. 109–125). Thousand Oaks, CA: Sage.

Frey, M. A., Rooke, L., Sieloff, C., Messmer, P. R., & Kameoka, T. (1995). King's framework and theory in Japan, Sweden, and the United States. *Image: Journal of Nursing Scholarship, 27*, 127–130.

Frey, M. A., & Sieloff, C. L. (Eds.). (1995). *Advancing King's systems framework and theory of nursing.* Thousand Oaks, CA: Sage.

Froman, D. (1995). Perceptual congruency between clients and nurses: Testing King's Theory of Goal Attainment. In M. A. Frey & C. L. Sieloff (Eds.), *Advancing King's systems framework and theory of nursing* (pp. 223–238). Thousand Oaks, CA: Sage.

Funghetto, S. S., Terra, M. G., & Wolff, L. R. (2003). Woman [sic] with breast cancer: Perception about the disease, family and society [Portuguese]. *Revista Brasilerira de Enfermagem, 56*, 528–532. Abstract in English retrieved May 18, 2007, from CINAHL Plus with Full Text database.

Gellatly-Frey, H. L. (1997). Women's perceptions of factors that contributed to weight loss and maintenance. *Masters Abstracts International, 35*(04), 998.

Gerstle, D. S. (2001). Relationships among registered nurses' moral judgment and their perception and judgment of pain, and selected nurse factors. *Dissertation Abstracts International, 62*(04B), 1803.

Gesell, A. (1952). *Infant development.* New York: Harper & Row. [out of print]

Gill, J., Hopwood-Jones, L., Tyndall, J., Gregoroff, S., LeBlanc, P., Lovett, C., et al. (1995). Incorporating nursing diagnosis and King's theory in O.R. documentation. *Canadian Operating Room Nursing Journal, 13*(1), 10–14.

Glasgow, V. M. (1998). Preconceptual health and its effect on pregnancy outcomes in African-Canadian Women and their partners. *Masters Abstracts International, 36*(06), 1585.

Glenn, C. J. (1989). The development of autonomy in nurses. *Dissertation Abstracts International, 50*(05B), 1852.

Gold, C., Haas, S., & King, I. (2000). Conceptual frameworks: Putting the nursing focus into core curricula. *Nurse Educator, 25*(2), 95–98.

Gulitz, E. A., & King, I. M. (1988). King's general systems model: Application to curriculum development. *Nursing Science Quarterly, 1,* 128–132.

Gunther, M. E. (2001). The meaning of high-quality nursing care derived from King's interacting systems. *Dissertation Abstracts International, 62*(04B), 1804.

Hampton, D. C. (1994). King's Theory of Goal Attainment as a framework for managed care implementation in a hospital setting. *Nursing Science Quarterly, 7,* 170–173.

Hanna, K. M. (1990). Effect of nurse–client transaction on female adolescents' contraceptive perceptions and adherence. *Dissertation Abstracts International, 51*(07B), 3323.

Hanna, K. (1993). Effect of nurse–client transaction on female adolescents' oral contraceptive use. *Image, 25,* 285–290.

Hanucharunkui, S., & Vinya-nguag, P. (1991). Effects of promoting patient's participation in self-care on postoperative recovery and satisfaction with care. *Nursing Science Quarterly, 4,* 14–20.

Harman, B. J. (1998). The effects of a paraprofessional preceptor program for certified nursing assistants in dementia special care units. *Dissertation Abstracts International, 59*(11B), 5786.

Harrity, M. C. (1992). The characteristics of the military retirees who volunteered as civilians for a U.S. Army family support system during Operation Desert Shield/Storm. *Masters Abstracts International, 31*(01), 273.

Havinghurst, R. (1953). *Human development and education.* New York: McKay. [out of print]

Hobdell, E. F. (1995). Using King's interacting systems framework for research on parents of children with neural tube defect. In M. A. Frey & C. L. Sieloff (Eds.), *Advancing King's systems framework and theory of nursing* (pp. 126–136). Thousand Oaks, CA: Sage.

Husband, A. (1988). Application of King's theory of nursing to the care of the adult with diabetes. *Journal of Advanced Nursing, 13,* 484–488.

Husting, P. M. (1997). A transcultural critique of Imogene King's Theory of Goal Attainment. *Journal of Multicultural Nursing and Health, 3*(3), 15–20.

Inhelder, B. F., & Piaget, J. (1964). *The early growth of logic in the child.* New York: Norton. [out of print]

Jersild, A. T. (1952). *In search of self.* New York: Columbia University Teachers College Press. [out of print]

Johnson, T. (2005). Job satisfaction recruitment and retention of public health nurses. *Masters Abstracts International, 43*(05), 1701.

Jolly, M. L., & Winker, C. K. (1995). Theory of Goal Attainment in the context of organizational structure. In M. A. Frey & C. L. Sieloff (Eds.), *Advancing King's systems framework and theory of nursing* (pp. 305–316). Thousand Oaks, CA: Sage.

Jonas, C. M. (1987). King's goal attainment theory: Use in gerontological nursing practice. *Perspectives, 11*(4), 9–12.

Jones, S., Clark, V. B., Merker, A., & Palau, D. (1995). Changing behaviors: Nurse educators and clinical nurse specialists design a discharge planning program. *Journal of Nursing Staff Development, 11,* 291–295.

Kameoka, T. (1995). Analyzing nurse–patient interactions in Japan. In M. A. Frey & C. L. Sieloff (Eds.), *Advancing King's systems framework and theory of nursing* (pp. 251–260). Thousand Oaks, CA: Sage.

Kaminski, L. A. (1999). Perceptions of homecare nurses as facilitators of discussions and advance directives. *Masters Abstracts International, 37*(04), 1179.

Kemppainen, J. K. (1990). Imogene King's theory: A nursing case study of a psychotic client with human immunodeficiency virus infection. *Archives of Psychiatric Nursing, 4,* 384–388.

Kennedy, M. S. (2008). In Memoriam: Imogene King, December 24, 2007. *American Journal of Nursing, 108,* 87.

Keyworth, C. A. (1998). Responses of visiting nurses to sexual harassment by clients. *Masters Abstracts International, 36*(03), 782.

Khowaja, K. (2006). Utilization of King's interacting systems framework and Theory of Goal Attainment with new multidisciplinary model: Clinical pathway. *Australian Journal of Advanced Nursing, 24*(2), 44–50. Abstract retrieved April 14, 2007, from CINAHL Plus with Full Text database.

Killeen, M. B. (1996). Patient-consumer perceptions and responses to professional nursing care: Instrument development. *Dissertation Abstracts International, 57*(04B), 2479.

Killeen, M. B. (2007). Viewpoint: Use of King's conceptual system, nursing informatics, and nursing classification systems for global communication. *International Journal of Nursing Terminologies and Classifications, 18*(2), 51–57.

King, I. M. (1964). Nursing theory: Problems and prospects. *Nursing Science, 2,* 394–403.

King, I. M. (1968). A conceptual frame of reference for nursing. *Nursing Research, 17,* 27–37.

King, I. M. (1971). *Toward a theory for nursing: General concepts of human behavior.* New York: Wiley. [out of print]

King, I. M. (1983). King's theory of nursing. In I. W. Clements & F. B. Roberts (Eds.), *Family health: A theoretical approach to nursing care.* New York: Wiley. [out of print]

King, I. M. (1986a). *Curriculum and instruction in nursing.* East Norwalk, CT: Appleton-Century-Crofts. [out of print]

King, I. M. (1986b). King's Theory of Goal Attainment. In P. Winstead-Fry (Ed.), *Case studies in nursing theory* (pp. 197–213) (Pub. No. 15-2152). New York: National League for Nursing.

King, I. M. (1987a). *King's theory.* Paper presented at Nurse Theorist Conference, Pittsburgh, PA. [cassette recording]

King, I. M. (1987b). King's Theory of Goal Attainment. In R. R. Parse, *Nursing science: Major paradigms, theories and critiques* (pp. 107–113). Philadelphia: Saunders.

King, I. M. (1988). Measuring health goal attainment in patients. In C. Waltz & O. Strickland (Eds.), *Measurement of nursing outcomes* (Vol. 1, pp. 109–117). New York: Springer.

King, I. M. (1989). King's general systems framework and theory. In J. Riehl-Sisca (Ed.), *Conceptual models for nursing practice* (3rd ed., pp. 149–58). Norwalk, CT: Appleton & Lange.

King, I. M. (1990a). *A theory for nursing: Systems, concepts, process.* Albany, NY: Delmar. (Originally published 1981, New York: Wiley)

King, I. M. (1990b). Health as a goal for nursing. *Nursing Science Quarterly, 3,* 123–128.

King, I. M. (1990c). King's conceptual framework and theory of goal of attainment. In M. E. Parker (Ed.), *Nursing theories in practice* (pp. 73–84) (Pub. No. 15-2350). New York: National League for Nursing.

King, I. M. (1992). King's Theory of Goal Attainment. *Nursing Science Quarterly, 5,* 19–26.

King, I. M. (1994). Quality of life and goal attainment. *Nursing Science Quarterly, 7,* 29–32.

King, I. M. (1995a). A systems framework for nursing. In M. A. Frey & C. L. Sieloff (Eds.), *Advancing King's systems framework and theory of nursing* (pp. 14–22). Thousand Oaks, CA: Sage.

King, I. M. (1995b). The Theory of Goal Attainment. In M. A. Frey & C. L. Sieloff (Eds.), *Advancing King's systems framework and theory of nursing* (pp. 23–32). Thousand Oaks, CA: Sage.

King, I. M. (1997). King's Theory of Goal Attainment in practice. *Nursing Science Quarterly, 10,* 180–185.

King, I. M. (1999). A Theory of Goal Attainment: Philosophical and ethical implications. *Nursing Science Quarterly, 12,* 292–296.

King, I. M. (2001). Theory of Goal Attainment. In M. Parker (Ed.), *Nursing theories and nursing practice* (pp. 275–286). Philadelphia: F. A. Davis.

King, I. M. (2006a). Imogene M. King's Theory of Goal Attainment In M. Parker (Ed.), *Nursing theories and nursing practice* (2nd ed., pp. 235–243). Philadelphia: F. A. Davis.

King, I. M. (2006b). A systems approach in nursing administration: Structure, process, and outcome. *Nursing Administration Quarterly, 30*(2), 100–104.

Kirkpatrick, N. C. (1992). A phenomenological study of adolescent females' perceptions of death and dying in light of the AIDS epidemic. *Masters Abstracts International, 31*(02), 765.

Konkle-Parker, D. J. (1996). Survey of nurse practitioners' health counseling strategies. *Masters Abstracts International, 35*(04), 1000.

Krassa, T. J. (1994). A study of political participation by registered nurses in Illinois. *Dissertation Abstracts International, 56*(02B), 743.

Laben, J. K., Dodd, D., & Sneed, L. (1991). King's Theory of Goal Attainment applied in group therapy for inpatient juvenile sexual offenders, maximum security state offenders, and community parolees, using visual aids. *Issues in Mental Health Nursing, 12*(1), 51–64.

Laben, J. K., Sneed, L. D., & Seidel, S. L. (1995). Goal attainment in short-term group psychotherapy settings: Clinical implications for practice. In M. A. Frey & C. L. Sieloff (Eds.), *Advancing King's systems framework and theory of nursing* (pp. 261–277). Thousand Oaks, CA: Sage.

Lane-Tillerson, C. (2007). Imaging practice in 2050: King's conceptual framework. *Nursing Science Quarterly, 20*, 140–143.

Lincoln, K. E. (1997). A comparison of postpartum clients' and nurses' perceptions of priority information needs for early discharge. *Masters Abstracts International, 36*(05), 1330.

Lockhart, J. S. (1992). Female nurses' perceptions regarding the severity of facial disfigurement in patients following surgery for head and neck cancer: A comparison based on experience in head and neck oncology. *Dissertation Abstracts International, 54*(02B), 745.

Lockhart, J. S. (2000). Nurses' perceptions of head and neck oncology patients after surgery: Severity of facial disfigurement and patient gender. *Plastic Surgical Nursing, 20*(2), 68–80. Abstract retrieved July 11, 2007, from CINAHL Plus with Full Text database.

Lockhart, J. S., & Goodfellow, L. M. (2009). The effect of a 5-week head and neck surgical oncology practicum on nursing students' perceptions of facial disfigurement: Part I. *ORL-Head and Neck Nursing, 27*(3), 7–12.

Lott, C. E. (1996). Perceptions of acceptance and recognition among professional Black nurses. *Masters Abstracts International, 34*(04), 1551.

Machado, M. F. A., & Vieira, N. F. C. (2004). The mother's participation in the child malnutrition program [Portuguese]. *Revista Latino-Americana de Enfermagem, 12*(1), 76–82. Abstract in English retrieved May 18, 2007, from CINAHL Plus with Full Text database.

Mann, C. M. (1997). Home care nurses' perceptions of continuing their education. *Masters Abstracts International, 35*(04), 1000.

Marasco, G. (1990). Parents' perceptions of the effects of early postpartum discharge on family adjustment. *Masters Abstracts International, 29*(01), 95.

May, B. A. (2000). Relationships among basic empathy, self-awareness, and learning styles of baccalaureate pre-nursing students within King's personal system. *Dissertation Abstracts International, 61*(06B), 2991.

McGeein, M. L. S. (1992). A descriptive study of community health nurses' perceptions of elder maltreatment. *Masters Abstracts International, 31*(01), 278.

McGirr, M., Rukholm, E., Salmoni, A., O'Sullivan, P., & Koren, I. (1990). Perceived mood and exercise behaviors of cardiac rehabilitation program referras. *Canadian Journal of Cardiovascular Nursing, 1*(4), 14–19.

McKay, T. A. (1999). An examination of case management nurses' role strain, participative decision-making, and their relationships to patient satisfaction: Utilization of King's Theory of Goal Attainment in a managed care environment. *Dissertation Abstracts International, 60*(09B), 4522.

Meighan, M. M. (1998). Testing a nursing intervention to enhance paternal–infant interaction and promote paternal role assumption. *Dissertation Abstracts International, 60*(07B), 3204.

Messmer, P. R. (1995). Implementation of theory-based nursing practice. In M. A. Frey & C. L. Sieloff (Eds.), *Advancing King's systems framework and theory of nursing* (pp. 294–304). Thousand Oaks, CA: Sage.

Messner, R., & Smith, M. N. (1986). Neurofibromatosis: Relinquishing the masks; a quest for quality of life. *Journal of Advanced Nursing, 11*, 459–464.

Monna, K. A. (1989). The perception of job satisfaction of baccalaureate-prepared and diploma-prepared community health nurses. *Masters Abstracts International, 28*(04), 579.

Monti, A. (1992). Members' perceptions of the transactions within their psychosocial club. *Masters Abstracts International, 30*(04), 1296.

Moreira, T. M. M., & Araújo, T. L. (2002a). The conceptual model of interactive open systems and the Theory of Goal Attainment by Imogene King [Portuguese]. *Revista Latino-Americana de Enfermagem, 10*(1), 97–103. Abstract in English retrieved May 18, 2007, from CINAHL Plus with Full Text database.

Moreira, T. M. M., & Araújo, T. L. (2002b). Interpersonal system of Imogene King: The relationships among patient with no-compliance to the treatment of the hypertension and professionals of health [Portuguese]. *Acta Paulista de Enfermagem, 15*(3), 35–43. Abstract in English retrieved May 18, 2007, from CINAHL Plus with Full Text database.

Morris, G. L. (1996). Client satisfaction with nursing care in the home. *Masters Abstracts International, 34*(06), 2348.

Norgan, G. H., Ettipio, A. M., & Lasome, C. E. M. (1995). A program plan addressing carpal tunnel syndrome: The utility of King's goal attainment theory. *AAOHN Journal, 43,* 407–411.

Norris, D. M., & Hoyer, P. J. (1993). Dynamism in practice: Parenting within King's framework. *Nursing Science Quarterly, 6,* 79–85.

Oates, S. J. (1994). Nurses' perceptions of participation in shaping the workplace. *Masters Abstracts International, 33*(03), 874.

Olsson, H., & Forsdahl, T. (1996). Expectations and opportunities of newly employed nurses at the University Hospital, Tromso, Norway. *Social Sciences in Health, 2*(1), 14–22. Abstract retrieved July 12, 2007, from CINAHL Plus with Full Text database.

Omar, M. A. (1989). Relationship of family processes to family life satisfaction in stepfamilies and biological families during pregnancy. *Dissertation Abstracts International, 51*(03B), 1196.

O'Shall, M. L. (1988). The relationship of congruency of role conception between head nurse and staff nurse and staff nurse job satisfaction. *Masters Abstracts International, 27*(03), 379.

Parsons, A. E., & Ricker, V. J. (1993). Critique of practices used by Massachusetts nurse practitioners to promote breastfeeding. *Nursing Scan in Research, 6*(5), 4–5.

Petrich, B. E. A. (2000). Medical and nursing students' perceptions of obesity. *Journal of Addictions Nursing, 12*(1), 3–16.

Phillips, E. L. (1995). Diploma nursing students' attitudes toward poverty. *Masters Abstracts International, 33*(06), 1846.

Porter, H. B. (1991). A Theory of Goal Attainment and ambulatory care oncology nursing: An introduction. *Canadian Oncology Nursing Journal, 1*(4), 124–126.

Quirk, S. E. (1995). A study to determine if working on self-directed teams increases job satisfaction among home health registered nurses. *Masters Abstracts International, 34*(01), 283.

Rawlins, P. S., Rawlins, T. D., & Horner, M. (1990). Development of the family needs assessment tool. *Western Journal of Nursing Research, 12,* 201–214.

Rexford, D. S. (2001). Quality of life in a heart failure population. *Masters Abstracts International, 40*(01), 152.

Rhodes, E. R. (1995). Perceptions of health among low-income African-Americans and utilization of health services. *Masters Abstracts International, 34*(03), 1153.

Richard-Hughes, S. (1997). Attitudes and beliefs of Afro-Americans related to organ and tissue donation. *International Journal of Trauma Nursing, 3*(4), 119–123. Abstract retrieved July 12, 2007, from CINAHL Plus with Full Text database.

Rooda, L. A. (1992). The development of a conceptual model for multicultural nursing. *Journal of Holistic Nursing, 10,* 337–347.

Rooke, L. (1995a). The concept of space in King's systems framework: Its implications for nursing. In M. A. Frey & C. L. Sieloff (Eds.), *Advancing King's systems framework and theory of nursing* (pp. 79–96). Thousand Oaks, CA: Sage.

Rooke, L. (1995b). Focusing on King's theory and systems framework in education by using an experiential learning model: A challenge to improve the quality of nursing care. In M. A. Frey & C. L. Sieloff (Eds.), *Advancing King's systems framework and theory of nursing* (pp. 278–93). Thousand Oaks, CA: Sage.

Rosendahl, P. B., & Ross, V. (1982). Does your behavior affect your patient's response? *Journal of Gerontological Nursing, 8,* 572–575.

Scott, L. D. (1998). Perceived needs of parents of critically ill children. *Journal of the Society of Pediatric Nurses, 3*(1), 4–12. Abstract retrieved July 12, 2007, from CINAHL Plus with Full Text database.

Sharts-Engel, N. C. (1984). On the vicissitudes of health appraisal. *Advances in Nursing Science, 7,* 12–23.

Sharts-Hopko, N. C. (1995). Using health, personal, and interpersonal system concepts within the King's systems framework to explore perceived health status during the menopause transition. In M. A. Frey & C. L. Sieloff (Eds.), *Advancing King's systems framework and theory of nursing* (pp. 147–160). Thousand Oaks, CA: Sage.

Shea, H., Rogers, M., Ross, E., Tucker, D., Fitch, M., & Smith, I. (1989). Implementation of nursing conceptual models: Observations of a multisite research team. *Canadian Journal of Nursing Administration, 2*(1), 15–20.

Sieloff, C. L. (1996). Development of an instrument to estimate the actualized power of a nursing department. *Dissertation Abstracts International, 57*(04B), 2484.

Sieloff, C. L. (2003). Measuring nursing power within organizations. *Journal of Nursing Scholarship, 35,* 183–187.

Sink, K. K. (2001). Perceptions, informational needs, and feelings of competency of new parents. *Dissertation Abstracts International, 62*(01B), 166.

Skariah, R. A. (1999). Analysis of first nation children's drawings of their perceptions of health. *Masters Abstracts International, 37*(04), 1184.

Smith, M. C. (1988). King's theory in practice. *Nursing Science Quarterly, 1,* 145–146.

Sowell, R. L., & Lowenstein, A. (1994). King's theory as a framework for quality: Linking theory to practice. *Nursing Connections, 7*(2), 19–31.

Talosi, R. (1993). Puppetry simulation: The health education vehicle to goal attainment in children with asthma. *Masters Abstracts International, 32*(04), 1172.

Tawil, T. M. P. (1993). Gender differences in frequency of assistance and perceived elderly patients' level of need by spouse primary caregivers with the activities of daily living: Dressing and bathing. *Masters Abstracts International, 32*(04), 1172.

Temple, A., & Fawdry, K. (1992). King's Theory of Goal Attainment: Resolving filial caregiver role strain. *Journal of Gerontological Nursing, 18*(3), 11–15.

Theobald, S. K. (1992). Clinical teaching characteristics of baccalaureate and associate degree nursing faculty: A comparative study. *Masters Abstracts International, 31*(01), 284.

Tritsch, J. M. (1998). Application of King's Theory of Goal Attainment and the Carondelet St. Mary's case management model. *Nursing Science Quarterly, 11,* 69–73.

Ventresca, A. R. (1994). Job satisfaction: Goal attainment of community health nurses. *Masters Abstracts International, 33*(04), 1232.

Villanueva-Noble, N. S. (1998). Cross-cultural analysis of perceptions of health in children's drawings: A replicate study. *Masters Abstracts International, 36*(04), 1070.

West, P. (1991). Theory implementation: A challenging journey. *Canadian Journal of Nursing Administration, 4*(1), 29–30.

White-Linn, V. M. (1994). Perceived quality of life of adults aged 30 to 50 years with type I and II diabetes. *Masters Abstracts International, 33*(05), 1496.

Wicks, M. L. N. (1992). Family health in chronic illness. *Dissertation Abstracts International, 53*(12B), 6228.

Williams, L. A. (2001). Imogene King's interacting systems theory—Application in emergency and rural nursing. *Online Journal of Rural Nursing & Health Care, 2*(1). Retrieved May 18, 2007, from http://www.rno.org/journal/issues/Vol-2/issue-1/Williams.htm.

Winker, C. K. (1996). A descriptive study of the relationship of interaction disturbance to the organizational health of a metropolitan general hospital. *Dissertation Abstracts International, 57*(07B), 4306.

Woods, E. C. (1994). King's theory in practice with elders. *Nursing Science Quarterly, 7,* 65–69.

Zurakowski, T. L. (1990). Interpersonal factors and nursing home resident health. *Dissertation Abstracts International, 51*(09B), 4281.

Annotated Bibliography

Glasgow, V. M. (1998). Preconceptual health and its effect on pregnancy outcomes in African-Canadian women and their partners. *Masters Abstracts International, 36*(06), 1585.

A sample of 30 African Canadian women and their partners completed questionnaires about their perceptions of preconceptual health and these perceptions were related to pregnancy outcomes. Overall, the data supported a strong relationship between the perceptions of both partners and improved pregnancy outcomes.

Harman, B. J. (1999). The effects of a paraprofessional preceptor program for certified nursing assistants in dementia special care units. *Dissertation Abstracts International, 59*(11B), 5786.

This study utilized a multisite, repeated measures, quasi-experimental design to investigate the outcomes of a newly instituted paraprofessional mentor program for certified nursing assistants (CNAs) in dementia special care units. Participating CNAs attended a six-hour educational program to prepare them to serve as preceptors. Sixteen new CNAs were enrolled in the study with 11 completing the data collection. Of these 11, six had preceptors and five participated in the usual program or served as the control group. Because of the sample size, statistical significance was not found. However, 100% of the experimental group continued employment as compared to 56% in the control group.

Quirk, S. E. (1995). A study to determine if working on self-directed teams increases job satisfaction among home health registered nurses. *Masters Abstracts International, 34*(01), 283.

This descriptive study investigated job satisfaction in 30 home health registered nurses in two agencies. In one agency, nurses participated in self-directed teams, while in the other, nurses did not have access to self-directed teams. Those who worked on self-directed teams exhibited higher levels of job satisfaction.

Sieloff, C. L. (1996). Development of an instrument to estimate the actualized power of a nursing department. *Dissertation Abstracts International, 57*(04B), 2484. and

Sieloff, C. L. (2003). Measuring nursing power within organizations. *Journal of Nursing Scholarship, 35,* 183–187.

Sieloff originally developed and tested the Sieloff–King Assessment of Departmental Power (SKADP) instrument. Tests of the SKADP supported content and construct validity. However, because of feedback from study participants and psychometric analysis, the instrument was revised and became the Sieloff–King Assessment of Group Power Within Organizations (SKAGPO). Factor analysis supported subscales of controlling the effects of environmental forces, position, power perspective, resources, role, power competency, communication competency, and goal and outcome competency. Initial reliability and validity have been established and Sieloff recommends both further study of reliability and validity and use of the SKAGPO in future studies of nursing power in organizations.

West, P. (1991). Theory implementation: A challenging journey. *Canadian Journal of Nursing Administration, 4*(1), 29–30.

Describes the implementation of King's conceptual system for theory-based practice in a large metropolitan hospital. Identifies that more time spent in educating the staff about the framework would have helped the staff understand and accept the value of theory-based practice.

CHAPTER 12

Science of Unitary Human Beings

Martha E. Rogers

Maryanne Garon

Martha Elizabeth Rogers (May 12, 1914–March 13, 1994) was an influential and visionary nurse theorist, an innovative thinker, and an articulate spokesperson for professional nursing education. Her conceptual system has had a profound impact on practice, theory development, and research in the profession. But, in addition to all that, Martha Rogers was a warmly regarded and honored human being. She had a rich family life and was much loved by her family members, from her sisters and brother to innumerable nieces, nephews, and grandnieces, as well as by her many friends and colleagues in nursing. Some of this respect and affection is reflected in her recognition as a fellow in the American Academy of Nursing and her induction into the American Nurses Association Hall of Fame.

Martha Rogers was born in Dallas, Texas, on May 12, 1914. She attended the University of Tennessee, Knoxville, from 1931 to 1933. Her broad academic and scientific interests were manifested early, as she took a science-med course that she characterized as more substantial than pre-med, including French, zoology, genetics, embryology, and many other courses (Hektor, 1989). However, at some point during this period, she and her parents concluded that medicine was an inappropriate career for a woman (Garon, 1992). She decided to enter the Knoxville General Hospital School of Nursing, Tennessee, because one of her friends was planning to attend there. Being an independent and intelligent young woman, Martha Rogers found the routines of the hospital school to be restrictive. At one point she even left the school briefly but returned to complete her nurses training with her class (personal interview with M. Rogers, 1991). She received her nursing diploma in 1936. Rogers continued her education at George Peabody College in Nashville, Tennessee, receiving a bachelor of science degree in Public Health. After receiving her B.S. degree, Rogers's first position was as a public health nurse in rural Michigan. She remained there for two years, until she returned to study for her first master's degree, an M.A. in public health supervision from Teachers College, Columbia University, New York, New York, in 1945 (Hektor, 1989). Rogers also worked as a staff nurse, supervisor, and education director for a visiting nurse agency in Hartford, Connecticut. After advancing to the position of acting director of education, she moved to Phoenix, Arizona, where she established and became the executive director of the first Visiting Nursing Service in Phoenix, Arizona (Martha E. Rogers: A Short Biography, n.d., para. 3). She later returned to the East Coast to continue her education. She earned a master's degree in public health in 1952 and a doctor of science degree in 1954, both from Johns Hopkins University, Baltimore, Maryland. Rogers's career in academia began when she was appointed chairperson of the Department of Nursing Education at New York University in 1954. She officially retired in 1979 but continued as Professor Emerita. After retiring, she moved back to Phoenix, where she lived until her death in 1994.

"Ahead of her time, in and out of this world" (Ireland, 2000, p. 59)

Rogers's view of nursing as a separate and essential discipline and a unique field of study was influential in her life's work. She focused much of her writing, particularly prior to 1970, on working for the establishment of nursing in higher education. She believed that there was a unique body of knowledge in nursing that had not yet been identified or written about. In her books and articles that argued the need for higher education for nurses, Rogers developed and wrote about this unique body of knowledge that would eventually become her conceptual system, the Science of Unitary Human Beings (SUHB) (Garon, 1992).

Rogers's first book, published in 1961, *Educational Revolution in Nursing*, was a call for a broad liberal university education for nurses. It also contained the beginnings of her conceptual system. Further evidence of the development of the conceptual system is found in her second book, *Reveille in Nursing*, published in 1964. In this book, she proposed a professional curriculum for nursing. As a focus of the curriculum, Rogers developed several assumptions that later became central to her conceptual system. Meleis (1985) credited these writings as the first comments on the theoretic basis of the nursing process. Rogers continued to refine her thinking about her conceptual system and published *An Introduction to the Theoretical Basis of Nursing* in 1970. This book contains the basis for her conceptual system. While Rogers never revised the 1970 book, she wrote a number of updates. It was in these updates and refinements that newer views of her conceptual system were introduced. The concepts and principles presented in this section will include the later explications presented by Rogers as well as references to the original work. While reading the 1970 book is necessary to better understand Rogers's conceptual system, knowledge of Rogers would be incomplete without including the revisions presented in her later publications.

Throughout her life, Rogers was consistent in identifying nursing as a science with a unique body of knowledge (Malinski, 2006). Nursing focuses on unitary human beings and their world. Rogers used the word *unitary* to connote human beings as unified wholes, greater than the sum of their parts. Rogers abandoned the word *holism* because of its widespread and often inaccurate use to describe everything from dietary regimens to massages to the use of colonics (Malinski, 1994). Unitary human beings and their environments cannot be understood or studied by looking at their parts. Gathering information about physiological indices or a person's social context may be helpful for nurses in some of their collaborative functions, but this information would not lead to an understanding of the unitary human being.

Rogers (1990b/1994) argued that every discipline has many theories and that she was presenting an abstract or conceptual system, an abstract worldview from which theories could be derived. She "identified the body of her work as the basic science of nursing" (Malinski, 2006, p. 7). She emphasized that this is a new product, rooted in a different paradigm. The word *paradigm* has been noted to have many different meanings (Guba, 1990). A paradigm may be defined as the way that scientists or persons in a given field approach the problems or areas of interest in their field (Briggs & Peat, 1984). It is a particular perspective of reality and has been likened to a worldview. Thomas Kuhn (1970) wrote about scientific paradigms and how they change. He believed that knowledge advances through revolutions, or leaps in knowledge, that he called paradigm shifts. However, it is difficult for someone who has been rooted in one paradigm to shift to viewing things in the new paradigm. The shift is said to take place all at once—the old information is suddenly seen differently, as though the person were wearing a different shade of lenses. One example that has been used to demonstrate this shift in paradigm view is with the sketch shown in Figure 12-1.

Viewed from one perspective, the drawing appears to be a rabbit. But, by shifting the view—just rotating the page—one can suddenly see the duck. Once you make the shift, you can easily see both. It is difficult to go back to where you were before, when you could see only one animal. This is likened to a paradigm shift. At first, you see things only from the old paradigm. But once you have made the shift—it is difficult to go backwards and not view things from the new paradigm while still including the old one.

Many nurses are accustomed to viewing people and the practice of nursing from a biomedical perspective that is based on reductionism. Nurses who practice from a reductionistic perspective or the biomedical model need to make a paradigm shift to begin to understand the SUHB. The words and concepts are very different from those that most nurses use in everyday practice.

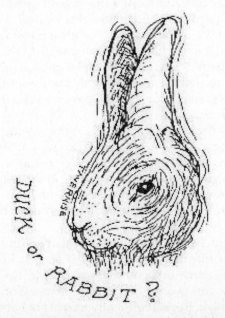

FIGURE 12-1 Drawing by Cindy Tavernise. *(Used with permission.)*

The conceptual system developed by Martha Rogers requires a paradigm shift similar to that illustrated in Figure 12-1. Initially, it is hard to "see," as the old views are paramount. After reading her conceptual system and applying it to practice, the paradigm shift may occur. Suddenly, the "duck" appears. The new views make sense—and it is difficult to ever go back to the old or previous view of reality. This does not mean that the old views are discarded; rather, they are now incorporated within the newer worldview.

ROGERS'S CONCEPTUAL SYSTEM

In her 1970 book *An Introduction to the Theoretical Basis of Nursing Science,* Rogers outlined five assumptions that provide the foundation for the discipline of nursing:

1. Man [Rogers used "man" in place of person or human being in 1970] is a unified whole possessing his own integrity and manifesting characteristics that are more than and different from the sum of his parts. (p. 47)
2. Man [as an open system] and environment are continuously exchanging matter and energy with one another. (p. 54)
3. The life process evolves irreversibly and unidirectionally along the space-time continuum. (p. 59)
4. Pattern and organization identify man and reflect his innovative wholeness. (p. 65)
5. Man is characterized by the capacity for abstraction and imagery, language and thought, sensation and emotion. (p. 73)

Rogers drew upon her readings from the arts, the sciences, and philosophy, as well as her scientific education, to develop this conceptual system for nursing. In deducing her conceptual system, she used terminology from the general system theory of Von Bertalanffy to support her conceptions of a universe of open systems and the continuous interaction of human and environmental fields (Meleis, 2007). She also drew upon both physics and electrodynamic theory as underpinnings for some of her concepts. Other influences included early Greek philosophers, Lewin's field theory, and the works of theologian Teilhard de Chardin and of Polanyi (Garon, 1992). In later writings, Rogers refined and condensed the assumptions, finally settling on the five building blocks of the conceptual system (Rogers, 1992): *energy fields, pandimensionality, pattern, unitary persons,* and *environment.*

The first concept is that of *energy field.* An energy field is defined as "the fundamental unit of the living and the non-living" (Rogers, 1990b, p. 109; 1994, p. 252). Understanding Rogers's view of energy fields is essential to understanding her conceptual system. *Energy* signifies the dynamic nature of the field; a *field* is in continuous motion and is infinite (Rogers, 1990b/1994, 1994). Both human beings and their environment are conceptualized as energy fields in this system. Because both are infinite, their boundaries do not end at the physical body.

The concept of energy field seems to be particularly difficult for many nurses to understand. Because of this difficulty, they may either dismiss Rogers as "too abstract" or question how they can see, touch, or identify an energy field. Reeder (1999) acknowledged the questions that many nurses have and raised the possibility of energy field in the Rogerian system as metaphor. Rogers constantly referred to human beings and their environments as energy fields but gave little further elaboration. Her explanations revolved around the nature of energy fields as dynamic and unified. "Field is a unifying concept. Energy signifies the dynamic nature of the field; a field is in continuous motion and is infinite" (Rogers, 1990b, p. 109; 1994, p. 252). Reeder wrote that it is possible that "Rogers deliberately chose the metaphor *energy field* as a figure of speech to evoke the imagination and wonderment of possibilities . . . to represent the revolutionary, fully pandimensional human being rather than . . . a literal entity connoting Newtonian three dimensionality" (p. 7). Understanding the concept of energy fields becomes easier when they are viewed as metaphors. While it may be difficult for some nurses to look at a person and see him or her as something like a Kirlian field photograph or a *Star Trek* version of an evolved alien, most every nurse can agree that people are incredibly dynamic yet integral beings. Because it is difficult to measure or visualize energy fields, this perspective can be a good starting point for making the switch to viewing things in the Rogerian conceptual system.

Pattern, the next concept, received increasing importance in Rogers's writings in later years (Sarter, 1987). This concept arises both from systems thinking and views from quantum physics. *Pattern* is defined as "the distinguishing characteristic of an energy field perceived as a single wave" (Rogers, 1990b, p. 109; 1994, p. 252). Rogers used the concept of pattern to emphasize that unitary human beings cannot be understood by studying or summing their parts. Each human being instead has a unique identifiable pattern. Pattern is the unique configuration of relationships characteristic of a particular system. Capra, in *The Web of Life,* emphasized that the "study of pattern is essential to the understanding of living systems" (1996, p. 81). In systems thinking, it is not the structure or the physical parts that are important but the pattern of relationships. Systemic properties *are* properties of a pattern. The irreducible, nonmaterial aspect of life is the pattern. One of the difficulties in operationalizing Rogers's model has been deciding on means to assess the patterning of the human energy field. Several nurse researchers have attempted to develop means to better identify and measure human field patterns. Examples of such research include that by Bays (1995, 2001), Bernardo (1993, 1996), Brown (1992), Butcher (1994a, 1996), Matas (1997), Rapacz (1991), Yarcheski & Mahon (1995), and others included in Malinski's (1986) *Explorations on Martha Rogers' Science of Unitary Human Beings,* Barrett's (1990b) *Visions of Rogers' Science-Based Nursing,* and Madrid and Barrett's (1994) *Rogers' Scientific Art of Nursing Practice.* Areas of human field patterns that have been explored include adolescents, chronic pain, hope, injury-associated behaviors and life events, repatterning, and time and creativity.

The next concept is *pandimensionality.* In her earliest writings, Rogers referred to this concept as space-time. Later, she refined it to four-dimensionality, then multidimensionality. She finally settled on pandimensionality in 1992. Pandimensionality refers to an infinite domain without limit. Rogers drew upon changes in knowledge from 20th-century physics that theorized space-time dimensions beyond three dimensions. Human and environmental fields, and all reality, are believed to be pandimensional (Rogers, 1992). This is a way of perceiving reality, of moving beyond the standard view of the world as three-dimensional. When we move beyond the three-dimensional view of the world as one that we can experience with our five senses, there is no limit on the realm of possibility. The pandimensional nature of reality can explain a number of phenomena thought to be paranormal, such as déjà vu, precognition, and clairvoyance. A standard way to help with understanding of these concepts can be found in Abbott's (1992) *Flatland.* In that book a resident of a two-dimensional world finds his way into a three-dimensional world. He had never imagined a reality beyond his two dimensions and is both overwhelmed and enlightened by the idea of another dimension. Just as the protagonist of *Flatland* has difficulty in conceptualizing a third dimension, so do we have difficulty imaging a reality *beyond* three dimensions. Yet theories from modern physics lend support to Rogers's conceptualization of multiple dimensions (Capra, 1983). Our words and understandings lag behind reality in this case.

The *unitary human being* is defined by Rogers as "an irreducible, indivisible, pandimensional energy field identified by pattern and manifesting characteristics that are specific to the whole and which cannot be predicted from knowledge of the parts" (Rogers, 1992, p. 29). Unitary human beings and their environments are the focus of nursing science and give nursing its unique perspective and area of practice.

The *environment or environmental energy field* is defined as "an irreducible, pandimensional energy field identified by pattern and integral with the human field" (Rogers, 1992, p. 29).

In addition to these basic building blocks or concepts, Rogers (1992) proposed three principles. These principles express the nature of change in human and environmental fields. Like other aspects of her conceptual system, these have evolved and been refined over the years. Rogers was very concerned with language and the precise meanings of words. When she found that a word was not appropriate to the meaning of a concept or principle, she clarified by refining, revising, or replacing the term. In regard to the principles, earlier writings will have different names for them. In the most current conceptualizations the principles are the *principle of resonancy, principle of helicy,* and *principle of integrality*.

The *principle of resonancy* is defined as the "continuous change from lower to higher frequency wave patterns in human and environmental fields" (Rogers, 1992, p. 31). Human beings are perceived as wave patterns, and a variety of life rhythms can be likened to wave patterns. These include things such as sleep–wake rhythms, hormone levels, and fluctuating emotional states (waves of joy or pain or loneliness). The changes that occur to these patterns of human beings are from lower- to higher-frequency patterns. Some examples of these changes are shown in Table 12-1, which illustrates the principle of resonancy. These changes are postulated to express the continuous creative change in the flow of human/environmental field patterning.

The *principle of helicy* is defined as "continuous, innovative, unpredictable, increasing diversity of human and environmental field patterns" (Rogers, 1992, p. 31). Rogers saw helicy as "an ordering of man's evolutionary emergence" (1970, p. 100). This principle underlies the fact that humans do not regress but become increasingly diverse and complex. Rogers frequently used the Slinky toy to illustrate the nature of human change as spiral-like, continually progressing toward increased diversity (see Figure 12-2). She emphasized

TABLE 12-1   Manifestation of Field Patterning in Unitary Human Beings

Lower Frequency	Higher Frequency	Highest Frequency
Pragmatic	Imaginative	Visionary
Time experienced as slower	Time experienced as faster	Timelessness
Lesser diversity		Greater diversity
Longer sleeping	Longer waking	Beyond waking
Longer rhythms	Shorter rhythms	Seems continuous
Slower motion	Faster motion	Seems continuous

Modified from Rogers, M. (1992). *Nursing science and the space age.* Nursing Science Quarterly, 5, 31.

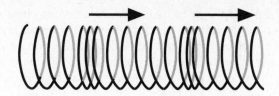

FIGURE 12-2   Slinky toy as a representation of helicy.

that this eliminates the idea of homeostasis. Human development is not static, and humans do not ever return to exactly the same place where they were before. Following a path along the Slinky, the person may have spiraled to a place that is similar to where he or she was before but is just one circuit or turn on the Slinky from that place. Unitary persons, in their development, do not go backward. This view of human development places a positive light on aging. Humans are becoming more diverse and complex as they age.

The *principle of integrality* is defined as "continuous mutual human field and environmental field process" (Rogers, 1992, p. 31). *Integrality* is derived from the word *integral* to explain the essential relationship between the human and environmental fields. Rogers emphasized the continuous mutual nature of the human–environmental field relationship by the deliberate use of the word *process* instead of *interaction*. Interaction implies an episodic or even causal relationship. To illustrate this, imagine a child playing outside in the sun on a bright summer day. The child gets a sunburn. This might be perceived as an interaction between the child and the sun. However, consider the mutual process between the child and the sun as occurring simultaneously and continuously over a lifetime. Included in the process is everything from the necessity of the sun for life on this planet to vitamin D absorption by the child to ongoing effects of radiation on the skin to the child's impact on the ozone layer. This ongoing mutual *process* is the nature of human beings and their environment.

ROGERS'S WORK AND THE FOUR MAJOR NURSING METAPARADIGM CONCEPTS

Rogers addressed each of the four major nursing metaparadigm concepts in her writings, but she did not view them as the building blocks of the SUHB. She defined and described *human beings* as unitary persons, being irreducible, pandimensional energy fields identified by pattern and integral with the environment (Rogers, 1992). *Environment* is also defined as an irreducible, pandimensional energy field that is identified by pattern and is integral with the human field. Rogers repeatedly emphasized that *nursing* is a noun and referred to the body of knowledge and area of study that is unique to this profession. However, she also emphasized that nursing is both a science and an art. She wrote eloquently and passionately of the role of nursing in society:

Nursing's story is a magnificent epic of service to mankind. It is about people: How they are born, and live and die; in health and in sickness; in joy and in sorrow. Its mission is the translation of knowledge into human service.

Nursing is compassionate concern for human beings. It is the heart that understands and the hand that soothes. It is the intellect that synthesizes many learnings into meaningful ministrations. (Rogers, 1966, cited in Barrett, 1990b, p. 31)

Furthermore, Rogers defined the purpose of nursing as promoting "symphonic interaction between man and environment, to strengthen the coherence and integrity of the human field, and to direct and redirect patterning of the human and environmental fields for realization of maximum health potential" (1970, p. 122) and "to promote human betterment wherever people are, on planet earth or in outer space"(Rogers, 1992, p. 33).

Rogers viewed *health* as a value term. She stated that "unitary human health signifies an irreducible human field manifestation (1990a, p. 10; 1994, p. 248) and "disease and pathology are value terms applied when the human field manifests characteristics that may be deemed undesirable" (1992, p. 33). Rogers believed that health is relative and infinite. She viewed health and illness not as dichotomous but as expressions of the life process. Nurses participate in the process of helping people to achieve their maximum health or well-being, according to each person's own definitions and potentials. The concept of health is not as important in the Rogerian conceptual system as the concepts of unitary human beings and their mutual process with the environment.

Rogerian Practice Methodology

Rogers described nursing practice as "the process by which the body of scientific knowledge (nursing science) is used for the purpose of assisting human beings to move in the direction of maximum well-being" (Rogers, 1994, p. 64). She described this process as subsumed under two categories: (1) evaluative and diagnostic and (2) interventive. The evaluative/diagnostic phase is "the process of determining the position of an individual, family or group on the continuum of minimum to maximum well-being" (Rogers, 1994, p. 64). The interventive category is "the process of determining and initiating . . . processes characterized by ongoing modification, alteration, revision, and change" (p. 64). While Rogers was a participant in early conferences of the North American Nursing Diagnosis Association, she later stated some clear opposition to the use of nursing diagnoses:

> Diagnosis is not appropriate. Rather, nursing is dealing with all of the potentials of human beings. . . . Diagnosis is not something to hang onto simply because it's a word that has been around, and the worst group to copy is the medical profession. We don't deal with the same phenomena as medicine does. I am not going to study medicine: I am not going to study law. The concern of nursing is with people. (as quoted in an interview, in M. J. Smith, 1988, p. 84)

Because of the inconsistency of the nursing process and nursing diagnosis with the SUHB, Barrett (1990a) developed a practice methodology within the framework of the SUHB. She named this practice methodology the health patterning practice method. Barrett derived the method from Rogers's descriptions of health and nursing's role as well as from her own experience in working with clients and developing a health patterning practice.

In the health patterning practice method there are two major processes. The processes are *pattern manifestation knowing* (originally pattern manifestation appraisal) and *voluntary mutual patterning* (originally deliberative mutual patterning). The processes are neither sequential nor separable. In the first, knowing includes to come to know, to recognize the nature of, and to discern. Barrett (1998) changed the term from *appraisal* to *knowing* because she believed that appraisal implied an inequality between the nurse and client, as well as a suggestion of measurement, while knowing implies a more egalitarian view.

The second process, voluntary mutual patterning, acknowledges the client's free choice in making decisions about health. However, the nurse does have the obligation to encourage "the client to discover whether he/she is making choices without being fully aware or feeling free" (Barrett, 1998, p. 137). Barrett emphasized that clients are full participants in these processes. She suggested posing questions to clients such as "What do you want?" or "What choices are open to you now?"

Use in Actual Practice Situations

Rogers's SUHB has appealed to many groups of nurses because of its emphasis on viewing human beings and environments as integral wholes. Both individuals and institutions have adopted it as their basis for nursing practice. An experience with an individual client will be presented next, followed by a discussion of use in nursing leadership and nursing education.

Use in Clinical Practice

The first is an example of the use of Rogers's theory in clinical practice with an individual client.

Ms. X. is an experienced nurse, who has worked for nearly six years in a medical-surgical unit. She has just returned to school to earn her B.S.N. and is learning about the nursing theories. During her shift, she admits a patient, Mr. G. Mr. G. is a 66-year-old patient with type II diabetes mellitus. Ms. X. has cared for Mr. G. many times over the past five years. When she first met him, Mr. G. was an energetic, vibrant man, working full-time as a salesman. He lives in his own home in a nearby community with his wife and two high school–aged daughters. His first admission had been for initiation of insulin therapy for his poorly controlled diabetes with acute hyperglycemia and hyperlipidemia. Now, after five years, Mr. G. has experienced numerous complications. He has had a cardiac bypass surgery and a left below-the-knee amputation, he is nearly blind, and his kidneys are failing. Today, he is being admitted with a pleural effusion and an elevated temperature.

Because Ms. X. has been studying Rogers's SUHB, she begins the process of pattern manifestation knowing. She enters Mr. G.'s room and is surprised to see his condition. His color is gray and pasty, his face sad and lined, and he seems to be staring into the distance. Ms. X. realizes that he doesn't see her, so she moves closer to him to touch his hand and reintroduce herself. She notes that his wife and daughters are also in the room, sitting quietly. The room appears dark, and there are many chairs and pieces of equipment cluttering the room. She begins to talk with him about why he is in the hospital (from his perspective), what his life has been like, and what his goals are. As they talk, Mr. G. becomes more animated, and Ms. X. sees the "old Mr. G." in him. He is discouraged by this new development but is eager to return to his home, his family, and his hobbies. He has a new computer, with voice-recognition software that he has learned to use, and, on pleasant days, he loves to sit outside as his wife gardens.

By learning more about his current life and his goals, Ms. X. facilitates Mr. G. to be a full participant in his care and achieve his goals. Ms. X. is surprised how her new Rogerian worldview has influenced her views of Mr. G. She realized that she used to consider patients like Mr. G. as deteriorating and somehow being less than their former selves. She also had to admit to herself that she could be judgmental in her view of patients with chronic illnesses who did not care for themselves as she or others in the healthcare system thought they should.

Now, she recognizes, under the principle of helicy, that Mr. G., like everyone else, is becoming more complex and diverse. She sees his connection with the people and places in his integral environment. She realizes that he is still developing new skills (his computer) and enjoying his environment (his garden). She also sees that Mr. G. is more than his disabilities or his illness; he is still the vibrant man she always knew. Recognizing this changes the way she talks to and interacts with him.

As the physicians work up Mr. G.'s medical problems, Ms. X. works with him and his family to prepare him to go home. It is found that he has coccidiomycosis and will need six weeks of IV therapy with Amphotericin B. Ms. X. works with the discharge planner to arrange for him to get the antibiotics in his home. She helps Mr. G. and family identify needs: prosthetic adjustment, in-home equipment, dietician consultation, and others.

> *After several days off, Ms. X. returns to her unit and finds Mr. G. in his wheelchair, with his family surrounding him, being discharged. She stops to talk with him—and he turns in her direction and reaches for her hand. "You know," he says, "of all the people that work here, Ms. X., you are the one who has made the most difference for me . . . thank you!" Ms. X. smiles to herself, as she starts her shift. . . pleased with the difference in her attitude and her care for patients that the SUHB has made!*

Using Barrett's practice methodology, the nurse first used *pattern manifestation knowing*. She was able to understand Mr. G. as a whole human being—his pattern, his values, his beliefs about what is important to him in life. She had to redefine the meaning of health from the patient's perspective, not what she thought it was. In the other phase (which may actually occur simultaneously), *voluntary mutual patterning*, the nurse discussed Mr. G.'s health needs from his perspective. She determined his current values and knowledge levels. Mr. G. and his family were very eager to learn and sought out Internet information about cocciodiomycosis. Because it is important for him to go home, he and his family actively participated in working with staff to ready their home for Mr. G.'s discharge. They also planned to learn to give his therapy with the help of the home health nurse. Mr. G. has suffered from a devastating chronic illness, but using the practice methodology as defined by Barrett helps nurses to focus their care on individual patients and their perspective.

Use in Nursing Leadership and Education

Rogers's conceptual model can also be used in administration and in education. Her conceptual system requires a view of human beings as "sentient and creative and held in high regard" (Gueldner, 1989, p. 114). Using the conceptualization of power that Barrett (1989) derived from Rogers, people have choice to knowingly create change. Nurse leaders (whether administrator or educator) utilize knowledge to create evolutionary change. Leaders must both practice and provide role models within the Rogerian conceptual system by being open in communication patterns and appreciating the unique and unitary nature of each individual with whom they interact. Nurse leaders also understand that the nursing and health care systems (or educational systems) are highly complex and continuously evolving toward higher-frequency diversifying wholeness.

When nurse leaders create environments characterized by acceptance for openness, creativity, and diversity, nurses and others are able to grow, evolve, improve, and shape their practices or educational experiences in ways that benefit them, their institutions, and their clients. The experience of implementing Rogers's model in practice at the San Diego Veterans Administration Medical Center has been described in Heggie, Schoenmehl, Greico, and Chang (1989) and Heggie, Garon, Kodiath, and Kelly (1994). These authors demonstrated that the paradigm shift required to use the SUHB does not occur quickly, and they described the change process they employed, including modeling the use of Rogers's ideas. Administrative modeling resulted in the staff nominating their manager for a nursing service award for caring. The staff identified her Rogerian approach as having created a major, positive difference for them.

In the same way, the SUHB can be applied to students and teachers in an online course. In this example, the process occurs between students and instructors who are separated physically and temporally. Yet their energy fields are definitely interacting. In pattern manifestation knowing, the instructor views the students as more than just physical beings and more than just names entering postings in the online course. The instructor recognizes that the students are each unitary human beings—complex, dynamic and diverse, and much more than the sum of their parts. Besides being students, they each have their individual pattern. They enter their educational program with their own history, culture, families, and various experiences that have led them to become the people they are today. In the voluntary mutual patterning process, the students are active *participants* in the education in an online course. They are knowingly participating in change. They have chosen to be in a BSN program and to participate in an online course. Other choices include how they schedule their time to be online, select the resources they will access and utilize, and, to some extent, set their own pace. The instructor's role is to work in conjunction with the students and to facilitate in this *knowing participation in change*.

These examples demonstrate how vastly different areas of nursing practice can be reframed using the Rogers worldview (SUHB). From the unitary perspective, there is a focus on the integrality of person and environment, the individual's active participation in change, and each person's individual pattern. The value in this approach lies in the shift in focus from the nurse or leader to the recipient of care and to the focus on choice, participation, mutuality, and wholeness. In an era of nurse shortages, burnout, and retention issues, this worldview provides a focus for nursing that is innovative and transformative for the nurse as well as the client.

SCIENCE OF UNITARY HUMAN BEINGS AND THEORY CRITIQUE QUESTIONS

1. *What is the historical context of the theory?*   Rogers began to conceptualize her view of nursing in the mid-1950s and continued to develop her thinking until her death in 1994. She had studied sciences before becoming a nurse and earned a doctorate in science. She was very interested in the changes in science and approaches to knowledge development in the 20th century. She drew upon knowledge from fields as diverse as physics to theology (Garon, 1992). Rogers was one of the first nurses to think and write about the conceptual bases for nursing (Meleis, 1985). Among other areas, the content of her work has been found to be consistent with Tao Te Ching and Buddhist thought (Hanchett, 1992; Overman, 1994).

The SUHB is not in itself a theory, but a number of theories have been derived from it. Rogers derived three theories from the SUHB: the theory of accelerating evolution/change, the emergence of the paranormal, and manifestations of field patterning (Malinski, 2006). Examples of derived theories include enfolding health-as-wholeness-and-harmony (Carboni, 1995b), power (Barrett, 1983, 1989; Caroselli, 1995; Caroselli & Barrett, 1998; Caroselli-Dervan, 1991), and spirituality (D. W. Smith, 1994). Concept analyses include integrated awareness (Phillips & Bramlett, 1994), healing (Wendler, 1996), and beyond-waking experience (Watson, 1998). Some writers have labeled the theories of Parse and Newman as derived from Rogers's SUHB, as they share the unitary worldview. Malinski (2006) stated that "each used different theoretical perspectives not necessarily consistent with Rogers to produce their own creative syntheses and new emergents that share the newer worldview with Rogers, thus expanding its presence in nursing" (p. 7).

Since her death in 1996, a devoted group of scholars have continued to develop the SUHB. Their work can be found mainly in *Nursing Science Quarterly*; on websites; through the Society of Rogerian Scholars and its journal, *Visions*; and at annual conferences. Their contributions have helped the SUHB to continue to grow and for nurses to continue to explore, expand on, and work on the emergent unfolding of knowledge first presented by Rogers. The influence of Martha Rogers continues in all nurses who met her and who have been touched by her work. Reeder (2002) stated it so well: "Most of all, Martha wanted to wake up nursing and desired that nurses 'think' and know why they live and work as they do" (para. 2).

2. *What are the basic concepts and relationships presented by the theory?* The basic concepts are energy field, pandimensionality, pattern, unitary human beings, and environment. The relationships are defined in the principles of resonancy, helicy, and integrality. The concepts of the theory are defined and used in a consistent fashion. Rogers was meticulous about use of language and would refine word usage to appropriately present her meanings. The relationships among concepts are logical and are based upon the stated assumptions. However, the concepts and the relationship are stated in language that is not familiar to most nurses and is difficult to read and understand without substantial background information.

3. *What major phenomena of concern to nursing are presented? (These phenomena may include* but are not limited to *human beings, environment, health, interpersonal relations, caring, goal attainment, adaptation, and energy fields.)* Rogers wrote that the major phenomena of interest to nursing were unitary human beings and their environment. Her definition of unitary human beings and their environments is that they are unitary, indivisible energy fields. She also wrote of nursing as a compassionate concern for human beings and that its purpose is to promote human health and well-being (Rogers, 1988).

4. *To whom does the theory apply? In what situations? In what ways?* Since humans are integral with their environment, Rogers's work is applicable wherever humans are located—including outer space. The SUHB has been applied in all aspects of nursing. It has been labeled a "grand" theory. Any limitations to the use of SUHB lie more within the practitioner than within the SUHB.

Use of the SUHB in nursing practice requires both critical thinking and ability to take a systems approach to knowledge. Using the Rogers conceptual system directs nurses to consider a wide variety of interventions in their work with unitary human be-ings. Rogers (1970) emphasized that nursing interventions are focused not on disease states but on wholeness. Interventions focusing on wholeness would include guided imagery, relaxation and stress reduction techniques, therapeutic touch, motion therapy, meditation, and aromatherapy, among others. The nurse who utilizes Rogers's work in practice needs to be able to suspend judgment and accurately assess human beings from their own perspective as well as support them in making decisions.

   5. *By what method or methods can the theory be tested?*   Rogers's conceptual sys-tem has been utilized as the underlying framework for multiple nursing studies. These research studies have used multiple modes of inquiry but have remained consistent to Rogers's epistemological holism (Barrett, 1990a). Rawnsley (1977) is credited with being the first nurse researcher to frame her study solely within the SUHB (Ference, 1986a). A number of nursing dissertations emerged from New York University (NYU) framed within the Rogerian system and developing particular aspects into theory, including Bernardo (1993), Bray (1989), Caroselli-Dervan (1991), de Sevo (1991), Doyle (1995), Hastings-Tolsoma (1992), McNiff (1995a), Mersmann (1993), Moulton (1994), Rizzo (1990), Schneider (1995b), Schodt (1989), Sherman (1993), and D. W. Smith (1992). Two early examples are Ference (1979) and Barrett (1983). Ference studied time experience, creativity traits, differentiation, and human field motion. From her study, she devel-oped the Human Field Motion tool. Barrett studied human field motion and power. From her study, she developed a theory of power as knowing participation in change.

   From these studies and others, there has been some support for a number of Rogers's propositions. The continual mutual process of human and environmental fields has been supported in some of the studies (Meleis, 1997). However, there are also methodological difficulties in finding ways to do research that remain consistent with the Rogerian frame-work. Other approaches to knowledge generation, including philosophical explorations, have also added to the growth of knowledge within this conceptual system.

   Both qualitative and quantitative methods have been used to test theories derived from the SUHB. Examples of descriptive research include Abu-Realh, Magwood, Narayan, Rupprecht, and Suraci (1996), Allen (1988), Alligood (1991), Alligood and McGuire (2000), Bray (1989), Donahue and Alligood (1995), Doyle (1995, 1998), Ireland (1996), MacNeil (1996), McNiff (1995a, 1995b), Morris (1991), Moulton (1994), Orshan (1996), Richard (1993), Rush (1997), Sherman (1993, 1996), D. W. Smith (1992, 1995); Examples of phenomenological research include Dominguez (1996), Kells (1995), Klebanoff (1994), C. T. Smith (1989), Sullivan (1994), and Thomas (1993). Examples of quasi-experimental studies include Biley (1996a), Bramlett and Gueldner (1993), Krause (1991), and Meehan (1993). Experimental studies include Butcher and Parker (1988), Girardin (1990), Lewandowsdki (2004), Mersmann (1993), Samarel, Fawcett, Ryan, and Davis (1998), Straneva (1992), Thornton (1996a, 1996b), and Wall (2000). Daingerfield (1993) used ethnography, and Halkitis and Kirton (1999) used focus groups. Grounded theory methodology was used by Krause (1991), Quinn (1988), and Schneider (1995a, 1995b). Pohl (1992) reported using both quantitative and qualitative methods in her study.

   Obviously, no one methodology is identified as the "best" for studying and testing Rogers's conceptual system and the theories derived from that system. Alligood and Fawcett (1999) argued that rational interpretive hermeneutics methodology is compati-ble with the SUHB. They utilized this method to explore Rogers's conception of pattern in three of her publications (2004). Butcher (1994a, 1994b, 1998) has developed the

Unitary Field Pattern Portrait Research Method (a phenomenological-hermeneutical method), and Carboni (1995a) described a qualitative methodology called the Rogerian process of inquiry. Cowling (1998) argues for the use of case studies (unitary case inquiry), while Sherman (1997) supported the use of quantitative research methods, and M. C. Smith and Reeder (1998) discussed how clinical outcomes research can be reconciled with the SUHB. One review of Rogerian research can be found in Dykeman and Loukissa (1993) and another in Kim (2008). Malinski (2008) continues to support a diversity of research methods for Rogerian science.

A number of tools have been developed for the SUHB. These include the following:

Power as Knowing Participation in Change Tool (Barrett & Caroselli, 1998)

Human Field Image Metaphor Scale (Johnston, 1993, 1994)

Person-Environment Participation Scale (Leddy, 1999)

Human Field Motion Tool (Ference, 1979, 1986b)

McCanse Readiness for Death Instrument (McCanse, 1995)

Mutual Exploration of the Healing Human Field–Environmental Field Relationship (Carboni, 1992)

Diversity of Human Field Pattern Scale (Hastings-Tolsma, 1992)

Temporal Experiences Scale (Paletta, 1990)

Assessment of Dream Experiences (Watson, 1999)

Time Metaphor Test (Allen, 1988; Hastings-Tolsma, 1992; Watson, Sloyan, & Robalino, 2000)

6. Does this theory direct nursing actions that lead to favorable outcomes? Rogers would view this question as value laden—it would depend on whose outcomes are being questioned and who defines favorable. The emphasis in health care has definitely been on outcomes recently, but in a Rogerian practice model the person would provide the leadership in deciding which would be favorable outcomes to be sought. While Barrett (1998) indicated that her Rogerian practice model, health patterning practice method, does not seek to identify or anticipate consequences, M. C. Smith and Reeder (1998) argued that clinical outcomes research can be reconciled with Rogerian science.

7. How contagious is this theory? Rogers's SUHB has definitely been contagious. There is a Society for Rogerian Scholars, a Rogerian newsletter, and an annual conference. Numerous graduates of NYU and other universities continue to research, write about, and apply the Rogerian conceptual system. Furthermore, it has been identified as the starting point for the development of other nursing theories, such as those of Fitzpatrick, Parse, and Margaret Newman. Sarter (1988) wrote that the profession would be at a very different point if not for Martha Rogers. Her ideas have brought a paradigm change to nursing and opened the door for ideas on alternative means of healing, Eastern philosophy, and philosophical explorations. Furthermore, her views of unitary human beings as irreducible wholes probably helped bring consensus to the profession about its holistic focus as the basis for practice (Garon, 1992).

Multiple areas of study have investigated specific principles. Research in relation to the principle of integrality includes studies of spirituality as integrality in chronic heart failure patients (Hardin, Hussey, Wolford, & Steele, 2003); guided imagery and parent-fetal attachment (Kim, 1990); hardiness, uncertainty, power, and environment in adults waiting for kidney transplant (Stoeckle, 1993); health choices in older women (Johnson, 1996); human field pattern, risk taking, and time experience (Hastings-Tolsma, 1992); leadership styles (Kilker, 1994); life satisfaction, purpose in life, and power in those over 65 years of age (Rizzo, 1990); lightwave frequency and sleep–wakefulness frequency (Girardin, 1990); music and dyspnea (McBride, Graydon, Sidani, & Hall (1999); music and human field motion (Edwards, 1991); music and perception of environment (Biley, 1996a); parent–fetus attachment and couvade (Schodt, 1989); rest and harmonics (M. J. Smith, 1986); sleep patterns and environment change (Dixon, 1994); temporal experience and musical sequence complexity (de Sevo, 1991); and unitary field practice modalities through use of complementary therapies by people with cancer (Abu-Realh et al., 1996). Research in relation to the principle of resonancy includes studies of guided imagery (Butcher & Parker, 1988; Lewandowski, 2004) and tension headache (MacNeil, 1996). Research in relation to helicy includes studies of creativity, time experience, and mystical experience (Bray, 1989); the theory of aging, including time, sleep patterns, and activity (Alligood & McGuire, 2000); the theory of accelerating change (Alligood, 1991; Biley, 1992a); and time experience, human field motion, and creativity (Allen, 1988). More recently, researchers have realized that Rogers's principles are more appropriately studied from a unitary perspective, encompassing all three principles. Wright (2004) studied trust and power in adults, Lewandowski (2004) studied the patterning of pain and power with guided imagery, and Yarcheski, Mahon, and Yarcheski (2004) studied health and well-being in early adolescents. Todaro-Franceschi (2008) sought to clarify the enigma of energy.

Therapeutic touch is one of the most widely known interventions associated with the SUHB. Research on therapeutic touch includes studies on the experience of receiving therapeutic touch (Samarel, 1992), in vitro erythropoiesis (Straneva, 1992), milk letdown (Mersmann, 1993), pain and anxiety in burn patients (Turner, Clark, Williams, & Gautheir, 1998), pain in elders with degenerative arthritis (Peck, 1997, 1998), postoperative pain (Meehan, 1993), and stress reduction and immune function (Garrard, 1995).

Use of the SUHB has been discussed in multiple areas of practice. These areas include addiction/drug abuse (Compton, 1989; Conti-O'Hare, 1998; Rushing, 2008), approaches to aging (Butcher, 2003), awareness (Phillips & Bramlett, 1994/2008; Sharts-Hopko, 2008), cardiac care (Contrades, 1987), care of the terminally ill (Buczny, Speirs, & Howard, 1989), caring (M. C. Smith, 1999), community health (Ruka, Brown, & Procope, 1997), dreaming (Repede, 2009), family nursing (Winsted-Fry, 2000), healing (Schneider), health in older women (Shearer, Fleury, & Reed, 2009), home health (Heggie et al., 1994), innovative imagery as a health patterning modality (Barrett, 1992), menopause (Novak, 1999), oncology (Farren, 2009; Feber, 1996), pain (Baumann, 2009); pet therapy (Coakley & Mahoney, 2009), postpartum assessment (Tettero, Jackson, & Wilson, 1993), preventing teen pregnancy (Porter, 1998), post-mastectomy care (Biley, 1993), psychiatric care (Thompson, 1990), Reiki (2009b), spirituality (Malinski, 1991), staffing (Douglas & Kerfoot, 2008), therapeutic touch (Benor, 1996; Biley, 1996b; Green, 1998; Griffin, Moore, Ruge, & Weiler-Crespo, 1996; Kenosian, 1995; Mills, 1996; Samarel, 1997), time (Ring, 2009a; Watson, 2008), unitary pattern appreciation (Cowling, 2000), use in the future (Barrett, 2000), and use of the Personalized Nursing LIGHT model (Andersen & Smereck, 1989).

The SUHB has also been used in education. Batra (1995, 1996) discusses its use in baccalaureate and graduate nursing education. Hellwig and Ferrante (1993) describe the use of SUHB as a framework for an associate degree nursing education program. Klemm and Stashinko (1997) described a method for teaching Rogers's work, and Patty (1999) presented a use of SUHB in teaching surgical technologists.

In addition to the widespread use of the SUHB in the United States, it has influenced nursing in many other countries. These include Australia (Powell, 1997), Canada

(Chapman, Mitchell, & Forchuk, 1994), and China (Sheu, Shiau, & Hung, 1997), Germany (Ammende, 1996a, 1996b; Madrid, 1996; Richter, 1998), Korea (Kim, Kim, Park, Park, & Lee, 2008), Spain (Tejero, 1998), and the United Kingdom and Ireland (Benor, 1996; Biley, 1992a, 1992b, 1993, 1996a, 1996b, 1998, 1999; Feber, 1996; Green, 1998; Mills, 1996; Mills & Biley, 1994; Tettero et al., 1993; Wendler, 1996).

STRENGTHS AND LIMITATIONS

Rogers presented an optimistic conceptual system that views human beings as unique, developing, "becoming" systems rather than compilations of mechanistic parts subject to breakdown. She offered a view of nurses and the people for whom they provide care as partners in care, as equal participants in ever-changing life processes. She has helped nurses refocus on the importance of the ever-developing environment in continual process with human beings (Garon, 1992, p. 71).

Rogers's conceptual system is most often criticized for its abstractness and difficulty in application. Rogers herself recognized that she was oft criticized and stated, "People either think I'm great or that I should have died a long time ago!" (Safier, 1977). Cerilli and Burd (1989) critiqued the abstractness and difficulty in application to practice and contended that the terminology is difficult to understand and apply. The experience of the nursing service at the San Diego Veterans Affairs Health Care System lends some support to these critiques. While individual nurses were enthusiastic and supportive, others were frustrated with the model's abstractness and difficulty of application. It was time consuming to continuously educate nurses about this way of thinking. In the end, it may be not Rogers's conceptual model that is the problem but rather the readiness of nurses and health care systems for this innovative thinking.

Summary

Rogers's conceptual system is acknowledged as being broad in scope and applicable in all nursing practice settings. The Rogerian conceptual system has been applied in education and practice settings. It has led to the growth of nursing research and the development of further theoretical knowledge. Her emphasis on viewing human beings and their environment as irreducible wholes has brought some consensus to nursing in regard to a focus on holism (Meleis, 1985). Her writings have given rise to explorations in nursing of new paradigm views consistent with the received view of science, feminist theory, and Eastern cultures and philosophy (Garon, 1992). Despite some difficulty in operationalizing some of her concepts, nurses will undoubtedly continue to explore her ideas and utilize them in practice.

Thought Questions

1. Rogers's worldview encourages nurses to assess patients from a perspective other than biomedical. How might you use her worldview to know more about the patterning of a patient in your settings?
2. How does Rogers's view of the environment differ from Nightingale's? In planning care for the patient, Mr. G., in the scenario, what sort of things might the nurse do to create a better healing environment in the hospital?
3. If you are selected as a new manager of a troubled unit, how could you use Rogers's SUHB to improve the work environment?

4. With its focus on the nursing as a separate and independent discipline, might Rogers's SUHB provide a more positive future for nursing? Why or why not?

5. If you were assigned to convince other nurses that Rogers's SUHB would be the ideal nursing theory on which to base their practice, what would be your three most compelling reasons?

6. Review the research areas derived from Rogers's SUHB. What one area would best be developed for your practice area and why?

PEARSON

EXPLORE mynursingkit™

MyNursingKit is your one stop for online chapter review materials and resources. Prepare for success with additional NCLEX®-style practice questions, interactive assignments and activities, web links, animations and videos, and more!

Register your access code from the front of your book at
www.mynursingkit.com.

References

Abbott, E. (1992). *Flatland*. New York: Dover.

Abu-Realh, M. H., Magwood, G., Narayan, M. C., Rupprecht, C., & Suraci, M. (1996). The use of complementary therapies by cancer patients. *Nursing Connections, 9*(4), 3–12.

Allen, V. L. R. (1988). The relationship of time experience, human field motion, and clairvoyance: An investigation in the Rogerian conceptual framework. *Dissertation Abstracts International, 50* (1B), 121.

Alligood, M. R. (1991). Testing Rogers's theory of accelerating change: The relationships among creativity, actualization, and empathy in persons 18 to 92 years of age. *Western Journal of Nursing Research, 13*(1), 84–96.

Alligood, M. R., & Fawcett, J. (1999). Acceptance of the invitation to dialogue: Examination of an interpretive approach for the Science of Unitary Human Beings. *Visions: The Journal of Rogerian Nursing Science, 7*(1), 5–13.

Alligood, M. R., & Fawcett, J. (2004). An interpretive study of Martha Rogers' conception of pattern. *Visions: The Journal of Rogerian Nursing Science, 12*(1), 8–13.

Alligood, M. R., & McGuire, S. L. (2000). Perception of time, sleep patterns, and activity in senior citizens: A test of a Rogerian theory of aging. *Visions: The Journal of Rogerian Nursing Science, 8*(1), 6–14.

Ammende, M. (1996a). Changes of paradigm in nursing. Part 1: Theory of Martha Rogers [German]. *Pflege, 9*, 5–11.

Ammende, M. (1996b). Changes of paradigm in nursing: Part 2: Elizabeth Barrett's "Theory of power" [German]. *Pflege, 9*, 98–104.

Andersen, M. D., & Smereck, G. A. D. (1989). Personalized Nursing LIGHT model. *Nursing Science Quarterly, 2*, 120–130.

Barrett, E. A. M. (1983). An empirical investigation of Martha E. Rogers' principle of helicy: The relationship of human field motion and power. *Dissertation Abstracts International, 45*(2A), 615.

Barrett, E. A. M. (1989). A nursing theory of power for nursing practice: Derivation from Rogers' paradigm. In J. Riehl-Sisca (Ed.), *Conceptual models for nursing practice* (3rd ed., pp. 207–217). Norwalk, CT: Appleton & Lange.

Barrett, E. A. M. (1990a). Rogers' science-based nursing practice. In E. A. M. Barrett (Ed.), *Visions of Rogers' science based nursing* (pp. 31–44). New York: National League for Nursing.

Barrett, E. A. M. (Ed.). (1990b). *Visions of Rogers' science based nursing*. New York: National League for Nursing.

Barrett, E. A. M. (1992). Innovative imagery: A health-patterning modality for nursing practice. *Journal of Holistic Nursing, 10*, 154–166.

Barrett, E. A. M. (1998). A Rogerian practice methodology for health patterning. *Nursing Science Quarterly, 11*, 136–138.

Barrett, E. A. M. (2000). Speculations on the unpredictable future of the Science of Unitary Human Beings. *Visions: The Journal of Rogerian Nursing Science, 8*, 15–25.

Barrett, E. A. M., & Caroselli, C. (1998). Methodological ponderings related to the Power as Knowing Participation in Change Tool. *Nursing Science Quarterly, 11*, 17–22.

Batra, C. (1995). Theory based curricula and utilization of Martha Rogers framework in undergraduate and graduate programs. *Rogerian Nursing Science News, 8*(2), 8–9.

Batra, C. (1996). Developing a baccalaureate curriculum based on Martha Rogers' framework. *Rogerian Nursing Science News, 9*(1), 10–11.

Baumann, S. (2009). A nursing approach to pain in older adults. *MEDSURG Nursing, 18*(2), 77–82.

Bays, C. L. (1995). Older adults' descriptions of hope after a stroke. *Dissertation Abstracts International, 56*(10B), 5412.

Bays, C. L. (2001). Older adults' descriptions of hope after a stroke. *Rehabilitation Nursing, 26*(1), 18–20, 23–27.

Benor, R. (1996). Innovations in practice. Therapeutic touch. *British Journal of Community Health Nursing, 1*, 203–208.

Bernardo, L. M. (1993). Parent-reported injury-associated behaviors and life events among injured, ill, and well preschool children. *Dissertation Abstracts International, 54*(7B), 3548.

Bernardo, L. M. (1996). Parent-reported injury-associated behaviors and life events among injured, ill, and well preschool children. *Journal of Pediatric Nursing: Nursing Care of Children and Families, 11*, 100–110.

Biley, F. C. (1992a). The perception of time as a factor in Rogers' Science of Unitary Human Beings: A literature review. *Journal of Advanced Nursing, 17*, 1141–1145.

Biley, F. (1992b). The Science of Unitary Human Beings: A contemporary literature review. *Nursing Practice, 5*(4), 23–26.

Biley, F. C. (1993). Energy fields nursing: A brief encounter of a unitary kind. *International Journal of Nursing Studies, 30*, 519–525.

Biley, F. C. (1996a). An exploration of the Science of Unitary Human Beings and the principle of integrality: The effects of background music on patients and their perception of the environment. *Rogerian Nursing Science News, 9*, 9.

Biley, F. C. (1996b). Rogerian science, phantoms, and therapeutic touch: Exploring potentials. *Nursing Science Quarterly, 9*, 165–169.

Biley, F. C. (1998). The Beat Generation and beyond: Popular culture and the development of the Science of Unitary Human Beings. *Visions: The Journal of Rogerian Nursing Science, 6*, 5–12.

Biley, F. (1999). The impact of the beat generation and popular culture on the development of Martha Rogers's Theory of the Science of Unitary Human Beings. *International History of Nursing Journal, 5*(1), 33–39.

Bramlett, M. H., & Gueldner, S. H. (1993). Reminiscence: A viable option to enhance power in elders. *Clinical Nurse Specialist, 7*(2), 68–74.

Bray, J. D. (1989). The relationships of creativity, time experience and mystical experience. *Dissertation Abstracts International, 50*(8B), 3394.

Briggs, J. P., & Peat, F. D. (1984). *The looking glass universe: The emerging science of wholeness.* New York: Cornerstone.

Brown, P. W. (1992). Sibling relationship qualities following the crisis of divorce. *Dissertation Abstracts International, 53*(11B), 5639.

Buczny, B., Speirs, J., & Howard, J. R. (1989). Nursing care of a terminally ill client: Applying Martha Rogers' conceptual framework. *Home Healthcare Nurse, 7*(4), 13–18.

Butcher, H. K. (1994a). A unitary field pattern portrait of dispiritedness in later life. *Dissertation Abstracts International, 55*(11B), 4784.

Butcher, H. K. (1994b). The unitary field pattern portrait method: Development of research method within Rogers' scientific art of nursing practice. In M. Madrid & E. A. M. Barrett (Eds.), *Rogers' scientific art of nursing practice* (pp. 397–429). New York: National League for Nursing.

Butcher, H. K. (1996). A unitary field pattern portrait of dispiritedness in later life. *Visions: The Journal of Rogerian Nursing Science, 4*, 41–58.

Butcher, H. K. (1998). Crystallizing the processes of the Unitary Field Pattern Portrait research method. *Visions: The Journal of Rogerian Nursing Science, 6*, 13–26.

Butcher, H. K. (2003). Aging as emerging brilliance: Advancing Rogers's unitary theory of aging. *Visions: The Journal of Rogerian Nursing Science, 11*(1), 55–66.

Butcher, H. K., & Parker, N. I. (1988). Guided imagery within Rogers' Science of Unitary Human Beings: An experimental study. *Nursing Science Quarterly, 1*, 103–110.

Capra, F. (1983). *The turning point.* Toronto: Bantam Books.

Capra, F. (1996). *The web of life: A new scientific understanding of living systems.* New York: Anchor Books, Doubleday.

Carboni, J. T. (1992). Instrument development and the measurement of unitary constructs. *Nursing Science Quarterly, 5,* 134–142.

Carboni, J. T. (1995a). The Rogerian process of inquiry. *Nursing Science Quarterly, 8,* 22–37.

Carboni, J. T. (1995b). Enfolding health-as-wholeness-and-harmony: A theory of Rogerian nursing practice. *Nursing Science Quarterly, 8,* 71–78.

Caroselli, C. (1995). Power and feminism: A nursing science perspective. *Nursing Science Quarterly, 8,* 115–119.

Caroselli, C., & Barrett, E. A. M. (1998). A review of the power as knowing participation in change literature. *Nursing Science Quarterly, 11,* 9–16.

Caroselli-Dervan, C. (1991). The relationship of power and feminism in female nurse executives in acute care hospitals. *Dissertation Abstracts International, 52*(6B), 2990.

Cerilli, K., & Burd, S. (1989). An analysis of Martha Rogers' nursing as a Science of Unitary Human Beings. In J. Riehl-Sisca (Ed.), *Conceptual models for nursing practice* (3rd ed., pp. 189–195). Norwalk, CT: Appleton & Lange.

Chapman, J. S., Mitchell, G. J., & Forchuk, C. (1994). A glimpse of nursing theory-based practice in Canada. *Nursing Science Quarterly, 7,* 104–112.

Coakley, A. M., & Mahoney, E. K. (2009). Creating a therapeutic and healing environment with a pet therapy program. *Complementary Therapies in Clinical Practice, 15,* 141–146.

Compton, M. A. (1989). A Rogerian view of drug abuse: Implications for nursing. *Nursing Science Quarterly, 2,* 98–105.

Conti-O'Hare, M. (1998). Examining the wounded healer archetype: A case study in expert addictions nursing practice. *Journal of the American Psychiatric Nurses Association, 4*(3), 71–76.

Contrades, S. (1987). Altered cardiac output: An assessment tool. *DCCN: Dimensions of Critical Care Nursing, 6,* 274–282.

Cowling, W. R. (1998). Unitary case inquiry. *Nursing Science Quarterly, 12,* 139–141.

Cowling, W. R. (2000). Healing as appreciating wholeness. *Advances in Nursing Science, 22*(3), 16–32.

Daingerfield, M. A. F. (1993). Communication patterns of critical care nurses. *Dissertation Abstracts International, 54*(4B), 1888.

de Sevo, M. R. (1991). Temporal experience and the preference for musical sequence complexity: A study based on Martha Rogers' conceptual system. *Dissertation Abstracts International, 52*(6B), 2991.

Dixon, D. S. (1994). An exploration of the sleep patterns of individuals when their environment changes from home to the hospital. *Dissertation Abstracts International, 55*(11B), 4785.

Dominguez, L. M. (1996). The lived experience of women of Mexican heritage with HIV/AIDS. *Dissertation Abstracts International, 57*(4B), 2475.

Donahue, L., & Alligood, M. R. (1995). A description of the elderly from self-selected attributes. *Visions: The Journal of Rogerian Nursing Science, 3,* 12–19.

Douglas, K., & Kerfoot, K. (2008). Applying a systems thinking model for effective staffing. *Nurse Leader, 6*(5), 52–55.

Doyle, M. B. (1995). Mental health nurses' imagination, power, and empathy: A descriptive study using Rogerian nursing science. *Dissertation Abstracts International, 56*(11B), 6033.

Doyle, M. B. (1998). Mental health nurses' imagination, power, and empathy: A descriptive study using Rogerian nursing science. *Rogerian Nursing Science News, 10*(4), 8.

Dykeman, M. C., & Loukissa, D. (1993). The Science of Unitary Human Beings: An integrative review. *Nursing Science Quarterly, 6,* 179–188.

Edwards, J. V. (1991). The relationship of contrasting selections of music and human field motion. *Dissertation Abstracts International, 52*(6B), 2992.

Farren, A. T. (2009). An oncology case study demonstrating the use of Rogers's Science of Unitary Human Beings and standardized nursing languages. *International Journal of Nursing Terminologies and Classifications, 20*(1), 34–39.

Feber, T. (1996). Promoting self-esteem after laryngectomy. *Nursing Times, 92*(30), 37–39.

Ference, H. M. (1979). The relationship of time experience, creativity traits, differentiation, and human field motion: An empirical investigation of Rogers' correlates of synergistic human development. *Dissertation Abstracts International, 40*(11B), 5206.

Ference, H. (1986a). Foundations of a nursing science and its evolution: A perspective. In V. M. Malinski (Ed.), *Explorations on Martha Rogers'*

Science of Unitary Human Beings (pp. 35–44). Norwalk, CT: Appleton-Century-Crofts.

Ference, H. M. (1986b). The relationship of time experience, creativity traits, differentiation, and human field motion. In V. M. Malinski (Ed.), *Explorations on Martha Rogers' Science of Unitary Human Beings* (pp. 95–106). Norwalk, CT: Appleton-Century-Crofts.

Garon, M. (1992). Contributions of Martha Rogers to the development of nursing science. *Nursing Outlook, 40*(2), 67–72.

Garrard, C. T. (1995). The effect of therapeutic touch on stress reduction and immune function in persons with AIDS. *Dissertation Abstracts International, 56*(7B), 3692.

Girardin, B. W. (1990). The relationship of light-wave frequency to sleepwakefulness frequency in well, full-term, Hispanic neonates. *Dissertation Abstracts International, 52*(2B), 748.

Green C. A. (1998). Critically exploring the use of Rogers' nursing theory of Unitary Human Beings as a framework to underpin therapeutic touch practice. *European Nurse, 3,* 158–169.

Griffin, W. M., Moore, P., Ruge, C., & Weiler-Crespo, W. (1996). Martha E. Rogers' nursing science: Application to Therapeutic Touch. *Rogerian Nursing Science News, 8*(3), 9–12.

Guba, E.G. (Ed.). (1990). *The paradigm dialog.* Newbury Park, CA: Sage.

Gueldner, S. H. (1989). Applying Rogers' model to nursing administration: Emphasis on client and nursing. In B. Henry, C. Arndt, M. DiVincenti, & A. Marriner-Tomey (Eds.), *Dimensions of nursing administration* (pp. 113–119). Boston: Blackwell Scientific.

Halkitis, P. N., & Kirton, C. (1999). Self-strategies as means of enhancing adherence to HIV antiretroviral therapies: A Rogerian approach. *Journal of the New York State Nurses Association, 30,* 22–27.

Hanchett, E. S. (1992). Concepts from Eastern philosophy and Rogers' Science of Unitary Human Beings. *Nursing Science Quarterly, 5,* 164–170.

Hardin, S. R., Hussey, L., Wolford, N. R., & Steele, L. (2003). Spirituality as integrality among heart failure patients: A pilot study. *Visions: The Journal of Rogerian Nursing Science, 11*(1), 43–49.

Hastings-Tolsma, M. T. (1992). The relationship of diversity of human field pattern to risk-taking and time experience: An investigation of Rogers' principles of homeodynamics. *Dissertation Abstracts International, 53*(8B), 4029.

Heggie, J., Garon, M., Kodiath, M., & Kelly, A. (1994). Implementing the Science of Unitary Human Beings at the San Diego VA Medical Center. In M. Madrid & E. A. M. Barrett (Eds.), *Rogers' scientific art of nursing practice* (pp. 285–304). New York: National League for Nursing.

Heggie, J. R., Schoenmehl, P. A., Grieco, C., & Chang, M. K. (1989). Selection and implementation of Dr. Martha Rogers' nursing conceptual model in an acute care setting. *Clinical Nurse Specialist, 3,* 143–147.

Hektor, L. M. (1989). Martha E. Rogers: A life history. *Nursing Science Quarterly, 2,* 63–73.

Hellwig, S. D., & Ferrante, S. (1993). Martha Rogers' model in associate degree education. *Nurse Educator, 18*(5), 25–27.

Ireland, M. (1996). Death anxiety and self-esteem in children four, five and six years of age: A comparison of minority children who have AIDS with minority children who are healthy. *Rogerian Nursing Science News, 8*(4), 16.

Ireland, M. (2000). Martha Rogers' odyssey. *American Journal of Nursing, 100*(10), 59.

Johnson, E. E. (1996). Health choice-making: The experience, perception, expression of older women. *Dissertation Abstracts International, 57*(11B), 6851.

Johnston, L. W. (1993). The development of the Human Field Image Metaphor Scale. *Dissertation Abstracts International, 54*(4B), 1890.

Johnston, L. W. (1994). Psychometric analysis of Johnston's Human Field Image Metaphor Scale. *Visions: The Journal of Rogerian Nursing Science, 2,* 7–11.

Kells, K. J. (1995). Sensing presence as open or closed space: A phenomenological inquiry on blind individuals' experiences of obstacle detection. *Dissertation Abstracts International, 57*(1B), 239.

Kenosian, C. V. (1995). Wound healing with non-contact therapeutic touch used as an adjunct therapy. *Journal of WOCN, 22,* 95–99.

Kilker, M. J. (1994). Transformational and transactional leadership styles: An empirical investigation of Rogers' principle of integrality (abstract). *Rogerian Nursing Science News, 7*(2), 1.

Kim, H. (1990). Patterning of parent-fetal attachment during the experience of guided imagery: An experimental investigation of Martha Rogers human-environment integrality. *Dissertation Abstracts International, 51*(10B), 4778.

Kim, T. S. (2008). Science of Unitary Human Beings: An update on research. *Nursing Science Quarterly, 21,* 294–299.

Kim, T. S., Kim, C., Park, K. M., Park, Y. S., & Lee, B. S. (2008). The relation of power and well-being in Korean adults. *Nursing Science Quarterly, 21,* 247–254.

Klebanoff, N. A. (1994). Menstrual synchronization. *Dissertation Abstracts International, 56*(2B), 742.

Klemm, P. R., & Stashinko, E. E. (1997). Martha Rogers' Science of Unitary Human Beings: A participative teaching-learning approach. *Journal of Nursing Education, 36,* 341–345.

Krause, D. A. B. (1991). The impact of an individually tailored nursing intervention on human field patterning in clients who experience dyspnea. *Dissertation Abstracts International, 53*(3B), 1293.

Kuhn, T. (1970). *The structure of scientific revolutions* (2nd ed.). Chicago: University of Chicago Press.

Leddy, S. K. (1999). Further exploration of the psychometric properties of the Person-Environment Participation Scale: Differentiating instrument reliability and construct stability. *Visions: The Journal of Rogerian Nursing Science, 7,* 55–57.

Lewandowski, W. A. (2004). Patterning of pain and power with guided imagery. *Nursing Science Quarterly, 17*(3), 233 – 241.

MacNeil, M. (1996). Therapeutic Touch and pain in tension headache. *Rogerian Nursing Science News, 8*(3), 13.

Madrid, M. (1996). The participating process of human field patterning in an acute-care environment [German]. *Pflege, 9,* 246–254.

Madrid, M., & Barrett, E. A. M. (Eds.). (1994). *Rogers' scientific art of nursing practice.* New York: National League for Nursing.

Malinski, V. M. (1986). *Explorations on Martha Rogers' Science of Unitary Human Beings.* Norwalk, CT: Appleton-Century-Crofts.

Malinski, V. M. (1991). Spirituality as integrality: A Rogerian perspective on the path of healing. *Journal of Holistic Healing, 9*(1), 54–64.

Malinski, V. M. (1994). Highlights in the evolution of nursing science: Emergence of the Science of Unitary Human Beings. In V. M. Malinski & E. A. M. Barrett (Eds.), *Martha E. Rogers: Her life and her work* (pp. 197-204). Philadelphia: F. A. Davis.

Malinski, V. M. (2006). Rogerian science-based nursing theories. *Nursing Science Quarterly, 19,* 7–12.

Malinski, V. M. (2008). Research diversity from the perspective of the science of unitary human beings. *Nursing Science Quarterly, 21,* 291–293.

Martha E. Rogers: A short biography. (n.d.). Retrieved July 6, 2006, from http://medweb .uwcm.ac.uk/martha.

Matas, K. E. (1997). Human patterning and chronic pain. *Nursing Science Quarterly, 10,* 88–96.

McBride, S., Graydon, J., Sidani, S., & Hall, L. (1999). The therapeutic use of music for dyspnea and anxiety in patients with COPD who live at home. *Journal of Holistic Nursing, 17,* 229–250.

McCanse, R. P. (1995). The McCanse Readiness for Death Instrument (MRDI): A reliable and valid measure for hospice care. *Hospice Journal: Physical, Psychosocial, and Pastoral Care of the Dying, 10*(1), 15–26.

McNiff, M. A. (1995a). A study of the relationship of power, perceived health, and life satisfaction in adults with long-term care needs based on Martha E. Rogers' Science of Unitary Human Beings. *Dissertation Abstracts International, 56*(11B), 6037.

McNiff, M. A. (1995b). A study of the relationship of power, perceived health, and life satisfaction in adults with long-term care needs based on Martha E. Rogers' Science of Unitary Human Beings. *Rogerian Nursing Science News 8*(2), 1–2.

Meehan, T. C. (1993). Therapeutic touch and postoperative pain: A Rogerian research study. *Nursing Science Quarterly, 6,* 69–78.

Meleis, A. (1985). *Theoretical nursing: Development and progress.* Philadelphia: Lippincott.

Meleis, A. (1997). *Theoretical nursing: Development and progress* (3rd ed.). Philadelphia: Lippincott.

Meleis, A. (2007). *Theoretical nursing: Development and progress* (4th ed.). Philadelphia: Lippincott, Williams & Wilkins.

Mersmann, C. A. (1993). Therapeutic touch and milk letdown in mothers of non-nursing preterm infants. *Dissertation Abstracts International, 54*(4B), 4602.

Mills, A. (1996). Nursing. Therapeutic touch— Case study: The application, documentation and outcome. *Complementary Therapies in Medicine, 4,* 127–132.

Mills, A., & Biley, F. C. (1994). A case study in Rogerian nursing. *Nursing Standard, 9*(7), 31–34.

Morris, D. L. (1991). An exploration of elders' perceptions of power and well-being. *Dissertation Abstracts International, 52*(8B), 4125.

Moulton, P. J. (1994). An investigation of the relationship of power and empathy in nurse executives. *Dissertation Abstracts International, 55*(4B), 1379.

Novak, D. M. (1999). Perception of menopause and its application to Rogers' Science of Unitary Human Beings. *Visions: The Journal of Rogerian Nursing Science, 7,* 24–29.

Orshan, S. A. (1996). The relationships among perceived social support, self-esteem, and acculturation in pregnant and non-pregnant Puerto Rican teenagers—abstract of doctoral dissertation. *Rogerian Nursing Science News, 9*(1), 9–10.

Overman, B. (1994). Lessons from the Tao for birthing practice. *Journal of Holistic Nursing, 12,* 142–147.

Paletta, J. L. (1990). The relationship of temporal experience to human time. In E. A. M. Barrett (Ed.), *Visions of Rogers' science based nursing* (pp. 239–253). New York: National League for Nursing.

Patty, C. M. (1999). Teaching affective competencies to surgical technologists. *AORN Journal, 70,* 776, 778–781.

Peck, S. D. E. (1997). The effectiveness of therapeutic touch for decreasing pain in elders with degenerative arthritis. *Journal of Holistic Nursing, 15,* 176–198.

Peck, S. D. (1998). The efficacy of therapeutic touch for improving functional ability in elders with degenerative arthritis. *Nursing Science Quarterly, 11,* 123–132.

Phillips, B. B., & Bramlett, M. H. (1994). Integrated awareness: A key to the pattern of mutal process. *Visions: The Journal of Rogerian Nursing Science, 2,* 19–34.

Pohl, J. M. (1992). Mother-daughter relationships and adult daughters' commitment to caregiving to their aging disabled mothers. *Dissertation Abstract International, 53*(12B), 6225.

Porter, L. S. (1998). Reducing teenage and unintended pregnancies through client-centered and family-focused school-based family planning programs. *Journal of Pediatric Nursing: Nursing Care of Children and Families, 13,* 158–163.

Powell, G. M. (1997). The new physics: Health and nursing. *Australian Journal of Holistic Nursing, 4*(1), 17–23.

Quinn, A. A. (1988). Integrating a changing me: A grounded theory of the process of menopause for perimenopausal women. *Dissertation Abstracts International, 50*(1B), 126.

Rapacz, K. E. (1991). Human patterning and chronic pain. *Dissertation Abstracts International, 52*(9B), 4670.

Rawnsley, M. (1977). *Relationships between the perception of the speed of time and the process of dying: An empirical investigation of the holistic theory of nursing proposed by Martha Rogers.* Unpublished doctoral dissertation, Boston University.

Reeder, F. (1999). Energy: Its distinctive meanings. *Nursing Science Quarterly, 12,* 6–7.

Reeder, F. (March, 2002). Remembrances of Martha E. Rogers. *Rogerian Nursing Science News Online, 1*(2). Retrieved June 25, 2006, from http://medweb.uwcm.ac.uk/martha.

Repede, E. J. (2009). Participatory dreaming: A conceptual exploration from a unitary appreciative inquiry perspective. *Nursing Science Quarterly, 22,* 360–368.

Richard, M. A. (1993). Staff nurses' perception of power as a function of organizational factors. *Dissertation Abstracts International, 54*(2A), 466.

Richter, D. (1998). Holistic nursing—Do nurses take on too much? [German]. *Pflege, 11,* 255–262.

Ring, M. E. (2009a). An exploration of the perception of time from the perspective of the science of unitary human beings. *Nursing Science Quarterly, 22,* 8–12.

Ring, M. E. (2009b). Reiki and changes in pattern manifestations. *Nursing Science Quarterly, 22,* 250–258.

Rizzo, J. A. (1990). An investigation of the relationships of life satisfaction, purpose in life, and power in individuals sixty-five years and older. *Dissertation Abstracts International, 51*(9B), 4280.

Rogers, M. E. (1961). *Educational revolution in nursing.* New York: Macmillan.

Rogers, M. E. (1964). *Reveille in nursing.* Philadelphia: F. A. Davis.

Rogers, M. E. (1970). *An introduction to the theoretical basis of nursing.* Philadelphia: F. A. Davis.

Rogers, M. E. (1988). Nursing science and art: A prospective. *Nursing Science Quarterly, 1,* 99–102.

Rogers, M. E. (1990a). Nursing: Science of Unitary, Irreducible, Human Beings: Update 1990. In E. A. M. Barrett (Ed.), *Visions of Rogers' science-based nursing* (pp. 5–11). New York: National League for Nursing. (Reprinted in 1994 in V. M. Malinski & E. A. M. Barrett [Eds.], *Martha E. Rogers: Her life and her work* [pp. 244–249]. Philadelphia: F. A. Davis)

Rogers, M. E. (1990b). Space-age paradigm for new frontiers in nursing. In M. E. Parker (Ed.), *Nursing theories in practice* (pp. 105–113). New York: National League for Nursing. (Reprinted in 1994 in V. M. Malinski & E. A. M. Barrett [Eds.], *Martha E. Rogers: Her life and her work* [pp. 250–255]. Philadelphia: F. A. Davis)

Rogers, M. E. (1992). Nursing science and the space age. *Nursing Science Quarterly, 5,* 27–34.

Rogers, M. E. (1994). Educating the nurse for the future. In V. M. Malinski & E. A. M. Barrett

(Eds.), *Martha E. Rogers: Her life and her work* (pp. 61–68). Philadelphia: F. A. Davis.

Ruka, S. M., Brown, J. A., & Procope, B. (1997). Clinical exemplar: A blending of health strategies in a community-based nursing center. *Clinical Nurse Specialist, 11*, 179–187.

Rush, M. M. (1997). A study of the relations among perceived social support, spirituality, and power as knowing participation in change among sober female alcoholics within the Science of Unitary Human Beings. *Journal of Addictions Nursing, 9*, 146–155.

Rushing, A. M. (2008). The unitary life pattern of persons experiencing serenity in recovery from alcohol and drug addiction. *Advances in Nursing Science, 31* (3), 198–210.

Safier, G. (1977). *Contemporary American leaders in nursing: An oral history.* New York: McGraw-Hill.

Samarel, N. (1992). The experience of receiving therapeutic touch. *Journal of Advanced Nursing, 17*, 651–657.

Samarel, N. (1997). Therapeutic touch, dialogue, and women's experiences in breast cancer surgery. *Holistic Nursing Practice, 12*(1), 62–70.

Samarel, N., Fawcett, J., Ryan, F. M., & Davis, M. M. (1998). Effects of dialogue and therapeutic touch on preoperative and postoperative experiences of breast cancer surgery: An exploratory study. *Oncology Nursing Forum, 25*, 1369–1376.

Sarter, B. (1987). Philosophical sources of nursing theory. *Nursing Science Quarterly, 1*, 52–57.

Sarter, B. (1988). *The stream of becoming: A study of Martha Rogers's theory.* New York: National League for Nursing.

Schneider, P. E. (1995a). Focusing awareness: The process of extraordinary healing from a Rogerian perspective. *Visions: The Journal of Rogerian Nursing Science, 3*, 32–43.

Schneider, P. E. (1995b). A model of alternative healing: A comparative case analysis. *Dissertation Abstracts International, 56*(4B), 1938.

Schodt, C. M. (1989). Patterns of parent-fetus attachment and the couvade syndrome: An application of human-environment integrality as postulated in the Science of Unitary Human Beings. *Dissertation Abstracts International, 50*(10B), 4455.

Sharts-Hopko, N. (2008). Integrated awareness: A commentary fifteen years later. *Visions: The Journal of Rogerian Nursing Science, 15*(2), 56–59.

Shearer, N. B. C., Fleury, J. D., & Reed, P. G. (2009). The rhythm of health in older women with chronic illness. *Research and Theory for Nursing Practice, 23*(2), 148–160.

Sherman, D. W. (1993). An investigation of the relationships among spirituality, perceived social support, death anxiety, and nurses' willingness to care for AIDS patients. *Dissertation Abstracts International, 55*(5B), 1808.

Sherman, D. W. (1996). Nurses' willingness to care for AIDS patients and spirituality, social support, and death anxiety. *Image: Journal of Nursing Scholarship, 28*, 205–213.

Sherman, D. W. (1997). Rogerian science: Opening new frontiers of nursing knowledge through its application in quantitative research. *Nursing Science Quarterly, 10*, 131–135.

Sheu, S. L., Shiau, S. J., & Hung, C. H. (1997). The application of Rogers' Science of Unitary Human Beings to an adolescent with mental illness [Chinese]. *Journal of Nursing (China), 44*(2), 51–57.

Smith, C. T. (1989). The lived experience of staying healthy in rural Black families. *Dissertation Abstracts International, 50*(9B), 3925.

Smith, D. W. (1992). A study of power and spirituality in polio survivors using the nursing model of Martha E. Rogers. *Dissertation Abstracts International, 53*(4B), 1791.

Smith, D. W. (1994). Toward developing a theory of spirituality. *Visions: The Journal of Rogerian Nursing Science, 2*, 35–43.

Smith, D. W. (1995). Power and spirituality in polio survivors: A study based on Rogers' science. *Nursing Science Quarterly, 8*, 133–139.

Smith, M. C. (1999). Caring and the Science of Unitary Human Beings. *Advances in Nursing Science, 21*(4), 14–28.

Smith, M. C., & Reeder, F. (1998). Clinical outcomes research and Rogerian science: Strange or emergent bedfellows? *Visions: The Journal of Rogerian Nursing Science, 6*, 27–38.

Smith, M. J. (1986). Human-environment process: A test of Rogers' principle of integrality. *Advances in Nursing Science, 9*(1), 21–28.

Smith, M. J. (1988). Perspectives on nursing science. *Nursing Science Quarterly, 1*(2), 80–85.

Stoeckle, M. L. (1993). Waiting for a second chance at life: An examination of health-related hardiness, uncertainty, power, and the environment in adults on the kidney transplant waiting list. *Dissertation Abstracts International, 54*(6B), 3000.

Straneva, J. A. E. (1992). Therapeutic touch and in vitro erythropoiesis. *Dissertation Abstracts International, 54*(3B), 1338.

Sullivan, L. M. (1994). The meaning and significance of homelessness to a child: A phenomenological inquiry. *Dissertation Abstracts International, 56*(2B), 746.

Tejero, M. C. (1998). Reflections on Martha E. Rogers' theory [Spanish]. *Revista Rol de Enfermeria, 21*(238), 43–46.

Tettero, I., Jackson, S., & Wilson, S. (1993). Theory to practice: Developing a Rogerian based assessment tool. *Journal of Advanced Nursing, 18,* 776–782.

Thomas, D. J. (1993). The lived experience of people with liver transplants. *Dissertation Abstracts International, 54*(2B), 747.

Thompson, J. E. (1990). Finding the borderline's border: Can Martha Rogers help? *Perspectives in Psychiatric Care, 26*(4), 7–10.

Thornton, L. M. (1996a). A study of Reiki, an energy field treatment, using Rogers' science. *Rogerian Nursing Science News, 8*(3), 14–15.

Thornton, L. M. (1996b). A study of Reiki using Rogers' science, part II. *Rogerian Nursing Science News, 8*(4), 13–14.

Todaro-Franceschi, V. (2008). Clarifying the enigma of energy, philosophically speaking. *Nursing Science Quarterly, 21,* 285-290.

Turner, J. G., Clark, A. J., Williams, M., & Gautheir, D. K. (1998). The effect of therapeutic touch on pain and anxiety in burn patients. *Journal of Advanced Nursing, 28*(1), 10–20.

Wall, L. M. (2000). Changes in hope and power in lung cancer patients who exercise. *Nursing Science Quarterly, 13,* 234–242.

Watson, J. (1998). Exploring the concept of beyond waking experience. *Visions: The Journal of Rogerian Nursing Science, 6,* 39–46.

Watson, J. (1999). Measuring dreaming as a beyond waking experience in Rogers' conceptual model. *Nursing Science Quarterly, 12,* 245–250.

Watson, J. (2008) Issues with measuring time experience in Rogers' conceptual model. *Visions: The Journal of Rogerian Nursing Science, 15*(2), 79–90.

Watson, J., Sloyan, C. M., & Robalino, J. E. (2000). The Time Metaphor Test re-visited: Implications for Rogerian research. *Visions: The Journal of Rogerian Nursing Science, 8,* 32–45.

Wendler, M. C. (1996). Understanding healing: A conceptual analysis. *Journal of Advanced Nursing, 24,* 836–842.

Winsted-Fry, P. (2000). Rogers' conceptual system and family nursing. *Nursing Science Quarterly, 13,* 278–280.

Wright, B. W. (2004). Trust and power in adults: An investigation using Rogers' science of unitary human beings. *Nursing Science Quarterly, 17,* 139–146.

Yarcheski, A., & Mahon, N. E. (1995). Rogers' pattern manifestations and health in adolescents. *Western Journal of Nursing Research, 17,* 383–397.

Yarcheski, A., Mahon, N. E., & Yarcheski, T. J. (2004). Health and well-being in early adolescents using Rogers' science of unitary human beings. *Nursing Science Quarterly, 17,* 72–29.

Selected Annotated Bibliography (Nursing)

Alligood, M. R., & Fawcett, J. (2004). An interpretive study of Martha Rogers' conception of pattern. *Visions: The Journal of Rogerian Nursing Science, 12*(1), 8–13.

This rational hermeneutic interpretive study reviewed three of Rogers's publications to seek a better understanding of her conceptualization of pattern. They concluded that "patterning" is the observable active dynamic process of unitary human beings and that "pattern" is more of an abstraction. They believe that "patterning" is a more useful term in actual nursing practice. This study raises interesting questions about one of the key concepts in the SUHB.

Barrett, E. A. M. (Ed.). (1990). *Visions of Rogers' science-based nursing.* New York: National League for Nursing.

This book is a compilation of materials from scholars and clinicians who have worked with Rogerian science. One of the noteworthy contributions of this book is Rogers's 1990 update. In addition, it is divided into sections on practice, research, and education.

Butcher, H. K. (2003). Aging as emerging brilliance: Advancing Rogers's unitary theory of aging. *Visions: The Journal of Rogerian Nursing Science, 11*(1), 55–66.

Butcher starts this article stating that "every 50 seconds, another baby boomer celebrates their

50th birthday" (p. 55). As people live longer, and an increased percentage of the population is in the older age-group, it is essential that we examine our understanding and views of aging and the aged. Butcher confronts some of the common negative stereotypes of the aged and helps to reframe the view of aging in Rogers's original notion as "a negentropic process of increasing diversity, creativity and innovation" (p. 55). This article is essential for nurses working with older persons as well as for anyone with aging family members or who may themselves join the ranks of the "elderly" one day.

Lewandowski, W. A. (2004). Patterning of pain and power with guided imagery. *Nursing Science Quarterly, 17,* 233–241.

Lewandowski used Rogers's SUHB to study changes in pain and power using a guided imagery modality in a quasi-experimental, randomized design. She used Barrett's definition of power and the Power as Knowing Participation in Change Tool. Chronic pain patients were randomly assigned to two groups, with the experimental group being taught to use guided imagery. The guided imagery technique was "effective for reducing pain, but it did not have a significant impact on their sense of power" (p. 241). While not demonstrating the desired links with the Power-as-Knowing Participation in Change, this study provides valuable information on a treatment modality consistent within the SUHB.

Madrid, M. (Ed.). (1997). *Patterns of Rogerian knowing.* New York: National League for Nursing.

The most recent compilations of writings from scholars and clinicians who share their applications of the Science of Unitary Human Beings.

Malinski, V. M. (2006). Rogerian science-based nursing theories. *Nursing Science Quarterly, 19,* 7–12.

In this article, Malinski provides an overview of relevant theories and research derived from Rogers's Science of Unitary Human Beings. It is an excellent overview of both recent and classic work in this paradigm and can serve as a starting point for nurses interested in developing their own research based in the SUHB.

Malinski, V. M., & Barrett, E. A. M. (1994). *Martha E. Rogers: Her life and her work.* Philadelphia: F. A. Davis.

One of the most comprehensive reviews of Martha Rogers's life and her writings. In addition to chapters devoted to Rogers's work, this book also includes a comprehensive bibliography of citations about Rogers and the Science of Unitary Human Beings, a review of her life history, and even her family geneaology provided by her sister. Just as the book was being prepared for press, the publishers received word of Martha Rogers's death and included the following tribute as a publisher's note:

> I climbed aboard her spacecraft a long time ago.
> It wasn't made of metal or plastic, and it had no
> rigid form. It was the web of the mind that carries
> us beyond our expectations. She brought a Slinky
> along to demonstrate "The Spiral of Life."
>
> I cannot visualize Martha at rest. She is out there
> somewhere discovering, developing, and nurturing ideas
> to challenge us when next we meet.
>
> Robert H. Craven, Sr. (p. iv)

Matas, K. E. (1997). Human patterning and chronic pain. *Nursing Science Quarterly, 10,* 88–96.

This study investigated pattern manifestations of chronic pain through comparing adults in chronic pain management programs and adults living in the community who did not report chronic pain. Findings included lower scores on human field motion and power as knowing participation measurements for the chronic pain group as compared to those without such pain, showing continued support for Rogers's abstract conceptual system. The author speculates that chronic pain may slow movement to higher-frequency patterns.

O'Mathuna, D. P., Pryjmachuk, S., Spencer, W., Stanwick, M., & Matthiesen, S. (2002). A critical evaluation of the theory and practice of therapeutic touch. *Nursing Philosophy, 3,* 163–176.

The authors critically scrutinize the practice of therapeutic touch (TT). They point out the incongruities between Rogers's work and conceptualization of energy fields and the original theoretical base of Krieger and Kunz. They conclude that "TT is a questionable intervention, underpinned by a very weak, theoretical, clinical and research base" (p. 163). Whatever the reader's beliefs about the subject, it is a well-done critique that looks seriously at the theories involved.

Phillips, B. B., & Bramlett, M. H. (1994). Integrated awareness: A key to the pattern of mutual process. *Visions: The Journal of Rogerian Nursing Science, 2,* 19–34.

This theoretical exploration sought to analyze the concept of integrated awareness in its relationship with the Science of Unitary Human Beings. Integrated awareness has direct relevance to the nature of human-to-human mutual process, involves creating a matrix recognizing cognition of a greater awareness of self and environment, implies an abstract sense of connection in the evolution of the human and environmental fields, and may be seen as a unifying schema of inner peace, serenity, well-being, and power.

Sarter, B. (1987). Philosophical sources of nursing theory. *Nursing Science Quarterly, 1,* 52–59.

Sarter's thoughtful and well-written article helps to explain some of the philosophical underpinnings of Rogers's writings (and of others).

Smith, M. C. (1999). Caring and the Science of Unitary Human Beings. *Advances in Nursing Science, 21*(4), 14–28.

This concept clarification sought to elucidate ambiguity about the concept of caring. By examining points of congruence between the literature on caring and the Science of Unitary Human Beings, five constitutive meanings of caring were identified. These are manifesting intentions, appreciating pattern, attuning to dynamic flow, experiencing the infinite, and inviting creative emergence. The article includes narratives to ground the abstract in concrete human experiences.

Selected Annotated Bibliography—Non-Nursing

Abbott, E. (1992). *Flatland.* New York: Dover.

This book, written at least a century ago, is an account of an intelligent creature from a two-dimensional world who finds his way to a three-dimensional world. It is an easy and quick read and is considered one of the best things of its kind that has ever been written. It is also a good introduction to the idea of dimensions beyond three.

Briggs, J. P., & Peat, F. D. (1984). *The looking glass universe: The emerging science of wholeness.* New York: Cornerstone.

A book about the science of wholeness, written for the general public. Dr. John Briggs is a science writer and Dr. David Peat a physicist. Together they produced an entertaining and enlightening book that helps explain many of the concepts underlying the Rogerian conceptual system.

Capra, F. (1996). *The web of life: A new scientific understanding of living systems.* New York: Anchor Books, Doubleday.

The most recent book by Fritjof Capra (author of *The Tao of Physics* and *The Turning Point*). Capra is a theoretical physicist who is able to write about new conceptions of science for the general public. His writings are quite consistent with the Rogerian conceptual system and provide both support and explanation for some of her views. His two earlier books are also helpful in understanding Rogers's conceptual system.

Websites

http://www.societyofrogerianscholars.org
A comprehensive website filled with useful information about the SUHB, research, references, conferences, and multiple links.

http://www.nyu.edu/nursing/centers/martharogerscenter.html
Information about the Martha E. Rogers center at New York University.

http://www.sandiego.edu/academics/nursing/theory
Website devoted to nursing theorists, Martha Rogers included.

http://www.twu.edu/cns
A website devoted to nonlinear science, defined as "one of a number of emerging methodological and theoretical constructs that make up what is often called the 'science of complexity.' The popular name for this new science is 'chaos theory.'"

CHAPTER 13

Roy Adaptation Model

Sister Callista Roy

Julia Gallagher Galbreath

Sister Callista Roy, RN, Ph.D. (b. 1939), is professor and nurse theorist at the William F. Connell School of Nursing, Boston College, Massachusetts. Roy is known worldwide for her work with the Roy Adaptation Model (RAM). In addition to teaching, she is involved in scholarly thinking, research, and writing related to the development of nursing knowledge and nursing practice. Her conceptual work includes philosophic conceptualization of the nature of knowledge as Universal Cosmic Imperative and how this worldview affects the development of nursing knowledge and nursing practice (Roy & Jones, 2007). Roy has worked to conceptualize and develop measurements of coping (Roy & Chayaput, 2004). Along with colleagues she formed the Boston-Based Adaptation Research in Nursing Society, now called the Roy Adaptation Association. Before her appointment to the Connell School of Nursing, Roy was a postdoctoral fellow and Robert Wood Johnson Clinical Nurse Scholar at the University of California, San Francisco, and had served in many leadership positions, including chair of the Department of Nursing, Mount Saint Mary's College, Los Angeles, California; adjunct professor, Graduate Program, School of Nursing, University of Portland, Oregon; and acting director and nurse consultant, Saint Mary's Hospital, Tucson, Arizona.

Sister Roy earned her B.S. in nursing in 1963 from Mount Saint Mary's College, Los Angeles; her M.S. in nursing in 1966; and her doctorate in sociology in 1977 from the University of California, Los Angeles. She is a fellow of the American Academy of Nursing. She is the author, coauthor, and contributing author of numerous works, including Introduction to Nursing: An Adaptation Model *(Roy, 1976, 1984),* Essentials of the Roy Adaptation Model *(Andrews & Roy, 1986),* Theory Construction in Nursing: An Adaptation Model *(Roy & Roberts, 1981),* The Roy Adaptation Model: The Definitive Statement *(Roy & Andrews, 1991),* The Roy Adaptation Model *(Roy & Andrews, 1999),* Roy Adaptation Model-Based Research: Twenty-Five Years of Contributions to Nursing Science *(Roy et al., 1999), and* Nursing Knowledge Development and Clinical Practice *(Roy & Jones, 2007).*

The Roy Adaptation Model (RAM) has evoked much interest and respect since its 1964 inception by Sister Roy as part of her graduate work under the guidance of Dorothy E. Johnson at the University of California, Los Angeles. In 1970, the faculty of Mount Saint Mary's College in Los Angeles adopted the RAM as the conceptual framework of the undergraduate nursing curriculum. That same year Roy first published her ideas about adaptation (Roy, 1970).

A text, written by Roy and fellow faculty, described the RAM and presented nursing assessment and intervention reflective of the distinctive focus of the model (Roy, 1976). In 1991 Roy and Andrews presented *The Roy Adaptation Model: The Definitive Statement*, which included the collective experiences of several contributing authors who taught and practiced using the Roy model for over two decades. Based on four earlier books, this text included the diagrammatic conceptualizations of the model developed at the Royal Alexandra Hospital's School of Nursing, Edmonton, Alberta, Canada. In 1999, Roy redefined elements in the RAM in preparation for nursing in the 21st century (Roy & Andrews, 1999).

Further, Roy and Roberts (1981) wrote *Theory Construction in Nursing: An Adaptation Model* to discuss the use of the RAM to construct nursing theory. Overall, 74 propositions related to the theory were offered.

In 1991, Roy and a group of fellow researchers formed the Boston-Based Adaptation Research in Nursing Society, now called the Roy Adaptation Society (RAA). The objectives of the society include the following:

1. advancing nursing practice by developing nursing knowledge based on the RAM;
2. providing scholarly colleagueship needed for knowledge and research;
3. enhancing networks for dissemination and utilization of research for nursing practice; and
4. promoting the development of expert nurse scientists. (Pollock, Frederickson, Carson, Massey, & Roy, 1994, p. 362)

Additionally, this group of nurse scholars undertook the task of gathering, reviewing, and analyzing research studies related to the RAM to create a critical analysis and synthesis of research conducted over the 25 years from 1970 to 1995. To collect the research studies searchers used the key words *research and adaptation, Roy Adaptation Theory, Adaptation Model*, and *Roy* in the following databases: Cancer, CINAHL, Dissertation Abstracts International, Educational Resources Index Citations (ERIC), Health Planning, Medline, Psychological Abstracts (Psyc Lit), and Social Science Citation Index (SSCI) (Roy et al., 1999). Works related to the model were collected from North American, South American, Asian, African, and European countries as well as Australia. The resulting publication is titled *Roy Adaptation Model-Based Research: Twenty Years of Contributions to Nursing Science* (Roy et al., 1999).

In *Nursing Knowledge Development and Clinical Practice*, Roy and coeditor Dorothy A. Jones gather the writings of nursing leaders to look at the practice of nursing as it emerges into the next century. In the book, Roy contributes to the philosophical discussion of knowledge as Universal Cosmic Imperative, the philosophic view underpinning the RAM, a discussion she began in 1997 (Roy, 1997b). This philosophic perspective places emphasis on the purposefulness of life and the creative potential of the adaptive person (Roy & Jones, 2007).

THE ROY ADAPTATION MODEL

Roy credits the works of von Bertalanffy's (1968) general system theory and Helson's (1964) adaptation theory as forming the original basis of the scientific assumptions underlying the RAM. The assumptions flow from the initial philosophical and scientific perspectives. The philosophical assumptions were based in humanism perspectives of creativity, purposefulness, holism, and interpersonal process relating to the RAM concept of veritivity, including purposefulness of existence, unity of purpose, activity and creativity, and the value and meaning of life. The scientific assumptions were based in systems theory perspectives of holism, interdependence, control processes, information feedback, and complexity of living systems relating to adaptation-level theory assumptions that behavior is adaptive, adaptation is a function of stimuli and adaptation level, adaptation levels are individual and dynamic, and the processes of responding are positive and active (Roy & Andrews, 1999).

In response to the 25th anniversary of the model's publication, Roy restated the assumptions that form the basis of the model and redefined adaptation. *Adaptation* is defined as "the process and outcome whereby thinking and feeling persons, as individuals or in groups, use conscious awareness and choice to create human and environmental integration" (Roy & Andrews, 1999, p. 30). In expanding her philosophic statements in 1997, Roy drew on the richness found in a diversity of cultures (Roy, 1997a). The philosophic assumptions flow, according to Roy, from humanism and veritivity. The term *veritivity* is used by Roy to "identify a philosophical assumption that connotes the richness of rootedness in an absolute truth that leads to values of conviction, commitment, and caring" (Roy & Jones, 2007, p. 236).

The philosophic premise is stated as "nursing sees persons as co-extensive with their physical and social environments. Nurse scholars take a value-based stance. Rooted in beliefs and hopes about the nature of the human person, they fashion a discipline that participates in the well-being of persons" (Roy, 1997a, p. 42). Roy drew on the characteristics of creation spirituality (Swimme & Berry, 1992) as she redefined the philosophic assumptions of the model. Within this framework there is the following:

- A focus on awareness and the notion of eliminating false consciousness.
- Enlightenment to reach self-control, balance, and quietude.
- The reclamation of earthly creation as the core of faith. (Roy & Andrews, 1999, p. 35)

Roy discussed her philosophic assumptions in 1988 and in 1999 continues her development of them to include a focus on a person's mutuality with others, the world, and God (Roy & Andrews, 1999). A human system is viewed more from the perspective of purposefulness within a creative universe than as a static system with a limited focus on stability (Roy & Jones, 2007). A more complete discussion of the philosophic and scientific assumptions underpinning the model is found in *Nursing Knowledge Development and Clinical Practice* (Roy & Jones, 2007). Table 13-1 lists the most recent scientific and philosophic assumptions (Roy & Jones, 2007).

The four major concepts of the RAM are the following:

1. Humans as adaptive systems as both individuals and groups
2. The environment
3. Health
4. The goal of nursing (Roy & Andrews, 1999, p. 35)

The model presents concepts related to these four areas, clarifying each and defining their interrelationships.

TABLE 13-1   Vision Basic to Concepts for the 21st Century

Scientific Assumptions

Systems of matter and energy progress to higher levels of complex self-organization.

Consciousness and meaning are constitutive of person and environment.

Awareness of self and environment is rooted in thinking and feeling.

Human decisions are accountable for the integration of creative processes.

Thinking and feeling mediate human action.

System relationships include acceptance, protection, and fostering of interdependence.

Persons and the earth have common patterns and integral relationships.

Persons and environment transformations are created in human consciousness.

Integration of human and environment meanings results in adaptation.

Philosophic Assumptions Based on the Worldview of Knowledge as Universal Cosmic Imperative

Persons have mutual relationships with the world and with a God figure.

Human meaning is rooted in an omega point convergence of the universe.

God is intimately revealed in the diversity of creation and is the common destiny of creation.

Persons use human creative abilities of awareness, enlightenment, and faith.

Persons are accountable for entering the process of deriving, sustaining, and transforming the universe.

Source: Roy, C., & Jones, D. A. (2007). *Nursing knowledge development and clinical practice.* New York: Springer.

Humans as Adaptive Systems

The first area of focus is humans as adaptive systems, both as individuals and in groups. The model offers a point of view or paradigm for shaping nursing activities. The focus of nursing relationships and interactions can be at the level of the individual, groups, organizations, communities, and societies in which they are included (Roy & Andrews, 1999, p. 35). Any of these may be considered a human system, and each is considered by the nurse as a holistic adaptive system. The idea of an adaptive system combines the concepts of system and adaptation.

HUMAN ADAPTIVE SYSTEM.   Roy conceptualizes the human system in a holistic perspective, as holism stems from the underlying philosophic assumption of the model. Holism is the aspect of unified meaningfulness of human behavior in which the human system is greater than the sum of individual parts (Roy & Andrews, 1999, p. 35). As living systems, persons are in constant interaction with their environments. Characteristics of a system include inputs, outputs, controls, and feedback.

H. L. Dunn (1971), a system theorist, calls our attention to the smallest unit of life, the cell. The cell is a living open system. The cell has its inner and outer worlds. From its outer world, it must draw forth the substances it needs to survive; within itself, the cell must maintain order over its vast number of molecules. System openness, therefore, implies the constant exchange of information, matter, and energy between the system and the environment. These system qualities are held by the individual as well as by groups or aggregates of humans. Figure 13-1 illustrates a simple system.

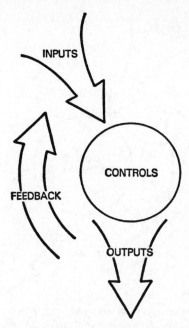

FIGURE 13-1   Diagrammatic representation of a simple system. (*From Roy, C., & Andrews, H. A. (Eds.).* *(1991). The Roy Adaptation Model: The definitive statement (p. 7). Norwalk, CT: Appleton & Lange.* *Used with permission.)*

ADAPTATION.   Figure 13-2 is used by Roy to represent humans as adaptive systems. The human adaptive system has inputs of stimuli and adaptation level, outputs as behavioral responses that serve as feedback, and control processes known as coping mechanisms. The human adaptive system has input coming from the external environment as well as from within the system. Roy identifies inputs as *stimuli* and *adaptation level* (a particular internal pooling of stimuli). Stimuli are conceptualized as falling into three classifications: focal, contextual, and residual. The stimulus most immediately confronting the human system is the *focal stimulus*. The focal stimulus demands the highest awareness from the human system. It is the center of the system's consciousness. *Contextual stimuli* are all other stimuli of the human system's internal and external worlds that can be identified as having a positive or negative influence on the situation. *Residual stimuli* are those internal or external factors whose current effects are unclear. In nursing practice, the nurse considers general knowledge related to the event or situation that has possible but unknown influences as residual stimuli. Along with stimuli, the adaptation level of the human system acts as an important internal input to that system as an adaptive system. *Adaptation level* is the combining of stimuli that represents the condition of life processes for the human adaptive system. The three levels defined by Roy are integrated, compensatory, and compromised life processes. *Integrated* processes are present when the adaptation level is working as a whole to meet the needs of the human system. *Compensatory* processes occur when the human's response systems have been activated, and *compromised* processes occur when the compensatory and integrated processes are not providing for adaptation. Integrated life process can change to compromised processes, which activates the system's compensatory processes (Roy & Andrews, 1999, pp. 36–43).

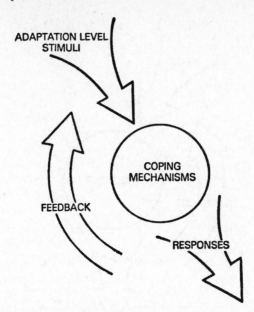

FIGURE 13-2 The person as a system. (*From Roy, C., & Andrews, H. A. (Eds.). (1991).* The Roy Adaptation Model: The definitive statement *(p. 8). Norwalk, CT: Appleton & Lange. Used with permission.)*

Outputs of the human adaptive system are behavioral responses (see Figure 13-2). Output responses can be both external and internal; thus, these responses are the system's behaviors. They can be observed, intuitively perceived by the nurse, measured, and subjectively reported by the human system. Output responses become feedback to the system and to the environment. Roy categorizes outputs of the system as either adaptive responses or ineffective responses. *Adaptive responses* are those that promote the integrity of the human system. The system's integrity, or wholeness, is behaviorally demonstrated when the system is able to meet the goals in terms of survival, growth, reproduction, mastery, and transformations of the system and the environment (Roy & Andrews, 1999, p. 44). In turn, the families, groups, communities, and society of which the individual is a member must sense and respond to changes in the person. An example of family adaptation might include reporting of ability to establish, and satisfaction with, breastfeeding a newborn. *Ineffective responses,* on the other hand, do not support the goals of humans as adaptive systems. Ineffective responses can immediately or gradually threaten the system's survival, growth, reproduction, mastery, or transformations (Roy & Andrews, 1999, p. 44). Ineffective responses can occur also at the higher system level such as in the family or in a group. In a clinical situation, an ineffective response might be defined as a family's lack of ability to establish and dissatisfaction with, breastfeeding a newborn.

For the human adaptive system, complex internal dynamics act as control processes. Roy has used the term *coping mechanisms* to describe the control processes of the human as an adaptive system. Some coping mechanisms are inherited or genetic, such as the white blood cell defense system against bacteria that seek to invade the body or shivering in response to hypothermia. Other mechanisms are learned, such as the use of antiseptics to cleanse a wound. Roy presents a unique nursing science concept of control mechanisms: the *regulator* and the *cognator*. Roy's model considers the regulator and cognator coping mechanisms to be subsystems of the person as an adaptive system and the *innovator* and *stabilizer* as control mechanisms inherent to the functioning of groups (Roy & Anway, 1989).

The *regulator subsystem* has the components of input, internal process, and output. Input stimuli may originate externally or internally to the person. The transmitters of the regulator system are chemical, neural, or endocrine in nature. Autonomic reflexes, which are neural responses originating in the brain stem and spinal cord, are generated as output responses of the regulator subsystem. Target organs and tissues under endocrine control also produce regulator output responses. Finally, Roy presents psychomotor responses originating from the central nervous system as regulator subsystem responses (Roy & Roberts, 1981). Many physiological processes can be viewed as regulator subsystem responses. For example, several regulatory feedback mechanisms of respiration have been identified. One of these is increased carbon dioxide, the end product of metabolism, which stimulates chemoreceptors in the medulla to increase the respiratory rate. Strong stimulation of these centers can increase ventilation six- to sevenfold (Guyton, 1971). An example of a regulator process is when a noxious external stimulus is visualized and transmitted via the optic nerve to higher brain centers and then to lower brain autonomic centers. The sympathetic neurons from these origins have multiple visceral effects, including increased blood pressure and increased heart rate. Roy's schematic representation of the regulator processes is seen in Figure 13-3.

When considering the individual, the other control subsystem original to the RAM is the *cognator subsystem* (Roy & Andrews, 1999). Stimuli to the cognator subsystem are also both external and internal in origin. Output responses of the regulator subsystem can be feedback stimuli to the cognator subsystem. Cognator control processes are related to the higher brain functions of perception or information processing, learning, judgment, and emotion. Perception, or information processing, is related to the internal processes of selective attention, coding, and memory. Learning is correlated to the processes of imitation, reinforcement, and insight. Problem solving and decision making are examples of the internal processes related to judgment. Finally, emotion has the processes of defense to seek relief, affective appraisal, and attachment. A schematic presentation by Roy of the cognator subsystem is presented in Figure 13-4. In maintaining the integrity of the person, the regulator and cognator are postulated as interrelated and acting together.

INDIVIDUAL SITUATION.   A decrease in the oxygen supply to Albert Smith's heart muscle stimulates pain receptors that transmit the message of pain along sympathetic afferent nerve fibers to his central nervous system. The autonomic centers of his lower brain then stimulate the sympathetic efferent nerve fibers, and there is an increase in heart and respiratory rates. The result is an increase in the oxygen supply to the heart muscle. This increase can be viewed as regulator subsystem action.

The cognator subsystem also receives the internal pain stimuli as input. Mr. Smith has learned from past experiences that the left chest and arm pain are related to his heart. His judgment is activated in deciding what action to take. He decides to go inside to air-conditioning, to sit with his legs elevated, and to take slow, deep breaths. He also decides not to call for emergency help. Certainly, he believes that an adaptive response secondary to these actions will occur. However, he may be increasingly alert for further regulator subsystem output responses that might cause him to question his decision. This represents the cognator process of selective attention and coding. Following the

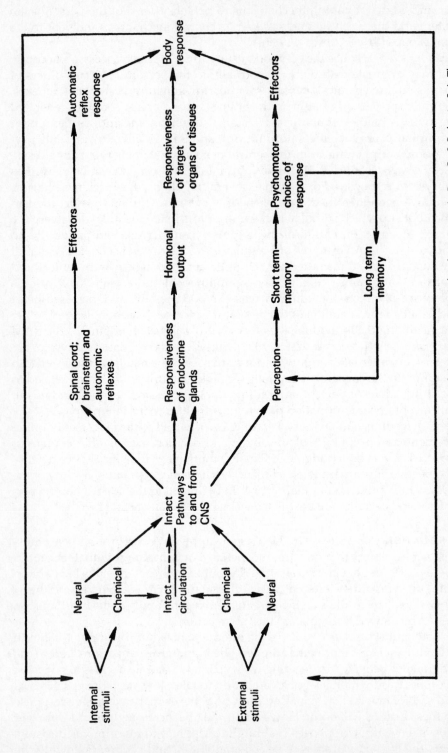

FIGURE 13-3 The regulator. (*From Roy, C., & McLeod, D. (1984). Theory of the person as an adaptive system. In Roy, C., & Roberts, S. L. Theory construction in nursing: An adaptation model (p. 61). Upper Saddle River, NJ: Prentice-Hall. Used with permission.*)

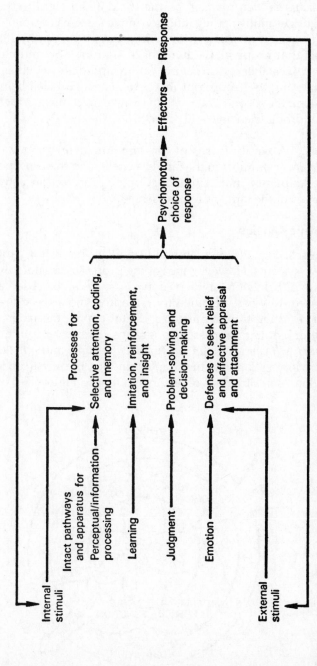

FIGURE 13-4 The cognator. (*From Roy, C., & McLeod, D. (1984). Theory of the person as an adaptive system. In Roy, C., & Roberts, S. L. Theory construction in nursing: An adaptation model (p. 64). Upper Saddle River, NJ: Prentice-Hall. Used with permission.*)

episode of pain, Mr. Smith may attempt to gain further insight into the cause of the episode. He may decide that the 90° F weather was causal and remember to limit his activities during extreme heat. In this example, Mr. Smith used the cognator subsystem processes of perception, learning, and judgment.

Control mechanisms are proposed by the RAM as inherent to the functioning of groups. Roy categorizes family, group, and collective system control mechanisms as the *stabilizer* and the *innovator subsystems* (Roy & Andrews, 1999, pp. 47–48). This conceptualization suggests that groups have two goals: stabilization and change. Stabilizer processes are those of established structure, values, and daily activities where the work of the group is done and the group contributes to the general well-being of society. The innovator subsystem, the second of the group control mechanisms, identifies structures and processes that promote change and growth.

GROUP SITUATION.   A family learns of the unplanned pregnancy of a 15-year-old daughter. This is a focal stimulus in the family system, and there is a potential for effective or ineffective adaptation in the situation. Coping processes are activated in the family and the responses of the family can be assessed.

The Four Adaptive Modes

The coping processes, cognator-regulator and stabilizer-innovator, promote adaptation in human adaptive systems. However, the coping processes are not directly observable. Only the responses or behaviors of the person or group can be observed, measured, or subjectively reported. Roy has identified four adaptive modes as categories for assessment of behavior resulting from regulator-cognator coping mechanisms in persons or stabilizer-innovator coping processes in groups. These adaptive modes are the *physiological-physical, self-concept-group identity, role function*, and *interdependence* modes. By observing behavior in relation to the adaptive modes, the nurse can identify adaptive or ineffective responses in situations of health and illness. Figure 13-5 diagrammatically

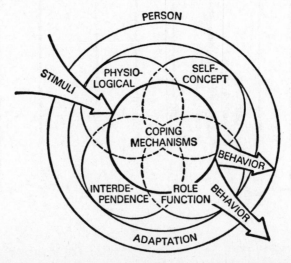

FIGURE 13-5   The person as an adaptive system. (*From Roy, C., & Andrews, H. A. (Eds.). (1991). The Roy Adaptation Model: The definitive statement (p. 17). Norwalk, CT: Appleton & Lange. Used with permission.*)

conceptualizes the human system as an adaptive system that includes the four adaptive modes for assessment. Further explanation of the four adaptive modes follows.

PHYSIOLOGICAL-PHYSICAL MODE.   The physiological mode represents the human system's physical responses and interactions with the environment (Roy & Andrews, 1999). For the individual, the underlying need of this mode is physiologic integrity, which is composed of the basic needs associated with oxygenation, nutrition, elimination, activity and rest, and protection. The complex processes of this mode are associated with the senses; fluid, electrolyte, and acid–base balance; neurological function; and endocrine function. These needs and processes may be defined as follows:

- Oxygenation   The processes of ventilation, gas exchange, and transport of gases by which cellular oxygen supply is maintained by the body (p. 126)

- Nutrition   The series of processes by which a person takes in nutrients, then assimilates and uses them to maintain body tissue, promote growth, and provide energy (p. 149)

- Elimination   Expulsion from the body of undigested substances, fluid wastes, and excess ions (p. 171)

- Activity and rest   Body movement that serves various purposes and changes in such movement so energy requirements are minimal (pp. 192–193)

- Protection   Nonspecific (surface membrane barriers and chemical and cellular defenses) and specific (immune system) defense processes to protect the body from foreign substances (p. 233)

- Senses   The processes by which energy (light, sound, heat, mechanical vibration, and pressure) changes to neural activity and becomes perception (p. 259)

- Fluid, electrolyte, and acid–base balance   The complex process of maintaining a stable internal environment of the body (p. 295)

- Neurological function   Key neural processes and the complex relationship of neural function to regulator and cognator coping mechanisms (p. 313)

- Endocrine function   Patterns of endocrine control and regulation that act in conjunction with the autonomic nervous system to maintain control of all physiologic processes (p. 355)

The physical is the focus of assessment in the first adaptive mode for a family, group, or collective human adaptive system. The need underlying this mode is resource adequacy or wholeness. For groups, the mode relates to basic operating resources such as participants, physical facilities, and fiscal resources (Roy & Andrews, 1999, p. 49).

SELF-CONCEPT-GROUP IDENTITY MODE.   For individuals, the self-concept mode relates to the basic need for psychic and spiritual integrity or a need to know the self with a sense of unity. Self-concept is central to the person's behavior because it consists of a person's beliefs or feelings about himself or herself at any given time (Roy & Andrews, 1999, p. 49). Self-concept has the components of physical self and personal self. The physical self includes body sensation and body image; the personal self includes self-consistency, self-ideal, and the moral-ethical-spiritual self. Body sensation is how the person experiences the physical self, and body image is how the person views the physical self. Self-consistency represents the person's efforts to maintain self-organization and avoid disequilibrium, self-ideal represents what the person expects to be and do, and the moral-ethical-spiritual self represents the person's belief system and self-evaluator (pp. 379–382). The need underlying the group identity mode for a family, group, or a collective is identity integrity. In collectives, "the mode consists of interpersonal relationships, group self-image, social milieu, and culture" (p. 49).

ROLE FUNCTION MODE.   Role function mode is a category of behavior for both individuals and groups. A role consists of a set of expectations of how a person in a particular position will behave in relation to a person who holds another position. The need underlying this mode is social integrity. More specifically, Roy states that social integrity is knowing who one is in relation to others so that one can act appropriately. For the individual this mode focuses on the roles of the individual in society. Role behavior in groups is the means through which the social system achieves goals and functions. The need underlying the role function mode in groups is termed *role clarity*. The mode includes functions of members of the administration and staff, information management, decision-making systems, systems to maintain order, or the need for group members to understand and commit to fulfilling expected responsibilities (Roy & Andrews, 1999, pp. 49–50).

INTERDEPENDENCE MODE.   The interdependence mode applies to adaptive behavior for both individuals and groups. Behavior is assessed as it relates to interdependent relationships of individuals and groups. For individuals, the underlying need of this mode is relational integrity or security in nurturing relationships. The mode focuses on the giving and receiving of love, respect, and value with significant others and support systems. Significant others are those persons who are of greatest importance to the person. Support systems are identified as those who help the person meet the needs for love, respect, and value. For groups, interdependence relates to social context, including both public and private contacts within and outside the group. The components are context, infrastructure, and resources (Roy & Andrews, 1999, p. 50).

Environment

According to Roy, stimuli from within the human adaptive system and stimuli from around the system represent the element of internal and external environment. Roy specifically defines environment as "all conditions, circumstances, and influences that surround and affect the development and behavior of humans as adaptive systems, with particular consideration of person and earth resources" (Roy & Andrews, 1999, p. 52).

Health

Roy defines health as "a state and a process of being and becoming an integrated and whole human being" (Roy & Andrews, 1999, p. 54). The integrity of the person is expressed as the ability to meet the goals of survival, growth, reproduction, mastery, and person and environment transformation. Roy states that the term *integrity* is used to mean "soundness or an unimpaired condition leading to wholeness" (p. 54). One's sense of purpose in life and the meaning of life, according to Roy, are significant factors relating to integration and wholeness. This view of health transcends a simple absence of disease. In fact health, as viewed in this perspective, can exist for persons with physical, emotional, or other changes. More important than the existence of a condition, illness, or change is the response of the person. Health in the RAM is a state and a process of integration that indicates successful adaptation. The aim of the nurse practicing under the RAM is to promote the health of the human by promoting adaptive responses in all life processes, including dying with dignity.

Goal of Nursing

Roy defines the goal of nursing as the promotion of adaptive responses in relation to the four adaptive modes: physiological-physical, self-concept-group identity, role function, and interdependence. Adaptive responses are those that positively affect health, that is, support the integrity of the human adaptive system. In the perspective of the RAM, human responses include not only problems, needs, and deficiencies but also capacities, assets, knowledge, skills, abilities, and commitments (Roy & Andrews, 1999). All responses are behavior. Nursing activities support adaptive responses and seek to reduce ineffective responses. The nurse may anticipate that the human system has a potential for ineffective responses secondary to stimuli likely to be present in a particular situation. The nurse acts to prepare the human system through anticipatory guidance. Nursing actions suggested by the model include approaches aimed at maintaining adaptive responses.

> In the example of the person experiencing chest pain, the stimulus immediately confronting Albert Smith (the focal stimulus) is the deficit of oxygen supply to his heart muscle. The contextual stimuli include, but are not limited to, the 90° F temperature, the sensation of pain, and Mr. Smith's age, weight, blood sugar level, degree of coronary artery patency, and his perception of health. The residual stimuli include his history of cigarette smoking and work-related stress.
>
> For Mr. Smith, the stimuli, adaptation level, and coping processes have resulted in an ineffective response. The deficit of oxygen to his heart is a threat to his physiologic integrity and will not maintain his survival. This response became feedback to the system and a focal stimulus. Mr. Smith used the cognator mechanism to adjust the total stimuli by going indoors to a cooler room and decreasing his oxygen needs by sitting down and elevating his legs. After the adjustment of the stimuli, the oxygen needs of his heart muscle were met, and the pain stopped. His coping would be further supported by a changing perception of his abilities in relation to his potential for chest pain.

THE NURSING PROCESS

The nursing process is a vehicle or decision-making method compatible with the practice of nursing using the RAM. After making a behavioral assessment and a nursing judgment, nurses assess stimuli affecting responses, make a nursing diagnosis, set goals, and implement interventions to promote adaptation (Roy & Andrews, 1999, p. 55). Roy offers the following broad aims for nursing in response to the assumptions written for the 21st century: "nurses aim to enhance system relationships through acceptance, protection, and fostering of interdependence and to promote personal and environmental transformations" (p. 55).

The RAM offers guidelines to the nurse in application of the *nursing process*. The elements of the Roy nursing process include assessment of behavior, assessment of stimuli, nursing diagnosis, goal setting, intervention, and evaluation (Roy & Andrews, 1999).

Assessment of Behavior

Assessment of behavior is considered to be the gathering of responses or output behaviors of the human system as an adaptive system in relation to each of the four adaptive modes: physiological-physical, self-concept-group identity, role function, and interdependence. Roy defines behavior as "actions or reactions under specified circumstances. It can be observable or nonobservable" (Roy & Andrews, 1999, p. 67). The nurse, through the processes of observation, careful measurement, and skilled interview techniques, gathers the specific data.

Assessment of the client in each of the four adaptive modes enhances a systematic and holistic approach. Such assessment clarifies the focus that the nurse or nursing team will use in caring for the client. In the ideal situation, thoroughly conducted and recorded nursing assessment in the four adaptive modes sets the tone for understanding the particular situation of a client for an entire health care team. Proficiency in the practice of nursing requires skilled assessment of behaviors and the knowledge to compare the person to specific criteria to evaluate behavioral responses as adaptive or ineffective. Figure 13-6 shows a Nursing History/Assessment developed by the nurses at Upper Valley Medical Center in Troy, Ohio. This form uses the four adaptive modes of the RAM. Guide questions related to each adaptive mode can be developed to reflect the age or acuity of the client population being assessed. Information collected includes subjective, objective, and measurement data. Extensive discussion of assessment of behavior related to the four adaptive modes can be found in *The Roy Adaptation Model* (Roy & Andrews, 1999) and *Nursing Manual: Assessment Tool According to the Roy Adaptation Model* (Cho, 1998).

Assessment of Stimuli

After gathering behavioral assessment data, the nurse analyzes the emerging themes and patterns of client behavior to identify ineffective responses or adaptive responses requiring nurse support with continual involvement of the human system receiving care. Behavior that varies from expectations, norms, and guidelines frequently represents ineffective responses. Roy has identified frequently occurring signs of pronounced regulator activity and cognator ineffectiveness (Roy & Andrews, 1999). Pronounced regulator activity may be indicated by elevated heart rate or blood pressure, excitement, loss of appetite, tension, or an increase in serum cortisol. Cognator ineffectiveness may be indicated by flawed perception and information processing, unsuccessful learning, poor judgment, or inappropriate affect. The presence of these behaviors suggests ineffective responses.

When ineffective behaviors or adaptive behaviors requiring support are present, the nurse assesses internal and external stimuli that may be affecting behavior. In this phase of assessment, the nurse collects data about the focal, contextual, and residual

UPPER VALLEY MEDICAL CENTERS
PMMC STOUDER
ADMISSION NURSING ASSESSMENT

INSTRUCTIONS: Check all boxes that apply. For Surgical Admissions: complete white area at P.A.T. and grey area day of admission. *See Care Plan / 24 HR Nursing Assessment & Care Record. N/A-Not Applicable

INTERDEPENDENCE – ROLE FUNCTION – SELF-CONCEPT

Date	Time	Received From: ☐ ER ☐ ____ ☐ admitting ☐ doctor's office	VIA ☐ w/c ☐ ambulatory ☐ cart	Room	Family Physician	☐ male ☐ female	Age

Temp.	Pulse	☐ Regular ☐ Irregular / ☐ Regular ☐ Irregular	Resp.	BP (LA)	BP (RA)	Height	Weight

Informant: ☐ patient ☐ family member ☐ friend ☐ transfer form ☐ prior medical record / date: ________ ☐ interview per phone
☐ current ER record ☐ other ________

History and present status of chief complaint: ________

Pain Present: ☐ no ☐ yes / location	Intensity Scale 1 (mild) – 10 (severe)	When did pain start?	How was pain managed at home?

Allergies: (describe reaction) ☐ Medications ☐ food ☐ environment ☐ None — Allergy band on? ☐ yes ☐ N/A

PATIENT HISTORY:

No Yes
- ☐ ☐ Heart disease (MI, angina, CHF, arrhythmia, murmur, mitral valve, prolapse, pacemaker)
- ☐ ☐ High Blood Pressure
- ☐ ☐ Stroke
- ☐ ☐ Respiratory (asthma, emphysema, bronchitis)
- ☐ ☐ Kidney (stones, infection, hemodialysis)
- ☐ ☐ Liver (hepatitis, mono, jaundice)
- ☐ ☐ Cancer
- ☐ ☐ Blood Disorder (bleeding, clots, anemia, phlebitis)

No Yes
- ☐ ☐ Blood Transfusion
- ☐ ☐ Diabetes
- ☐ ☐ Thyroid Disease
- ☐ ☐ Seizures/Fainting
- ☐ ☐ Muscle Disease
- ☐ ☐ Neck/Back Disorder, Arthritis
- ☐ ☐ Depression, Mental Illness
- ☐ ☐ Alcohol/Drug Abuse
- ☐ ☐ Communicable disease (TB, STD, ...)
- ☐ ☐ Other ________

Past Surgeries: ☐ none Pt/Family Reactions to anesthesia: ☐ N/A ☐ no ☐ yes ________

Past Medical Hospitalizations: ☐ none Recent xrays: ☐ no ☐ yes ________ Recent lab: ☐ no ☐ yes

FAMILY HEALTH HISTORY: (Check conditions that apply) ☐ none
☐ cancer ☐ diabetes ☐ stroke ☐ high blood pressure ☐ heart disease ☐ muscle disease ☐ other ________

Medications: (prescription, O.T.C., recreational) Include dose and frequency. Admission Nurse, note time last dose taken.
☐ None

Are medications taken as prescribed: ☐ yes ☐ no ☐ N/A

Home Situation: (marital status, children, significant others, living environment – stairs, etc.)

NSG-001 **Admission Nursing Assessment** (page 1) UVMC 3/88 Rev. 3/92

(a)

FIGURE 13-6 Upper Valley Medical Center Admission Nursing Assessment. *(From C. Mikolajewski, J. Frantz, C. Garber, J. Snyder, J Boles, S. Deslich, et al. Used with permission.* Braden Scale © *Braden, B. J., & Bergstrom, N. Used with permission.)*

INTERDEPENDENCE ROLE-SELF CONCEPT (cont.)

Occupation:

Social History: (education, special learning needs, religion, hobbies)

Utilization of community resources: ☐ no ☐ home care ☐ hospice ☐ Meals on Wheels ☐ church group ☐ support groups ☐ other _____
Personal Concerns: _____
Do you have any religious special requests? ☐ no ☐ yes _____
Emotional Status: ☐ calm ☐ anxious ☐ angry ☐ quiet ☐ talkative ☐ sad ☐ agitated ☐ other _____
Life changes in past 1-2 years? ☐ none ☐ change in health ☐ new baby ☐ marriage / divorce ☐ death someone close
☐ job / business related change ☐ other _____
Do you feel you deal successfully with stress? ☐ yes ☐ no ☐ depends on circumstance   Describe:

NEUROLOGICAL

Mental Status: ☐ alert ☐ oriented ☐ disoriented ☐ restless ☐ drowsy ☐ unresponsive ☐ memory loss
☐ other

Speech: ☐ clear ☐ slurred ☐ garbled ☐ aphasic ☐ hoarse   barriers/ ☐ foreign language _____

2 3 4 5 6 7 8 9   + - Reactive
                         – - Nonreactive
                         ± - Sluggish

Right Eye: ___ mm   Left Eye: ___ mm

Ability to Move Extremities to Command
0 (no movement)   1 (weak)   2 (strong)
RA: LA: RL: LL:

SENSES

Vision Impairment: ☐ no ☐ yes   ☐ glasses / contacts   ☐ artificial eye   ☐ cataracts   ☐ glaucoma ☐ blind ☐ R ☐ L

Hearing Impairment: ☐ no ☐ yes   partial deaf ☐ R ☐ L   total deaf ☐ R ☐ L   hearing aid ☐ R ☐ L

ACTIVITY / REST

Sleep: (Usual time of day and hours) _____
Sleep problems: ☐ none ☐ unrested after sleep ☐ insomnia ☐ nightmares ☐ other _____

SELF-CARE ABILITY (Check appropriate column)

ACTIVITY	0	1	2	3	4	5
Eating / Drinking						
Bathing						
Dressing / Grooming						
Toileting						
Bed mobility						
Transferring						
Ambulating						
Stair Climbing						
Shopping						
Cooking						
Home Maintenance						

0 - Independent
1 - Assistive Device
2 - Assistance from person
3 - Assistance from person & equipment
4 - Dependent/ unable
5 - Change in last week

FALL RISK EVALUATION

Age <3 or >75	10 points	
Confused and disoriented, hallucinating, senile	15 points	
History of falls	15 points	
Recent history of loss of consciousness, seizure disorder	15 points	
Unsteady on feet / amputation	10 points	
Poor eyesight	5 points	
Poor hearing	5 points	
Drug / alcohol problem, sedatives	5 points	
Postop condition / sedated	5 points	
Language barrier	5 points	
Attitude (resistant, belligerent, combative, fearful)	10 points	
Postural hypotension	5 points	
15 or more indicates risk. Fall precautions started:	TOTAL POINTS	

Fall Band on ☐

Assistive Devices: ☐ none ☐ crutches ☐ bedside commode ☐ walker ☐ cane ☐ splint / brace ☐ wheelchair ☐ prosthesis
☐ other _____
Activity Tolerance: ☐ no problem ☐ weakness ☐ vertigo ☐ unsteady gait ☐ angina ☐ dyspnea ☐ dyspnea at rest
☐ other _____

Admission Nursing Assessment (page 2)

(b)

FIGURE 13-6   (Continued)

OXYGENATION - SKIN INTEGRITY

Skin: ☐ Warm ☐ Hot ☐ Cool ☐ Dry ☐ Diaphoretic ☐ Clammy　　Skin Color: ☐ Normal ☐ Pale ☐ Cyanotic ☐ Jaundiced ☐ Mottled ☐ Flushed

Edema: ☐ none ☐ yes / location:

Pedal Pulses: ☐ Present ☐ Abormal / Explain:

Skin Lesions: (mark location of skin lesions by number on diagram)
☐ none ☐ scar (1) ☐ rash (2) ☐ wound or open area (3) ☐ bruise (4) ☐ incision (5) ☐ sutures / staples (6)
☐ abrasions (7) ☐ discolorations (8) ☐ other (9)

Describe

Dressings: ☐ no ☐ yes / location:

Monitor pattern: ☐ N/A

Respirations: ☐ nonlabored ☐ labored ☐ rapid ☐ shallow

Heart sounds: ☐ audible ☐ abnormal

Cough: ☐ no ☐ yes ☐ non-productive ☐ productive / color:

Oxygen: ☐ no ☐ yes - method / amt.:

Tobacco Use: ☐ no ☐ yes / type: _____
_____ pkg/day x _____ years

Breath Sounds: ☐ clear ☐ abnormal / describe:

BRADEN SCALE

RISK PREDICTORS FOR SKIN BREAKDOWN*

SENSORY PERCEPTION	1. COMPLETELY LIMITED	2. VERY LIMITED	3. SLIGHTLY LIMITED	4. NO IMPAIRMENT	
MOISTURE	1. CONSTANTLY MOIST	2. VERY MOIST	3. OCCASIONALLY MOIST	4. RARELY MOIST	
ACTIVITY	1. BEDFAST	2. CHAIRFAST	3. WALKS OCCASIONALLY	4. WALKS FREQUENTLY	
MOBILITY	1. COMPLETELY IMMOBILE	2. VERY LIMITED	3. SLIGHTLY LIMITED	4. NO LIMITATIONS	
NUTRITION	1. VERY POOR	2. PROBABLY INADEQUATE	3. ADEQUATE	4. EXCELLENT	
SHEAR & FRICTION	1. PROBLEM	2. POTENTIAL PROBLEM	3. NO APPARENT PROBLEM		

* Refer to Braden Scale for description of each subscale category
Score of 15 or less indicates that patient is a risk. Refer to SKIN CARE DECISION TREE.　　TOTAL

ELIMINATION

Abdomen ☐ soft ☐ firm ☐ distended / girth _____ ☐ non-distended ☐ tender / location:

Bowel Sounds: ☐ present ☐ absent　　Last BM / color / character:

Bowel Pattern: ☐ diarrhea ☐ constipation ☐ blood in stool ☐ hemorrhoids
☐ no problem ☐ incontinence ☐ laxative / enema Use/List:

Bladder Pattern: ☐ burning ☐ nocturia (No. times/night) ☐ difficulty starting flow ☐ frequency
☐ no problem ☐ incontinence - ☐ total ☐ daytime ☐ night time ☐ occasional ☐ urgency ☐ hematuria

Drainage Tubes: ☐ none ☐ indwelling catheter (1) ☐ intermittant catheterization (2) _____ ☐ N/G (3) ☐ G-tube (4)
☐ chest tube (5) ☐ T-tube (6) ☐ penrose (7) ☐ ostomy (8) type: _____
☐ other (9)

Describe Drainage:

LYTES - NUTRITION

Current Diet/Restrictions: ☐ Regular　　Is diet followed: ☐ yes ☐ no　　Last fluid / food intake　　Appetite: ☐ good ☐ fair ☐ poor

Recent weight change last 6 months: ☐ no ☐ yes / describe:

Fluid Intake: ☐ restricted ☐ 0 - 5 glasses / day ☐ 5 - 10 glasses / day ☐ > 10 glasses / day

☐ Caffeine use: Amt. _____　　☐ Alcohol use: Type/Amt. _____

Eating disorders: ☐ none ☐ nausea ☐ emesis ☐ chewing / swallowing difficulty ☐ sore mouth ☐ taste alterations ☐ mouth ulcers
☐ indigestion ☐ ulcer ☐ mouth-white patches ☐ erythema ☐ other

Dentures: ☐ no ☐ yes/ ☐ upper: ☐ full ☐ partial ☐ lower: ☐ full ☐ partial ☐ caps ☐ bridges ☐ loose teeth ☐ retainer ☐ crowns

IV: ☐ no ☐ yes – solution - rate - site - cath no.　　☐ IML　　☐ vascular access device

Admission Nursing Assessment (page 3)

(c)

FIGURE 13-6 (Continued)

ENDOCRINE	☐ N/A	**ADMISSION NURSING ASSESSMENT**		
		Last Menstrual Period Problems: ☐ none ☐ abnormal bleeding ☐ breast lump history ☐ vaginal drainage ☐ other ☐ breast feeding		Breast self-exam done: ☐ no ☐ yes Frequency
		Pap smear requested during hospitalization: ☐ no ☐ yes* *See sticker on front of chart		Last Pap Exam:
	☐ N/A	Last Rectal Exam Rectal exam requested during hospitalization ☐ no ☐ yes* *see sticker on front chart		
		Concerns about current or future effects of illness / surgery / treatment on: ☐ appearance ☐ male / female roles ☐ other _____		

NOTES: _____

_____

(numerous blank ruled lines)

Admission Nursing Assessment (page 4)

(d)

FIGURE 13-6   (Continued)

stimuli challenging the person's coping. For groups, ineffective responses may be indicated by increased stabilizer activity associated with innovator ineffectiveness. For example, the announcement of an unplanned teen pregnancy could result in frenzied housecleaning by the rest of the family (increased stabilizer activity) along with refusal to discuss the pregnancy or to ask for help in coping with the issue (innovator ineffectiveness). Adaptive responses requiring nursing support include behaviors related to promoting, maintaining, or improving adaptive responses that will not continue

TABLE 13-2   Common Stimuli Affecting Adaptation

Culture. Socioeconomic status, ethnicity, belief system.
Family/aggregate participants. Structure and tasks.
Developmental stage. Age, sex, tasks, heredity, genetic factors, longevity of aggregate, vision.
Integrity of adaptive modes. Physiologic (including disease pathology): physical (including basic operating resources); self-concept-group identity; role function; interdependence modes.
Cognator–Innovator effectiveness. Perception, knowledge, skill.
Environmental considerations. Change in internal or external environment; medical management; use of drugs, alcohol, tobacco; political or economic stability.

From Roy, C., & Andrews, H. A. (1999). *The Roy Adaptation Model* (2nd ed., p. 72). Stamford, CT: Appleton & Lange. Used with permission.

to be effective with the occurrence of anticipated future changes. They may also include behaviors that are adaptive but that could be strengthened through education or antici-patory guidance.

The assessment of stimuli uses the same skills as assessment of behavior and clarifies the nature of the focal stimulus; that is, the focal stimulus makes the greatest demand on the human system or provides the most immediate cause of the behavior. In identifying the focal stimulus, it should be remembered that behavior in one mode can serve as a focal stimulus for another mode and that a given focal stimulus may influence more than one mode. The first priority is given to behaviors that indicate a threat to the integrity of the system (ineffective responses). The nurse identifies significant contextual and residual stimuli. Common influencing stimuli have been identified by Roy and her colleagues and are listed in Table 13-2.

The nurse assesses the *adaptation level* (a pooling of internal stimuli), a significant internal stimulus, to assess *life processes* as integrated, compensated, or compromised. In *The Roy Adaptation Model*, the life processes and indicators of integration, compromise, and compensation are discussed in detail by chapter authors (Roy & Andrews, 1999). Other areas of stimuli to be considered include the acquired coping processes of the cognator and innovator mechanisms and changes in the environment.

NURSING DIAGNOSIS   A nursing diagnosis is an interpretative statement that represents a judgment that the nurse makes in relation to the adaptation status of the human adaptive system (Roy & Andrews, 1999, p. 77). The method suggested by Roy is stating the observed behavior along with the most influential stimuli. Using this method, a diagnosis for Mr. Smith could be stated as "Chest pain caused by a deficit of oxygen to the heart muscle associated with an overexposure to hot weather." A nursing diagnosis can also be a statement of adaptive responses that the nurse wishes to support. For example, if Mr. Smith is seeking help through vocational counseling to adapt to his physical limitation, the nurse may diagnose a need to support this behavior. In this case, an appropriate diagnosis would be "Adaptation to role failure by seeking an alternative career." Roy and others also have developed a typology of indicators of positive adaptation (see Table 13-3). Roy indicates that the NANDA diagnostic categories may be related to adaptation problems and refers to these categories as clinical classifications (Roy & Andrews, 1999) (see Table 13-4).

TABLE 13-3 **Typology of Indicators of Positive Adaptation**

Physiologic-Physical Mode

Individuals	Groups
Oxygenation	
Stable processes of ventilation	Adequate fiscal resources
Stable pattern of gas exchange	Member capability
Adequate transport of gases	Availability of physical facilities
Adequate processes of compensation	
Nutrition	
Stable digestive processes	
Adequate nutritional pattern for body requirements	
Metabolic and other nutritive needs met during altered means of ingestion	
Elimination	
Effective homeostatic bowel processes	
Stable pattern of bowel elimination	
Effective processes of urine formation	
Stable pattern of urine elimination	
Effective coping strategies for altered elimination	
Activity and Rest	
Integrated processes of mobility	
Adequate recruitment of compensatory movement processes during inactivity	
Effective pattern of activity and rest	
Effective sleep pattern	
Effective environmental changes for altered sleep conditions	
Protection	
Intact skin	
Effective healing response	
Adequate secondary protection for changes in integrity and immune status	
Effective processes of immunity	
Effective temperature regulation	
Senses	
Effective processes of sensation	
Effective integration of sensory input into information	
Stable patterns of perception, interpretation, and appreciation of input	
Effective coping strategies for altered sensation	
Fluid, Electrolyte, and Acid–Base Balance	
Stable processes of water balance	
Stability of electrolytes in body fluids	
Balance of acid–base system	
Effective chemical buffer regulation	

TABLE 13-3   (Continued)

Physiologic-Physical Mode

Individuals	Groups

Neurologic Function

Effective processes of arousal and attention; sensation and perception; coding, concept formation, memory, language; planning, motor response

Integrated thinking and feeling processes

Plasticity and functional effectiveness of developing, aging, and altered nervous system

Endrocrine Function

Effective hormonal regulation of metabolic and body processes

Effective hormonal regulation of reproductive development

Stable patterns of closed-loop negative feedback hormone systems

Effective coping strategies for stress

Self-Concept-Group Identity Mode

Individuals	Groups
Physical Self	
Positive body image	Effective interpersonal relationships
Effective sexual function	Supportive culture
Psychic integrity with physical growth	Positive morale
Adequate compensation for bodily changes	Group acceptance
Effective coping strategies for loss	Principle-based relationships
Effective process of life closure	Value-driven relationships
Personal Self	
Stable pattern of self-consistency	
Effective integration of self-ideal	
Effective processes of moral-ethical-spiritual growth	
Functional self-esteem	
Effective coping strategies for threats to self	

Role Function Mode for Individuals and Groups

Role clarity

Effective processes of role transition

Integration of instrumental and expressive role behaviors

Integration of primary, secondary, and tertiary roles

Effective pattern of role performance

Effective processes for coping with role changes

Role performance accountability

Effective group role integration

Stable pattern or role mastery

(*continued*)

TABLE 13-3 (Continued)	
Interdependence Mode for Individuals and Groups	
Individuals	**Groups**
Affectional adequacy	
Stable pattern of giving and receiving	
Effective pattern of dependency and independency	
Effective coping strategies for separation and loneliness	
Developmental adequacy	
Resource adequacy	

Source: Roy, Sr. C., & Andrews, H. A. (1999). *The Roy Adaptation Model* (2nd ed., pp. 79–81). Stamford, CT: Appleton & Lange. Used with permission.

TABLE 13-4 Typology of Commonly Recurring Problems	
Physiologic-Physical Mode	
Individuals	**Groups**
Oxygenation	
Hypoxia	Inadequate fiscal resources
Shock	Capability deficits
Ventilatory impairment	Inadequate physical facilities
Inadequate gas exchange	
Inadequate gas transport	
Altered tissue perfusion	
Poor recruitment of compensatory process for changing oxygen need	
Nutrition	
Weight 20–25% above or below average	
Nutrition more or less than body requirements	
Anorexia	
Nausea and vomiting	
Ineffective coping strategies for altered means of ingestion	
Elimination	
Diarrhea	
Bowel incontinence	
Constipation	
Urinary incontinence	
Urinary retention	
Flatulence	
Ineffective coping strategies for altered elimination	
Activity and Rest	
Immobility	
Activity intolerance	
Inadequate pattern of activity and rest	

TABLE 13-4   (Continued)

Physiologic-Physical Mode

Individuals	Groups

Restricted mobility, gait, and/or coordination
Disuse syndrome
Sleep deprivation
Potential for sleep pattern disturbance

Protection
Disrupted skin integrity
Pressure sores
Itching
Delayed wound healing
Infection
Potential for ineffective coping with allergic reaction
Ineffective coping with changes in immune status
Ineffective temperature regulation
Fever
Hypothermia

Senses
Impairment of a primary sense
Potential for injury
Loss of self-care abilities
Sensory monotony or distortion
Sensory overload or deprivation
Potential for distorted communication
Acute pain
Chronic pain
Perceptual impairment
Ineffective coping strategies for sensory impairment

Fluid and Electrolytes
Dehydration
Edema
Intracellular water retention
Shock
Hyper- or hypocalcemia, kalemia, or natremia
Acid–base imbalance
Ineffective buffer regulation for changing pH

Neurologic Function
Decreased level of consciousness
Defective cognitive processing
Memory deficits
Instability of behavior and mood
Ineffective compensation for cognitive deficit
Potential for secondary brain damage

(continued)

TABLE 13-4 (Continued)	
Physiologic-Physical Mode	
Individuals	**Groups**
Endocrine Function	
Ineffective hormone regulation	
Ineffective reproductive development	
Instability of hormone system loops	
Instability of internal cyclical rhythms	
Stress	
Self-Concept-Group Individual Identity Mode	**Groups**
Physical Self	
Body image disturbance	Ineffective interpersonal relationships
Sexual dysfunction	Oppressive culture
Rape trauma syndrome	Low morale
Unresolved loss	Stigma
Personal Self	
Anxiety	Abusive relationships
Powerlessness	Valueless relationships
Guilt	
Low self-esteem	
Role Function Mode for Individuals and Groups	
Ineffective role transitions	
Prolonged role distance	
Role conflict—intrarole and interrole	
Role failure	
Role ambiguity	
Outgroup stereotyping	
Interdependent Mode for Individuals and Groups	
Ineffective pattern of giving	
Ineffective pattern of dependency and independency	
Separation anxiety	
Loneliness	
Ineffective development of relationships	
Inadequate resources	

From Roy, Sr. C., & Andrews, H. A. (1999). *The Roy Adaptation Model* (2nd ed., pp. 82–84). Stamford, CT: Appleton & Lange. Used with permission.

Goal Setting

The goal of nursing intervention is to maintain and enhance adaptation and to change ineffective behavior to adaptive behavior. Goal setting involves making clear statements of the desired behavioral outcomes of nursing care. These outcomes will reflect adaptation. Roy suggests that goal statements be in terms of the desired behavior of the human system. A complete statement is described as one that includes the behavior desired, the change expected, and a time frame (Roy & Andrews, 1999, p. 85). Goals may be short term or long term relative to the situation.

> In the case of Mr. Smith presented in this chapter, the short-term goal would read, "Mr. Smith will proceed with daily activities (*behavior*) with no chest pain (*change*) after 30 minutes of rest (*time frame*). The long-term goal statement would read: Mr. Smith will be able to resume work (*behavior*) in a new field (*change*) in 6 months (*time frame*)."

Intervention

Nursing interventions are planned with the person or group for the purpose of altering stimuli or strengthening adaptive processes. The nurse plans specific activities to alter the selected stimuli appropriately (Roy & Andrews, 1999). Nursing activities manage stimuli by "altering, increasing, decreasing, removing, or maintaining them" as most appropriate to the situation (p. 86). By using these strategies, the nurse adjusts stimuli so that the total stimuli fall within that person's ability to cope. The coping processes of the person are the usual means of adaptation for the human adaptive system. It is when the coping processes are unable to respond effectively that the integrity of the person is compromised.

> Consider Mr. Smith, previously discussed, who has chest pain. The nurse might identify needs for information related to heart disease, low-fat diet information, and cooking classes, as well as a need for a program of cardiac rehabilitation exercises to increase cardiac strength and endurance, and a need for vocational counseling. These plans of care seek to alter the contextual stimuli and assist Mr. Smith in reaching the long-term goal of resuming productive work.

Because many alternatives may be available to the nurse to modify the focal and contextual stimuli in any situation, Roy suggests the use of a nursing judgment method developed by McDonald and Harms in 1966. First, relevant stimuli and coping processes are identified. Then nursing intervention alternatives are considered in terms of the anticipated *consequences* of changing each stimulus, the *probability* of the occurrence of the consequences (high, moderate, or low), and the *value* of the change (desirable or undesirable). The use of this judgment method includes collaboration with the members of the human adaptive system (Roy & Andrews, 1999, p. 87).

> In the case of Mr. Smith, the nurse judges the consequences of taking a cooking class as increasing the likelihood of maintaining a low-fat diet. The probability of success is rated high. This rating is based on a class being available at no cost at a community agency close to the client's home. In addition, the value is seen as desirable. The nurse and Mr. Smith select this intervention strategy along with others for implementation. The implementation requires that the nurse work with the patient, the family, the doctor, and the community agency. On the other hand, the nurse may find that the community does not have such a program to help Mr. Smith. While exploring the alternatives with Mr. Smith, the nurse may also identify a community need to enhance the health of community members. The nurse then works with community agencies and groups, using the nursing judgment method to change this ineffective community response. In either situation, the identified actions must be initiated.

Evaluation

Evaluation occurs to establish the effectiveness of the actions taken. The nurse and the involved individual(s) look collaboratively at the behaviors to see if the behavioral goals have been reached. Goal behaviors are compared to the client's output responses, and movement toward or away from goal achievement is determined. If the goals have not been achieved, the nursing process continues with additional questions relating to the accuracy and completeness of the assessment data, the match between identified goals and the client system's wishes, and the ways in which interventions were carried out. Readjustments to goals and interventions are made on the basis of evaluation data (Roy & Andrews, 1999).

The Roy Nursing Process Applied to Nursing Practice

INDIVIDUAL SITUATION. In a recovery room, the RAM can be applied to nursing assessment and interventions in various clinical situations. In the following case study, the RAM is applied to a person during the period of immediate recovery from surgery and anesthesia.

Assessment of behavior focuses on the physiologic mode responses during the first hour of recovery time after a person experiences surgery and general anesthesia. By applying the RAM, significant behaviors can be conceptualized as regulator output responses. Increased sympathetic or parasympathetic system activity can signal regulator system activity. Regulator output responses that vary from baseline values determined for the person may be the first warning of an ineffective response to postoperative stimuli. Key baseline values are the person's presurgery measures of heart rate, blood pressure, and respiratory rate. Immediately upon observation of changes from the baseline, assessment of stimuli is done. Goals are set, with the basic survival of the person as a priority. Interventions are taken so that focal and contextual stimuli are altered and adaptation is promoted. The evaluation of goal achievement is made, and further actions are taken as necessary.

Mrs. Reed is received from surgery after a major abdominal operation. Before surgery, her baseline vital signs were heart rate, 80 beats per minute; blood pressure, 120/80 mm Hg; and respiratory rate, 16 per minute. After 45 minutes in recovery, her vital signs are heart rate, 150 beats per minute; blood pressure, 90/60 mm Hg; and respiratory rate, 32 per minute. Increased regulator output response is signaled by sympathetic nervous system stimulation of the heart in response to decreased blood pressure. The nurse decides that Mrs. Reed is showing an ineffective response. Therefore, assessment of stimuli is done.

The focal stimulus is a decrease in arterial blood pressure secondary to an unknown underlying cause. The contextual stimuli are age 45 years, cool extremities, poor nail blanching, no food or drink for 12 hours, and intravenous infusion (IV) of dextrose 5% in water with lactated Ringer's solution at 100 cc per hour. Also, contextual stimuli include 200 cc of IV fluids infused during surgery, 10 cc of urine excreted during the first 45 minutes in recovery, 1.5 hours of general anesthesia, estimated blood loss of 500 cc during surgery, no operative site bleeding, and level of consciousness slow to respond to tactile stimuli after 45 minutes in recovery. The residual stimuli include history of renal infections.

The nursing diagnosis of a decreased arterial blood pressure secondary to fluid volume deficit is made. A fluid volume loss is suggested both by the contextual data and by the changes in the baseline heart rate, blood pressure, and urine output. The nurse then intervenes by altering contextual stimuli so that an adaptive response is promoted. The goal of a circulatory volume adequate to maintain a blood pressure of plus or minus 20 mm Hg of baseline levels within 15 minutes is set. The nurse plans and then takes the following intervention steps. The IV rate is increased to 300 cc per hour. The foot of the bed is elevated to increase venous return. Forty percent oxygen is given by mask. Mrs. Reed is verbally and tactilely stimulated and told to take slow deep breaths. The nurse prepares vasopressor medications for immediate use and applies an external continuous blood pressure cuff for constant blood pressure monitoring. The nurse also consults with other team members as to Mrs. Reed's clinical presentation.

A constant evaluation of the effectiveness of the nursing actions is made. The nurse holds Mrs. Reed in recovery until the goal of adequate circulation volume is met. Evaluation criteria include urine output greater than 30 cc per hour, mental alertness, rapid nail bed blanching, blood pressure plus or minus 20 mm Hg of presurgery levels, pulse plus or minus 20 beats per minute of baseline, and respirations plus or minus 5 per minute of presurgery levels.

GROUP SITUATION.   A school nurse surveys the members of the 10th grade in her school about personal substance use and finds that 30% of the teens are smoking more than two cigarettes a day. The students state that smoking is "cool," gives them a "buzz," and is a way to "break away from control by parents" and that the health risk is "almost none." Stimuli are assessed as lack of positive role modeling in the media that present smoking as "cool," lack of adaptive coping by students to control developmental anxieties, lack of involvement by parents in building parent–teen communication, and lack of knowledge related to the health risk of smoking. The nursing diagnoses include ineffective use of substance to create sense of self-worth and self-esteem, ineffective use of substance to control developmental anxieties, ineffective use of substance in separation issues with the family, and inadequate knowledge of health risks of smoking. The nurse sets the following goals: Within three months, the students will state the myths related to the image of smoking created by the media. Within four months, the 10th-grade students will state the health risks of cigarette smoking. Within six months, the rate of cigarette use by 10th graders will decrease by 50%. Within one year, students will identify positive coping strategies to deal with developmental anxieties, and parents will increase involvement in teen activities. The nurse creates a core group of concerned teens, parents, and teachers to plan strategies. The team decides to alter stimuli related to lack of positive role modeling in the media that presents smoking as "cool." Plans include use of posters that show a "different" image of the smoker and talks by nonsmoking college nursing students about setting life goals and building self-esteem without substance use or abuse. The group members secure resources including funding, space, and scheduling assistance. The team that the nurse has assembled develops many other strategies. One year later, smoking has decreased to 17% of the teens.

CRITIQUE OF THE ROY ADAPTATION MODEL

1. *What is the historical context of the theory?*   The RAM has been a phenomena in nursing since the mid-1960s and continues to grow in use in practice, educational, and research settings. The underlying assumptions are well detailed and have been expanded to meet the challenges of nursing in the 21st century. The scientific assumptions initially were drawn from von Bertalanffy's (1968) general system theory, Helson's (1964) view of adaptation as a pooled effect with three categories of stimuli, Davies's (1988) discussion of the ability to self-organize, and Swimme and Berry's (1992) concepts to accept, protect, and foster. Roy has added unity and meaningfulness of the created universe. The philosophical assumptions originated from humanism with emphasis on mutuality with

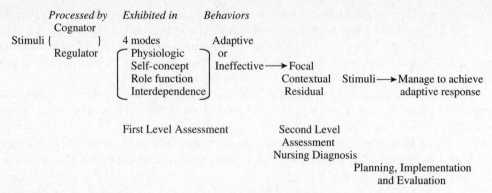

FIGURE 13-7   Relationship of concepts in the Roy Adaptation Model. *(From Julia B. George, California State University, Fullerton, 1997. Used with permission.)*

others, work, and God. Roy considers the place of the human system in creation and the meaning of human existence. She indicates human decisions are accountable for the integration of the creative processes and draws on Fox (1983) and deChardin (1966, 1969) in relation to creation spirituality. Roy states that "new knowledge can be developed related to higher levels of complex self-organization; consciousness and meaning; integration of creative processes; common person and earth patterns; diversity and destiny; convergence and transformation of the universe; and human creative abilities of awareness, enlightenment, and faith" (Roy & Andrews, 1999, p. 44).

2. *What are the basic concepts and relationships presented by the theory?*   The RAM offers a conceptual path to aid in the understanding of human behavior that is of interest to nursing and the identification of interventions that promote the well-being of people and society. The concepts are presented in Figure 13-7. The sequence of concepts in the RAM follows logically. In the presentation of each of the key concepts there is the recurring idea of adaptation to maintain integrity. The definition of health is based on the idea of integrity, which in turn is operationalized to mean responses that meet the person's goals of survival, growth, reproduction, mastery, and person and environment transformations. Promoting coping and adaptive processing is a primary activity of nursing. The RAM offers a breadth of vision that is reflective of the human experience and fits well with the practice of nursing even as knowledge is refined through research to increase the understanding of underlying concepts and the relationship between concepts. In particular, the broad philosophic framework of Universal Cosmic Imperative is joined with scientific assumptions related to system theory and adaptation-level theory to offer a value-based view of humans purposefully responding to and shaping the universe.

3. *What major phenomena of concern to nursing are presented? (These phenomena may include* but are not limited to *human beings, environment, health, interpersonal relations, caring, goal attainment, adaptation, and energy fields.)*   The RAM considers the phenomena of individuals and of groups. It concerns itself with the coping and adaptation processing of the person through the regulator and cognator subsystems\and of enhancing adaptation processing in groups through the stabilizer and innovator coping processes. It concerns itself with the behavioral focus of nursing assessment and guides the development of extensive guidelines for each area of assessment. It suggests a

scientific and philosophic perspective for nursing interaction with human systems based on the concepts of wholeness, veritivity, and cosmic openness. It presents adaptation of the human adaptive system as the reflection of health and the concept of wholeness as the system's process of meeting the goals of survival, growth, reproduction, mastery, and person–environment transformation. It concerns itself with the integration of the human system and the universe.

4. *To whom does the theory apply? In what situations? In what ways?* The RAM has broad implications for the practice of nursing. The concepts of the model have application for individuals across the life span and for families, groups, and other collective human adaptive systems. No age or situation is particularly outside the scope of the model. Portions of the model may be of greater concern to the nurse at different times. For example, if an automobile has hit a child, the physiological integrity of the child is assessed, and nursing activities that support regulator subsystems coping and the goal of survival are most important. As priorities shift in a given situation, the model continues to give the practicing nurse direction and guidance. As the nurse cares for the injured child, the nurse begins to care for the family. The group identity of the family is now affected by having an injured child and the nurse assesses the contextual stimuli related to this change. The model helps the nurse organize and apply the vast body of knowledge of nursing science and related sciences and arts to promote adaptation of individuals and groups.

5. *By what method or methods can this theory be tested?* Quantitative and qualitative research as well as instrument development has been substantial to date in relation to the RAM. Roy herself has participated in over 35 research studies related to development of nursing knowledge. Fredrickson (2000) reviewed research conducted using the RAM and concluded that both theoretically and empirically there is support for the person as an adaptive system and for health as an outcome of adaptation as conceptualized by Roy. Fredrickson recommended further research on environment and nursing, as conceptualized in the RAM. Yoder (2005) reported on RAM-based studies, both completed and ongoing, conducted at Brooke Army Medical Center and the United States Army Institute of Surgical Research in San Antonio, Texas. She concluded that the RAM has "served as an excellent guide" for these studies on quality of life among those with chronic illness or requiring long-term rehabilitation following burn injuries. Additional discussions of the RAM and research can be found in Fawcett (2005) and Roy, Whetsell, and Frederickson (2009).

Roy and Zhan (2006) offer that the structure of knowledge development in nursing falls into two broad categories: basic nursing science and the clinical science of nursing:

> Basic nursing science discovers knowledge about persons and groups from a nursing perspective that can provide understandings for practice. . . . Within the basic science, the investigator studies the person or group as an adaptive system, including (1) the adaptive processes; that is, cognator and regulator activity, stabilizer and innovator activity, stability of adaptation level patterns, and dynamics of evolving adaptive patterns; (2) the adaptive modes; that is, their development, interrelatedness, and cultural and other influences, and (3) adaptation related to health, particularly person and environment interaction and integration of the adaptive modes. (pp. 270–271)

The clinical science of nursing investigates specifically the role of the nurse in promoting adaptation and human and environment transformations. . . . Topics for research in the clinical science of nursing include (1) changes in cognator-regulator or stabilizer-innovator effectiveness; (2) changes within and among the adaptive modes; and (3) nursing care to promote adaptive processes, particularly in times of transition, during environmental changes, and during acute and chronic illness, injury , treatment, and technologic threats. (pp. 270–271)

Along with colleagues, Roy formed the Boston-Based Adaptation Research in Nursing Society, now called the Roy Adaptation Association (RAA). In a monumental undertaking, this group of nurse scholars reviewed 163 research studies related to the model for critical analysis and synthesis. Research studies were reviewed to determine linkage to the RAM, the strength and weaknesses of the study design and methods, linkage to propositions derived from the RAM, and application to nursing practice. Further, application to practice was considered for each study as falling into one of three categories: having high potential for implementation, needing further clinical evaluation before implementation, and warranting further research before implementation (Roy et al., 1999).

Barone, Roy and Frederickson (2008) evaluated the instruments used to measure concepts in the RAM. They reviewed 231 studies conducted over a 30-year period in which 123 instruments were used. Of these, 20 were found to meet the criteria for secondary analysis. Results included 14 instruments with high usefulness, three with moderate usefulness, one with limited usefulness, and two that the authors do not recommend be used with the RAM.

Because the model is an umbrella that can link concepts, it offers the opportunity for middle-range theory development as well. Examples of such middle-range theories include coping with hemodialysis (Burns, 1997), adaptation to chronic pain (Dunn, 2004), theory of chronic pain (Tsai, Tak, Moore, & Palencia, 2003), Tsai's (2003) theory of caregiver stress, theory synthesis about adapting to diabetes mellitus (Whittemore & Roy, 2002) theory on adaptation as a mediator in battered women (Woods, 2001) and theory on cognitive adaptation in hearing-impaired older persons (Zahn, 2000). Weinert, Cudney, and Spring (2008) report the development of a conceptual model for adaptation to chronic illness.

Examples of areas covered in studies using the RAM include the following:

By age: Children	Hovey, 2005; Katz, 2002; Knipp, 2006; Newman, 2005
Adolescents	Modrcin-Talbott, Pullen, Ehrenberger, Zandstra, & Muenchen, 1998; Modrcin-Talbott, Pullen, Zandstra, Ehrenberger, & Muenchen, 1998
College students	Gipson-Jones, 2009
Older adults	Chen, 2005; Flood, 2005/2006; Lee & Ellenbecker, 1998;
and elderly	Nicholson, 2009; Shyu, Liang, Lu, & Wu, 2004; Taylor, 1997; Zhan, 2000
By clinical area:	
Anesthesia induction	Mayne & Bagaoisan, 2009
Alzheimer patients	Santana, Almeida, & Savoldi, 2009
Battered women	Woods, 2001
Cardiac care	Kan, 2009
Childbearing	Fawcett et al., 2005; Shin, Park, & Kim, 2006; Weiss, Fawcett, & Aber, 2009

Chronic illness/pain	K. S. Dunn, 2004, 2005; Pollock, 1993; Tsai et al., 2003
Death and dying	Dobratz, 2004a, 2004b, 2005
Diabetes mellitus	Scollan-Koliopoulos, 2004; Whittemore & Roy, 2002
Hospice	Raleigh, 2006
HIV/AIDS	Orsi, Grandy, Tax, & McCorkle, 1997
Mental health	Bigelow et al., 2006
Multiple sclerosis	Gagliardi, 2003; Gagliardi, Frederickson, & Shanley, 2002
Neonatal intensive care	Raeside, 1997, 2000; Modrcin-Talbott, Harrison, Groer, & Younger, 2003
Oncology	Chen, Ma, Kuo, & Shyr, 1999; Coleman, 2005; Ezer et al., 2006; Grimes, 1997; John, 2007; P. D. Morgan, 2006, Nuamah, Cooley, Fawcett & McCorkle, 1999; Phuphaibul & Muensa, 1999; Samarel et al., 1998; Samarel, Fawcett, & Tulman, 1997; Samarel et al., 1999; Samarel, Tulman, & Fawcett, 2002
Orthopedics	Hsiao & Hsieh, 2009
Spinal cord injury	Chen, Boore, & Mullan, 2005; DeSanto-Madeya, 2006, 2009
Urinary incontinence	Gallagher, 1998; Johnson, 1997
Groups:	
Children/families	Bournaki, 1997; Van Riper, 2007
Combat veterans	Nayback, 2009
Grieving families	O'Mallon, 2009
Parenting	Niska, 1999; Niska, Lia-Hoagberg, & Snyder, 1997; Niska, Snyder, & Lia-Hoagberg, 1999
Psychosocial determinants	Ducharme, Ricard, Duquette, Levesque, & Lachance, 1998; Levesque, Ricard, Ducharme, Duquette, & Bonin, 1998
Tool development	DeSanto-Madeya & Fawcett, 2009; Modrcin-McCarthy, McCue, & Walker, 1997; Newman, 1997; Pollock & Duffy, 1990

6. *Does this theory direct nursing actions that lead to favorable outcomes?* Perhaps the most important question that one can consider is the usefulness of the RAM in directing nursing interventions. The model suggests that nurses alter, increase, decrease, remove, or maintain the focal stimulus or, if that is not possible, manage the contextual stimuli to promote adaptation. The search for nursing knowledge lies in greater understanding of the relative impact of contextual stimuli and the coping mechanisms in human adaptive systems. For example, should the nurse *teach* (contextual stimuli being lack of information) teens about the physiologic risks of smoking or guide a group discussion on the *perception* (cognator coping mechanism) the media creates to make smoking look "cool"?

The model sets the goal of promoting adaptation for human adaptive systems—a favorable outcome. Consider again the philosophical assumptions for the 21st century (Table 13-1). When the nurse promotes survival, growth, reproduction, mastery, and person and environment transformation, the well-being of the individual and the society of which he or she is a member is enhanced. The role of the person in creating and driving his or her life decisions is strongly respected.

7. *How contagious is this theory?* In the process of teaching, the RAM has been used to organize curriculum by the faculty at Mount Saint Mary's College in Los Angeles. Similarly, extensive use of the model, as well as pictorial representations of it, has been made by the faculty and students of the Royal Alexandra Hospital's School of Nursing (Andrews & Roy, 1986).

Few can fail to be excited by the explosive use of the RAM in clinical practice, nursing administration, nursing education, and scholarly research. A review of the literature since 1997 indicates widespread use around the world in practice, administration, research, and education. Please see the separate bibliography for dissertations and master theses. Examples of use of the RAM around the world may be found in the following:

Asia: *adolescent childbearing,* Wang & Kuo, 2006; *care analysis,* Dey, 2005; *concept mapping,* Hsu, 2004; Hsu & Hsieh, 2005; *chronic illness,* Sung, Jong, & Lu, 2006; *geriatric health education,* Sengupta, 2007; *infertility,* Ko & Chen, 2005; *intensive care,* Chan, 2003, 2004; *intrauterine death,* Shih, 2004; *multiple role adaptation,* Lin, 2005; *post-surgery care,* Chen & Chang, 2004; Kan, 2009; *spinal cord injury,* Chen et al., 1999;

Australia: *childbearing,* Fawcett et al., 2005

Colombia: *nursing education,* Moreno, Durán, & Hernandez, 2009; *renal transplant,* de Carvalho Lira, Cavalcante, & de Oliveira, 2005;

Brazil: *Alzheimers,* Santana et al, 2009; *access to health services,* Pagliuca, de Araújo, & de Araújo, 2006; *chronic illness,* da Rocha & da Silva, 2004; Guedes & de Araújo, 2005; da Silva Rocha, Moreira, & Rodrigues, 2005; *concept analysis,* Lopes, Pagliuca, & Araujo, 2006; *mothers of children with congenital heart disease,* Rocha, & Zagonel, 2009; *obstetrics,* Rodrigues, Pagliuca, & da Silva, 2004; *oncology,* Caetano & Soares, 2005; Castro Montenegro, de Araújo, Diniz, & Marques, 2005; *ostomy care,* Monge & Avelarm, 2009; *well-being,* Salvodi, Neves, dos Santos, & Mauro, 2003

Canada: *children,* Pejic, 2005; *elderly,* Thelot & Guimond-Papai, 2000; *psychosocial determinants of adaptation,* Ducharme et al., 1998; Levesque et al., 1998;

France: *elderly and social support,* Paul & Robichaud-Ekstrand, 2002; *transplant,* Baert et al., 2000

India: *hemodialysis,* Fathima, 2004

Italy: *oncology,* Vellone et al., 2004

Mexico: *elderly,* Salazar Gonzalez & Jirovec, 2001

Slovenia: *family,* Hitejc, 2001; *quality of life,* Dornik, 2001

Spain: *groups,* Guedes, Lopes, & de Araujo, 2005; *home care,* Madina Lizarraide, 2001; *intensive care,* Hernández Gil, 2002; *mothers' adaptation* de Mondonça Gondim, de Figueiredo Carvalho, & Di Ciero Miranda, 2009; *nursing models,* Roy, 2000; *parenting,* Fortes & Lopes, 2005; *service-learning,* Martínez Riera, Cibanal Juan, & Pérez, 2009

Sweden: *neonatal intensive care,* Nyqvist & Karlsson, 1997;

Thailand: *children,* Phuphaibul & Muensa, 1999; *oncology,* Sirapo-ngam, Putwatana, Kitrungroj, & Piratchavet, 2002

Turkey: *cancer,* Ozkan & Ogce, 2009

United Kingdom: *community health,* Lankester & Sheldon, 1999; *elderly,* Dawson, 1998; *neonatal intensive care,* Raeside, 1997, 2000; *oncology,* Cook, 1999

United States: *adolescents,* Hennessey-Harstad, 1999; *caregivers,* Newman, 2005; *community health,* Dixon, 1999; *concept analysis,* Duquette, 1997; *hemodialysis,* Keen et al., 1998; *managing work groups,* Hanna, 2006; *menopause,* Cunningham, 2002; *multicultural nursing,* M. G. Morgan, 1997; *parenting,* Niska, 2001; *spinal cord injury,* Harding-Okimoto, 1997; *theory based practice,* Frederickson et al., 1997;

Zimbabwe: *chronic illness,* Saburi, Mapanga, & Mapanga, 2006

STRENGTHS AND WEAKNESSES OF THE ROY ADAPTATION MODEL

The RAM offers a variety of strengths for all areas of nursing. First is the focus on, and inclusion of, the whole person or group. The four modes provide an opportunity for consideration of multiple aspects of the human adaptive system and support gaining an understanding of the whole system. The importance of the spiritual aspects of the human adaptive system, often omitted from nursing assessment, is included in a manner that allows for incorporation of spirituality without imposition of the nurse's beliefs. It is evident from the amount of research using the RAM reported in the literature and through the formation of RAA that research is supported. Because of this research connection, the RAM is evolving rather than static. It is logically organized and draws on the nurse's observational and interviewing skills.

Weaknesses have been identified in relation to research and to practice. One is the need for consistent definitions of the concepts and terms within the RAM as well as for more research based on such consistent definitions. Also, in a practice arena that is increasingly challenged with time constraints, the amount of time required to fully implement the two areas of RAM assessment may be viewed as insurmountable. This is particularly true as one begins to use the RAM; a nurse more experienced in the use of the RAM may find the time constraints less compelling.

Summary

The Roy Adaptation Model identifies the essential concepts relevant to nursing as the human adaptive system, the environment, health, and nursing. The human adaptive system is viewed as constantly interacting with internal and external environmental stimuli. The human adaptive system is active and reactive to these stimuli. Stimuli are defined as focal, contextual, and residual. The *focal stimulus* is that most immediately confronting the human system and demanding the greatest awareness or consciousness of the system. *Contextual stimuli* are internal and/or external factors that can be identified as having a positive or negative effect. *Residual stimuli* are those factors in the internal or external environment whose effect on the present situation is not known. The model suggest that nurses seek to identify influencing stimuli and intervention strategies center around the changing stimuli or strengthening adaptive responses. For example, if the contextual stimulus of *lack of transportation to prenatal care* is identified by the nurse through community assessment, then community-based strategies to address the concern can be developed. The internal coping processes of regulator and cognator for the individual and stabilizer and innovation for collective human adaptive systems are phenomena of concern to nursing. Support of coping processes may be the focus of nursing intervention. The four adaptive modes—physiological-physical, self-concept-group identity, role function, and interdependence—are areas for *behavioral* assessment. The four adaptive modes may be the first aspect of the model that the student or nurse is able to assimilate. Based on nursing tradition, assessment of behavior related to fluid and electrolytes, elimination, oxygenation, self-concept, role, and such evoke familiar images. Roy and colleagues offer extensive direction to behavioral assessment in *The Roy Adaptation Model* (Roy & Andrews, 1999). By observing behavior in relation to the adaptive modes, the nurse can identify adaptive or ineffective responses in life situations. *Nursing diagnoses* are judgments that the nurse makes in relation to the adaptation status of the human adaptive system. The goal of nursing is to promote adaptation in each of the adaptive modes. The nurse changes stimuli or strengthens adaptive responses to promote the integrity of wholeness in the human adaptive system. The model suggests that nurses alter, increase, decrease, remove, or maintain the focal stimulus or, if that is not possible, change the contextual stimuli so that the purposeful adaptation and transformation between the person and environment is promoted. Health is defined as being or becoming an integrated whole person (Roy & Andrews, 1999).

Thought Questions

1. In caring for clients in your area of expertise, what critical focal stimuli might be a common factor for clients? Would experiencing a particular illness or having significant pain, fluid loss, hyperglycemia, hypothermia, hypoxia, or other stimuli be a focal stimulus commonly affecting your client population?
2. What is the impact of this focal stimulus on your client's behavior in the four adaptive modes?
3. Is there a particular mode being most significantly affected?
4. Are there ways to assess the most commonly occurring focal and contextual stimuli that are occurring for patients in your care setting?
5. Is there research related to your area of care that helps direct nursing actions that support coping processes?
6. What factors are most frequently present in families that cope effectively with a significant health issue or illness?
7. How can nurses help support self-management (a coping process) for people and families?

 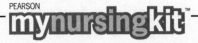
References

Andrews, H. A., & Roy, C. (1986). *Essentials of the Roy Adaptation Model*. Norwalk, CT: Appleton-Century-Crofts.

Baert, C., Cocula, N., Delran, J., Faubel, E., Foucaud, C., & Martins, V. (2000). Comparative study of transplant or pending patient's needs [French]. *Recherche en Soins Infirmiers, Dec* (63), 26-51. Abstract retrieved July 3, 2005, from EBSCOhost database.

Barone, S. H., Roy, C. L., & Frederickson, K. C. (2008). Instruments used in Roy Adaptation Model-based research: Review, critique, and future directions. *Nursing Science Quarterly, 21,* 353–362.

Bigelow, N. O., Turner, B. M., Andreasen, N. C., Paulsen, J. S., O'Leary, D. S., & Ho, B-C. (2006). Prism adaptation in schizophrenia. *Brain and Cognition, 61,* 235–242.

Bournaki, M. (1997). Correlates of pain-related responses to venipunctures in school-age children. *Nursing Research, 46,* 147–154.

Burns, D. P. (1997). *Coping with hemodialysis: A midrange theory deduced from the Roy Adaptation Model.* (Online) Dissertation abstract from CINAHL Accession No. 2000013715.

Caetano, J. Á., & Soares, E. (2005). Mastectomized women facing the physical-self and the personal-self adaptation process [Portuguese]. *Revista*

Enfermagem, 13, 210–216. Abstract retrieved July 3, 2005, from EBSCOhost database.

Castro Montenegro, S. M., de Araújo, S. E., Diniz, de Oliveira, F., & Marques Moraes, K. (2005). The nursing process in a patient with brain tumor based in Roy's Adaptation Model: A case study [Portuguese]. *Enfermagem Atual, 5*(30), 32–36. Abstract retrieved July 3, 2005, from EBSCOhost database.

Chan, D. (2003). Applying Roy Adaptation Model in assessing health in a patient with severe acute respiratory syndrome in ICU. *Hong Kong Nursing Journal, 39*(2). Abstract retrieved July 3, 2005, from EBSCOhost database.

Chan, D. (2004). Using the Roy Adaptation Model to guide the assessment of patients in an intensive care setting in Hong Kong. *Connect: The World of Critical Care Nursing, 3*(4), 106–110. Abstract retrieved July 3, 2005, from EBSCOhost database.

Chen, C. C. (2005). Dynamics of nutritional health in a community sample of American elders: A multidimensional approach using Roy Adaptation Model. *Advances in Nursing Science, 28,* 376–389.

Chen, H., Ma, F., Kuo, B., & Shyr, Y. (1999). Physical and psychological adjustment in women with mastectomy: Based on Roy's Adaptation Model [Chinese]. *Nursing Research (China), 7,* 321–332.

Chen, H-Y., Boore, J. R. P., & Mullan, F. D. (2005). Nursing models and self-concept in patients with spinal cord injury—A comparison between UK and Taiwan. *International Journal of Nursing Studies, 42,* 255–272.

Chen, Y., & Chang, P. (2004). Nursing care for a post coronary artery bypass graft patient [Chinese]. *Journal of Nursing, 51*(6), 80–86. Abstract retrieved July 3, 2005, from EBSCOhost database.

Cho, J. (1998). *Nursing manual: Assessment tool according to Roy Adaptation Model.* Glendale, CA: Polaris.

Coleman, E. A. (2005). The effect of telephone social support and education on adaptation to breast cancer during the year following diagnosis. *Oncology Nursing Forum, 32,* 822–829.

Cook, N. F. (1999). Clinical. Self-concept and cancer: Understanding the nursing role. *British Journal of Nursing, 8,* 318–324.

Cunningham, D. A. (2002). Application of Roy's Adaptation Model when caring for a group of women coping with menopause. *Journal of Community Health Nursing, 19*(1), 49–60.

da Rocha, L. A., & de Silva, L. F. (2004). Living with high blood pressure: Physiological adaptative [*sic*] way and the necessity of health education [Portuguese]. *Revista Paulista de Enfermagem, 23*(2), 144–152. Abstract retrieved July 3, 2005, from EBSCOhost database.

da Silva Rocha, J. M., Moreira, T. M. M., & Rodrigues, D. P. (2005). Adaptation of the patient suffering from diabetes mellitus type 2 to the disease and to the treatment [Portuguese]. *Revista da Rede de Enfermagem do Nordeste, 6*(1), 20–28. Abstract retrieved July 3, 2005, from EBSCOhost database.

Davies, P. (1988). *The cosmic blueprint.* New York: Simon and Schuster.

Dawson, S. (1998). Adult/elderly care nursing. Pre-amputation assessment using Roy's Adaptation Model. *British Journal of Nursing 7,* 536, 538–542.

de Carvalho Lira, A. L. B., Cavalcante Guedes, M. V., & de Oliveira Lopes, M. V. (2005). Psicosocial [*sic*] adaptation of post-renal transplanted [*sic*] adolescents according to the Roy theory [Spanish]. *Invetigacion y Educacion en Enfermeria, 23*(1), 68–77. Abstract retrieved July 3, 2005, from EBSCOhost database.

deChardin, P. T. (1966). *Man's place in nature.* New York: Harper & Row.

deChardin, P. T. (1969). *Human energy.* New York: Harcourt Brace Jovanovich.

De Mendonça Gondim, K., de Figueriredo Carvalho, Z. M., & Di Ciero Miranda, M. (2009). Mothers' adaptation of children with cerebral paralysis—Application of Roy's Model [Spanish]. *Nure Investigación, 40,* 13 pp. Abstract in English retrieved November 30, 2009, from CINAHL Plus with Full Text database.

DeSanto-Madeya, S. A. (2006). A secondary analysis of the meaning of living with spinal cord injury using Roy's Adaptation Model. *Nursing Science Quarterly, 19,* 240–246.

DeSanto-Madeya, S. (2009). Adaptation to spinal cord injury for families post-injury. *Nursing Science Quarterly, 22,* 57–66.

DeSanto-Madeya, S., & Fawcett, J. (2009). Toward understanding and measuring adaptation level in the context of the Roy Adaptation Model. *Nursing Science Quarterly, 22,* 355–359.

Dey, M. (2005). Application of Roy's Adaptation Model in care analysis. *Asian Journal of Cardiovascular Nursing, 13*(2), 14–20. Abstract retrieved July 3, 2005, from EBSCOhost database.

Dixon, E. L. (1999). Community health nursing practice and the Roy Adaptation Model. *Public Health Nursing, 16,* 290–300.

Dobratz, M. C. (2004a). Life-closing spirituality and the philosophic assumptions of the Roy Adaptation Model. *Nursing Science Quarterly, 17,* 335–338.

Dobratz, M. C. (2004b). The Life Closure Scale: Additional psychometric testing of a tool to measure psychological adaptation in death and dying. *Research in Nursing and Health, 27*(1), 52–62.

Dobratz, M.C. (2005). A comparative study of life-closing spirituality in home hospice patients. *Research and Theory for Nursing Practice, 19,* 243–256.

Dornik, E. (2001). Quality of life of a tetraplegic—case study [Slovene]. *Obzornik Zdravstvene Nege, 35,* 205–211. Abstract retrieved July 3, 2005, from EBSCOhost database.

Ducharme, F., Ricard, N., Duquette, A., Levesque, L., & Lachance, L. (1998). Empirical testing of a longitudinal model derived from the Roy Adaptation Model. *Nursing Science Quarterly, 11,* 149–159.

Dunn, H. L. (1971). *High level wellness.* Arlington, VA: Beatty.

Dunn, K. S. (2004). Toward a middle-range theory of adaptation to chronic pain. *Nursing Science Quarterly, 17,* 78–84.

Dunn, K. S. (2005). Testing a middle-range theoretical model of adaptation to chronic pain. *Nursing Science Quarterly, 18,* 146–156.

Duquette, A. M. (1997). Adaptation: A concept analysis. *Journal of School Nursing, 13*(3), 30–33.

Ezer, H., Ricard, N., Bouchard, L., Souhami, L., Saad, F., Aprikian, A., et al. (2006). Adaptation of wives to prostate cancer following diagnosis and 3 months after treatment: A test of family adaptation theory. *International Journal of Nursing Studies, 43,* 827–838.

Fathima, L. (2004). The effect of information booklet provided to caregivers of patients undergoing haemodialysis on knowledge of home care management. *Nursing Journal of India, 95*(4), 81–82. Abstract retrieved July 3, 2005, from EBSCOhost database.

Fawcett, J. (2005). Using the Roy Adaptation Model to guide nursing research. *Nursing Science Quarterly, 18,* 320–320.

Fawcett, J., Aber, C., Weiss, M., Haussler, S., Myers, S. T., King, C., et al. (2005). Adaptation to cesarean birth: Implementation of an international multisite study. *Nursing Science Quarterly, 18,* 204–210.

Flood, M. (2005/2006). A mid-range nursing theory of successful aging. *Journal of Theory Construction and Testing, 9*(2), 35–39.

Fortes, A. N., & Lopes, M. V. O. (2005). Psychosocial adaptation problems in mothers of children carrying Down syndrome [Spanish]. *Cultura de los Culdados, 9*(17), 68–73. Abstract retrieved July 3, 2005, from EBSCOhost database.

Fox, M. (1983). *Original blessing: A primer in creation spirituality.* Santa Fe, NM: Bear & Co.

Fredrickson, K. (2000). Research issues. Nursing knowledge development through research: Using the Roy Adaptation Model. *Nursing Science Quarterly, 13,* 12–17.

Frederickson, K., Williams, J. K., Mitchell, G. J., Bernardo, A., Bournes, D., & Smith, M. C. (1997). Nursing theory—Guided practice. *Nursing Science Quarterly, 10,* 53–58.

Gagliardi, B. A. (2003). The experience of sexuality for individuals living with multiple sclerosis. *Journal of Clinical Nursing, 12,* 571–578.

Gagliardi, B. A., Frederickson, K., & Shanley, D. A. (2002). Living with multiple sclerosis: A Roy Adaptation Model-based study. *Nursing Science Quarterly, 15,* 230–236.

Gallagher, M. S. (1998). Urogenital distress and the psychosocial impact of urinary incontinence on elderly women . . . including commentary by Baggerly, J. *Rehabilitation Nursing, 23*(4), 192–197.

Gipson-Jones, T. (2009). Perceived work and family conflict among African American nurses in college. *Journal of Transcultural Nursing, 20,* 304-312.

Grimes, C. E. (1997). The relationship of daily hassles, life change events, and pain to hopelessness in the ambulatory cancer patient. *Dissertation Abstracts International, 58*(02), 632B. Abstract retrieved July 5, 2007, from Dissertation Abstracts Online.

Guedes, M. V. C., & de Araújo, T. L. (2005). Hypertensive crisis: Case study with use of the nursing interventions classification in order to reach adaptive responses based in the Roy's Theoretic Model [Portuguese]. *Acta Paulista de Enfermagem, 18,* 241–246. Abstract retrieved July 3, 2005, from EBSCOhost database.

Guedes, M. V. C., Lopes, M. V. O., & de Araujo, T. L. (2006). Studying the evidence in the concept of group in Roy's Adaptation Model [Spanish]. *Cultura de los Cuidados, 9*(17), 82–87. Abstract retrieved July 3, 2005, from EBSCOhost database.

Guyton, A. C. (1971). *Basic human physiology: Normal function and mechanisms of disease.* Philadelphia: Saunders.

Hanna, D. R. (2006). Using the Roy Adaptation Model in management of work groups. *Nursing Science Quarterly, 19,* 226–227.

Harding-Okimoto, M. B. (1997). Pressure ulcers, self-concept and body image in spinal cord injury patients. *SCI Nursing, 14*(4), 111–117.

Helson, H. (1964). *Adaptation level theory.* New York: Harper & Row.

Hennessey-Harstad, E. B. (1999). Empowering adolescents with asthma to take control through adaptation. *Journal of Pediatric Health, 13,* 273–277.

Hernández Gil, E. (2002). The Callista Roy Adaptation Model: Caring for the patient with an acute myocardial infarction [Spanish]. *Metas de Enfermeria, 5*(44), 52–58. Abstract retrieved July 3, 2005, from EBSCOhost database.

Hitejc, K. (2001). Practical application of the theory of Caliste Roy in the process of adaptation of the family to a mentally retarded child [Slovene]. *Obzornik Zdravstvene Nege, 35*(5), 185–191. Abstract retrieved July 3, 2005, from EBSCOhost database.

Hovey, J. K. (2005). Fathers parenting chronically ill children: Concerns and coping strategies. *Issues in Comprehensive Pediatric Nursing, 28*(2), 83–95.

Hsiao, T., & Hsieh, H. (2009). Nurse's experience of using music therapy to relieve acute pain in a post-orthopedic surgery patient [Chinese]. *Journal of Nursing, 56*(4), 105–110.

Hsu, L. (2004). Developing concept maps from problem-based learning scenario discussions. *Journal of Advanced Nursing, 48,* 510–518. Abstract retrieved July 3, 2005, from EBSCOhost database.

Hsu, L., & Hsieh, S. (2005). Concept maps as an assessment tool in a nursing course. *Journal of Professional Nursing, 21*(3), 141–149. Abstract retrieved July 3, 2005, from EBSCOhost database.

John, L. (2007). Pilot study of a seated exercise intervention for lung cancer patients. *Oncology Nursing Forum, 34*(1), 190.

Johnson, V. Y. (1997). Effects of a submaximal exercise protocol to recondition the circumvaginal musculature in women with genuine stress urinary incontinence. *Dissertation Abstracts International, 58*(03), 1213B. Abstract retrieved July 5, 2007, from Dissertation Abstracts Online.

Kan, E. Z. (2009). Perceptions of recovery, physical health, personal meaning, role function, and social support after first-time coronary artery bypass graft surgery. *Dimensions of Critical Care Nursing, 28*(4), 189–195.

Katz, S. (2002). Gender differences in adapting to a child's chronic illness: A causal model. *Journal of Pediatric Nursing, 17,* 257–269.

Keen, M., Breckenridge, D., Frauman, A. C., Hartigan, M. F., Smith, L., Butera, E., et al. (1998). Nursing assessment and intervention for adult hemodialysis patients: Application of Roy's Adaptation Model. *ANNA Journal, 25,* 311–319.

Knipp, D. K. (2006). Teens' perceptions about attention deficit/hyperactivity disorder and medications. *Journal of School Nursing, 22*(2), 120–125.

Ko, H., & Chen, S. (2005). An experience nursing a patient with ovarian hyperstimulation syndrome who has undergone artificial fertilization treatment [Chinese]. *Journal of Nursing, 52*(3), 90–96. Abstract retrieved July 3, 2005, from EBSCOhost database.

Lankester, K., & Sheldon, L. M. (1999). Health visiting with Roy's model: A case study. *Journal of Child Health Care, 3*(1), 28–34.

Lee, A. A., & Ellenbecker, C. H. (1998). The perceived life stressors among elderly Chinese immigrants: Are they different from those of other elderly Americans? *Clinical Excellence for Nurse Practitioners, 2*(2), 96–101.

Levesque, L., Ricard, N., Ducharme, F., Duquette, A., & Bonin, J. (1998). Empirical verification of a theoretical model derived from the Roy Adaptation Model: Findings from five studies. *Nursing Science Quarterly, 11,* 31–39.

Lin, L. (2005). Multiple role adaptation among women who have children and re-enter nursing school in Taiwan. *Journal of Nursing Education, 44*(3), 116–123. Abstract retrieved July 3, 2005, from EBSCOhost database.

Lopes, M. V., Pagliuca, L. F., & Araujo, T. L. (2006). Historical evolution of the concept environment proposed in the Roy Adaptation Model. *Revista Latino-Americana de Enfermagem, 14,* 259–265. Abstract retrieved July 3, 2005, from EBSCOhost database.

Madina Lizarraide, E. (2001). A study of a case of homecare in accordance with Roy's Adaptation Model [Spanish]. *Metas de*

Enfermeria, 4(33), 18–25. Abstract retrieved July 3, 2005, from EBSCOhost database.

Martinez Riera, J. R., Cibanal Juan, L., & Pérez Mora, M. J. (2009). Teaching integration into the service-learning process [Spanish]. *Metas de Enfermería, 12*(6), 50–55.

Mayne, I. P., & Bagaoisan, C. (2009). Social support during anesthesia induction in an adult surgical population. *AORN Journal, 89,* 307–310, 313–315.

McDonald, F. J., & Harms, M. (1966). Theoretical model for an experimental curriculum. *Nursing Outlook, 14*(8), 48–51

Modrcin-McCarthy, M. A., McCue, S., & Walker, J. (1997). Preterm infants and STRESS: A tool for the neonatal nurse. *Journal of Perinatal and Neonatal Nursing, 10*(4), 62–71.

Modrcin-Talbott, M. A., Harrison, L. L., Groer, M. W., & Younger, M. S. (2003). The biobehavioral effects of gentle human touch on preterm infants. *Nursing Science Quarterly, 15,* 60–67.

Modrcin-Talbott, M. A., Pullen, L., Ehrenberger, H., Zandstra, K., & Muenchen, B. (1998). Self-esteem in adolescents treated in an outpatient mental health setting. *Issues in Comprehensive Pediatric Nursing, 21,* 159–171.

Modrcin-Talbott, M. A., Pullen, L., Zandstra, K., Ehrenberger, H., & Muenchen, B. (1998). A study of self-esteem among well adolescents: Seeking a new direction. *Issues in Comprehensive Pediatric Nursing, 21,* 229–241.

Monge, R. A., & Avelar, M. C. Q. (2009). Nursing care of patients with intestinal stoma: Nurse's perceptions. *OnlineBrazilian Journal of Nursing, 8*(1), 1 p.

Moreno, M. E., Durán, M. M., & Hernandez, Á. (2009). Nursing care for adaptation. *Nursing Science Quarterly, 22,* 67–73.

Morgan, M. G. (1997). The Roy Adaptation Theory and multicultural nursing. *Journal of Multicultural Nursing and Health, 3*(3), 10–14

Morgan, P. D. (2006). Spiritual well-being, religious coping, and the quality of life of African American breast cancer treatment: A pilot study. *ABNF Journal, 17*(2), 73–77.

Nayback, A. M. (2009). PTSD in the combat veteran: Using Roy's Adaptation Model to examine the combat veteran as a human adaptive system. *Issues in Mental Health Nursing, 30,* 304–310.

Newman, D. M. L. (1997). Responses to caregiving: A reconceptualization using the Roy Adaptation Model. *Holistic Nursing Practice, 12*(1), 80–88.

Newman, D. M. L. (2005). Functional status, personal health, and self-esteem of caregivers of children in a body cast: A pilot study. *Orthopaedic Nursing, 24,* 416–425.

Nicholson, N. R., Jr. (2009). Social isolation in older adults: An evolutionary concept analysis. *Journal of Advanced Nursing, 65,* 1342–1352.

Niska, K. J. (1999). Family nursing interventions: Mexican American early family formation . . . third part of a three-part study. *Nursing Science Quarterly, 12,* 335–340.

Niska, K. J. (2001). Mexican American family survival, continuity, and growth: The parental perspective. *Nursing Science Quarterly, 14,* 322–329.

Niska, K. J., Lia-Hoagberg, B., & Snyder, M. (1997). Parental concerns of Mexican American first-time mothers and fathers. *Public Health Nursing, 14,* 111–117.

Niska, K. J., Snyder, M., & Lia-Hoagberg, B. (1999). The meaning of family health among Mexican American first-time mothers and fathers. *Journal of Family Nursing, 5,* 218–233.

Nuamah, I. F., Cooley, M. E., Fawcett, J., & McCorkle, R. (1999). Testing a theory for health-related quality of life in cancer patients: A structural equation approach. *Research in Nursing and Health, 22,* 231–242.

Nyqvist, K. H., & Karlsson, K. H. (1997). A philosophy of care for a neonatal intensive care unit: Operationalization of a nursing model. *Scandinavian Journal of Caring Sciences, 11*(2), 91–96.

O'Mallon, M. (2009). Vulnerable populations: Exploring a family perspective of grief. *Journal of Hospice and Palliative Nursing, 11*(2), 91–100.

Orsi, A. J., Grandy, C., Tax, A., & McCorkle, R. (1997). Nutritional adaptation of women living with HIV: A pilot study. *Holistic Nursing Practice, 12*(1), 71–79.

Ozkan, S., & Ogce, F. (2009). Psychometric analysis of the Inventory of Functional Status—Cancer (IFS-CA) in Turkish women. *Journal of Transcultural Nursing, 20*(2), 187–193.

Pagliuca, L. M. F., de Araújo, T. L., & de Araújo Aragão, A. E. (2006). The limp amputee person and the access to health services: Nursing care based on Roy [Portuguese]. *Revista Enfermagem, 14*(1), 100–106. Abstract retrieved July 3, 2005, from EBSCOhost database.

Paul, R., & Robichaud-Ekstrand, S. (2002). Expected and received assistance from the informal social support network by older persons undergoing heart surgery [French]. *Recherche en Soins Infirmiers, Dec*(71), 38–55. Abstract retrieved July 3, 2005, from EBSCOhost database.

Pejic, A. R. (2005). Verbal abuse: A problem for pediatric nurses. *Pediatric Nursing, 31,* 271–281. Abstract retrieved July 3, 2005, from EBSCOhost database.

Phuphaibul, R., & Muensa, W. (1999). International pediatric nursing: Negative and positive adaptive behaviors of Thai school-aged children who have a sibling with cancer. *Journal of Pediatric Nursing: Nursing Care of Children and Families, 14,* 342–348.

Pollock, S. E. (1993). Adaptation to chronic illness: A program of research for testing nursing theory. *Nursing Science Quarterly, 6,* 86–92.

Pollock, S. E., & Duffy, M. E. (1990). The health-related hardiness scale: Development and psychometric evaluation. *Nursing Research, 39,* 218–222.

Pollock, S. E., Frederickson, K., Carson, M. A., Massey, V. H., & Roy, C. (1994). Contributions to nursing science: Synthesis of findings from adaptation model research. *Scholarly Inquiry for Nursing Practice, 8,* 361–374.

Raeside, L. (1997). Clinical. Perceptions of environmental stressors in the neonatal unit. *British Journal of Nursing, 6,* 914–916.

Raeside, L. (2000). Caring for dying babies: Perceptions of neonatal nurses. *Journal of Neonatal Nursing, 6*(3), 93–99.

Raleigh, E. D. H. (2006). Family caregiver perception of hospice support. *Journal of Hospice and Palliative Nursing, 8*(1), 25–33.

Rocha, D. L. B., & Zagonel, I. P. S. (2009). Model of maternal transitional care in mothers of a child with congenital heart disease [Portuguese]. *Acta Paulista de Enfermagem, 22,* 243–249. Abstract in English retrieved November 30, 2009, from CINAHL Plus with Full Text database.

Rodrigues, D. P., Pagliuca, L. M. F., & da Silva, R. M. (2004). Roy's Model in obstetric nursing: Analysis from Meleis' point of view [Portuguese]. *Revista Gaucha de Enfermagem, 25*(2), 165–175. Abstract retrieved July 3, 2005, from EBSCOhost database.

Roy, C. (1970). Adaptation: A conceptual framework for nursing. *Nursing Outlook, 18,* 43–45.

Roy, C. (1976). *Introduction to nursing: An adaptation model.* Upper Saddle River, NJ: Prentice Hall. [out of print]

Roy, C. (1984). *Introduction to nursing: An adaptation model* (2nd ed.). Upper Saddle River, NJ: Prentice Hall. [out of print]

Roy, C. (1988). An explication of the philosophical assumptions of the Roy Adaptation Model. *Nursing Science Quarterly, 1,* 26–24.

Roy, C. (1997a). Future of the Roy model: Challenge to redefine adaptation. *Nursing Science Quarterly, 10,* 42–48.

Roy, C. (1997b). Knowledge as universal cosmic imperative. *Proceedings of Nursing Knowledge Impact Conference 1996* (pp. 95–118). Chestnut Hill, MA: BC Press.

Roy, C. (2000). The Roy Adaptation Model in the context of nursing models with examples of application and difficulties [Spanish]. *Cultura de los Cuidados, 4*(7/8), 139–159. Abstract retrieved July 3, 2005, from EBSCOhost database.

Roy, C., & Andrews, H. A. (1991). *The Roy Adaptation Model: The definitive statement.* Norwalk, CT: Appleton & Lange.

Roy, C., & Andrews, H. A. (1999). *The Roy Adaptation Model* (2nd ed.). Stamford, CT: Appleton & Lange.

Roy, C., & Anway, J. (1989). Roy's Adaptation Model: Theories and propositions for administration. In B. Henry, C. Arndt, M. DeVincenti, & A. Marriner-Tomey (Eds.), *Dimensions and issues of nursing administration* (pp. 75–88). St. Louis: Mosby.

Roy, C., & Chayaput, P. (2004). Coping and Adaptation Processing Scale—English and Thai versions. *RAA Review Newsletter, 6*(2), 4, 6.

Roy, C., & Jones, D. A. (2007). *Nursing knowledge development and clinical practice.* New York: Springer.

Roy, C., Pollock S., Massey, V., Lauchner, K., Whetsel, V., Frederickson, K., et al. (1999). *Roy Adaptation Model-based research: Twenty-five years of contributions to nursing science.* Indianapolis: Sigma Theta Tau International.

Roy, C., & Roberts, S. (1981). *Theory construction in nursing: An adaptation model.* Upper Saddle River, NJ: Prentice Hall.

Roy, C., Whetsell, M. V., & Frederickson, K. (2009). The Roy Adaptation Model and research. *Nursing Science Quarterly, 21,* 209–211.

Roy, C., & Zahn, L. (2006). Sister Callista Roy's Adaptation Model and its applications. In M. E. Parker (Ed.), *Nursing theories and nursing practice* (2nd ed., pp. 268–280). Philadelphia: F. A. Davis.

Saburi, G. L., Mapanga, K. G., & Mapanga, M. B. (2006). Perceived family reactions and quality of life of adults with epilepsy. *Journal of Neuroscience*

Nursing, 38(3), 158–165. Abstract retrieved July 3, 2005, from EBSCOhost database.

Salazar Gonzalez, B. C., & Jirovec, M. M. (2001). Elderly Mexican women's perceptions of exercise and conflicting role responsibilities. *International Journal of Nursing Studies, 38*(1), 45–49. Abstract retrieved July 3, 2005, from EBSCOhost database.

Salvodi, N. A., Neves, E. P., dos Santos, I., & Mauro, M. Y. C. (2003). Searching for the well being and being healthy as a worker [Portuguese]. *Escola Anna Nery Revista de Enfermagem, 7*, 413–423. Abstract retrieved July 3, 2005, from EBSCOhost database.

Samarel, N., Fawcett, J., Krippendorf, K., Piacentino, J. C., Eliasof, B., Hughes, P., et al. (1998). Women's perceptions of group support and adaptation to breast cancer. *Journal of Advanced Nursing, 28*, 1259–1268.

Samarel, N., Fawcett, J., & Tulman, L. (1997). Effect of support groups with coaching on adaptation to early stage breast cancer. *Research in Nursing and Health, 20*(1), 15–26.

Samarel, N., Fawcett, J., Tulman, L., Rothman, H., Spector, L., Spillane, P. A., et al. (1999). Patient education: A resource kit for women with breast cancer: Development and evaluation. *Oncology Nursing Forum, 26*, 611–618.

Samarel, N., Tulman, L., & Fawcett, J. (2002). Effects of two types of social support and education on adaptation to early-stage breast cancer. *Research in Nursing and Health, 25*, 459–470.

Santana, R. F., Almeida, K. S., & Savoldi, N. A. M. (2009). Indicators of the applicability of nursing instructions in the daily lives of Alzheimer patient caregivers [Portuguese]. *Revista de Escola de Enfermagem da USP, 43*, 459–464. Abstract in English retrieved November 30, 2009, from CINAHL Plus with Full Text database.

Scollan-Koliopoulos, M. (2004). Theory-guided intervention for preventing diabetes-related amputations in African Americans. *Journal of Vascular Nursing, 22*(4), 126–133.

Sengupta, M. (2007). An evaluative study to assess the effectiveness of health education on prevention and management of constipation among geriatric cardiac clients. *Asian Journal of Cardiovascular Nursing, 15*(1), 19–24. Abstract retrieved July 3, 2005, from EBSCOhost database.

Shih, H. (2004). Nursing experience in helping a primipara with intrauterine fetal death adapt to labor induction in hospital [Chinese]. *Journal of Nursing, 51*(5), 101–107. Abstract retrieved July 3, 2005, from EBSCOhost database.

Shin, H., Park, Y-J., & Kim, M. J. (2006). Predictors of maternal sensitivity during the early postpartum period. *Journal of Advanced Nursing, 55*, 425–434.

Shyu, Y-I. L., Liang, J., Lu, J. R., & Wu, C-C. (2004). Environmental barriers and mobility in Taiwan: Is the Roy Adaptation Model applicable? *Nursing Science Quarterly, 17*, 165–170.

Sirapo-ngam, Y., Putwatana, P., Kitrungroj, L., & Piratchavet, V. (2002). Factors influencing role adaptation of patients with cervical cancer receiving radiation therapy. *Thai Journal of Nursing Research, 6*(4), 163–176. Abstract retrieved July 3, 2005, from EBSCOhost database.

Sung, R., Jong, S., & Lu, P. (2006). Nursing experience with an [*sic*] lymphangioleiomyomatosis patient with chylothorax [Chinese]. *Journal of Nursing, 53*(4), 96–105. Abstract in English retrieved July 3, 2005, from EBSCOhost database.

Swimme, S. A., & Berry, T. (1992). *The universe story*. San Francisco: Harper.

Taylor H. J. (1997). Self-esteem, coping, and attitude toward menopause among older rural Southern women. *Dissertation Abstracts International, 58*(05), 2359B. Abstract retrieved July 5, 2007, from Dissertation Abstracts Online.

Thelot, W., & Guimond-Papai, P. (2000). Physical restraints and older adults [French]. *Canadian Nurse, 96*(2), 36–40.

Tsai, P-F. (2003). A middle-range theory of caregiver stress, *Nursing Science Quarterly, 16*, 137–145.

Tsai, P-F., Tak, S., Moore, C., & Palencia, I. Testing a theory of chronic pain. *Journal of Advanced Nursing, 43*, 158–169.

Van Riper, M. (2007). Families of children with Down syndrome: Responding to "A change in plans" with resilience. *Journal of Pediatric Nursing, 22*, 116–128.

Vellone, E., Sinapi, N., Piria, P., Bernardi, F. M., Dario, L., & Brunetti, A. (2004). Anxiety and depression of cancer patient hospitalized and at home [Italian]. *Professioni Infermieristiche, 57*(2), 93–101. Abstract retrieved July 3, 2005, from EBSCOhost database.

von Bertalanffy, L. (1968). *General system theory*. New York: Braziller.

Wang, Y., & Kuo, H. (2006). The nursing experience in helping an unmarried adolescence [*sic*] girl to care for her premature infant [Chinese]. *Journal of Nursing, 53*(5), 76–83. Abstract retrieved July 3, 2005, from EBSCOhost database.

Weinert, C., Cudney, S., & Spring, A. (2008). Evolution of a conceptual model for adaptation to chronic illness. *Journal of Nursing Scholarship, 40,* 364–372.

Weiss, M., Fawcett, J., & Aber, C. (2009). Adaptation, postpartum concerns, and learning needs in the first two weeks after caesarean birth. *Journal of Clinical Nursing, 18,* 2938-2948.

Whittemore, R., & Roy, C. (2002). Adapting to diabetes mellitus: A theory synthesis. *Nursing Science Quarterly, 15,* 311–317.

Woods, S. J. (2001). Adaptation as a mediator of intimate abuse and traumatic stress in battered women. *Nursing Science Quarterly, 14,* 215–21.

Yoder, L. H. (2005). Using the Roy Adaptation Model: A program of research in a military nursing research service. *Nursing Science Quarterly, 18,* 321–323.

Zhan, L. (2000). Cognitive adaptation and self-consistency in hearing-impaired older persons: Testing Roy's Adaptation Model. *Nursing Science Quarterly, 13,* 158–165.

Selected Bibliography of Dissertations Using Ram

Arcamone, A. A. (2005). The effect of prenatal education on adaptation to motherhood after vaginal childbirth in primiparous women as assessed by Roy's four adaptive modes. *Dissertation Abstracts International, 66*(09), 4722B. Abstract retrieved July 2, 2007, from Dissertation Abstracts Online.

Armentrout, D. C. (2005). Holding a place: A grounded theory of parents bringing their infant forward in their daily lives following the removal of life support and subsequent infant death. *Dissertation Abstracts International, 66*(03), 1387B. Abstract retrieved July 5, 2007, from Dissertation Abstracts Online.

Beck-Little, R. (2000). Sleep enhancement interventions and the sleep of institutionalized older adults. *Dissertation Abstracts International, 61*(07), 3503B. Abstract retrieved July 2, 2007, from Dissertation Abstracts Online.

Black, K. D. (2004). Physiologic responses, sense of well-being, self-efficacy for self-monitoring role, perceived availability of social support, and perceived stress in women with pregnancy-induced hypertension. *Dissertation Abstracts International, 65*(04), 1773B. Abstract retrieved July 2, 2007, from Dissertation Abstracts Online.

Bufe, G. M. (1996). A study of opinions of children about mental illness and associated predictor variables. *Dissertation Abstracts International, 58*(01), 133B. Abstract retrieved July 5, 2007, from Dissertation Abstracts Online.

Burns, D. P. (1997). Coping with hemodialysis: A mid-range theory deduced from the Roy Adaptation Model. *Dissertation Abstracts International, 58*(03), 1206B. Abstract retrieved July 2, 2007, from Dissertation Abstracts Online.

Cacchione, P. Z. (1998). Assessment of acute confusion in elderly persons who reside in long term care facilities. *Dissertation Abstracts International, 59*(01), 156B. Abstract retrieved July 2, 2007, from Dissertation Abstracts Online.

Carson, M. A. (1991). The effect of discrete muscle activity on stress response. *Dissertation Abstracts International, 52*(11), 5757B. Abstract retrieved July 5, 2007, from Dissertation Abstracts Online.

Chayaput, P. (2004). Development and psychometric evaluation of the Thai version of the Coping and Adaptation Processing Scale. *Dissertation Abstracts International, 65*(06), 2864B. Abstract retrieved July 2, 2007, from Dissertation Abstracts Online.

Chen, Y. (2005). The influence of physiological factors, psychological factors, and informal social support on hospital readmission in discharged patients with chronic obstructive pulmonary disease (COPD) in Taiwan. *Dissertation Abstracts International, 66*(04), 1976B. Abstract retrieved July 2, 2007, from Dissertation Abstracts Online.

Cheng, S. (2002). A multi-method study of Taiwanese children's pain experiences. *Dissertation Abstracts International, 63*(03), 1265B. Abstract retrieved July 2, 2007, from Dissertation Abstracts Online.

Chiou, C-P. (1997). Correlates of functional status of hemodialysis patients in Taiwan. *Dissertation Abstracts International, 58*(11), 5887B. Abstract retrieved July 2, 2007, from Dissertation Abstracts Online.

Ciambelli, M. M. (1996). Adaptation in marital partners with fertility problems: Testing a midrange theory derived from Roy's Adaptation Model. *Dissertation Abstracts International, 57*(12), 7448B. Abstract retrieved July 5, 2007, from Dissertation Abstracts Online.

Collins, J. M. (1992). Functional health, social support, and morale of older women living alone in Appalachia. *Dissertation Abstracts International, 53*(04), 1781B. Abstract retrieved July 5, 2007, from Dissertation Abstracts Online.

Corbett, R. W. (1995). The relationship among trace elements, pica, social support and infant birthweight. *Dissertation Abstracts International, 56*(06), 3125B. Abstract retrieved July 5, 2007, from Dissertation Abstracts Online.

Domico, V. D. (1997). The impact of social support and meaning and purpose in life on quality of life of spousal caregivers of persons with dementia. *Dissertation Abstracts International, 58*(12), 6485B. Abstract retrieved July 2, 2007, from Dissertation Abstracts Online.

Dunn, K. S. (2001). Adaptation to chronic pain: Religious and non-religious coping in Judeo-Christian elders. *Dissertation Abstracts International, 62*(12), 5640B. Abstract retrieved July 2, 2007, from Dissertation Abstracts Online.

Ellison, K. J. (1993). Focal and contextual stimuli influencing caregiving in spouses of older adults with diabetes. *Dissertation Abstracts International, 55*(04), 1377B. Abstract retrieved July 5, 2007, from Dissertation Abstracts Online.

Flaugher, M. (2002). The intervention of music on perceptions of chronic pain, depression, and anxiety in ambulatory individuals with cancer. *Dissertation Abstracts International, 63*(10), 4593B. Abstract retrieved July 2, 2007, from Dissertation Abstracts Online.

Frame, K. R. (2002). The effect of a support group on perceptions of scholastic competence, social acceptance and behavioral conduct in preadolescents diagnosed with attention deficit hyperactivity disorder. *Dissertation Abstracts International, 63*(02), 737B. Abstract retrieved July 2, 2007, from Dissertation Abstracts Online.

Giedt, J. F. (1999). The psychoneuroimmunological effects of guided imagery in patients on hemodialysis for end-stage renal disease. *Dissertation Abstracts International, 61*(01), 192B. Abstract retrieved July 2, 2007, from Dissertation Abstracts Online.

Gipson-Jones, T. L. (2005). The relationship between work-family conflict, job satisfaction and psychological well-being among African American nurses. *Dissertation Abstracts International, 66*(05), 2512B. Abstract retrieved July 2, 2007, from Dissertation Abstracts Online.

Haines, S. A. (2000). Relative bioavailability of estradiol and norethindrone after a single application of an estradiol progestin matrix transdermal system. *Dissertation Abstracts International, 61*(10), 5234B. Abstract retrieved July 2, 2007, from Dissertation Abstracts Online.

Hamid, A. Y. S. (1993). Child-family characteristics and coping patterns of Indonesian families with a mentally retarded child. *Dissertation Abstracts International, 54*(03), 1332B. Abstract retrieved July 5, 2007, from Dissertation Abstracts Online.

Harner, H. M. (2001). Obstetrical outcomes of teenagers with adult and peer age partners. *Dissertation Abstracts International, 62*(05), 2256B. Abstract retrieved July 2, 2007, from Dissertation Abstracts Online.

Hay, C. G. (2005). Predictors of quality of life of elderly end-state renal disease patients: An application of Roy's model. *Dissertation Abstracts International, 66*(03), 1395B. Abstract retrieved July 2, 2007, from Dissertation Abstracts Online.

Henderson, P. D. (2002). African-American women coping with breast cancer. *Dissertation Abstracts International, 63*(12), 5764B. Abstract retrieved July 2, 2007, from Dissertation Abstracts Online.

Higgins, K.M. (1996). The entrepreneurial nurse-midwife: A profile of successful business practice. *Dissertation Abstracts International, 58*(03), 1211B. Abstract retrieved July 5, 2007, from Dissertation Abstracts Online.

Hinkle, J. L. (1999). A descriptive study of variables explaining functional recovery following stroke. *Dissertation Abstracts International, 60*(12), 6021B. Abstract retrieved July 2, 2007, from Dissertation Abstracts Online.

Huang, C-M. (2002). Sleep and daytime sleepiness in first-time mothers during early postpartum in Taiwan. *Dissertation Abstracts International, 64*(07), 3189B. Abstract retrieved July 2, 2007, from Dissertation Abstracts Online.

Jarczewski, P. A. H. (1995). Social support, self-esteem, symptom distress, and anxiety of adults with acquired immune deficiency syndrome. *Dissertation Abstracts International, 56*(04), 1936B. Abstract retrieved July 5, 2007, from Dissertation Abstracts Online.

Jenkins, B. E. (2006). Emotional intelligence of faculty members, the learning environment, and empowerment of baccalaureate nursing students. *Dissertation Abstracts International, 67*(07), 3701B. Abstract retrieved July 2, 2007, from Dissertation Abstracts Online.

Jensen, K. A. (1996). Stress and coping of caregivers to individuals with dementia. *Dissertation Abstracts International, 57*(04), 2478B. Abstract retrieved July 5, 2007, from Dissertation Abstracts Online.

Khanobdee, C. (1994). Hope and social support of Thai women experiencing a miscarriage. *Dissertation Abstracts International, 55*(11), 4786B. Abstract retrieved July 5, 2007, from Dissertation Abstracts Online.

Kittiwatanapaisan, W. (2002). Measurement of fatigue in myasthenia gravis patients. *Dissertation Abstracts International, 63*(10), 4595B. Abstract retrieved July 2, 2007, from Dissertation Abstracts Online.

Klein, G. J. M. (2000). The relationships among anxiety, self-concept, the imposter phenomenon, and generic senior baccalaureate nursing students' perceptions of clinical competency. *Dissertation Abstracts International, 61*(10), 5236B. Abstract retrieved July 2, 2007, from Dissertation Abstracts Online.

Kochniuk, L. (2004). We never buy green bananas: The oldest old. A phenomenological study. *Dissertation Abstracts International, 65*(06), 2318A. Abstract retrieved July 2, 2007, from Dissertation Abstracts Online.

Kruszewski, A. Z. (1999). Psychosocial adaptation to termination of pregnancy for fetal anomaly. *Dissertation Abstracts International, 61*(01), 194B. Abstract retrieved July 2, 2007, from Dissertation Abstracts Online.

Lefaiver, C. A. (2006). Quality of life: The dyad of caregivers and lung transplant candidates. *Dissertation Abstracts International, 67*(09), 4978B. Abstract retrieved July 2, 2007, from Dissertation Abstracts Online.

Lin, L. (2003). Juggling between maternal and student role: Multiple role adaptation among women who are re-entering school in Taiwan. *Dissertation Abstracts International, 64*(12), 6014B. Abstract retrieved July 2, 2007, from Dissertation Abstracts Online.

Lu, Y. (2001). Caregiving stress effects on functional capacity and self-care behavior for elderly caregivers of persons with Alzheimer's disease. *Dissertation Abstracts International, 62*(04), 1807B. Abstract retrieved July 2, 2007, from Dissertation Abstracts Online.

Mahoney, E. T. (2000). The relationships among social support, coping, self-concept, and stage of recovery in alcoholic women. *Dissertation Abstracts International, 61*(04), 1872B. Abstract retrieved July 2, 2007, from Dissertation Abstracts Online.

Martin, B. P. (1995). An analysis of common postpartum problems and adaptation strategies used by women during the first two to eight weeks following delivery of a full-term healthy newborn. *Dissertation Abstracts International, 56*(06), 3128B. Abstract retrieved July 5, 2007, from Dissertation Abstracts Online.

McLeod-Fletcher, C. (1996). Appraisal and coping with vaso-occlusive crisis in adolescents with sickle cell disease. *Dissertation Abstracts International, 57*(12), 5308A. Abstract retrieved July 5, 2007, from Dissertation Abstracts Online.

Murphy, K. P. (1993). Relationships between biopsychosocial characteristics and adaptive health patterns in elder women. *Dissertation Abstracts International, 55*(03), 822B. Abstract retrieved July 5, 2007, from Dissertation Abstracts Online.

Newman, A. M. (1991). The effect of the arthritis self-help course on arthritis self-efficacy, perceived social support, purpose and meaning in life, an arthritis impact in people with arthritis. *Dissertation Abstracts International, 52*(06), 2995B. Abstract retrieved July 5, 2007, from Dissertation Abstracts Online.

Patterson, J. E. (1995). Responses of institutionalized older adults to urinary incontinence: Managing the flow. *Dissertation Abstracts International, 56*(05), 2563B. Abstract retrieved July 5, 2007, from Dissertation Abstracts Online.

Phahuwatanakorn, W. (2004). The relationships between social support, maternal employment, postpartum anxiety, and maternal role competencies in Thai primiparous mothers. *Dissertation Abstracts International, 64*(11), 5451B. Abstract retrieved July 2, 2007, from Dissertation Abstracts Online.

Phillips, J. A. (1991). Adaptation and injury status of industrial workers on a rotating shift pattern. *Dissertation Abstracts International, 52*(06), 2995B. Abstract retrieved July 5, 2007, from Dissertation Abstracts Online.

Phillips, K. D. (1994). Testing biobehavioral adaptation in persons living with AIDS using Roy's theory of the person as an adaptive system. *Dissertation Abstracts International, 56*(02), 745B. Abstract retrieved July 5, 2007, from Dissertation Abstracts Online.

Rees, B. S. (1995). Influences of coronary artery disease knowledge, anxiety, social support, and self-efficacy on adaptive health behaviors of patients treated with a percutaneous transluminal coronary angioplasty. *Dissertation Abstracts International, 56*(07), 3696B. Abstract retrieved July 5, 2007, from Dissertation Abstracts Online.

Sabatini, M. (2003). Exercise and adaptation to aging in older women. *Dissertation Abstracts International, 64*(08), 3748B. Abstract retrieved July 2, 2007, from Dissertation Abstracts Online.

Saint-Pierre, C. (2003). Elaboration et verification d'un modele predictif de l'adaptation aux roles associes de mere et de travailleuse a statut precaire [French text]. *Dissertation Abstracts International, 65*(03), 1252B. Abstract retrieved July 2, 2007, from Dissertation Abstracts Online.

Sander, R. A. (2004). Measurement of functional status in the spinal cord injured patient. *Dissertation Abstracts International, 65*(04), 1783B. Abstract retrieved July 2, 2007, from Dissertation Abstracts Online.

Senesac, P. M. (2004). The Roy Adaptation Model: An action research approach to the implementation of a pain management organizational change project. *Dissertation Abstracts International, 65*(06), 2872B. Abstract retrieved July 2, 2007, from Dissertation Abstracts Online.

Shuler, P. J. (1990). Physical and psychosocial adaptation, social isolation, loneliness, and self-concept of individuals with cancer. *Dissertation Abstracts International, 51*(05), 2289B. Abstract retrieved July 5, 2007, from Dissertation Abstracts Online.

Sirapo-Ngam, Y. (1994). Stress, caregiving demands, and coping of spousal caregivers of Parkinson's patients. *Dissertation Abstracts International, 55*(04), 1381B. Abstract retrieved July 5, 2007, from Dissertation Abstracts Online.

Smith, B. J. A. (1989). Caregiver burden and adaptation in middle-aged daughters of dependent, elderly parents: A test of Roy's model. *Dissertation Abstracts International, 51*(05), 2290B. Abstract retrieved July 2, 2007, from Dissertation Abstracts Online.

Stevens, K. A. (2005). Preoxygenation practices prior to tracheal suctioning by nurses caring for individuals with spinal cord injury. *Dissertation Abstracts International, 66*(05), 2518B. Abstract retrieved July 2, 2007, from Dissertation Abstracts Online.

Taival, A. S. (1998). The older person's adaptation and the promotion of adaptation in home nursing care: Action research of intervention through training based on the Roy Adaptation Model. *Dissertation Abstracts International, 60*(01), 113C. Abstract retrieved July 2, 2007, from Dissertation Abstracts Online.

Thomas-Hawkins, C. (1998). Correlates of changes in functional status in chronic in-center hemodialysis patients. *Dissertation Abstracts International, 59*(11), 5792B. Abstract retrieved July 2, 2007, from Dissertation Abstracts Online.

Toughill, E. H. (2001). Quality of life: The impact of age, severity of urinary incontinence and adaptation. *Dissertation Abstracts International, 61*(10), 5240B. Abstract retrieved July 2, 2007, from Dissertation Abstracts Online.

Tsai, P-F. (1998). Development of a middle-range theory of caregiver stress from the Roy Adaptation Model. *Dissertation Abstracts International, 60*(01), 133B. Abstract retrieved July 2, 2007, from Dissertation Abstracts Online.

Velos Weiss, J. C. (1998). Lifestyle and angina in the elderly following elective coronary artery bypass graft surgery. *Dissertation Abstracts International, 59*(04), 1589B. Abstract retrieved July 2, 2007, from Dissertation Abstracts Online.

Wildblood, R. A. (2001). Helping siblings cope when a child has cancer. *Dissertation Abstracts International, 66*(09), 5110B. Abstract retrieved July 2, 2007, from Dissertation Abstracts Online.

Willoughby, D. F. (1995). The influence of psychosocial factors on women's adjustment to diabetes. *Dissertation Abstracts International, 56*(08), 4247B. Abstract retrieved July 5, 2007, from Dissertation Abstracts Online.

Wood, A. F. (1998). An investigation of stimuli related to baccalaureate nursing students' transition toward role mastery. *Dissertation Abstracts International, 59*(08), 4023B. Abstract retrieved July 2, 2007, from Dissertation Abstracts Online.

Woods, S. J. (1997). Predictors of traumatic stress in battered women: A test and explication of the Roy Adaptation Model. *Dissertation Abstracts International, 58*(03), 1220B. Abstract retrieved July 5, 2007, from Dissertation Abstracts Online.

Wunderlich, R. J. (2003). An exploratory study of physiological and psychological variables that predict weaning from mechanical ventilation. *Dissertation Abstracts International, 64*(08), 3750B. Abstract retrieved July 2, 2007, from Dissertation Abstracts Online.

Zbegner, D. K. (2003). An exploratory retrospective study using the Roy Adaptation Model:

The adaptive mode variables of physical energy level, self-esteem, marital satisfaction, and parenthood motivation as predictors of coping behaviors in infertile women. *Dissertation Abstracts International, 64*(08), 3751B. Abstract retrieved July 2, 2007, from Dissertation Abstracts Online.

Zhang, W. (2004). Factors influencing end-of-life decisions regarding the living will and durable power of attorney: An application of Roy's Adaptation Model. *Dissertation Abstracts International, 65*(06), 2874B. Abstract retrieved July 2, 2007, from Dissertation Abstracts Online.

Selected Bibliography of Master's Theses Using RAM

Baden, T. M. (2004). Roy's Adaptation Model and parental grief of adult children who died a traumatic death. *Masters Abstracts International, 42*(02), 566. Abstract retrieved July 2, 2007, from Dissertation Abstracts Online.

Blamer, K. (1999). A comparative study of women's perceptions of vaginal and cesarean births. *Masters Abstracts International, 37*(04), 1175. Abstract retrieved July 2, 2007, from Dissertation Abstracts Online.

Clark, E. D. (2001). The lived experience of mothers coping with their child's cancer. *Masters Abstracts International, 39*(05), 1379. Abstract retrieved July 2, 2007, from Dissertation Abstracts Online.

Gaines, G. (1997). A qualitative study of the levels of adaptation of African-American males who are recovering from crack addiction. *Masters Abstracts International, 35*(06), 1774. Abstract retrieved July 2, 2007, from Dissertation Abstracts Online.

Garris, T. M. (2006). Investigation of self-reported transitional health care needs of the adolescent with congenital heart disease. *Masters Abstracts International, 45*(02), 817. Abstract retrieved July 2, 2007, from Dissertation Abstracts Online.

Gorney, P. A. (1997). Nurses' beliefs and perceptions about children in pain. *Masters Abstracts International, 35*(06), 1774. Abstract retrieved July 2, 2007, from Dissertation Abstracts Online.

Lazenby, L. M. (2001). The experiences of Mexican mothers in a neonatal intensive care nursery. *Masters Abstracts International, 40*(05), 1219. Abstract retrieved July 2, 2007, from Dissertation Abstracts Online.

Lonobile, C. J. (1999). An exploratory study of victimization of emergency department nurses: Types encountered and coping mechanisms. *Masters Abstracts International, 37*(04), 1180. Abstract retrieved July 2, 2007, from Dissertation Abstracts Online.

Martin, J. L. (2003). Spousal grief in older adults: The lived experience of surviving spouses during the second year of bereavement. *Masters Abstracts International, 42*(04), 1242. Abstract retrieved July 2, 2007, from Dissertation Abstracts Online.

Moore, L. A. (2005). The lived experience of being a mother of a child with severe cerebral palsy. *Masters Abstracts International, 43*(06), 2197. Abstract retrieved July 2, 2007, from Dissertation Abstracts Online.

Moulton, S. A. (2005). Black Canadians' perceptions of hypertension control. *Masters Abstracts International, 44*(05), 2277. Abstract retrieved July 2, 2007, from Dissertation Abstracts Online.

Short, J. K. (2004). The lived experience of mothers coping with the birth of a stillborn infant. *Masters Abstracts International, 42*(06), 2167. Abstract retrieved July 2, 2007, from Dissertation Abstracts Online.

Annotated Bibliography of Selected Articles

Calvillo, E. R., & Flaskerud, J. H. (1993). The adequacy and scope of Roy's Adaptation Model to guide cross-cultural pain research. *Nursing Science Quarterly, 6*, 118–129.
This research investigated the operational, empirical, and pragmatic adequacy and scope of the RAM, in conjunction with the gate control theory of pain, in studying pain in 60 Mexican-American and Anglo-American women undergoing elective cholecystectomy. Operational adequacy was demonstrated through the reliability and validity of the empirical indicators used

(Spielberger State-Trait Anxiety Inventory, Acculturation Scale, Pain Rating Index, Self-Esteem Inventory, Sense of Coherence Scale, Index of Activities of Daily Living, and Support Scale). Empirical adequacy was evaluated by comparing actual findings to hypothesized results. Only partial support was found. Pragmatic adequacy was supported through the development of several innovative practice strategies. Scope was determined to be adequate.

Ducharme, F., Ricard, N., Duquette, A., Levesque, L., & Lachance, L. (1998). Empirical testing of a longitudinal model derived from the Roy Adaptation Model. *Nursing Science Quarterly, 11*, 149–159.

This article reports the results of four studies to test a theoretical longitudinal model of the psychosocial determinants of adaptation in different target groups vulnerable to mental health problems. In cross-sectional testing the model was found to be relatively stable over time. Longitudinal data indicated little consistency in relationship patterns across the studies. Important relationships were identified as those between perceived stress, passive/avoidance coping strategies, and psychological distress. Nursing interventions need to be aimed at perceived stress, conflicts in the exchange of support, and passive and avoidance coping strategies.

Fredrickson, K., Jackson, B. S., Strauman, T., & Strauman, J. (1991). Testing hypotheses derived from the Roy Adaptation Model. *Nursing Science Quarterly, 4*, 168–174.

This study hypothesized that the translation of physiological stimuli through the cognator mechanism of perception alters biopsychosocial responses. Subjects were 45 patients who were entering an aggressive chemotherapy program. Results supported that perception of symptoms correlates positively with both psychosocial adaptation and actual physiological status. Also, perception of symptoms and psychosocial adaptation correlated with six month survival but not with actual physiological status.

Lee, A. A., & Ellenbecker, C. H. (1998). The perceived life stressors among elderly Chinese immigrants: Are they different from those of other elderly Americans? *Clinical Excellence for Nurse Practitioners, 2*(2), 96–101.

This qualitative study investigated the type and amount of stressors experienced by 30 elderly people from two Chinese churches in a northeastern metropolitan city and compared the findings with those of a similar study conducted on other elderly Americans. Findings indicated elderly Chinese immigrants in the United States report amounts and sources of stress that differ from those of other elderly Americans. While additional studies are needed to identify coping strategies, this study alerts the practicing nurse to the importance of carefully categorizing stimuli from the perspective of the person who is experiencing them.

Levesque, L., Ricard, N., Ducharme, F., Duquette, A., & Bonin, J. (1998). Empirical verification of a theoretical model derived from the Roy Adaptation Model: Findings from five studies. *Nursing Science Quarterly, 11*, 31–39.

This article discusses a theoretical model and the findings of five studies conducted to verify that model. Subjects in the studies included informal caregivers of demented relatives and of psychiatrically ill relatives at home and professional caregivers of elderly institutionalized patients and of aged spouses in the community. Support was found for linking the focal stimulus of perceived stress with the contextual stimulus or conflicts in the exchange of social support and passive/avoidance coping strategies with psychological distress. Psychological distress was considered an indicator of adaptation in the self-concept mode.

Nuamah, I. F., Cooley, M. E., Fawcett, J., & McCorkle, R. (1999). Testing a theory for health-related quality of life in cancer patients: A structural equation approach. *Research in Nursing and Health, 22*, 231–242.

The study was a secondary analysis of data collected from 375 newly diagnosed cancer patients, aged 60 to 92. The analyses did not support that all four response modes are interrelated but did find a strong association between the severity of illness and adjuvant cancer treatment and biopsychosocial responses, including a reduction in health-related quality of life. Thus, the RAM proposition that environmental stimuli influence the biopsychosocial responses was supported. Findings suggest that nursing should seek to identify the needs of those receiving adjuvant cancer treatments and to help manage the severity of the illness.

Sabatine, M. (2003). Exercise and adaptation to aging in older women. *Dissertation Abstracts*

International, 64(08), 3748B. Abstract retrieved July 2, 2007, from Dissertation Abstracts Online. This study tested an assumption from the RAM: that exercise has a positive relationship to each of the adaptive modes (physiological: health status; role function: functional status; self-concept: self-esteem; interdependence: interpersonal relationship) and that the four modes are interrelated. Findings included positive relationships between exercise and health status, functional status and self-esteem, as well as support for the interrelatedness of the four modes. The relationship between exercise and interpersonal relationships was not statistically significant. The importance of this study includes its support for exercise as a positive adaptation factor in aging.

Smith, B. J. A. (1989). Caregiver burden and adaptation in middle-aged daughters of dependent, elderly parents: A test of Roy's model. *Dissertation Abstracts International*, 51(05), 2290B. Abstract retrieved July 2, 2007, from Dissertation Abstracts Online.

This longitudinal study sought to detect changes in caregiver burden and in the four modes of adaptation in a convenience sample of 30 40- to 60-year-old daughters who were caring for a dependent elderly parent. Caregiving had begun at some time before the beginning of the study. Caregiver burden scores were consistently at a high moderate perception throughout the six weeks of the study. Therefore, changes in physical symptoms (physiological mode), self-esteem, role function, and interdependence could not be assessed. It was noted that measures of physiological dysfunction were higher than established norms throughout the study. Self-concept and interdependence scores also remained high for the duration of study, and role scores were positive. It was recommended that the study be repeated with subjects entering the study at the beginning of the caregiving process.

Velos Weiss, J. C. (1998). Lifestyle and angina in the elderly following elective coronary artery bypass graft surgery. *Dissertation Abstracts International*, 59(04), 1589B. Abstract retrieved July 2, 2007, from Dissertation Abstracts Online. This study identified lifestyle as the focal stimulus and angina as the physiological mode response. Subjects were 166 males and females, 65 years of age or older, who were one year post-coronary-artery-bypass surgery. Correlational analyses supported weak relationships between the contextual stimuli of number of veins used for the surgery and the number of sequential vein grafts with the response of angina. Significant lifestyle predictors of angina were smoking tobacco products and being less than fully active. The study supported the RAM relationship between selected stimuli and physiological mode response.

Weiss, M. E., Hastings, W. J., Holly, D. C., & Craig, D. I. (1994). Using Roy's Adaptation Model in practice: Nurses' perspectives. *Nursing Science Quarterly*, 7, 80–86.

This qualitative study investigated the use of the RAM in hospital-based nursing practice. The RAM was found to be useful in focusing, organizing, and directing nurses' thoughts and actions in relation to patient care. Nurses who used the RAM perceived an improved quality of both nursing process and patient outcomes. However, the level of integration of the RAM into practice varied among the nurses in the study. Those with prior education in the RAM who also participated in professional advancement activities had higher levels of integration, while those who did not have such education and who were resistant to change were less likely to integrate the model into practice.

CHAPTER 14

The Neuman Systems Model
Betty Neuman

Julia B. George

Betty Neuman was born in 1924 on a 100-acre farm in Ohio. The middle of three children and the only daughter, she was 11 when her father died after six years of intermittent hospitalizations for treatment of chronic kidney disease. His praise of his nurses influenced Neuman's view of nursing and her commitment to becoming an excellent bedside nurse. Her mother's work as a rural midwife was also a significant influence.

After graduation from high school, Neuman could not afford nursing education. She worked as an aircraft instrument repair technician, as a draftsperson for an aircraft contracting company, and as a short-order cook in Dayton, Ohio, while saving for her education and helping support her mother and younger brother. The creation of the Cadet Nurse Corps Program expedited her entrance into a hospital school of nursing.

In 1947 Neuman graduated from the diploma program of Peoples Hospital (now Akron General Medical Center), Akron, Ohio. She received a B.S. in public health nursing (1957) and an M.S. as a public health–mental health nurse consultant (1966) from the University of California, Los Angeles. She has received honorary doctorates from Grand Valley State University, Allendale, Michigan, and Neumann College, Aston, Pennsylvania. In 1993 she became a fellow in the American Academy of Nursing.

She has practiced bedside nursing as a staff, head, and private-duty nurse in a wide variety of hospital settings. Her work in community settings has included school and industrial nursing, office nurse in her husband Kree's private practice, and counseling and crisis intervention in community mental health settings. In 1967, six months after completion of her M.S. degree, she became the faculty chair of the program from which she graduated and began her contributions as teacher, author, lecturer, and consultant in nursing and interdisciplinary health care.

In 1973 she and her family returned to Ohio. Since then she has worked as a state mental health consultant, provided continuing education programs, and continued the development of her model. She was one of the first nurses licensed in California as a marriage and family counselor (now marriage and family Therapist) and clinical fellow of the American Association of Marriage and Family Therapists and has maintained a limited private counseling practice. She is also a licensed real estate agent and obtained a private pilot's license in California. In addition to her professional activities, she has exercised her interest in personal property management and other investments as well as health maintenance and promotion activities.

The Neuman Systems Model (NSM) was originally developed in 1970 in response to the request of graduate students at the University of California, Los Angeles, for an introductory course that would provide an overview of the physiological, psychological, sociocultural, and developmental aspects of human beings (Neuman, 2002a). The model was developed as a teaching aid to provide structure for the integration of this material in a wholistic manner. After a two-year evaluation, the model was first published in *Nursing Research* (Neuman & Young, 1972). Since then it has become one of the most widely used nursing models in the world.

Neuman (1982b, 1989b, 1995, Neuman & Fawcett, 2002) has published four editions of *The Neuman Systems Model.* She also had chapters in all editions of *Conceptual Models for Nursing Practice* and in Parker's *Nursing Theories in Practice* (Neuman, 1974, 1980, 1989a, 1990b). Neuman continues work on the model but also incorporated the Neuman Systems Model Trustees Group in 1988. The trustees' agreement indicates that the trustees group was established for the perpetuation, preservation, and protection of the integrity of the model. Any future permanent changes in the original NSM diagram (see Figure 14-1) must have unanimous approval from the trustees (Neuman & Fawcett, 2002). The trustees provide consultation on the NSM; have established an NSM archive at Neumann College in Aston, Pennsylvania; maintain a NSM bibliography; and offer a biennial NSM symposium (Gigliotti, 2003). The NSM Trustees Group website can be located at http://www.neumansystemsmodel.org (recently changed from http://www.neumansystemsmodel.com).

DEVELOPMENT OF THE NEUMAN SYSTEMS MODEL

Neuman (2002a) says that her personal philosophy of *helping each other live* was supportive in developing the wholistic systems perspective of the NSM. She drew upon her clinical experiences from a variety of health care and community settings and the theoretical perspectives of stress and systems. Caplan's (1964) levels of prevention were also incorporated into the model. Others whose works were drawn upon include Beckstrand (1980), de Chardin (1955), Cornu (1957), Edelson (1970), Emery (1969), Laszlo (1972), Lazarus (1981), Oakes (1978), Putt (1972), Selye (1950), and von Bertalanffy (1968).

The original title of the model, "A Model for Teaching Total Person Approach to Patient Problems," reflected its origin as a teaching aid (Neuman & Young, 1972). As the model began to be recognized and utilized in clinical practice and research, as well as education, the title changed to "The Betty Neuman Health Care Systems Model: A Total Person Approach to Patient Problems" (Neuman, 1974, 1980). In 1982, while the book was titled *The Neuman Systems Model*, her chapter about the model was titled "The Neuman Health-Care Systems Model: A Total Approach to Client Care" (Neuman, 1982a, 1982b). In 1985, she used "The Neuman Systems Model" and has consistently used this title since then (Neuman, 1985).

In the NSM, nursing is considered a system because nursing practice contains elements in interaction with one another, and there is increasing diversity of nursing roles and functions (Neuman, 2002c). Advantages of an open-system perspective in nursing include the use of systems as a unifying force across various scientific fields, as well as

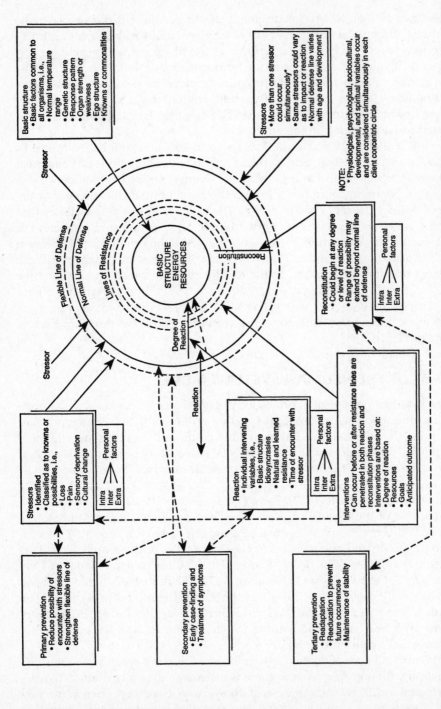

FIGURE 14-1 The Neuman Systems Model. *(From Neuman, B. & Fawcett, J. (2002). The Neuman Systems Model (4th ed., p. 13). Upper Saddle River, NJ: Prentice Hall. Used with permission.)*

the increasing complexity of nursing, which calls for an organizational system that can respond to change. A systems perspective supports recognition of the complex whole while valuing the importance of the parts. The relationships between the parts and the interactions of the parts or the whole with the environment provide a mechanism for viewing the system–environment exchanges, which support the dynamic and constantly changing nature of the system.

Neuman (2002c) views wholism as both a philosophical and a biological concept. *Wholism* includes relationships that arise from wholeness, dynamic freedom, and creativity as the system responds to stressors from the internal and external environments. Each component must be considered not as alone but as part of the whole and will influence one's perception of the whole.

THE NEUMAN SYSTEMS MODEL

The NSM is based on stress and the reaction/potential reaction to stress, with a philosophical basis in wholeness, wellness, client perception and motivation, energy, and environmental interaction (Neuman, 2002c). The key components are the client/client system composed of the physiological, psychological, sociocultural, developmental, and spiritual variables that interact with the internal and external environments and the three prevention-as-intervention levels (primary, secondary, and tertiary) with purpose of achieving optimal wellness (Neuman & Reed, 2007). The client in the NSM is viewed as an open system in which repeated cycles of input, process, output, and feedback constitute a dynamic organizational pattern. Using the systems perspective, the client may be an individual, a group, a family, a community, or any aggregate. In their development toward growth and survival, open systems continuously become more differentiated and elaborate or complex. As they become more complex, the internal conditions of regulation become more intricate. Exchanges with the environment are reciprocal; both the client and the environment may be affected either positively or negatively by the other. The system may adjust to the environment or adjust the environment to itself.

The ideal is to achieve optimal system stability. Neuman agrees with Heslin (1986) that when a system achieves stability, a revitalization occurs. As an open system, the client system has a propensity to seek or maintain a balance among the various factors, both within and outside the system, that seek to disrupt it (Neuman, 2002c). Neuman labels these forces as stressors and views them as capable of having either positive or negative effects. Reactions to the stressors may be possible (not yet occurring) or actual, with identifiable responses and symptoms.

The NSM diagram (see Figure 14-1) presents the major aspects of the model: the *basic structure and energy resources; physiological, psychological, sociocultural, developmental, and spiritual variables; lines of resistance; normal line of defense; flexible line of defense; stressors; reaction; primary, secondary, and tertiary prevention; intra-, inter-, and extrapersonal factors;* and *reconstitution.* The *environment, health,* and *nursing* are inherent parts of the model, although they are not labeled within the model. The client system is represented in the diagram by a basic structure surrounded by a series of concentric circles and is a living, open system.

Basic Structure and Energy Resources

The basic structure, or central core, is made up of those basic survival factors common to the species (Neuman, 2002c). These factors include the system variables (physiological, psychological, sociocultural, developmental, and spiritual), genetic features, and strengths and weaknesses of the components of the system. If the client system is a human being, the basic structure contains such features as the ability to maintain body temperature within a normal range, genetic characteristics such as hair color and response to stimuli, and the functioning of various body systems and their interrelationships. There are also the baseline characteristics associated with each of the five variables, such as physical strength, cognitive ability, cultural perspectives, developmental stage, and value systems.

Neuman (2002c) identifies system stability as occurring when the energy exchanges with the environment occur without disrupting the characteristics of the system. Since the system is an open system, stability is dynamic. As output becomes feedback and input, the system seeks to regulate itself. A change in one direction is countered by a compensating movement in the opposite direction. When the system is disturbed from its normal, or stable, state, there is a rapid surge in the amount of energy needed to deal with the disorganization that results from the disturbance. In stability, the system is able to cope with stressors to attain, retain, or maintain optimal health and integrity.

Client Variables

Neuman originally identified the recipient of nursing care as individual and patient (Neuman, 1974, 1980; Neuman & Young, 1972). In 1982 she used both client, in the chapter title, and patient, in the discussion (Neuman, 1982a). By 1989, she was using client/client system consistently in recognition of the movement toward collaborative client–caregiver relationships (Neuman, 2002c).

Neuman (2002c) views the individual client wholistically and considers the variables (physiological, psychological, sociocultural, developmental, and spiritual) simultaneously and comprehensively. The *physiological* variable refers to the structure and internal and external functions of the body; the *psychological* variable to mental processes and relationships; the *sociocultural* variable to system functions that relate to social and cultural expectations, activities, and influences; the *developmental* variable to those processes related to development over the life span; and the *spiritual* variable to the influence of spiritual beliefs. The spiritual variable was added in 1989. In the ideal situation, these variables function in harmony and stability in relation to internal and external environmental stressors. Each of the variables should be considered when assessing system reaction to stressors for each of the concentric circles in the model diagram. It is vital to avoid fragmentation if optimum stability of the client system is to be promoted through nursing care.

Neuman (2002c) indicates that the first four variables are commonly understood by nursing. Because the spiritual variable was added to the model more recently, she discusses it in more detail. This variable is viewed as an innate component of the basic structure that may or may not be acknowledged or developed by the client. Neuman views it as permeating all the other variables of the client system and existing on a developmental continuum from complete unawareness of the presence and potential of the variable to a highly developed spiritual understanding that supports optimal wellness. The continuum includes denial of the existence of the spiritual variable.

Spirituality has been incorporated into nursing care since Nightingale's time (Neuman & Reed, 2007). Neuman (2002c) likens the spiritual variable to a seed with enormous energy potential. When the appropriate environmental conditions occur, the seed becomes a living thing and offers sustenance. Life events such as experiencing humility or joy may engender this energy, which becomes recognized "as something whose truths must become known and tested in life situations" (p. 16). When the results of such testing have positive effects on thought patterns, the body is also positively affected. For example, happiness strengthens the immune system, while sadness or despair have the opposite effect. Neuman describes spiritual energy as being used "first by the mind and then by the body" (p. 16).

Lines of Resistance

The lines of resistance protect the basic structure and become activated when the normal line of defense is invaded by environmental stressors. An example of a response involving lines of resistance is the activation of the immune system mechanisms. If the lines of resistance are effective in their response, the system can reconstitute; if the lines of resistance are not effective, the resulting energy depletion may lead to death.

Normal Line of Defense

In terms of system stability, the normal line of defense represents stability over time (Neuman, 2002c). It is considered to be the usual level of stability for the system or the normal wellness state and is used as the baseline for determining deviation from wellness for the client system. For the system, the normal line of defense changes over time as a result of coping with a variety of stressors. The stability represented by the normal line of defense is actually a range of responses to the environment.

Any stressor may invade the normal line of defense when the flexible line of defense offers inadequate protection. When the normal line of defense is invaded or penetrated, the client system reacts. The reaction will be apparent in symptoms of instability or illness and may reduce the system's ability to withstand additional stressors.

Flexible Line of Defense

The flexible line of defense is represented in the model diagram as the outer boundary and initial response, or protection, of the system to stressors. The flexible line of defense serves as a cushion and is described as accordion-like as it expands away from or contracts closer to the normal line of defense (Neuman, 2002c). It protects the normal line of defense and acts as a buffer for the client system's usual stable state. Ideally, the flexible line of defense prevents stressors from invading the system. As the distance between the flexible and normal lines of defense increases, so does the degree of protection available to the system.

The flexible line of defense is dynamic rather than stable and can be altered over a relatively short period by factors such as inadequate nutrition, lack of sleep, or danger. Either single or multiple stressors may invade the flexible line of defense.

Environment

Neuman (2002c) defines environment as all the internal and external factors or influences that surround the client or client system. The influence of the client on the environment and the environment on the client may be positive or negative at any time. Variations in both the client system and the environment can affect the direction of the reaction. For example, individuals who experience sleep deprivation are more susceptible to viruses of the common cold from the environment than those who are well rested.

The *internal* environment exists within the client system and is intrapersonal. All forces and interactive influences that are exclusively within the boundaries of the client system make up this environment.

The external environment exists outside the client system and is inter- and extrapersonal. Those forces and interactive influences that are outside the system boundaries are identified as external.

In 1989, Neuman first identified a third environment, the *created environment*, which is intra-, inter-, and extrapersonal. The created environment is developed unconsciously by the client and is symbolic of system wholeness. It represents the open-system exchange of energy with both the internal and external environments. It is dynamic and depicts the unconscious mobilization of all system variables but particularly the psychological and sociocultural variables. The purpose of this mobilization is the integration, integrity, and stability of the system. Based on Lazarus's (1981) work, its function is seen as a protective coping shield that encompasses both the internal and external environments. Because it serves as an insulator, the created environment may change the client system's response to stressors. A major objective of the created environment is to provide a positive stimulus toward health for the client. Capers (1996) emphasizes that the created environment includes cultural factors that influence the state of wellness. The created environment is developed to be protective but may have a negative effect on the system if it uses energy needed to react to environmental stressors.

To assess the created environment, the caregiver needs to identify three aspects. First, what has been created, and what is the nature of the created environment? Second, to what extent is it used, what value does the client place on it, and what are the outcomes? Third, what protection is needed or is possible, and what is the ideal that is yet to be created? The created environment is a process-based concept of perpetual adjustment that may increase or decrease the client's state of wellness (Neuman, 2002c).

Stressors

Neuman (2002c) defines stressors as stimuli that produce tensions and have the potential for causing system instability. She views stressors, within themselves, as neutral; it is the client/client system's perception that determines the impact as positive or negative. The system may need to deal with one or more stressors at any given time. It is important to identify the type, nature, and intensity of the stressor; the time of the system's encounter with the stressor; and the nature of the system's reaction or potential reaction to that encounter, including the amount of energy needed. The reaction may occur in one or more subparts, or subsystems, of the system. A reaction in one subsystem may, in turn, affect the original stressor. Outcomes may be positive with the potential for beneficial system changes that may be temporary or permanent.

Stressors are present both within or outside of the system. Neuman (2002c) classifies stressors as intra-, inter-, or extrapersonal in nature. *Intrapersonal* stressors are those that occur within the client system boundary and correlate with the internal environment. An example for the individual client system is the autoimmune response. *Interpersonal* stressors occur outside the client system boundary, are proximal to the system, and have an impact on the system. An example is role expectations. *Extrapersonal* stressors also occur outside the system boundaries but are at a greater distance from the system than are interpersonal stressors. An example is social policy. Interpersonal and extrapersonal stressors correlate with the external environment. The created environment includes intra-, inter-, and extrapersonal stressors.

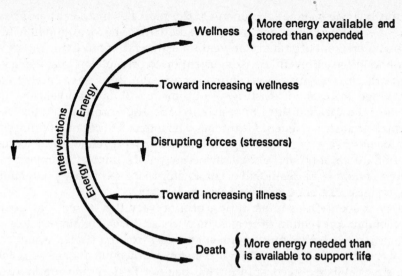

FIGURE 14-2 Neuman Systems Model wellness–illness continuum. (*From Neuman, B. & Fawcett, J. (2002). The Neuman Systems Model (4th ed., p. 23). Upper Saddle River, NJ: Prentice Hall. Used with permission.*)

Health

Neuman (2002c) identifies health as optimal system stability, harmony among the five variables, or the optimal state of wellness at a given time. Health is seen as a continuum from wellness to illness (see Figure 14-2). Health is also described as dynamic, with changing levels occurring within a normal range for the client system over time. The levels vary because of basic structure factors and the client system's response and adjustment to environmental stressors. Wellness may be determined by identifying the actual or potential effects of invading stressors on the system's available energy levels. The client system moves toward illness and death (entropy) when more energy is needed than is available and toward wellness (negentropy) when more energy is available, or can be generated, than is needed.

Reaction

Although reaction is identified within Figure 14-1, Neuman does not discuss it separately. She does point out that reactions and outcomes may be positive or negative, and she discusses system movement toward negentropy or entropy.

Prevention-as-Intervention

Primary, secondary, and tertiary prevention-as-interventions are used to retain, attain, and maintain system balance. More than one prevention-as-intervention mode may be used simultaneously.

   Primary prevention-as-intervention occurs before the system reacts to a stressor; it includes health promotion and maintenance of wellness. Primary prevention focuses on strengthening the flexible line of defense through preventing stress and reducing risk factors. This intervention occurs when the risk or hazard is identified but before a reaction occurs. Strategies that might be used include immunization, health education, exercise, and lifestyle changes. Neuman (2002c) indicates that health promotion is an area of major concern to client and caregiver and that, in the ideal situation, health promotion, as a component of primary prevention-as-intervention, should work with both secondary and tertiary prevention-as-intervention to promote optimal wellness.

Secondary prevention-as-intervention occurs after the system reacts to a stressor and is provided in terms of existing symptoms. Secondary prevention focuses on strengthening the internal lines of resistance and thus protects the basic structure through appropriate treatment of symptoms. The intent is to regain optimal system stability and to conserve energy in doing so. If secondary prevention is unsuccessful and reconstitution does not occur, the basic structure will be unable to support the system and its interventions, and death will occur. Examples of secondary prevention include the use of analgesics or of positioning to decrease pain.

Tertiary prevention-as-intervention occurs after the system has been treated through secondary prevention strategies. Its purpose is to maintain wellness or protect the client system reconstitution through supporting existing strengths and continuing to conserve energy. Tertiary prevention may begin at any point after system stability has begun to be reestablished (reconstitution has begun). Tertiary prevention tends to lead back to primary prevention. An example of tertiary prevention is participation in a cardiac rehabilitation program.

Reconstitution

Reconstitution begins at any point following initiation of treatment for invasion of stressors. Neuman (2002c) defines reconstitution as the return to and maintenance of system stability. Reconstitution may expand the normal line of defense beyond its previous level to a higher level of wellness, stabilize the system at a lower level of wellness, or return it to the level that existed before the illness. It depends on successful mobilization of client resources to prevent further reaction to the stressor and represents a dynamic state of adjustment.

Nursing

Neuman (2002c) also discusses nursing as part of the model. The major concern of nursing is to help the client system attain, maintain, or retain system stability. The goal of optimal wellness is achieved when the system has the greatest possible degree of stability at any given time. This may be accomplished through accurate assessment of both the actual and the potential effects of stressor invasion and assisting the client system to make those adjustments necessary for optimal wellness through primary, secondary, and tertiary prevention-as-intervention. In supporting system stability, the nurse provides the linkage between the client system, the environment, health, and nursing.

Unique Perspective of the Neuman Systems Model

In 1974, Neuman first presented the assumptions she identified as underlying the NSM. In 1995 she labeled these as propositions and in 2002 described them as summarizing the unique perspective of the NSM:

- Each individual client or group as a client system is unique; each system is a composite of common known factors or innate characteristics within a normal, given range of response contained within a basic structure.
- The client as a system is in dynamic, constant energy exchange with the environment.

- Many known, unknown, and universal environmental stressors exist. Each differs in its potential for disturbing a client's usual stability level, or normal line of defense. The particular interrelationships of client variables—physiological, psychological, sociocultural, developmental, and spiritual—at any point in time can affect the degree to which a client is protected by the flexible line of defense against possible reaction to a single stressor or a combination of stressors.
- Each individual client/client system has evolved a normal range of response to the environment that is referred to as a normal line of defense, or usual wellness/stability state. It represents change over time through coping with diverse stress encounters. The normal line of defense can be used as a standard from which to measure health deviation.
- When the cushioning, accordionlike effect of the flexible line of defense is no longer capable of protecting the client/client system against an environmental stressor, the stressor breaks through the normal line of defense. The interrelationships of variables—physiological, psychological, sociocultural, developmental, and spiritual—determine the nature and degree of the system reaction or possible reaction to the stressor.
- The client, whether in a state of wellness or illness, is a dynamic composite of the interrelationships of variables—physiological, psychological, sociocultural, developmental, and spiritual. Wellness is on a continuum of available energy to support the system in an optimal state of system stability.
- Implicit within each client system is a set of internal resistance factors known as lines of resistance, which function to stabilize and return the client to the usual wellness state (normal line of defense) or possibly to a higher level of stability following an environmental stressor reaction.
- Primary prevention relates to general knowledge that is applied in client assessment and intervention in identification and reduction or mitigation of possible or actual risk factors associated with environmental stressors to prevent possible reaction. The goal of health promotion is included in primary prevention.
- Secondary prevention relates to symptomatology following a reaction to stressors, appropriate ranking of intervention priorities, and treatment to reduce their noxious effects.
- Tertiary prevention relates to the adjustive processes taking place as reconstitution begins and maintenance factors move the client back in a circular manner toward primary prevention. (Neuman, 2002c, p. 14)

THE NEUMAN SYSTEMS MODEL AND NURSING'S METAPARADIGM

The four major concepts in nursing's metaparadigm are identified by Neuman as part of her model and have been discussed. A brief summary of each follows.

The *human being* is viewed as an open system that interacts with both internal and external environmental forces and stressors. The human is in constant change, moving toward a dynamic state of system stability or toward illness of varying degrees. This open system is comprised of the five variables with a central core and protective lines of defense.

The *environment* is a vital arena that is germane to the system and its function; it includes internal, external, and created environment (Neuman, 2002c). The environment may be viewed as all factors that affect and are affected by the system.

Health is defined as the condition or degree of system stability and is viewed as a continuum from wellness to illness (Neuman, 2002c) (see Figure 14-2). Stability occurs when all the system's parts and subparts are in balance or harmony so that the whole system is in balance. When system needs are met, optimal wellness exists. When needs are not satisfied, illness exists. When the energy needed to support life is not available, death occurs.

The primary concern of *nursing* is to define the appropriate action in situations that are stress related or in relation to possible reactions of the client or client system to stressors. Nursing interventions are aimed at helping the system adapt or adjust and to retain, restore, or maintain some degree of stability between and among the client system variables and environmental stressors, with a focus on conserving energy.

THE NEUMAN SYSTEMS MODEL IN CLINICAL PRACTICE

Neuman (1982b, 1995, 2002b) presents a three-step nursing process format, known as the Neuman Systems Model Nursing Process Format (see Table 14-1). The first step, titled "Nursing Diagnosis," includes the use of a database to identify variances from wellness and development of hypothetical interventions. The second step, "Nursing Goals," includes caregiver–client negotiation of intervention strategies to retain, attain, or maintain system stability. The third step, "Nursing Outcomes," includes nursing intervention using the prevention modes, confirming that the desired change has occurred or reformulating the nursing goals, using the outcomes of short-term goals to determine longer-term goals, and validating the nursing process through client outcomes.

Freese, Neuman, and Fawcett (2002) have provided guidelines for clinical practice based in the NSM:

- The purpose of clinical practice is to assist clients to retain, attain, or maintain optimal system stability.
- Clinical problems encompass actual or potential reactions to intrapersonal, interpersonal, and extrapersonal stressors.
- Clinical practice occurs in virtually any health care or community-based setting, such as clinics, hospitals, hospices, homes, and the streets and sidewalks of the community.
- Legitimate participants in clinical practice are those individuals, families, groups, and communities who are faced with actual or potential intrapersonal, interpersonal, and extrapersonal stressors.
- The process of clinical practice is the Neuman Systems Model Process Format, which encompasses three components—diagnosis, goals, and outcomes.
- The Neuman Systems Model Process Format engages the client system and the caregiver in a mutual partnership to determine diagnosis, goals, and outcomes.
- Diagnoses may be classified into a Neuman Systems Model diagnostic taxonomy that is organized according to client system (individual, family, group, community), level of response (primary, secondary, tertiary), client subsystem responding to the stressor (physiological, psychological, sociocultural, developmental, spiritual), source of the stressor (intrasystem, intersystem, extrasystem), and type of stressor (physiological, psychological, sociocutural, developmental, spiritual).
- Clinical interventions occur as primary, secondary, and tertiary prevention interventions, in accord with the degree to which stressors have penetrated the client system's lines of defense and resistance.

TABLE 14-1 Neuman Systems Model Nursing Process Format

Nursing Diagnosis

Variances from wellness are
determined by
correlations and
constraints

Data base

Hypothetical interventions
are determined for
prescriptive change

I. Nursing Diagnosis
 A. Data base—determined by:
  1. Identification and
   evaluation of potential
   or actual stressors that
   pose a threat to the
   stability of the client/
   client systems.
  2. Assessment of con-
   dition and strength of
   basic structure factors
   and energy resources.
  3. Assessment of characteristics of the flexible
   and normal lines of
   defense, lines of
   resistance, degree of
   potential reaction,
   reaction, and/or potential
   for reconstitution
   following a reaction.
  4. Identification, classification, and evaluation of
   potential and/or actual
   intra-, inter-, and extrapersonal interactions
   between the client and
   environment, considering
   all five variables.
  5. Evaluation of influence of
   past, present, and possible future life process
   and coping patterns on
   client system stability.
  6. Identification and calculation of actual and
   potential internal and
   external resources for
   optimal state of wellness.
  7. Identification and
   resolution of perceptual
   differences between
   caregivers and
   client/client system.
  Note: In all the above areas of
  consideration the caregiver simultaneously considers five variables
  (dynamic interactions in the client/
  client system)—physiological,
  psychological, sociocultural,
  developmental, and spiritual.

(continued)

TABLE 14-1 (Continued)

Nursing Diagnosis

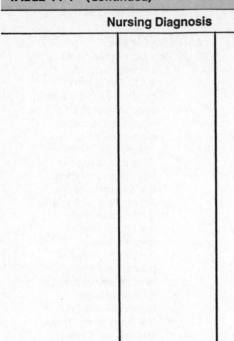

B. Variances from wellness—
   determined by
   1. Synthesis of theory with
      client data to identify the
      condition from which a
      comprehensive diag-
      nostic statement can
      be made. Goal prioritiza-
      tion is determined by
      client/client system
      wellness level, system
      stability needs, and total
      available resources to
      accomplish desired goal
      outcomes.
   2. Hypothetical goals and
      interventions postulated
      to reach the desired client
      stability or wellness level,
      that is, to maintain the
      normal line of defense
      and retain the flexible
      line of defense, thus
      protecting the basic
      structure.

Nursing Goals

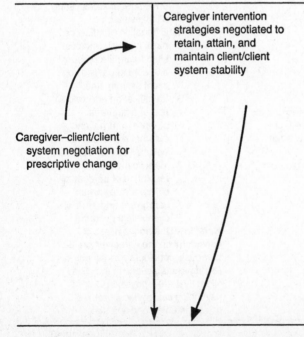

Caregiver intervention
strategies negotiated to
retain, attain, and
maintain client/client
system stability

Caregiver–client/client
system negotiation for
prescriptive change

II. Nursing goals—determined by
A. Negotiations with the client
   for desired prescriptive
   change or goal outcomes to
   correct variances from
   wellness, based on classified
   needs and resources
   identified in the nursing
   diagnosis.
B. Appropriate prevention as
   intervention strategies are
   negotiated with the client
   for retention, attainment,
   and/or maintenance of
   client system stability as
   desired outcome goals.
   Theoretical perspectives
   used for assessment and
   client data synthesis are
   analogous to those used
   for intervention.

TABLE 14-1 (Continued)

Nursing Outcomes

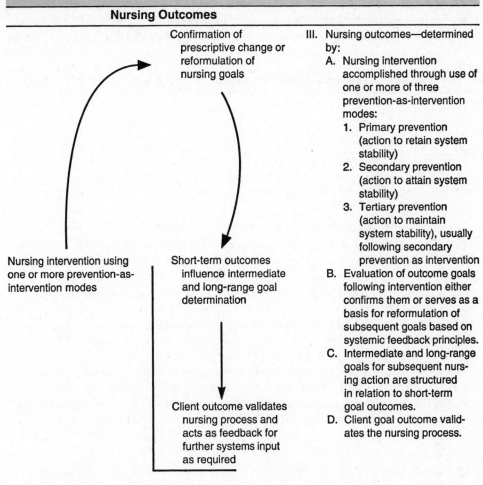

III. Nursing outcomes—determined by:
   A. Nursing intervention accomplished through use of one or more of three prevention-as-intervention modes:
      1. Primary prevention (action to retain system stability)
      2. Secondary prevention (action to attain system stability)
      3. Tertiary prevention (action to maintain system stability), usually following secondary prevention as intervention
   B. Evaluation of outcome goals following intervention either confirms them or serves as a basis for reformulation of subsequent goals based on systemic feedback principles.
   C. Intermediate and long-range goals for subsequent nursing action are structured in relation to short-term goal outcomes.
   D. Client goal outcome validates the nursing process.

- General outcomes are derived from the content of the Neuman Systems Model. Client-system-specific outcomes involve application of the general outcomes to particular clinical situations.
- Neuman Systems Model–based clinical practice contributes to client system well-being by facilitating the highest possible level of stability achievable at a given point in time.
- Clinical practice is linked to research through the use of research findings to direct practice. In turn, problems encountered in clinical practice give rise to new research questions. (p. 38)

In the diagnosis phase of the NSM process format, the nurse focuses on obtaining a comprehensive client database to determine the existing state of wellness and the actual or potential reaction to environmental stressors. A more specific guide to assessment is presented in Table 14-2. The collected data are prioritized and compared to or synthe-sized with relevant theories to explain the client's condition. Variances from the usual state of wellness are identified and a summary of impressions developed. The summary includes intra-, inter-, and extrapersonal factors. The synthesis of data with theory also

---

TABLE 14-2   An Assessment and Intervention Tool

A. Intake Summary
   1. Name _____
      Age _____
      Sex _____
      Marital status _____
   2. Referral source and related information _____

B. Stressors as Perceived by Client
   (If client is incapacitated, secure data from family or other resources.)
   1. What do you consider your major stress area, or areas, of health concern? (Identify these areas.)
   2. How do present circumstances differ from your usual pattern of living? (Identify lifestyle patterns.)
   3. Have you ever experienced a similar problem? If so, what was that problem and how did you handle it? Were you successful? (Identify past coping patterns.)
   4. What do you anticipate for yourself in the future as a consequence of your present situation? (Identify perceptual factors, that is, reality versus distortions—expectations, present and possible future coping patterns.)
   5. What are you doing and what can you do to help yourself? (Identify perceptual factors, that is, reality versus distortions—expectations, present and possible future coping patterns.)
   6. What do you expect caregivers, family, friends, or others to do for you? (Identify perceptual factors, that is, reality versus distortions—expectations, present and possible future coping patterns.)

C. Stressors as Perceived by Caregiver
   1. What do you consider to be the major stress area, or areas, of health concern? (Identify these areas.)
   2. How do present circumstances seem to differ from the client's usual pattern of living? (Identify lifestyle patterns versus distortions—expectations, present and possible future coping patterns).
   3. Has the client ever experienced a similar situation? If so, how would you evaluate what the client did? How successful do you think it was? (Identify past coping patterns.)
   4. What do you anticipate for the future as a consequence of the client's present situation? (Identify perceptual factors, that is, reality versus distortions—expectations, present and possible future coping patterns.)
   5. What can the client do to help himself? (Identify perceptual factors, that is, reality versus distortions—expectations, present and possible future coping patterns.)
   6. What do you think the client expects from caregivers, family, friends, or other resources? (Identify perceptual factors, that is, reality versus distortions—expectations, present and possible future coping patterns.)

Summary of Impressions
Note any discrepancies or distortions between the client's perception and that of the caregiver as relates to the situation.

TABLE 14-2 (Continued)

D. Intrapersonal Factors

    1. Physical (Examples: degree of mobility, range of body function)

    2. Psycho-sociocultural (Examples: attitudes, values, expectations, behavior patterns, and nature of coping patterns)

    3. Developmental (Examples: age, degree of normalcy, factors related to present situation)

    4. Spiritual belief system (Examples: hope and sustaining factors)

E. Interpersonal Factors

    Examples are resources and relationships of family, friends, or caregivers that either influence or could influence Area D.

F. Extrapersonal Factors

    Examples are resources and relationship of community facilities, finances, employment, or other area that either influence or could influence Areas D and E.

G. Formulation of a Comprehensive Nursing Diagnosis

    This is accomplished by identifying and ranking the priority of needs based on total data obtained from the client's perception, the caregiver's perception, or other resources, such as laboratory reports, other caregivers, or agencies. Appropriate theory is related to the above data.

    Reassessment is a continuous process and is related to the effectiveness of intervention based on the prior stated goals. Effective reassessment would include the following as they relate to the total client situation:

    a. Changes in nature of stressors and priority assignments

    b. Changes in intrapersonal factors

    c. Changes in interpersonal factors

    d. Changes in extrapersonal factors

    In reassessment it is important to note the change of priority of goals in relation to the primary, secondary, and tertiary prevention-as-intervention categories. An assessment tool of this nature should offer a current, progressive, and comprehensive analysis of the client's total circumstances and relationship of the five client variables (physiological, psychological, sociocultural, developmental, and spiritual) to environmental influences.

From Neuman, B. (1995). *The Neuman Systems Model* (pp. 59–61). Norwalk, CT: Appleton & Lange.

provides the basis for the *nursing diagnosis*. The diagnostic statement should reflect the entire client condition as reflected in the guidelines for use in clinical practice.

    The second phase, nursing goals, involves negotiation between the caregiver and the client, or recipient of care. The overall goal of the caregiver is to guide the client to conserve energy and to use energy as a force to move beyond the present, ideally in a way that preserves or enhances the client's wellness level. More specific outcomes will be derived from the nursing diagnoses. The perceptions of both the client and the caregiver must be considered in setting goals. Outcomes are specified under nursing goals in the NSM as goal outcomes to correct variances. These are to be based on the identified needs and the available resources. Outcomes are negotiated with the client.

    The third phase, nursing outcomes, begins with nursing interventions. According to Neuman (2002b), nursing actions are based on the synthesis of a comprehensive database about the client and the theory(ies) that are appropriate in light of the client's and caregiver's perceptions and possibilities for functional competence within the environment. The modes for identifying these actions are the levels of prevention-as-intervention. Table 14-3 presents a guide to nursing actions using prevention-as-intervention.

These nursing interventions-as-prevention are followed by evaluation to confirm that the anticipated or prescribed change has occurred. If this is not true, then goals are reformulated. Immediate and long-range goals are then structured in relation to the short-range outcomes.

A case study example of the application of the Neuman System Model Nursing Process Format may be found in Table 14-4.

TABLE 14-3 Format for Prevention-as-Intervention

Nursing Action		
Primary Prevention	**Secondary Prevention**	**Tertiary Prevention**
1. Classify stressors that threaten stability of the client/client system. Prevent stressor invasion.	1. Following stressor invasion, protect basic structure.	1. During reconstitution, attain and maintain maximum level of wellness or stability following treatment.
2. Provide information to retain or strengthen existing client/client system strengths.	2. Mobilize and optimize internal/external resources to attain stability and energy conservation.	2. Educate, reeducate, and/or reorient as needed.
3. Support positive coping and functioning.	3. Facilitate purposeful manipulation of stressors and reaction to stressors.	3. Support client/client system toward appropriate goals.
4. Desensitize existing or possible noxious stressors.	4. Motivate, educate, and involve client/client system in health care goals.	4. Coordinate and integrate health service resources.
5. Motivate toward wellness.	5. Facilitate appropriate treatment and intervention measures.	5. Provide primary and/or secondary preventive intervention as required.
6. Coordinate and integrate interdisciplinary theories and epidemiological input.	6. Support positive factors toward wellness.	
7. Educate or reeducate.	7. Promote advocacy by coordination and integration.	
8. Use stress as a positive intervention strategy.	8. Provide primary preventive intervention as required.	

Note: A first priority for nursing action in each of the areas of prevention-as-intervention is to determine the nature of stressors and their threat to the client/client system. Some general categorical functions for nursing action are initiation, planning, organization, monitoring, coordinating, implementing, integrating, advocating, supporting, and evaluating. An example of a limited classification system for stressors is illustrated by the following four categories: (1) deprivation, (2) excess, (3) change, and (4) intolerance. Copyright © 1980 by Betty Neuman. Revised 1987 by Betty Neuman.

TABLE 14-4 Case Study Using the Neuman Systems Model

Intake Summary
Name: Carolyn Miles
Age: 35 years
Sex: Female
Marital Status: Married
Referral Source: Self-referred

A. Stressors as Perceived by Client

 1. Major stress areas or areas of concern:
    a. Found out two weeks ago is two months pregnant—here for prenatal visit
    b. First child is 11 months old, wants another child, ambivalent about the timing of this pregnancy

 2. Lifestyle patterns
    a. Cares for home and daughter
    b. Active in church
    c. Participates in community groups related to parenting
    d. Has supportive family and friends
    e. What is different now?—experiencing nausea and fatigue

 3. Ever experienced similar problem?
    a. The nausea and fatigue are similar to the first pregnancy
    b. What helped then—crackers and lying down helped some; primarily just suffered through it

 4. Anticipations for the future
    a. Concerns about how to maintain a healthy pregnancy and care for an active toddler (concern greater because first pregnancy resulted in a premature delivery of a small-for-gestational-age baby)
    b. Also anticipating the demands of caring for two children under the age of two

 5. What is client doing to help herself?
    a. Talking with friends and family about their experiences
    b. Reading articles and books on childbearing and childrearing
    c. "I need to lower my expectations of myself and try not to do so much—for me that's HARD!!"

 6. What is expected of others?
    a. Family is visiting around the time the baby is due and will help with the children and the house
    b. Husband is doing more of the cooking and helping keep the house clean

B. Stressors as Perceived by Caregiver (primary care provider who provided prenatal care with the first pregnancy)

 1. Major stress area
    a. History of premature delivery
    b. Type A personality who has difficulty relaxing

 2. Present circumstances differing from usual pattern of living
    a. Fatigue and nausea of pregnancy
    b. Dealing with anticipation concerns about expanding family

(continued)

TABLE 14-4   (Continued)

3. Client's past experience with similar situation
   a. Experienced with nausea and fatigue of pregnancy
   b. Not experienced in having two children under age two

4. Future anticipations
   a. Client is capable of handling the situation—will need support and encouragement to do so

5. What can client do to help herself?
   a. Use her support systems
   b. Concentrate on getting needed rest
   c. Remember that the goal is a healthy child and things can be done later

6. Clients expectations of family, friends, and caregivers
   a. Accurate information
   b. Support and encouragement
   c. A listening ear

Summary of Impressions: No apparent discrepancies between perceptions of client and caregiver.

C. Intrapersonal factors
   1. Physical
      a. Height: five feet, five inches
      b. Weight: 125 lbs (no change from prepregnancy weight)
      c. TPR 98.4 F, 76, 12
      d. B/P 118/76
      e. Urine negative for sugar and albumin
      f. Care—perform all activities of daily living for self and toddler
      g. Is current with all immunizations
      h. Sleeps seven to eight hours per night
      i. Does not smoke or ingest alcohol
      j. Follows a low-fat, balanced diet; usually eats three meals per day
      k. Reports experiencing nausea and fatigue—a major stressor at this time

   2. Psycho-sociocultural
      a. 35-year-old female, married
      b. Caucasian
      c. Holds a master's degree in communications
      d. Sometimes concerned about feeling isolated—likes to have lots of friends and best friend will be moving in 6 to 12 months
      e. Knows needs to "slow down" but states that is hard for her to do, "I plan too much for any given day. I've always done this and I don't really know how to do less. The one good thing is that it doesn't bother me too much if I don't get all that I have planned done!"
      f. Lives in own home
      g. Fluent in English and Spanish

   3. Developmental
      a. "I have demonstrated my ability to be a good mother—that is reassuring that I can meet this new challenge."
      b. "How am I going to find the time to do everything?"

TABLE 14-4   (Continued)

4. Spiritual belief system
   a. This is an area of support, not an area of concern
   b. Active at church, regular attendance is important
   c. Has personal Bible study daily

D. Interpersonal Factors
   1. Has supportive family and friends
   2. Often speaks on the phone to family and friends, has lunch with friends regularly
   3. Shares toddler play days with friends
   4. Concerned about having two children under age two in the house
   5. Is working on a project at church to improve the nursery program
   6. Cannot rest at will with toddler at home—this is different from that with first pregnancy so previous coping responses are not as effective
   7. Will try to interest toddler in quiet activities on the days she is really tired
   8. Husband can work at home some days and help with the toddler

E. Extrapersonal Factors
   1. Community lacks good day care programs/facilities for toddlers so there is no real community support for when she needs a respite from child care
   2. Health care for all family members is readily available

Overall Summary:

Physiological: Normal pregnancy with associated stressors of nausea and fatigue

Psychosociocultural: Has supportive family and friends. Stressors related to self-expectations

Developmental: Normal for age

Spiritual: Belief system is a positive support

F. Formulation of a Comprehensive Nursing Diagnosis:
   1. Nursing Diagnoses
      a. Nausea and fatigue related to pregnancy (individual client, secondary intervention, physiological subsystem and stressor, intrasystem)
      b. Lack of knowledge related to parenting two children under the age of two (family as client system, primary intervention, developmental subsystem and stressor, intersystem for her but intrasystem for the family)
   2. Goals (mutually agreed-upon desired outcomes)
      a. Manage nausea and fatigue so can continue normal activities of daily living
      b. Plan strategies for coping with two children under the age of two
      c. Have a healthy outcome to the pregnancy—healthy mother, father, toddler, and infant
   3. Prevention-as-Intervention
      a. Manage nausea and fatigue
         i. primary—normal line of defense has been invaded—is having symptoms
         ii. secondary—plan daily activities to include rest periods when toddler naps; explore types of foods and eating patterns that decrease nausea
         iii. tertiary—continue to encourage rest whenever possible; husband helps out as he can; plan daily intake of appropriate nutrients; keep a journal listing daily plans to demonstrate ability to plan less for each day

(continued)

TABLE 14-4   (Continued)

b. Lack of knowledge about parenting two children under two

    i. primary—discuss current parenting strategies with husband, friends, family, caregiver and explore how these strategies may be adapted; caregiver encourages discussion with friend who has two small children and works full time

    ii. secondary and tertiary—not needed as yet; flexible and normal lines of defense have functioned effectively

c. Healthy outcome to the pregnancy

    i. The overall desired outcome—preventions as intervention listed in a and b.

4. Evaluation

Carolyn delivered a healthy six-pound, eight-ounce girl at 38 weeks' gestation after a pregnancy she described as "much better than I thought it would be." Husband/father and older daughter are delighted with the new baby. Carolyn states, "I'm still working on not planning too much for each day." Identified outcome was achieved.

CRITIQUE OF THE NEUMAN SYSTEMS MODEL

1. *What is the historical context of the theory?* The perspectives that provide the basis for the NSM are clearly explicated in the work and follow a logical order. Neuman identifies that she has drawn upon her own clinical experiences in nursing as well as information in the literature on stress, systems, levels of prevention, wholism within systems, coping, and gestalt theory. While study of this literature could enrich one's understanding of the relationships she has developed, such study is not vital to comprehension of the NSM.

The NSM was developed during a period when other developing nursing theories were based in general systems theory. Chronologically, it fits in the middle period of theory development in nursing during the 20th century. Based on Parse's (1987) description of the totality paradigm, the NSM best fits this paradigm. The model is wholistic but emphasizes the five variables of physiological, psychological, sociocultural, developmental, and spiritual. The system's interaction with the external environment is described as responses to stressors that adapt or seek to control the stressors or the environment. Health is described as dynamic with an objective assessment of the invasion, or potential for invasion, of the lines of defense. Reconstitution and the levels of preventions may be identified as maintenance or restoration of norms. The plan of care is designed by the nurse based on skilled assessment. However, the client is viewed as unique, decision making is shared, and the care is negotiated with the client. Louis, Neuman, and Fawcett (2002) support the use of both quantitative and qualitative methods of research for studying relationships identified by the model.

2. *What are the basic concepts and relationships presented by the theory?* and

3. *What major phenomena of concern to nursing are presented? (These phenomena may include but are not limited to **human being, environment, health, interpersonal relations, caring, goal attainment, adaptation, and energy fields.)*** The basic concepts of the NSM are the five variables (physiological, psychological, sociocultural, developmental, and spiritual), levels of prevention-as-intervention (primary, secondary, and tertiary), lines of defense (flexible line of defense, normal line of defense, and lines of resistance), environment (internal, external, and created), stressors (intrapersonal, interpersonal, and extrapersonal), health, reconstitution, system core, and nursing. All of these are defined. However, as Fitzpatrick and Whall (2005) identify, it would be useful to have operational definitions of the concepts to help ensure that everyone applies them in the same manner. The reactions to stressors are less clearly defined.

Neuman uses the concepts consistently and presents them in a pictorial model (see Figure 14-1). The relationships among the concepts are logical and clearly defined in the stated perspectives. While the pictorial model is rather overwhelming on first view, an orderly analysis supports that it logically presents the identified relationships.

4. *To whom does this theory apply? In what situations? In what ways?* This model was designed for health care and applies to all recipients of nursing care—individuals, groups, organizations, and communities. Neuman's use of the term *client/client system* allows for the client to be an individual or a collection of people. The system perspective allows the user to define the system (an individual, a family, an organization, and so on) and then to identify the core and lines of defense for that system. The wholistic system approach indicates the model is not situation specific but may be used in a variety of situations. It would be difficult to identify a setting where this model could not be applied.

The model explains and predicts phenomena. For example, if the lines of resistance have been activated and they are not effective and cannot be strengthened through secondary prevention-as-intervention strategies, then death is threatened. If the flexible lines of defense are effective, there is no immediate threat to the system, but the client may be in need of primary prevention-as-intervention strategies to enhance responses to potential stressors.

Fawcett (2005) questions the utility of the NSM for practice with a client who does not wish to participate. Certainly this is a challenging situation with the NSM emphasis on mutual involvement of caregiver and client. The caregiver's perceptions could become an even greater part of the NSM nursing process in such a situation. Also, the involvement of family members or other representatives of the client's interpersonal system would be of great value.

5. *By what method or methods can this theory be tested?* Louis et al. (2002) identify guidelines for research based on the NSM:

- One purpose of the Neuman Systems Model–based research is to predict the effects of primary, secondary, and tertiary prevention interventions on retention, attainment, and maintenance of client system stability. Another purpose of Neuman Systems Model–based research is to determine the cost, benefit, and utility of prevention interventions.
- The phenomena of interest encompass the physiological, psychological, sociocultural, developmental, and spiritual variables; the properties of the central core of the client/client system; the properties of the flexible and normal lines of defense and the lines of resistance; the characteristics of the internal, external, and created environments; the characteristics of intrapersonal, interpersonal, and extrapersonal stressors; and the elements of primary, secondary, and tertiary prevention interventions.
- The precise problems to be studied are those dealing with the impact of stressors on client system stability with regard to physiological, psychological, sociocultural, developmental, and spiritual variables, as well as the lines of defense and resistance.

- Research designs encompass both inductive and deductive research using qualitative and quantitative research approaches and associated instrumentation.
- Data encompass both the client system's and the investigator's perceptions, and may be collected in inpatient, ambulatory, home, and community settings.
- Study participants can be the client systems of individuals, families, groups, communities, organizations, or collaborative relationships between two or more individuals. The investigator also is a study participant.
- Data analysis techniques associated with both qualitative and quantitative research methodologies are appropriate.
- Quantitative methods of data analysis should consider the flexible line of defense as a moderator variable and the lines of resistance as a mediator variable.
- Neuman Systems Model–based research findings advance understanding of the influence of prevention interventions on the relation between stressors and client system stability.
- Research is linked to clinical practice through the use of research findings to direct practice. In turn, problems encountered in clinical practice give rise to new research questions. (p. 114)

Note particularly the fourth guideline that indicates that both quantitative and qualitative research methods may be used in testing relationships identified from the NSM.

The NSM is one of the most widely used nursing models for nursing research. In 1989, Louis and Koertvelyessy reported the model was one of the three most frequently used models in nursing research. Louis (1995) reports findings ranging from no significant relationships to "decisive results" (p. 478). She suggests it is important to evaluate the rigor of each study as well as the strength of the use of prevention-as-intervention—both in the strength of the prevention used and in the length of the time it was applied. In 1999, Fawcett reported finding 200 studies published between 1982 and 1997. However, most of these studies did not include conclusions about the usability or validity of the model.

Gigliotti (1999a) points out the difficulty in making comparisons across studies, as the lines of defense have not been described in a consistent manner. For example, in four cited studies, although all discussed a stressor with a specific intervention to strengthen the flexible line of defense, the associated outcome is defined differently in each. Ali and Khalil (1989) and Gigliotti (1999b) speak to the normal line of defense penetration or invasion, Louis (1989) uses the term *line of resistance not activated*, and Freiberger, Bryant, and Marino (1992) identify activated lines of resistance.

Research is active on relationships and theories derived from this model. Use of the terminology and findings is not yet consistent. Both Fawcett (1999) and Gigliotti (1999a) support the need for more consistent and explicit linkages between the concepts of the NSM and the variables being studied. Fawcett and Giangrande (2001, 2002) conducted an integrative review of NSM-based research. They speak to the need for systematic NSM-based research programs and the inability to do meta-analysis without such coherent programs of research, as well as provide suggestions for using the NSM to guide nursing research.

6. *Does this theory direct nursing actions that lead to favorable outcomes?* The NSM directs nursing actions that lead to favorable outcomes through the use of the levels of prevention as intervention. The purpose of the levels of prevention is reconstitution, or the return to wholeness, with functioning lines of defense to protect against stressors invading the system and leading to illness. A strength of the model is that there are three levels of prevention as intervention. The intent of having three levels of prevention is to allow nursing actions to be taken as appropriate to the needs of the client system. Nursing interventions may be used to promote or maintain health status, prevent disease, and help the client/client system return to a healthful state.

A wholistic approach and viewpoint are an important part of the model, so the nurse who uses the NSM as a guide to the development of therapeutic nursing interventions could be using all levels of prevention as intervention over the course of the nurse and client interaction. The use of the five variables will also contribute to consideration of the whole client. The use of the NSM for directing nursing prevention as intervention has been tested. The fourth edition of *The Neuman Systems Model* has several chapters that discuss the use of the model in curriculum, nursing practice, and nursing administration in the United States and internationally.

Nursing actions are determined by asking, "What are the stressors as perceived by the client system and what has been the system's reaction been to these stressors?" and by mutually setting goals with the client. By focusing on the cause and the reactions, it is possible to carry out nursing actions that are likely to lead to favorable outcomes. Because the NSM directs the nurse to consider the perceptions of the client and of the caregiver, when these perceptions are congruent, the frequency of favorable outcomes is enhanced. For example, Puetz (1990) found that when nurses did not conduct an individualized assessment, the perceptions of the client and the nurse were less likely to be congruent. This lack of congruency could then be a stressor for the client and outcomes would be less favorable, as the nurse has not followed the assessment guidelines of the NSM. Lowry, Beckman, Gehrling, and Fawcett (2007) support the importance of congruence in their discussion that client satisfaction is a valuable outcome in NSM-based practice due to the plan of care being client driven.

7. *How contagious is this theory?*   The NSM is one of the most contagious of the nursing theories or models. It is in use worldwide in direct clinical practice and nursing administration, nursing research, and nursing education. Examples of the use of the model in these areas around the world include the following:

- **Australia:** Use in **education** at the University of South Australia (McCulloch, 1995)
- **Brazil: Practice** in relation to *work-health-disease* (Silveira, 2000)
- **Canada:**
  Practice *in chronic care* (Felix, Hinds, Wolfe, & Martin, 1995); *community/public health* (Beynon, 1995; Beynon & Laschinger, 1993; Bunn, 1995; Drew, Craig, & Beynon, 1989; Mytka & Beynon, 1994); *gerontology* (Gibson, 1996); *HIV* (Mill, 1997); *nursing administration* (Beynon, 1995; Craig & Morris-Coulter, 1995; Drew et al., 1989; Neuman, 1995); *orthopedics* (Shaw, 1991); and *pediatrics* (Galloway, 1993; Maligalig, 1994)
  Research related to *back pain* (McMillan, 1995); *caregiver burden* (Semple, 1995); *critical care* (Lunario, 2004), *diabetes* (Robinson-Lewis, 2004); *gender identity disorder* (Janze, Watson, & Stevenson, 1999); *hip surgery patients* (Bowman, 1997); *oncology* (Cava, 1992); *latex allergy* (Cowperthwaite, LaPlante, Mahon, & Markowski, 1997); Nurses' Association Presidents (Johnson, 1995); *perceptions* (Sheridan, 2005); *public health nursing* (Mackenzie & Laschinger, 1995); *stress* (Montgomery & Craig, 1990; Samuels-Dennis, 2004); *theory-based care* (Laschinger & Duff, 1991)

Education in *postdiploma and baccalaureate programs* (Beddome, 1995; Craig, 1995; Crawford, Tarko, Ting, Gunderson, & Andrews, 1999; Neuman, 1995; Peternelj-Taylor & Johnson, 1996; Tarko & Crawford, 1999)

- **China: Research** in *oncology* (Lin, Ku, Leu, Chen, & Lin, 1996)
- **Denmark: Practice:** *rehabilitation* (Thygesen & Esbensen, 2008); **Teaching:** *community health nursing* (Neuman, 1995)
- **Egypt: Research** in *oncology* (Ali & Khalil, 1989)
- **United Kingdom:**
  Practice: *breastfeeding* (Evely, 1994); *community health* (Damant, 1995; Davies & Proctor, 1995); *Down syndrome* (Owens, 1995); *family nursing* (Picton, 1995); *gerontology* (Beckingham & Baumann, 1990; Haggart, 1993; Millard, 1992; Moore & Munro, 1990); *general patient care* (Goodman, 1995); *intensive care* (Black, Deeny, & McKenna, 1997; Wormald, 1995); *multiple sclerosis* (Knight, 1990); *perioperative care* (Parr, 1993); *rehabilitation* (Bowles, Oliver, & Stanley, 1995)
  Research: *Oncology* (Hinds, 1990)
  Nursing education (Ross, Bourbonnais, & Carroll, 1987; Vaughan & Gough, 1995)
- **Guam:** *Baccalaureate education* (Neuman, 1995)
- **Hong Kong: Research** *in oncology* (Molassiotis, 1997); **Education** (Cheung, 1997)
- **Iceland: practice** at St. Joseph's Hospital, Reykjavik (Neuman, 1995) and baccalaureate **education** at Akureye University (Neuman, 1995)
- **Israel: Research** in *spirituality* (Musgrave, 2001)
- **Netherlands:**
  Practice: in *mental health care* (Fawcett, 2004; Timmermans, 1999; Verberk, 1995)
  Research: *addiction* (Westrik, 1999)
  Education: *higher education* (de Meij & de Kuiper, 1999; Fawcett, 2004)
- **Saudi Arabia: Research** in *surgically induced menopause* (Al-Nagshabandi, 1993)
- **South Africa: Practice:** *pediatrics* (Orr, 1993), **Research** in *conscious awareness* (Moola, 2004), *critical care nurses and stress* (Moola, Ehlers, & Hattingh, 2008); *holistic care* (Norrish, 2001), *pediatric HIV care* (Orr, 1999)
- **Sweden:**
  Practice: *community health* (Engberg, Bjälming, & Bertilson, 1995); *contraception* (Lindell & Olsson, 1991); *hospital care* (Neuman, 1995); *occupational health* (McGee, 1995)
  Research in *gerontology* (Lindgren & Olsson, 1999); *humor* (Carras & Olsson, 1999; Olsson & Leadersh, 1999); *slimming* (Eilert-Petersson & Olsson, 1999); *stress in student nurses* (Àgren, Fröistedt, & Olsson, 1999; Backe & Olsson, 1999)
  Education: *college* (Engberg, 1995)
- **Taiwan:**
  Research: *quality of life* (Lee, F-P., 2005)
  Education: (Neuman, 1995)
- **Thailand: research** in *cardiac care* (Pothiban, 1993); *coordinating community resources* (Noonill, Sindhu, Hanucharurnkul, & Suwonnaroop, 2007); *perinatal risk assessment* (Lapvongwatana, 2000)
- **Turkey: Concept building** *burnout* (Günüsen, Ustün, & Gigliotti, 2009)
- **United States:**
  Practice: *adolescents* (Cazzell, 2008); *advanced practice* (Gigliotti, 2002; Russell & Hezel, 1994); *caregivers* (Skipwith, 1994); *case management* (Bittinger, 1995; Mann, Hazel, Geer, Hurley, & Podrapovic, 1993); *cardiac care* (Lile, 1990); *cognitive*

impairment (Chiverton & Flannery, 1995); *community nursing* (Cookfair, 1996; Gellner, Landers, O'Rourke, & Schlegel, 1994; Neuman, 1995; Newman, 2005); *concept analysis* (Reed, 1999); *critical care nursing* (Bueno & Sengin, 1995); *critical pathways* (Lowry, 1999); *culture* (Capers, 1996); *depression* (Hassell, 1996); *diabetes mellitus* (Baerg, 1991); *dialysis* (Breckenridge, 1997a; 1997b); *elderly* (Burnett, 1999; LaReau, 2000); *end stage kidney disease* (Graham, 2006); *family assessment/nursing* (Berkey & Hanson, 1991; Flannery, 1991; Kahn, 1992; Ume-Nwagbo, DeWan & Lowry, 2006; Reed, 1993; Ridgell, 1993); *gerontological nursing* (Delunas, 1990; Hiltz, 1990; Peirce & Fulmer, 1995); *health protection* (Bigbee & Jansa, 1991); *HIV care* (Miner, 1995; Pierce & Hutton, 1992; Simmons & Borgdon, 1991); *holistic care* (DiJoseph & Cavendish, 2005); *home caregivers* (Russell, Hileman, & Grant, 1995); *hospital-based care* (Davidson & Myers, 1999; Neuman, 1995; Scicchitani, Cox, Heyduk, Maglicco, & Sargent, 1995); *in-service education* (Roberts, A. G., 1994); *intensive care* (Fulbrook, 1991; Kido, 1991); *interstitial cystitis* (Kubsch, Linton, Handerson, & Wichowski, 2008); *long-term care* (Schlentz, 1993); *multisystem organ failure* (Bergstrom, 1992); *neonatal intensive care* (Ware & Shannahan, 1995); *neuroscience nursing* (Foote, Piazza, & Schultz, 1990); *nurse anesthesia* (Martin, 1996); *obstetrics/battered women* (Barnes-McDowell & Freese, 1999; Bullock, 1993); *oncology* (Piazza, Foote, Wright, & Holcombe, 1992; Weinberger, 1991); *perinatal nursing* (Gigliotti, 1998; Trépanier, Dunn, & Sprague, 1995); *psychiatric nursing* (Herrick, Goodykoontz, Herrick, & Hackett, 1991; Stuart & Wright, 1995); *spirituality* (Beckman, Boxley-Harges, Bruick-Sorge, & Salmon, 2007); *substance abuse* (Mynatt & O'Brien, 1993; Waters, 1993); *terminal illness* (Lile, Pase, Hoffman, & Mace, 1994); *theory-based practice* (Dale & Savala, 1990; Derstine, 1992; Neuman, 1990, 1998)

Research: *AIDS education* (F. A. Brown, 1994); *adolescent pregnancy* (Sabatini, 2003); *alcohol use* (Rohr, 2006); *antibiotic therapy* (Herald, 1993); *anxiety* (Wilkey, 1990); *asthma* (Levi, 2001); *baccalaureate education* (Fulton, 1992; Lamb, 1998; Mirenda, 1995; Peterson, 1997; Roggensack, 1994; Speck, 1990); *aromatherapy* (Tweed, 1999); *back injuries/pain* (K. C. Brown, Sirles, Hilyer, & Thomas, 1992; Koku, 1992; Radwanski, 1992); *blood pressure* (Picot, Zauszniewski, Debanne, & Holston, 1999; Young, 2000); *breastfeeding* (Cagle, 1996; Marlett, 1998); *burnout* (Collins, M. A., 1996; Hansen, 2000; Marsh, 1997); *caregivers* (Jones-Cannon & Davis, 2005; Rowe, 1989); *cardiovascular* (Geiger, 1996; Harper, 1992; Kazakoff, 1990; Lijauco, 1997; Micevski, 1996; Metzger, 2006; Riley-Lawless, 2000; Williamson, 1992); *caring* (M. C. Roberts, 2002); *cerebral vascular accident* (Gifford, 1996); *childbirth* (Poe, 2002); *chronic lung disease patients* (Narsavage, 1997); *conceptual frameworks in research* (Grant, Kinney, & Davis, 1993); *cognitive assessment* (Flannery, 1995); *critical/intensive care* (Gavigan, Kline-O'Sullivan, & Klumpp-Lybrand, 1990; Ramsey, 1999; Watson, 1991); *diabetes* (Barron, 1998; Casalenuovo, 2002); *dialysis* (A. M. Jones, 2002); *gerontology* (Butts, 1998; C. R. Collins, 1999; Dunn, 2007; Kottwitz & Bowling, 2003; Rodrigues-Fisher, Bourguignon, & Good, 1993); *grieving* (Reed, 2003); *head injury* (Grant & Bean, 1992; Henze, 1993; W. R. Jones, 1996; Neabel, 1998); *health promotion* (Fowler & Risner, 1994); *HIV* (Gulliver, 1997; Norman, 1990; Simpson, 2000); *home care* (Peoples, 1990); *homeless women* (Hemphill, 2005); *hospice* (Decker & Young, 1991); *humor* (Cullen, 1993); *hyperlipedemia* (Britt, 2006); *immunization* (Chilton, 1996); *infant exposure to smoke* (Flanders-Stepans & Fuller, 1999); *job stress or satisfaction* (P. A. Hanson, 1997; Moody, 1996; Morris, 1991; Peters, 1997); *long-term care* (Petock, 1990);

neonatal intensive care unit (Alliston, 2003; Bass, 1991); *nursing administration* (Rowles, 1992; Walker, 1994); *nursing education* (Nortridge, Mayeux, Anderson, & Bell, 1992; Payne, 1993); *nursing vigilance* (Geib, 2003); *nurse–patient relations and culture* (Butrin, 1992); *nurse practitioner practice* (Larino, 1997); *nurses' values* (Cammuso, 1994); *oncology* (Allen, 1997; Jennings, 1997; Lancaster, 1991, 2005; O'Neal, 1993; Sabo & Michael, 1996; South, 1995); *orthopedics* (Nicholson, 1995; Wright, 1996); *pain control* (Vitthuhn, 1999); *parenting* (Heaman, 1991; Krajewski, 2003); *patient satisfaction* (Fukuzawa, 1995); *pediatrics* (Bishop, 2001; Chun, 2006; Courchene, Patalski, & Martin, 1991; Freiberger, Bryant, & Marino, 1992; Gray, 1998; Rosenfeld, Goldsmith, & Madell, 1998); *perinatal care* (Annamunthodo-Allen, 2005; Higgs, 1994; Lowry, Saeger, & Barnett, 1997; Wullschleger, 1999); *postanesthesia care* (Heffline, 1991); *psychiatric and community care* (Chiverton, Tortoretti, LaForest, & Walker, 1999; P. L. Lee, 1995); *psychiatric care* (Waddell & Demi, 1993); *quality of life* (Robinson, 1998); *role strain or stress* (P. S. Brown, 2004; Gigliotti, 2007); *sexual abuse* (Barnes, 1993; Goble, 1991); *school nursing* (Mannina, 1997; Zavala-Onyett, 2001); *shared governance* (George, 1997); *spinal cord injury* (Hayes, 1994); *spirituality* (Poppe, 2005); *stress and hardiness in students and educators* (Cox, 1995; Hood, 1997); *stress and nurse managers* (Holloway, 1995); *stressors* (Skalski, DiGerolamo, & Gigliotti, 2006); *substance abuse* (Bemker, 1996; M. S. Hanson, 1995; Monahan, 1996; Poole, 1991); *sudden infant death syndrome* (Barnes-McDowell, 1997); *spiritual care* (Carrigg & Weber, 1997); *terminal illness* (Hainsworth, 1996); *trauma care* (Bueno, Redeker, & Norman, 1992); *ventilator-dependent patients* (Lowry & Anderson, 1993); *wellness program* (James, 2001); *women's health* (Parodi, 1997; Reeves, 2004; Scalzo-Tarrant, 1992; Taggart & Mattson, 1996; Tarmina, 1992)

Education: *associate* (Bloch & Bloch, 1995; Hilton & Grafton, 1995; Lowry & Newsome, 1995; Moscaritolo, 2009); *baccalaureate* (Bremner & Initili, 1999; Glazebrook, 1995; Klotz, 1995; Knox, Kilchenstein, & Yakulis, 1982; Kilchenstein & Yakulis, 1984; Madrid & Stefanson, 1999; McHolm & Geib, 1998; Neuman, 1995; Strickland-Seng, 1995; Walker, 1995); *baccalaureate and graduate* (Edwards & Kittler, 1991; Neuman, 1995; Stittich, Flores, & Nuttall, 1995); *interdisciplinary* (Toot, Amaya, & Memmott, 1999); and graduate (Neuman, 1995)

• **Yugoslavia: Practice** in *primary health care* (Neuman, 1995); baccalaureate **education** (Neuman, 1995)

This listing is not intended to present a comprehensive review of all use of the NSM but nevertheless provides impressive documentation of the widespead contagiousness of the model. Lowry et al. (2007) express confidence that the NSM will continue to be an effective model because of its "focus on wholism, dynamic interacting systems, noxious and beneficial stressors, and emphasis on wellness" (p. 227), especially as people will continue to need people. Neuman and Reed (2007) believe this is particularly true with the continued trend toward emphasizing wholistic health. They aver that contagiousness will continue to be supported by the ease in which the language of the NSM is understood by nurses across many cultures. Additionally, Neuman, Newman, and Holder (2000) support the importance of the use of the NSM in nursing leadership to avoid fragmenting services and to provide clear direction for the organization of nursing care.

STRENGTHS AND WEAKNESSES OF THE NEUMAN SYSTEMS MODEL

The major strength of the NSM is its flexibility for use in all areas of nursing—research, administration, education, and practice. The third and fourth editions of *The Neuman Systems Model* includes many chapters that discuss the use of the model in all of these areas throughout the United States and in Australia, Canada, England, Holland, Sweden, Thailand, and Wales. This widespread acceptance supports the essentially universal applicability of the model.

Neuman (2002) reports that the model was designed for nursing but can be used by other health disciplines, which can be viewed as either a strength or weakness. As a strength, if multiple health disciplines use the model, a consistent approach to client care will be facilitated. If all disciplines use similar data collection techniques based on the assessment tool presented by Neuman, perhaps the client would not have to tell his story so many different times—at least once to each health care discipline. As a weakness, if the model is useful to a variety of disciplines, it is not specific to nursing and thus may not differentiate the practice of nursing from that of other disciplines.

The major weakness of the model is the need for further clarification of terms used. Interpersonal and extrapersonal stressors need to be more clearly differentiated. It may be that interpersonal stressors occur between two people and extrapersonal stressors occur between a group or society and the person. This differentiation is not clearly made. Other areas that require greater specification are how to identify variances of wellness and levels of wellness. Reaction also needs to be defined.

There are some inconsistencies in the presentation of the NSM. The pictorial diagram includes reaction; reaction is not specifically discussed in the text. Conversely, the verbal presentation incorporates health, environment, and nursing, which do not appear in the diagram. It is inferred that the diagram is considered to be the most important representation of the model because it is changes in the diagram that require unanimous agreement of the Neuman Trustees. Logically, based on this inference, the concepts in the verbal presentation should be derived from the diagram.

Other inconsistencies relate to Neuman's emphasis on a wholistic approach and a comprehensive review of the client system and her discussion of health and illness. The wholistic and comprehensive view is associated with an open system. Health and illness are presented on a continuum, with movement toward health described as negentropic and toward illness as entropic. Entropy is a characteristic of a closed rather than an open system. She does speak of levels of wellness, rather than levels of illness, but does not make it clear if health and illness are dichotomous.

Summary

The NSM was developed to help teach graduate students an integrated approach to client care. The model is based in general system theory and views the client as an open system that responds to stressors in the environment. The client variables are physiological, psychological, sociocultural, developmental, and spiritual. The client system consists of a basic or core structure that is protected by lines of resistance. The usual level of health is identified as the normal line of defense that is protected by a flexible line of defense. Stressors are intra-, inter-, and extrapersonal in nature and arise from the internal, external, and created environments. When stressors break through the flexible line of defense, the system is invaded, the lines of resistance are activated, and the system is described as moving into illness on a wellness–illness continuum. If adequate energy is available or can be generated, the system will be reconstituted with the normal line of defense restored at, below, or above its previous level. Nursing interventions occur through three prevention modalities: primary prevention occurs before the stressor invades the system, secondary prevention occurs after the system has reacted to an invading stressor, and tertiary prevention occurs after secondary prevention as reconstitution is being established.

This model has been widely used in all areas of nursing around the world. Its flexibility and universality are documented in the many publications that describe its use in nursing education, research, administration, and direct patient care. Further definition of some of the concepts in the model will serve to strengthen it further.

Thought Questions

1. Identify examples of the five variables for the client/client systems as an individual, as a family, and as a community.
2. List up to 10 common stressors for client in a selected area of clinical practice.
3. Of the stressors listed in the previous question, which are most likely to penetrate the flexible line of defense and why do you believe this is so? (Use Neuman's terminology to respond, including if the stressors are intra-, inter-, or extrapersonal.)
4. Select an area of clinical practice and give examples of primary, secondary, and tertiary preventions-as-intervention for a client in this area of practice. What are the stressors most likely to lead to the need for these preventions as intervention? In what order might these preventions as intervention be carried out?
5. Is it possible for a prevention as intervention to be primary, secondary, and tertiary? Why or why not?
6. What aspects of the NSM make it most likely and least likely that you will use it to guide your nursing practice?

 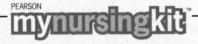

References

Ågren, C., Fröistedt, M., & Olsson, H. (1999, April 9). *Identifying stress in trainee psychiatric care nurses using the Neuman Systems Model.* Paper presented at The 7th Biennial International Neuman Systems Model Symposia, Vancouver, British Columbia, Canada.

Allen, K. S. (1997). The effect of cancer diagnosis information on the anxiety of patients with an initial diagnosis of first cancer. *Masters Abstracts International, 35*(04), 996. (University Microfilms No. AAG1384216)

Alliston, S. A. (2003). Neonatal nurses' attitudes, practices, and knowledge of skin care in the extremely low birth weight infant. *Masters Abstracts International, 41*(06), 1704. Abstract retrieved July 2, 2007, from Dissertation Abstracts Online database.

Al-Nagshabandi, E. A. H. (1993). An exploration of the physical and psychological responses of surgically-induced menopausal Saudi women using the Neuman Systems Model. *Dissertation Abstracts International, 55*(04B), 1374. (University Microfilms No. AAG941282)

Ali, N. S., & Khalil, H. Z. (1989). Effect of psychoeducational intervention on anxiety among Egyptian bladder cancer patients. *Cancer Nursing, 12*, 236–242.

Annamunthodo- Allen, M. (2005). The effects of a prenatal health teaching program. *Masters Abstracts International, 43*(05), 1698. Abstract retrieved July 2, 2007, from Dissertation Abstracts Online database.

Backe, H., & Olsson, H. (1999, April 9). *Stress amongst student nurses: An application of the Neuman Systems Model.* Paper presented at The 7th Biennial International Neuman Systems Model Symposia, Vancouver, British Columbia, Canada.

Baerg, K. L. (1991). Using Neuman's model to analyze a clinical situation. *Rehabilitation Nursing, 16*(1), 38–39.

Barnes, M. E. (1993). Knowledge, experiences, attitudes, and assessment practices of nurse practitioners with regard to stressors related to childhood sexual abuse. *Masters Abstracts International, 32*(01), 223. (University Microfilms No. AAG1353486)

Barnes-McDowell, B. M. (1997). Home apnea monitoring: Family functioning, concerns, and coping (Sudden Infant Death Syndrome, parents). *Dissertation Abstracts International, 58*(03B), 1205. (University Microfilms No. AAG9726731)

Barnes-McDowell, B. M., & Freese, B. (1999, April 9). *MEG's meeting: Dialog in diversity.* Paper presented at The 7th Biennial International Neuman Systems Model Symposia, Vancouver, British Columbia, Canada.

Barron, L. A. (1998). Diabetes self-management and psychosocial adjustment. *Masters Abstracts International, 37*(02), 587. (University Microfilms No. AAG1392504)

Bass, L. S. (1991). What do parents need when their infant is a patient in the NICU? *Neonatal Network: Journal of Neonatal Nursing, 10*(4), 25–38.

Beckingham, A. C., & Baumann, A. (1990). The ageing family in crisis: Assessment and decision-making models. *Journal of Advanced Nursing, 15*, 782–787.

Beckman, S., Boxley-Harges, S., Bruick-Sorge, C., & Salmon, B. (2007). Five strategies that heighten nurses' awareness of spirituality to impact client care. *Holistic Nursing Practice, 21*(3), 135–139.

Beckstrand, J. (1980). A critique of several conceptions of practice theory in nursing. *Research in Nursing and Health, 3*, 69–70.

Beddome, G. (1995). Community-as-client assessment: A Neuman-based guide for education and practice. In B. Neuman, *The Neuman Systems Model* (3rd ed., pp. 567–579). Stamford, CT: Appleton & Lange.

Bemker, M. A. (1996). Adolescent female substance abuse: Risk and resiliency factors (drug abuse, marijuana, learned helplessness, dependency). *Dissertation Abstracts International, 57*(12B), 7446. (University Microfilm No. AAG9714858)

Beynon, C. C. (1995). Neuman-based experiences of the Middlesex-London Health Unit. In B. Neuman, *The Neuman Systems Model* (3rd ed., pp. 537–547). Stamford, CT: Appleton & Lange.

Beynon, C. C., & Laschinger, H. K. (1993). Theory-based practice: Attitudes of nursing managers before and after educational sessions. *Public Health Nursing, 10*, 183–188.

Bergstrom, D. (1992). Hypermetabolism in multisystem organ failure: A Neuman systems perspective. *Critical Care Nursing Quarterly, 15*(3), 63–70.

Berkey, K. M., & Hanson, S. M. (1991). *Pocket guide to family assessment and intervention.* St. Louis: Mosby-Year Book.

Bigbee, J. L., & Jansa, N. (1991). Strategies for promoting health protection. *Nursing Clinics of North America, 26*, 895–913.

Bishop, B. D. (2001). Increasing parental knowledge in treatment of childhood fever. *Masters Abstracts International, 40*(06), 1500. Abstract retrieved July 2, 2007, from Dissertation Abstracts Online database.

Bittinger, J. P. (1995). Case management and satisfaction with nursing care of patients hospitalized with congestive heart failure. *Dissertation Abstracts International, 56*(07B), 3688. (University Microfilm No. AAI9537111)

Black, P., Deeny, P., & McKenna, H. (1997). Sensoristrain: An exploration of nursing interventions in the context of the Neuman systems theory. *Intensive and Critical Care Nursing, 13*, 249–258.

Bloch, C., & Bloch, C. (1995). Teaching content and process of the Neuman Systems Model. In B. Neuman, *The Neuman Systems Model* (3rd ed., pp. 175–182). Stamford, CT: Appleton & Lange.

Bowles, L., Oliver, N., & Stanley, S. (1995). A fresh approach . . . Staff in two wards formed a discussion group to create a new people-centred tool of assessment for rehabilitation. *Nursing Times, 91*(1), 40–41.

Bowman, A. M. (1997). Sleep satisfaction, perceived pain and acute confusion in elderly clients undergoing orthopedic procedures. *Journal of Advanced Nursing, 26*, 550–564.

Breckenridge, D. M. (1997a). Decisions regarding dialysis treatment modality: A holistic perspective. *Holistic Nursing Practice, 12*(1), 54–61.

Breckenridge, D. M. (1997b). Patients' perceptions of why, how, and by whom dialysis treatment modality was chosen . . . including commentary by Whittaker, A. A. and Locking-Cusolito, H. with author response. *ANNA Journal, 24*, 313–321.

Bremner, M. N., & Initili, H. (1999, April 8). *Development of an academic and community partnership using the Neuman Systems Model at a large urban hotel.* Paper presented at The 7th Biennial International Neuman Systems Model Symposia, Vancouver, British Columbia, Canada.

Britt, L. (2006). Investigating differences in management of hyperlipidemia: A comparison of nurse practitioners and physicians. *Masters Abstracts International, 44*(06), 2760. Abstract retrieved July 2, 2007, from Dissertation Abstracts Online database.

Brown, F. A. (1994). The effects of an eight-hour affective education program on fear of AIDS and homophobia in student nurses. *Masters Abstracts International, 33*(05), 1487. (University Microfilm No. AAI1361079)

Brown, K. C., Sirles, A. T., Hilyer, J. C., & Thomas, M. J. (1992). Cost-effectiveness of a back school intervention for municipal employees. *Spine, 17*, 1224–1228.

Brown, P. S. (2004). Relationships among life event stress, role and job strain, and sleep in middle-aged female shift workers. *Dissertation Abstracts International, 65*(04B), 1774. Abstract retrieved July 2, 2007, from Dissertation Abstracts Online database.

Bueno, M. M., Redeker, N., & Norman, E. M. (1992). Analysis of motor vehicle crash data in an urban trauma center: Implications for nursing practice and research. *Heart and Lung: Journal of Critical Care, 21*, 558–567.

Bueno, M. M., & Sengin, K. K. (1995). The Neuman Systems Model for critical care nursing. In B. Neuman, *The Neuman Systems Model* (3rd ed., pp. 275–291). Stamford, CT: Appleton & Lange.

Bullock, L. F. C. (1993). Nursing interventions for abused women on obstetrical units. *AWHONN's Clinical Issues in Perinatal and Women's Health Nursing, 4*, 371–377.

Bunn, H. (1995). Preparing nurses for the challenge of the new focus on community mental health nursing. *Journal of Continuing Education in Nursing, 26*(2), 55–59.

Burnett, H. M. (1999). An exploratory study on the perceived health status changes in criminally victimized older adults. *Masters Abstracts International, 38*(02), 418. Abstract retrieved July 2, 2007, from Dissertation Abstracts Online database.

Butrin, J. (1992). Cultural diversity in the nurse–client encounter. *Clinical Nursing Research, 1*, 238–251.

Butts, M. J. (1998). Outcomes of comfort touch in institutionalized elderly female residents (Nursing homes, women). *Dissertation Abstracts International, 59*(07B), 3344. (University Microfilm No. AAG9839828)

Cagle, R. (1996). The relationship between health care provider advice and the initiation of breast-feeding. *Dissertation Abstracts International, 57*(08B), 4974. (University Microfilm No. AAG9700009).

Cammuso, B. S. (1994). *Caring and accountability in nursing practice in Ireland and the United States:*

Helping Irish nurses bridge the gap when they choose to practice in the United States. Unpublished doctoral dissertation, Clark University, UMI PUZ9417668.

Capers, C. F. (1996, September/October). The Neuman Systems Model: A culturally relevant perspective. *The Association of Black Nursing Faculty Journal*, 113–117.

Caplan, G. (1964). *Principles of preventive psychiatry.* New York: Basic Books. [out of print]

Carras, C., & Olsson, H. (1999, April 8). *Exploratory study of student nurse attitudes to humour using Neuman Systems Model analysis.* Paper presented at The 7th Biennial International Neuman Systems Model Symposia, Vancouver, British Columbia, Canada.

Carrigg, K. C., & Weber, R. (1997). Development of the Spiritual Care Scale. *Image: Journal of Nursing Scholarship, 29,* 293.

Casalenuovo, G. A. (2002). Fatigue in diabetes mellitus: Testing a middle range theory of well-being derived from Neuman's theory of optimal client system stability and the Neuman Systems Model. *Dissertation Abstracts International, 63*(05B), 2301. Abstract retrieved July 2, 2007, from Dissertation Abstracts Online database.

Cava, M. A. (1992). An examination of coping strategies used by long-term cancer survivors. *Canadian Oncology Nursing Journal, 2*(3), 99–102.

Cazzell, M. (2008). Linking theory, evidence, and practice in assessment of adolescent inhalant use. *Journal of Addictions Nursing, 19*(1), 17–25.

Cheung, Y. L. (1997). Student forum: The application of Neuman System Model to nursing in Hong Kong. *Hong Kong Nursing Journal, 33*(4), 17–21.

Chilton, L. L. A. (1996). The influence of behavioral cues on immunization practices of elders (influenza). *Dissertation Abstracts International, 57*(09B), 5572. (University Microfilm No. AAG9704005)

Chiverton, P., & Flannery, J. C. (1995). Cognitive impairment: Use of the Neuman Systems Model. In B. Neuman, *The Neuman Systems Model* (3rd ed., pp. 249–261). Stamford, CT: Appleton & Lange.

Chiverton, P., Tortoretti, D., LaForest, M., & Walker, P. H. (1999). Bridging the gap between psychiatric hospitalization and community care: Cost and quality outcomes. *Journal of the American Psychiatric Nurses Association, 5*(2), 46–53.

Chun, A. U. (2006). Issues and concerns of transition from a pediatric healthcare facility to an adult healthcare facility for thalassemia patients. *Masters Abstracts International, 44*(05), 2273. Abstract retrieved July 2, 2007, from Dissertation Abstracts Online database.

Collins, C. R. (1999). The older widow-adult child relationship as an influence upon health promoting behaviors (Healthcare Decisions Questionnaire). *Dissertation Abstracts International, 60*(04B), 1527. (University Microfilm No. AAG9926389)

Collins, M. A. (1996). The relation of work stress, hardiness, and burnout among full-time hospital staff nurses. *Journal of Nursing Staff Development, 12*(2), 81–85.

Cookfair, J. M. (1996). *Nursing care in the community* (2nd ed.). St. Louis: Mosby-Year Book.

Cornu, A. (1957). *The origin of Marxist thought.* Springfield, IL: Thomas. [out of print]

Courchene, V. S., Patalski, E., & Martin, J. (1991). A study of the health of pediatric nurses administering cyclosporine A. *Pediatric Nursing 17,* 497–500.

Cowperthwaite, B., LaPlante, K., Mahon, B., & Markowski, T. (1997). Latex allergy in the nursing population. *Canadian Operating Room Nursing Journal, 15*(2), 23–24, 26–28, 30–32.

Cox, D. D. (1995). *The impact of stress, coping, constructive thinking and hardiness on health and academic performance of female registered nurse students pursuing a baccalaureate degree in nursing.* Unpublished doctoral dissertation, University of Pittsburgh, Pittsburgh, PA.

Craig, D. M. (1995). The Neuman Model: Examples of its use in Canadian educational programs. In B. Neuman, *The Neuman Systems Model* (3rd ed., pp. 521–527). Stamford, CT: Appleton & Lange.

Craig, D. M., & Morris-Coulter, C. (1995). Neuman implementation in a Canadian psychiatric facility. In B. Neuman, *The Neuman Systems Model* (3rd ed., pp. 397–406). Stamford, CT: Appleton & Lange.

Crawford, J., Tarko, M., Ting, B., Gunderson, J., & Andrews, H. (1999, April 8). *The Neuman Systems Model: A conceptual framework for advanced psychiatric/mental health nursing education.* Poster presented at The 7th Biennial International Neuman Systems Model Symposia, Vancouver, British Columbia, Canada.

Cullen, L. M. (1993). Nurses' perceptions of humor as a preventive intervention to promote the health of clients in a health care setting. *Masters Abstracts International, 32*(02), 592. (University Microfilm No. AAG1353482)

Dale, M. L., & Savala, S. M. (1990). A new approach to the senior practicum. *Nursing Connections, 3*(1), 45–51.

Damant, M. (1995). Community nursing in the United Kingdom: A case for reconciliation using the Neuman Systems Model. In B. Neuman, *The Neuman Systems Model* (3rd ed., pp. 607–620). Stamford, CT: Appleton & Lange.

Davidson, J., & Myers, J. (1999, April 8). *Neuman Systems Model: Application to organizational systems.* Poster presented at The 7th Biennial International Neuman Systems Model Symposia, Vancouver, British Columbia, Canada.

Davies, P., & Proctor, H. (1995). In Wales: Using the Model in community mental health nursing. In B. Neuman, *The Neuman Systems Model* (3rd ed., pp. 621–627). Stamford, CT: Appleton & Lange.

de Chardin, P. T. (1955). *The phenomenon of man.* London: Collins. [out of print]

Decker, S. D., & Young, E. (1991). Self-perceived needs of primary caregivers of home-hospice clients. *Journal of Community Health, 8*, 147–154.

Delunas, L. R. (1990). Prevention of elder abuse: Betty Neuman health care systems approach. *Clinical Nurse Specialist, 4*(1), 54–58.

de Meij, J., & de Kuiper, M. (1999, April 7). *The Neuman Systems Model as the basis for the curriculum of the Dutch Reformed College for Higher Education, Department of Nursing.* Paper presented at The 7th Biennial International Neuman Systems Model Symposia, Vancouver, British Columbia, Canada.

Derstine, J. B. (1992). Theory-based advanced rehabilitation nursing: Is it a reality? *Holistic Nursing Practice, 6*(2), 1–6.

DiJoseph, J., & Cavendish, R. (2005). Expanding the dialogue on prayer relevant to holistic care. *Holistic Nursing Practice, 19* (4), 147–154.

Drew, L. L., Craig, D. M., & Beynon, C. E. (1989). The Neuman Systems Model for community health administration and practice: Provinces of Manitoba and Ontario, Canada. In B. Neuman, *The Neuman Systems Model* (2nd ed., pp. 315–341). Norwalk, CT: Appleton & Lange.

Dunn, K. S. (2007). Predictors of self-reported health among older African-American central city adults. *Holistic Nursing Practice, 21*, 237–243.

Edelson, M. (1970). *Sociotherapy and psychotherapy.* Chicago: University of Chicago. [out of print]

Edwards, P. A., & Kittler, A. W. (1991). Integrating rehabilitation content in nursing curricula. *Rehabilitation Nursing, 16*, 70–73.

Eilert-Petersson, E., & Olsson, H. (1999, April 8). *Humor and slimming related to NSM.* Poster presented at The 7th Biennial International Neuman Systems Model Symposia, Vancouver, British Columbia, Canada.

Emery, F. (Ed.). (1969). *Systems thinking.* Baltimore: Penguin Books. [out of print]

Engberg, I. B. (1995). Brief abstracts: Use of the Neuman Systems Model in Sweden. In B. Neuman, *The Neuman Systems Model* (3rd ed., pp. 653–656). Stamford, CT: Appleton & Lange.

Engberg, I. B., Bjälming, E., & Bertilson, B. (1995). A structure for documenting primary health care in Sweden using the Neuman Systems Model. In B. Neuman, *The Neuman Systems Model* (3rd ed., pp. 637–651). Stamford, CT: Appleton & Lange.

Evely, L. (1994). A model for successful breast-feeding. *Modern Midwife, 4*(12), 25–27.

Fawcett, J. (1995). Constructing conceptual-theoretical-empirical structures for research: Future implications for use of the Neuman Systems Model. In B. Neuman, *The Neuman Systems Model* (3rd ed., pp. 459–471). Stamford, CT: Appleton & Lange.

Fawcett, J. (1999, April 9). *An integrative review of Neuman Systems Model-based research.* Paper presented at The 7th Biennial International Neuman Systems Model Symposia, Vancouver, British Columbia, Canada.

Fawcett, J. (2004). Conceptual models of nursing: International scope and substance? The case of the Neuman Systems Model. *Nursing Science Quarterly, 17*, 50–54.

Fawcett, J. (2005). Neuman's systems model. In *Contemporary nursing knowledge: Analysis and evaluation of nursing models and theories* (2nd ed., pp. 166–222). Philadelphia: F. A. Davis.

Fawcett, J., & Giangrande, S. K. (2001). Neuman Systems Model-based research: An integrative review project. *Nursing Science Quarterly, 14*, 231–238.

Fawcett, J., & Giangrande, S. K. (2002). The Neuman Systems Model and research: An integrative review. In B. Neuman, & J. Fawcett (Eds.), *The Neuman Systems Model* (4th ed., pp. 120–149). Upper Saddle River, NJ: Prentice Hall.

Fawcett, J., & Gigliotti, E. (2001). Using conceptual models of nursing to guide nursing research: The case of the Neuman Systems Model. *Nursing Science Quarterly, 14*, 339–345.

Felix, M., Hinds, C., Wolfe, S. C., & Martin, A. (1995). The Neuman Systems Model in a chronic care facility: A Canadian experience. In B. Neuman, *The Neuman Systems Model* (3rd ed., pp. 549–565). Stamford, CT: Appleton & Lange.

Fitzpatrick, J. J., & Whall, A. L. (2005). *Conceptual models of nursing: Analysis and application.* Upper Saddle River, NJ: Prentice Hall.

Flanders-Stepans, M. B., & Fuller, S. G. (1999). Physiological effects of infant exposure to environmental tobacco smoke: A passive observation study. *Journal of Perinatal Education, 8*(1), 10–21.

Flannery, J. (1991). FAMLI-RESCUE: A family assessment tool for use by neuroscience nurses in the acute care setting. *Journal of Neuroscience Nursing, 23,* 111–115.

Flannery, J. (1995). Cognitive assessment in the acute care setting: Reliability and validity of the Levels of Cognitive Functioning Assessment Scale (LOCFAS). *Journal of Nursing Measurement, 3*(1), 43–58.

Foote, A. W., Piazza, D., & Schultz, M. (1990). The Neuman Systems Model: Application to a patient with a cervical spinal cord injury. *Journal of Neuroscience Nursing, 22,* 302–306.

Fowler, B. A., & Risner, P. B. (1994). A health promotion program evaluation in a minority industry. *ABNF Journal, 5*(3), 72–76.

Freese, B. T., Neuman, B., & Fawcett, J. (2002). Guidelines for Neuman Systems Model-based clinical practice. In B. Neuman & J. Fawcett (Eds.), *The Neuman Systems Model* (4th ed., pp. 37–42). Upper Saddle River, NJ: Prentice Hall.

Freiberger, D., Bryant, J., & Marino, B. (1992). The effects of different central venous line dressing changes on bacterial growth in a pediatric oncology population. *Journal of Pediatric Oncology Nursing, 9,* 3–7.

Fulbrook, P. R. (1991). The application of the Neuman systems model to intensive care. *Intensive Care Nursing, 7*(1), 28–39.

Fulton, B. J. (1992). Evaluation of the effectiveness of the Neuman Systems Model as a theoretical framework for baccalaureate nursing program. *Dissertation Abstracts International, 53*(11B), 5641. (University Microfilm No. AAG9305991)

Fukuzawa, M. (1995). Nursing care behaviors which predict patient satisfaction. *Masters Abstracts International, 34*(04), 1547. (University Microfilm No. AAI1378670)

Galloway, D. A. (1993). Coping with a mentally and physically impaired infant: A self-analysis. *Rehabilitation Nursing, 18*(1), 34–36.

Gavigan, M., Kline-O'Sullivan, C., & Klumpp-Lybrand, B. (1990). The effect of regular turning on CABG patients. *Critical Care Nursing Quarterly, 12*(4), 69–76.

Geib, K. M. (2003). The relationships among nursing vigilance by nurses, patient satisfaction with nursing vigilance, and patient length of stay in a surgical cardiac care unit. *Dissertation Abstracts International, 64*(11B), 5448. Abstract retrieved July 2, 2007, from Dissertation Abstracts Online database.

Geiger, P. A. (1996). Participation in a Phase II cardiac rehabilitation program and perceived quality of life. *Masters Abstracts International, 34*(04), 1548. (University Microfilm No. AAI1378753)

Gellner, P., Landers, S., O'Rourke, D., & Schlegel, M. (1994). Community health nursing in the 1990s—Risky business? *Holistic Nursing Practice, 8*(2), 15–21.

George, J. (1997). Nurses' perceived autonomy in a shared governance setting. *Journal of Shared Governance, 3*(2), 17–21.

Gibson, M. (1996). Health promotion for a group of elderly clients. *Perspectives, 20*(3), 2–5.

Gifford, D. K. (1996). Monthly incidence of stroke in rural Kansas. *Kansas Nurse, 71*(5), 3–4.

Gigliotti, E. (1998). You make the diagnosis. Case study: Integration of the Neuman Systems Model with the theory of nursing diagnosis in postpartum nursing . . . including commentary by M. Lunney. *Nursing Diagnosis, The Journal of Nursing Language and Classification, 9*(1), 14, 34–38.

Gigliotti, E. (1999a, April 9) *The use of Neuman's lines of defense and resistance in the published nursing research literature.* Paper presented at The 7th Biennial International Neuman Systems Model Symposia, Vancouver, British Columbia, Canada.

Gigliotti, E. (1999b). Women's multiple role stress: Testing Neuman's flexible line of defense. *Nursing Science Quarterly, 12,* 36–44.

Gigliotti, E. (2002). A theory-based clinical nurse specialist practice exemplar using Neuman's Systems Model and nursing's taxonomies. *Clinical Nurse Specialist: The Journal for Advanced Nursing Practice, 16*(1), 10–16.

Gigliotti, E. (2003). The Neuman Systems Model Institute: Testing middle-range theories. *Nursing Science Quarterly, 16,* 201–206.

Gigliotti, E. (2007). Improving external and internal validity of a model of midlife women's maternal-student role stress. *Nursing Science Quarterly, 20*, 161–170.

Glazebrook, R. S. (1995). The Neuman Systems Model in cooperative baccalaureate nursing education: The Minnesota Inter collegiate Nursing Consortium experience. In B. Neuman, *The Neuman Systems Model* (3rd ed., pp. 227–230). Stamford, CT: Appleton & Lange.

Goble, D. S. (1991). A curriculum framework for the prevention of child sexual abuse (sexual abuse prevention, Neuman systems, Tyler's rationale). *Dissertation Abstracts International, 52*(06A), 2004. (University Microfilm No. AAG9133480)

Goodman, H. (1995). Patients' views count as well. *Nursing Standard, 9*(40), 55.

Graham, J. (2006). Nursing theory and clinical practice: How three nursing models can be incorporated into the care of patients with end stage kidney disease. *The CANNT Journal, 16*(4), 28–31.

Grant, J. S., & Bean, C. A. (1992). Self-identified needs of informal caregivers of head-injured adults. *Family and Community Health, 15*(2), 49–58.

Grant, J. S., Kinney, M. R., & Davis, L. L. (1993). Using conceptual frameworks or models to guide nursing research. *Journal of Neuroscience Nursing, 25*(1), 52–56.

Gray, R. (1998). The lived experience of children, ages 8–12 years, who witness family violence in the home. *Masters Abstracts International, 36*(05), 1327. (University Microfilm No. AAG1389149)

Gulliver, K. M. (1997). Hopelessness and spiritual well-being in persons with HIV infection (immune deficiency). *Masters Abstract International 35*(05), 1374. (University Microfilm No. AAG1385172)

Günüsen N. P., Ustün, B. & Gigliotti, E. (2009). Conceptualization of burnout from the perspective of the Neuman Systems Model. *Nursing Science Quarterly, 22*, 200–204.

Haggart, M. (1993). A critical analysis of Neuman's Systems Model in relation to public health nursing. *Journal of Advanced Nursing, 18*, 1917–1922.

Hainsworth, D. S. (1996). Research briefs. The effect of death education on attitudes of hospital nurses toward care of the dying. *Oncology Nursing Forum, 23*, 963–967.

Hansen, C. S. (2000). Is there a relationship between hardiness and burnout in full-time staff nurses versus per diem nurses? *Masters Abstracts International, 39*(01), 193. Abstract retrieved July 2, 2007, from Dissertation Abstracts Online database.

Hanson, M. S. (1995). *Beliefs, attitudes, subjective norms, perceived behavioral control, and cigarette smoking in white, African-American, and Puerto Rican-American teenage women.* Unpublished doctoral dissertation, University of Pennsylvania, Philadelphia, PA.

Hanson, P. A. (1997). An application of Bowen Family Systems Theory: Triangulation, differentiation of self and nurse manager job stress responses. *Dissertation Abstracts International, 58*(11B), 5889. (University Microfilm No. AAG9815103)

Harper, B. (1992). Nurses' beliefs about social support and the effect of nursing care on cardiac clients' attitudes in reducing cardiac risk factors. *Masters Abstracts International, 31*(01), 273. (University Microfilm No. AAG1349176)

Hassell, J. S. (1996). Improved management of depression through nursing model application and critical thinking. *Journal of the American Academy of Nurse Practitioners, 8*, 161–166.

Hayes, K. V. D. (1994). Diagnostic content validation and operational definitions of risk factors for the nursing diagnosis high risk for disuse syndrome (spinal cord injury). *Dissertation Abstracts International, 55*(12B), 5284. (University Microfilm No. AAI9511772)

Heaman, D. J. (1991). Perceived stressors and coping strategies of parents with developmentally disabled children (stressors). *Dissertation Abstracts International, 52*(12B), 6316. (University Microfilms No. AAG9208071)

Heffline, M. S. (1991). Second place: A comparative study of pharmacological versus nursing interventions in the treatment of postanesthesia shivering—Mary Hanna Memorial Journalism Award winner. *Journal of Post Anesthesia Nursing, 6*, 311–320.

Hemphill, J. C. (2005). Discovering strengths of homeless abused women. *Dissertation Abstracts International, 66*(07B), 3635. Abstract retrieved July 2, 2007, from Dissertation Abstracts Online database.

Henze, R. L. (1993). The relationship among selected stress variables and white blood count in severely head injured patients. *Dissertation Abstracts International, 55*(02B), 365. (University Microfilm No. AAG9419287)

Herald, P. A. (1993). Relationship between hydration status and renal function in patients receiving aminoglycoside antibiotics. *Dissertation Abstracts International, 55*(02B), 365. (University Microfilm No. AAF9419288)

Herrick, C. A., Goodykoontz, L., Herrick, R. H., & Hackett, B. (1991). Planning a continuum of care in child psychiatric nursing: A collaborative effort. *Journal of Child and Adolescent Psychiatric and Mental Health, 4*(2), 41–48.

Heslin, K. (1986). *A systems analysis of the Betty Neuman model.* Unpublished student paper. University of Western Ontario, London, Ontario, Canada.

Higgs, K. T. (1994). Preterm labor risk factors identified in an ambulatory perinatal setting with home uterine activity monitoring support. *Masters Abstracts International, 33*(05), 1490. (University Microfilm No. AAI1360323)

Hilton, S. A., & Grafton, M. D. (1995). Curriculum transition based on the Neuman Systems Model. In B. Neuman, *The Neuman Systems Model* (3rd ed., pp. 163–174). Stamford, CT: Appleton & Lange.

Hiltz, D. (1990). The Neuman Systems Model: An analysis of a clinical situation. *Rehabilitation Nursing, 15,* 330–332.

Hinds, C. (1990). Personal and contextual factors predicting patients' reported quality of life: Exploring congruency with Betty Neuman's assumptions. *Journal of Advanced Nursing, 15,* 456–462.

Holloway, C. (1995). Stress perceived among nurse managers in community health settings. *Masters Abstracts International, 33*(05), 1490. (University Microfilm No. AAI1361519)

Hood, L. J. (1997). The effects of nurse faculty hardiness and sense of coherence on perceived stress, scholarly productivity, and job satisfaction (stress). *Dissertation Abstracts International, 58*(09B), 4720. (University Microfilm No. AAG9809243)

James, B. R. (2001). Wellness program influence on health risk factors and medical costs among Seventh0day Adventist workers. *Dissertation Abstracts International, 62*(08B), 3566. Abstract retrieved July 2, 2007, from Dissertation Abstracts Online database.

Janze, T. R., Watson, D. B., & Stevenson, R. W. D. (1999, April 8). *Quality of life in patients with gender identity disorder.* Paper presented at The 7th Biennial International Neuman Systems Model Symposia, Vancouver, British Columbia, Canada.

Jennings, K. M. (1997). Predicting intention to obtain a pap smear among African-American and Latina women (cervical cancer, cancer prevention). *Dissertation Abstracts International, 58*(07B), 3557. (University Microfilm No. AAG9800878)

Johnson, K. M. (1995). Stressors of local Ontario Nurses' Association presidents. *Masters Abstracts International, 34*(03), 1149. (University Microfilm No. AAI1376934).

Jones, A. M. (2002). The effect of education on adherence with oral iron supplementation among hemodialysis patients. *Masters Abstracts International, 41*(01), 191. Abstract retrieved July 2, 2007, from Dissertation Abstracts Online database.

Jones, W. R. (1996). Stressors in the primary caregivers of traumatic head injured persons. *AXON, 18*(1), 9–11.

Jones-Cannon, S., & Davis, B. L. (2005). Coping among African-American daughters caring for aging parents. *The Association of Black Nursing Faculty Journal, 16*(6), 118–123.

Kahn, E. C. (1992). A comparison of family needs based on the presence or absence of DNR orders. *DCCN: Dimensions of Critical Care Nursing, 11,* 286–292.

Kazakoff, K. J. (1990). The evaluation of return to work and retention of employment of cardiac patients following cardiac rehabilitation programs. *Masters Abstracts International, 29*(03), 450. (University Microfilms No. AAG1343456)

Kido, L. M. (1991). Sleep deprivation and intensive care unit psychosis. *Emphasis: Nursing, 4*(1), 23–33.

Kilchenstein, L., & Yakulis, I. (1984). The birth of a curriculum: Utilization of the Betty Neuman Health Care Systems Model in an integrated baccalaureate program. *Journal of Nursing Education, 23,* 126–127.

Klotz, L. C. (1995). Integration of the Neuman Systems Model into the BSN curriculum at the University of Texas at Tyler. In B. Neuman, *The Neuman Systems Model* (3rd ed., pp. 183–195). Stamford, CT: Appleton & Lange.

Knight, J. B. (1990). The Betty Neuman Systems Model applied to practice: A client with multiple sclerosis. *Journal of Advanced Nursing, 15,* 447–455.

Knox, J. E., Kilchenstein, L., & Yakulis, I. M. (1982). Utilization of the Neuman Model in an integrated baccalaureate program: University of Pittsburgh. In B. Neuman, *The Neuman Systems Model: Application to nursing education and practice* (pp. 117–123). Norwalk, CT: Appleton-Century-Crofts.

Koku, R. V. (1992). Severity of low back pain: A comparison between participants who did and did not receive counseling. *AAOHN Journal, 40*(2), 84–89.

Kottwitz, D., & Bowling, S. (2003). A pilot study of the Elder Abuse Questionnaire. *Kansas Nurse, 78*(7), 4–6. Retrieved May 18, 2007, from the CINAHL Plus Full Text database.

Krajewski, L. L. (2003). Legislators' perceptions of respite care for children with special health care needs having tracheostomies with or without ventilator assistance. *Masters Abstracts International, 42*(05), 1682. Abstract retrieved July 2, 2007, from Dissertation Abstracts Online database.

Kubsch, S., Linton, S. M., Hankerson, C., & Wichowski, H. (2008). Holistic interventions protocol for interstitial cystitis symptom control: A case study. *Holistic Nursing Practice, 22* (4), 183–192.

Lamb, K. A. (1998). Baccalaureate nursing students' perception of empathy and stress in their interactions with clinical instructors: Testing a theory of optimal student system stability according to the Neuman Systems Model. *Dissertation Abstracts International, 60*(03B), 1028. (University Microfilms No. AAG9923301)

Lancaster, D. R. N. (1991). Coping with appraised threat of breast cancer: Primary prevention coping behaviors utilized by women at increased risk. *Dissertation Abstracts International, 53*(01B), 202. (University Microfilms No. AAG9215110).

Lancaster, D. R. N. (2005). Coping with appraised breast cancer risk among women with family histories of breast cancer. *Research in Nursing and Health, 28,* 144–158.

Lapvongwatana, P. (2000). Perinatal risk assessment for low birthweight in Thai mothers: Using the Neuman Systems Model. *Dissertation Abstracts International, 61*(03B), 1325. Abstract retrieved July 2, 2007, from Dissertation Abstracts Online database.

LaReau, R. M. (2000). The effect of an initial clinical nursing experience in a nursing home on associate degree nursing student attitudes toward the elderly. *Masters Abstracts International,*

38(02), 420. Abstract retrieved July 2, 2007, from Dissertation Abstracts Online database.

Larino, E. A. (1997). Determining the level of care provided by the family nurse practitioner during a deployment. *Masters Abstracts International, 35*(05), 1376. (University Microfilms No. AAG1385132)

Laschinger, H. K., & Duff, V. (1991). Attitudes of practicing nurses towards theory-based nursing practice. *Canadian Journal of Nursing Administration, 4*(1), 6–10.

Laszlo, E. (1972). *The systems view of the world: The natural philosophy of the new development in the sciences.* New York: Braziller. [out of print]

Lazarus, R. (1981). The stress and coping paradigm. In C. Eisdorfer, D. Cohen, A. Kleinman, & P. Maxim (Eds.), *Models for clinical psychopathology* (pp. 177–214). New York: SP Medical and Scientific Books.

Lee, F-P. (2005). The relationship of comfort and spirituality to quality of life among long-term care facility residents in southern Taiwan. *Dissertation Abstracts International, 66*(02B), 815. Abstract retrieved July 2, 2007, from Dissertation Abstracts Online database.

Lee, P. L. (1995). Caregiver stress as experienced by wives of institutionalized and in-home dementia husbands. *Dissertation Abstracts International, 56*(06B), 4241. (University Microfilms No. AAI9541861)

Leja, A. M. (1989). Using guided imagery to combat postsurgical depression. *Journal of Gerontological Nursing, 15*(4), 6–11.

Levi, C. (2001). School nurses' asthma knowledge and management, roles and functions. *Masters Abstracts International, 39*(06), 1558. Abstract retrieved July 2, 2007, from Dissertation Abstracts Online database.

Lijauco, C. C. (1997). Factors related to length of stay in coronary artery bypass graft patients. *Masters Abstracts International, 36*(02), 512.

Lile, J. L. (1990). A nursing challenge for the 90's: Reducing risk factors for coronary heart disease in women. *Health Values: Achieving High Level Wellness, 14*(4), 17–21.

Lile, J. L., Pase, M. N., Hoffman, R. G., & Mace, M. K. (1994). The Neuman Systems Model as applied to the terminally ill client with pressure ulcers. *Advances in Wound Care: The Journal for Prevention and Healing, 7*(4), 44–48.

Lin, M., Ku, N., Leu, J., Chen, J., & Lin, L. (1996). An exploration of the stress aspects, coping behaviors, health status and related aspects in family care-givers of hepatoma patients [Chinese]. *Nursing Research [China], 4*(2), 171–185.

Lindell, M., & Olsson, H. (1991). Can combined oral contraceptives be made more effective by means of a nursing care model? *Journal of Advanced Nursing, 16,* 475–479.

Lindgren, A., & Olsson, H. (1999, April 8). *Elderly and humour-An interview study with NSM as reference.* Poster presented at The 7th Biennial International Neuman Systems Model Symposia, Vancouver, British Columbia, Canada.

Loescher, L. J., Clark, L., Attwood, J. R., Leigh, S., & Lamb, G. (1990). The impact of cancer experience on long-term survivors. *Oncology Nursing Forum, 17,* 223–229.

Louis, M. (1989). An intervention to reduce anxiety levels for nurses working with long-term care clients using Neuman's model. In J. P. Riehl-Sisca (Ed.), *Conceptual models for nursing practice* (3rd ed., pp. 95–103). Norwalk, CT: Appleton & Lange.

Louis, M. (1995). The Neuman model in nursing research, an update. In B. Neuman, *The Neuman Systems Model* (3rd ed., pp. 473–495). Stamford, CT: Appleton & Lange.

Louis, M., & Koertvelyessy, A. (1989). The Neuman Model in nursing research. In B. Neuman (Ed.), *The Neuman Systems Model* (2nd ed., pp. 93–113). Norwalk, CT: Appleton & Lange.

Louis, M., Neuman, B., & Fawcett, J. (2002). Guidelines for Neuman Systems Model-based nursing research. In B. Neuman & J. Fawcett (Eds.), *The Neuman Systems Model* (4th ed., pp. 113–119). Upper Saddle River, NJ: Prentice Hall.

Lowry, L. W. (1999, April 8). *Critical pathways and the Neuman Systems Model.* Paper presented at The 7th Biennial International Neuman Systems Model Symposia, Vancouver, British Columbia, Canada.

Lowry, L. W., & Anderson, B. (1993). Neuman's framework and ventilator dependency: A pilot study. *Nursing Science Quarterly, 6,* 195–200.

Lowry, L., Beckman, S., Gehrling, K. R., & Fawcett, J. (2007). Imagining nursing practice: The Neuman Systems Model in 2050. *Nursing Science Quarterly, 20,* 226–229.

Lowry, L. W., & Newsome, G. G. (1995). Neuman-based associate degree programs: Past, present, and future. In B. Neuman, *The Neuman Systems Model* (3rd ed., pp. 197–214). Stamford, CT: Appleton & Lange.

Lowry, L. W., Saeger, J., & Barnett, S. (1997). Client satisfaction with prenatal care and pregnancy outcomes. *Outcomes Management for Nursing Practice, 1*(1), 29–35.

Lunario, R. A. (2004). The relationship between frequent suctioning and the risk of VAP. *Masters Abstracts International, 42*(05), 1682. Abstract retrieved July 2, 2007, from Dissertation Abstracts Online database.

Mackenzie, S. J., & Laschinger, H. K. (1995). Correlates of nursing diagnosis quality in public health nursing. *Journal of Advanced Nursing, 21,* 800–808.

Madrid, E., & Stafanson, D. (1999, April 7). *Diversity and dialogue: Use of the Neuman Systems Model in an RN-BSN curriculum.* Paper presented at The 7th Biennial International Neuman Systems Model Symposia, Vancouver, British Columbia, Canada.

Maligalig, R. M. (1994). Parents' perceptions of the stressors of pediatric ambulatory surgery. *Journal of Post Anesthesia Nursing, 9,* 278–282.

Mann, A. H., Hazel, C., Geer, C., Hurley, C. M., & Podrapovic, T. (1993). Development of an orthopaedic case manager role. *Orthopaedic Nursing, 12*(4), 23–27.

Mannina, J. (1997). Finding an effective hearing testing protocol to identify hearing loss and middle ear disease in school aged children. *Journal of School Nursing, 13*(5), 23–28.

Marlett, L. A. (1998). The breast feeding practices of women with a history of breast cancer. *Masters Abstracts International, 37*(04), 1180. (University Microfilm No. AAG1393760)

Marsh, V. (1997). Job stress and burnout among nurses: The mediational effect of spiritual well-being and hardiness. *Dissertation Abstracts International, 58*(08B), 4142. (University Microfilms No. AAG9804907)

Martin, S. A. (1996). Applying nursing theory to the practice of nurse anesthesia. *AANA Journal, 64,* 369–372.

McCulloch, S. J. (1995). Utilization of the Neuman Systems Model: University of South Australia. In B. Neuman, *The Neuman Systems Model* (3rd ed., pp. 591–597). Stamford, CT: Appleton & Lange.

McGee, M. (1995). Implications for use of the Neuman Systems Model in occupational health nursing. In B. Neuman, *The Neuman Systems Model* (3rd ed., pp. 657–667). Stamford, CT: Appleton & Lange.

McHolm, F. A., & Geib, K. M. (1998). Application of the Neuman Systems Model to teaching health assessment and nursing process. *Nursing Diagnosis: The Journal of Nursing Language and Classification, 9*(1), 23–33.

McMillan, D. E. (1995). Impact of therapeutic support of inherent coping strategies on chronic low back pain: A nursing intervention study. *Masters Abstracts International, 35*(02), 520. (University Microfilms No. AAGMM13363)

Metzger, M. E. (2006). The use of two peripheral intravenous sites in patients undergoing cardiac catheterization with possible percutaneous coronary intervention. *Masters Abstracts International, 45*(01), 285. Abstract retrieved July 2, 2007, from Dissertation Abstracts Online database.

Micevski, V. (1996). Gender differences in the presentation of physiological symptoms of myocardial infarction. *Masters Abstracts International, 35*(02), 520. (University Microfilms No. AAG1382268)

Mill, J. E. (1997). Clinical. The Neuman Systems Model: Application in a Canadian HIV setting. *British Journal of Nursing, 6*, 163–166.

Millard, J. (1992). Health visiting an elderly couple. *British Journal of Nursing, 1*, 772–773.

Miner, J. (1995). Incorporating the Betty Neuman Systems Model into HIV clinical practice. *AIDS Patient Care, 9*(1), 37–39.

Mirenda, R. M. (1995). A conceptual-theoretical strategy for curriculum development in baccalaureate nursing programs. *Dissertation Abstracts International, 56*(10B), 5421. (University Microfilms No. AAI9601825)

Molassiotis, A. (1997). A conceptual model of adaptation to illness and quality of life for cancer patients treated with bone marrow transplants. *Journal of Advanced Nursing, 26*, 572–579.

Monahan, G. L. (1996). A profile of pregnant drug-using female arrestees in California: The relationships among sociodemographic characteristics, reproductive and drug addiction histories, HIV/STD risk behaviors, and utilization of prenatal care services and substance abuse treatment programs (immune deficiency). *Dissertation Abstracts International, 57*(09B), 5576. (University Microfilms No. AAG9704608)

Montgomery, P., & Craig, D. (1990). Levels of stress and health practices of wives of alcoholics. *Canadian Journal of Nursing Research, 22*, 60–70.

Moody, N. B. (1996). Nurse faculty job satisfaction: A national survey. *Journal of Professional Nursing, 12*, 277–288.

Moola, S. (2004). Facilitating conscious awareness among critical care nurses. *Dissertation Abstracts International, 66*(08B), 4155. Abstract retrieved July 2, 2007, from Dissertation Abstracts Online database.

Moola, S., Ehlers, V. J., & Hattingh, S. P. (2008)., Critical care nurses' perceptions of stress and stress-related situations in the workplace. *Curationis, 31*(2), 77–86.

Moore, S. L., & Munro, M. F. (1990). The Neuman System Model applied to mental health nursing of older adults. *Journal of Advanced Nursing, 15*, 293–299.

Morris, D. C. (1991). Occupational stress among home care first line managers. *Masters Abstracts International, 29*(03), 443. (University Microfilms No. AAG1343455)

Moscaritolo, L. M. (2009). Interventional strategies to decrease nursing student anxiety in the clinical learning environment. *Journal of Nursing Education, 48*(1), 17–23.

Musgrave, C. F. (2001). Religiosity, spiritual well-being, and attitudes toward spiritual care of Israeli oncology nurses. *Dissertation Abstracts International, 61*(11B), 5799. Abstract retrieved July 2, 2007, from Dissertation Abstracts Online database.

Mynatt, S. L., & O'Brien, J. (1993). A partnership to prevent chemical dependency in nursing using Neuman's systems model. *Journal of Psychosocial Nursing and Mental Health Services, 31*(4), 27–34.

Mytka, S., & Beynon, C. (1994). A model for public health nursing in the Middlesex-London, Ontario schools. *Journal of School Health, 64*(2), 85–88.

Narsavage, G. L. (1997). Promoting function in clients with chronic lung disease by increasing their perception of control. *Holistic Nursing Practice, 12*(1), 17–26.

Neabel, B. (1998). A comparison of family needs perceived by nurses and family members of acutely brain-injured patients. *Masters Abstracts International, 37*(02), 592. (University Microfilms No. AAGMQ32546)

Neuman, B. (1974). The Betty Neuman health-care systems model: A total person approach to patient problems. In J. P. Riehl & C. Roy (Eds.) *Conceptual models for nursing practice* (pp. 99–114). New York: Appleton-Century-Crofts.

Neuman, B. (1980). The Betty Neuman Health-Care Systems Model: A total person approach to patient problems. In J. P. Riehl & C. Roy (Eds.), *Conceptual models for nursing practice* (2nd ed., pp. 119–134). New York: Appleton-Century-Crofts.

Neuman, B. (1982a). The Neuman health-care systems model: A total approach to client care. In B. Neuman, *The Neuman Systems Model: Application to nursing education and practice*. Norwalk, CT: Appleton-Century-Crofts. [out of print]

Neuman, B. (1982b). *The Neuman Systems Model: Application to nursing education and practice*. Norwalk, CT: Appleton-Century-Crofts.

Neuman, B. (1985). The Neuman Systems Model. *Senior Nurse, 3*(3), 20–23.

Neuman, B. (1989a). The Neuman Nursing Process Format: A family case study. In J. Riehl-Sisca (Ed.), *Conceptual models for nursing practice* (3rd ed., pp. 49–62). Norwalk, CT: Appleton & Lange.

Neuman, B. (1989b). *The Neuman Systems Model* (2nd ed.). Norwalk, CT: Appleton & Lange. [out of print]

Neuman, B. (1990b). Health on a continuum based on the Neuman Systems Model. *Nursing Science Quarterly, 3*, 129–135.

Neuman, B. (1990b). The Neuman Systems Model: A theory for practice. In M. E. Parker (Ed.), *Nursing theories in practice* (pp. 241–261). New York: National League for Nursing.

Neuman, B. (1995). *The Neuman Systems Model* (3rd ed.). Norwalk, CT: Appleton & Lange.

Neuman, B. (2002a). Appendix B: Betty Neuman's autobiography and chronology of the development and utilization of the Neuman Systems Model. In B. Neuman & J. Fawcett (Eds.), *The Neuman Systems Model* (4th ed., pp. 325–396). Upper Saddle River, NJ: Prentice Hall.

Neuman, B. (2002b). Appendix C: Assessment and intervention based on the Neuman Systems Model. In B. Neuman & J. Fawcett (Eds.), *The Neuman Systems Model* (4th ed., pp. 347–350). Upper Saddle River, NJ: Prentice Hall.

Neuman, B. (2002c). The Neuman Systems Model. In B. Neuman & J. Fawcett (Eds.), *The Neuman Systems Model* (4th ed., pp. 3–33). Upper Saddle River, NJ: Prentice Hall.

Neuman, B., & Fawcett, J. (2002). *The Neuman Systems Model* (4th ed.). Upper Saddle River: Prentice Hall.

Neuman, B., Newman, D. M. L., & Holder, P. (2000). Leadership-scholarship integration: Using the Neuman Systems Model for 21st-century professional nursing practice. *Nursing Science Quarterly, 13*, 60–63.

Neuman, B., & Reed, K. S. (2007). A Neuman Systems Model perspective on nursing in 2050. *Nursing Science Quarterly, 20*, 111–113.

Neuman, B. M., & Young, R. J. (1972). A model for teaching total person approach to patient problems. *Nursing Research, 21*, 264–269.

Newman, D. M. L. (2005). A community nursing center for the health promotion of senior citizens based on the Neuman Systems Model. *Nursing Education Perspectives, 26*, 221–223.

Nicholson, C. H. (1995). Clients' perceptions of preparedness for discharge home following total HIP or knee replacement surgery. *Masters Abstracts International, 33*(03), 873. (University Microfilms No. AAI1359739)

Noonill, N., Sindhu, S., Hanucharurnkul, S., & Suwonnaroop, N. (2007). An integrated approach to coordination of community resources improves health outcomes and satisfaction of care of Thai patients with COPD. *Thai Journal of Nursing Research, 11*(2), 118–131.

Norman, S. E. (1990). The relationship between hardiness and sleep disturbances in HIV-infected men. *Dissertation Abstracts International, 51*(10B), 4780. (University Microfilms No. AAG9104437)

Norrish, M. E. (2001). A holistic nursing care approach in an alcohol detoxification unit: A Neuman systems perspective. *Masters Abstracts International, 42*(04), 1243. Abstract retrieved July 2, 2007, from Dissertation Abstracts Online database.

Nortridge, J. A., Mayeux, V., Anderson, S. J., & Bell, M. L. (1992). The use of cognitive style mapping as a predictor for academic success of first-semester diploma nursing students. *Journal of Nursing Education, 31*, 352–356.

Oakes, K. L. (1978). A critique of general systems theory. In A. Putt (Ed.), *General systems theory applied to nursing*. Boston: Little, Brown.

Olsson, H., & Leadersh, E. (1999, April 7). *The retirement process and humor: A Swedish explorative study using Neuman Systems Model analysis*. Paper presented at The 7th Biennial International Neuman Systems Model Symposia, Vancouver, British Columbia, Canada.

O'Neal, C. A. S. (1993). Effects of BSE on depression/anxiety in women diagnosed with breast cancer. *Masters Abstracts International, 31*(04), 1747. (University Microfilms No. AAG1352556)

Orr, J. P. (1993). An adaptation of the Neuman Systems Model to the care of the hospitalized preschool child. *Curationis: South African Journal of Nursing, 16*(3), 37–44.

Orr, J. (1999, April 8). *Using the Neuman Systems Model to develop a training model for caregivers of abandoned children with HIV/AIDS.* Paper presented at The 7th Biennial International Neuman Systems Model Symposia, Vancouver, British Columbia, Canada.

Owens, M. (1995). Care of a woman with Down's syndrome using the Neuman Systems Model. *British Journal of Nursing, 4, British Journal of Disability Nursing,* 752–758.

Parodi, V. A. (1997). Neuman based analysis of women's health needs abroad a deployed Navy ship: Can nursing make a difference? *Dissertation Abstracts International, 58*(12B), 6491. (University Microfilms No. AAG9818848)

Parr, M. S. (1993). The Neuman Health Care Systems Model—An evaluation. *British Journal of Theatre Nursing, 3*(8), 20–27.

Parse, R. R. (1987). *Nursing science—Major paradigms, theories, and critiques.* Philadelphia: Saunders.

Payne, P. L. (1993). A study of the teaching of primary prevention competencies as recommended by the Report of the Pew Health Professions Commission in bachelor of science in nursing programs and associate in nursing programs. *Dissertation Abstracts International, 54*(07B), 3553.

Peirce, A. G., & Fulmer, T. T. (1995). Application of the Neuman Systems Model to gerontological nursing. In B. Neuman, *The Neuman Systems Model* (3rd ed., pp. 293–308). Stamford, CT: Appleton & Lange.

Peoples, L. T. (1990). The relationship between selected client, provider, and agency variables and the utilization of home care services. *Dissertation Abstracts International, 51*(08B), 3782.

Peternelj-Taylor, C. A., & Johnson, R. (1996). Custody and caring: Clinical placement of student nurses in a forensic setting. *Perspectives in Psychiatric Care: The Journal for Nurse Psychotherapists, 32*(4), 23–29.

Peters, M. R. (1997). An exploratory study of job stress and stressors in hospice administration. *Masters Abstracts International, 36*(02), 502. (University Microfilms No. AAG1387515)

Peterson, G. A. (1997). Nursing perceptions of the spiritual dimension of patient care: The Neuman Systems Model in curriculum formations. *Dissertation Abstracts International, 59*(02B), 605. (University Microfilms No. AAG9823988)

Petock, A. M. (1990). Decubitus ulcers and physiological stressors. *Masters Abstracts International, 29*(02), 267. (University Microfilms No. AAG1341348)

Piazza, D., Foote, A., Wright, P., & Holcombe, J. (1992). Neuman Systems Model used as a guide for the nursing care of an 8-year-old child with leukemia. *Journal of Pediatric Oncology Nursing, 9*(1), 17–24.

Picot, S. J., Zauszniewski, J. A., Debanne, S. M., & Holston, E. C. (1999). Mood and blood pressure in black female caregivers and noncaregivers. *Nursing Research, 48*, 150–161.

Picton, C. E. (1995). An exploration of family-centered care in Neuman's model with regard to the care of the critically ill adult in an accident and emergency setting. *Accident and Emergency Nursing, 3*(1), 33–37.

Pierce, J. D., & Hutton, E. (1992). Applying the new concepts of the Neuman Systems Model. *Nursing Forum, 27*(1), 15–18.

Poe, M. S. H. M. (2002). Predictors of spontaneous lacerations in primigravidae. *Dissertation Abstracts International, 63*(10B), 4598. Abstract retrieved July 2, 2007, from Dissertation Abstracts Online database.

Poole, V. L. (1991). Pregnancy wantedness, attitude toward pregnancy, and use of alcohol, tobacco and street drugs during pregnancy. *Dissertation Abstracts International, 52*(10B), 5193.

Poppe, C. A. (2005). A survey of senior level baccalaureate nursing students' beliefs about spirituality and spiritual care. *Masters Abstracts International, 44*(04), 1814. Abstract retrieved July 2, 2007, from Dissertation Abstracts Online database.

Pothiban, L. (1993). Risk factor prevalence, risk status, and perceived risk for coronary heart disease among Thai elderly. *Dissertation Abstracts International, 54*(03B), 1337. (University Microfilms No. AAG9319896)

Puetz, R. (1990). *Nurse and patient perception of stressors associated with coronary artery bypass surgery.* Unpublished thesis, University of Nevada, Las Vegas.

Putt, A. (1972). Entropy, evolution and equifinality in nursing. In J. Smith (Ed.), *Five years of cooperation to improve curricula in western schools of nursing.* Boulder, CO: Western Interstate Commission for Higher Education.

Radwanski, M. (1992). Self-medicating practices for managing chronic pain after spinal cord injury. *Rehabilitation Nursing, 17*, 312–318.

Ramsey, B. A. (1999). Can a multidisciplinary team decrease hospital length of stay for elderly trauma patients? *Masters Abstracts International, 37*(04), 1182.

Reed, K. S. (1993). Adapting the Neuman Systems Model for family nursing. *Nursing Science Quarterly, 6*, 93–97.

Reed, K. (1999, April 9). *Using Neuman's variables as a map for concept analysis.* Paper presented at The 7th Biennial International Neuman Systems Model Symposia, Vancouver, British Columbia, Canada.

Reed, K. S. (2003). Grief is more than tears. *Nursing Science Quarterly, 16*, 77–81.

Reeves, A. L. (2004). Childhood experiences of Appalachian women who have experienced intimate partner violence during adulthood. *Dissertation Abstracts International, 65* (10B), 5076. Abstract retrieved July 2, 2007, from Dissertation Abstracts Online database.

Ridgell, N. H. (1993). Home apnea monitoring: A systems approach to the family's home care needs. *Caring, 12*(12), 34–37.

Riley-Lawless, K. (2000). The relationship among characteristics of the family environment and behavioral and physiologic cardiovascular risk factors in parents and their adolescent twins. *Dissertation Abstracts International, 61*(03B), 1328. Abstract retrieved July 2, 2007, from Dissertation Abstracts Online database.

Roberts, A. G. (1994). Effective inservice education process. *Oklahoma Nurse, 39*(4), 11.

Roberts, M. C. (2002). The relationships among hospital staff nurses' occupational stress, caring behaviors, and spiritual well-being. *Dissertation Abstracts International, 63*(10B), 4598. Abstract retrieved July 2, 2007, from Dissertation Abstracts Online database.

Robinson, C. A. (1998). The difference in perception of quality of life in patients one year after an infrainguinal bypass for critical limb ischemia. *Masters Abstracts International, 37*(03), 914. (University Microfilms No. AAG13922664)

Robinson-Lewis, P. E. (2004). Middle to older West Indian Canadian adults diagnosed with type two diabetes: Perceptions of stressors related to complying with treatment regimen. *Masters Abstracts International, 43*(03), 823. Abstract retrieved July 2, 2007, from Dissertation Abstracts Online database.

Rodrigues-Fisher, L., Bourguignon, C., & Good, B. V. (1993). Dietary fiber nursing intervention: Prevention of constipation in older adults. *Clinical Nursing Research, 2*, 464–477.

Roggensack, J. (1994). The influence of perioperative theory and clinical in a baccalaureate nursing program on the decision to practice perioperative nursing. *Prairie Rose, 63*(2), 6–7.

Rohr, K. M. (2006). Alcohol use and injury-related outcomes in older rural trauma patients. *Dissertation Abstracts International, 67*(09B), 4982. Abstract retrieved July 2, 2007, from Dissertation Abstracts Online database.

Rosenfeld, R. M., Goldsmith, A. J., & Madell, J. R. (1998). How accurate is parent rating of hearing for children with otitis media? *Archives of Otolaryngology-Head Neck Surgery, 124*, 989–992.

Ross, M. M., Bourbonnais, F. F., & Carroll, G. (1987). Curricular design and the Betty Neuman Systems Model: A new approach to learning. *International Nursing Review, 34*(3/273), 75–79.

Rowe, M. L. (1989). The relationship of commitment and social support to the life satisfaction of caregivers to patients with Alzheimer's disease. *Dissertation Abstracts International, 51*(04B), 1747. Abstract retrieved July 2, 2007, from Dissertation Abstracts Online database.

Rowles, C. J. (1992). The relationship of selected personal and organizational variables and the tenure of directors of nursing in nursing homes. *Dissertation Abstracts International, 53*(09B), 4593. (University Microfilms No. AAG9302488)

Russell, J., & Hezel, L. (1994). Role analysis of the advanced practice nurse using the Neuman Health Care Systems Model as a framework. *Clinical Nurse Specialist, 8*, 215–220.

Russell, J., Hileman, J. W., & Grant, J. S. (1995). Assessing and meeting the needs of home caregivers using the Neuman Systems Model. In B. Neuman, *The Neuman Systems Model* (3rd ed., pp. 331–341). Stamford, CT: Appleton & Lange.

Sabatini, C. L. (2003). The meaning of the lived experience of adolescent pregnancy to women who gave birth during their teens: A phenomenological study. *Dissertation Abstracts International, 64*(02B), 987. Abstract retrieved July 2, 2007, from Dissertation Abstracts Online database.

Sabo, C. E., & Michael, S. R. (1996). The influence of personal message with music on anxiety and side effects associated with chemotherapy. *Cancer Nursing, 19*, 283–289.

Samuels-Dennis, J. A. (2004). Assessing stressful life events, psychological well-being and coping styles in sole-support parents. *Masters Abstracts International, 42* (05), 1685. Abstract retrieved July 2, 2007, from Dissertation Abstracts Online database.

Scalzo-Tarrant, T. (1992). Improving the frequency and proficiency of breast self examination. *Masters Abstracts International, 31*(03), 1211. (University Microfilms No. AAG1351247)

Scicchitani, B., Cox, J. G., Heyduk, L. J., Maglicco, P. A., & Sargent, N. A. (1995). Implementing the Neuman Model in a psychiatric hospital. In B. Neuman, *The Neuman Systems Model* (3rd ed., pp. 387–395). Stamford, CT: Appleton & Lange.

Schlentz, M. D. (1993). The Minimum Data Set and levels of prevention in the long-term care facility. *Geriatric Nursing: American Journal of Care for the Aging, 14,* 79–83.

Selye, H. (1950). *The physiology and pathology of exposure to stress.* Montreal, Quebec, Canada: ACTA.

Semple, O. D. (1995). The experiences of family members of persons with Huntington's Disease. *Perspectives, 19*(4), 4–10.

Shaw, M. C. (1991). A theoretical base for orthopaedic nursing practice: The Neuman Systems Model. *CONA Journal ACIIO, 13* (2), 19–21.

Sheridan, M. N. (2005). Students' perceptions of their learning experiences in a newly developed diploma program for practical nurses. *Masters Abstracts International, 43*(05), 1704. Abstract retrieved July 2, 2007, from Dissertation Abstracts Online database.

Silveira, D. T. (2000). Process of work-health-disease intervention based on Betty Neuman Systems Model [Portuguese]. *Revista Gaucha de Enfermagem, 21*(1), 31–43. Abstract retrieved May 18, 2007, from CINAHL Plus with Full Text database.

Simmons, L., & Borgdon, C. (1991). The clinical nurse specialists in HIV care. *Kansas Nurse, 66*(1), 6–7.

Simpson, E. M. (2000). Condom use among Black women: A theoretical basis for HIV prevention guide by Neuman Systems Model and Theory of Planned Behavior. *Dissertation Abstracts International, 61*(10B), 5240. Abstract retrieved July 2, 2007, from Dissertation Abstracts Online database.

Skalski, C. A., DiGerolamo, L., & Gigliotti, E. (2006). Stressors in five client populations: Neuman Systems Model-based literature review. *Journal of Advanced Nursing, 56*(1), 69–78.

Skipwith, D. H. (1994). Telephone counseling interventions with caregivers of elders. *Journal of Psychosocial Nursing and Mental Health Services, 32*(3), 7–12.

South, L. D. (1995). The relationship of self-concept and social support in school age children with leukemia. *Dissertation Abstracts International, 56*(04B), 1939. (University Microfilms No. AAI9527022)

Speck, B. J. (1990). The effect of guided imagery upon first semester nursing students performing their first injections. *Journal of Nursing Education, 29,* 346–350.

Stittich, E. M., Flores, F. C., & Nuttall, P. (1995). Cultural considerations in a Neuman-based curriculum. In B. Neuman, *The Neuman Systems Model* (3rd ed., pp. 147–162). Stamford, CT: Appleton & Lange.

Strickland-Seng, V. (1995). The Neuman Systems Model in clinical evaluation of students. In B. Neuman, *The Neuman Systems Model* (3rd ed., pp. 215–225). Stamford, CT: Appleton & Lange.

Stuart, G. W., & Wright, L. K. (1995). Applying the Neuman Systems Model to psychiatric nursing practice. In B. Neuman, *The Neuman Systems Model* (3rd ed., pp. 263–273). Stamford, CT: Appleton & Lange.

Taggart, L., & Mattson, S. (1996). Delay in prenatal care as a result of battering in pregnancy: Cross-cultural implications. *Health Care for Women International, 17*(1), 25–34.

Tarko, M., & Crawford, J. (1999, April 8). *Spirituality: The core dimension of the Neuman Systems Model applied to health assessment in psychiatric nursing education.* Paper presented at The 7th Biennial International Neuman Systems Model Symposia, Vancouver, British Columbia, Canada.

Tarmina, M. S. (1992). Self-selected diet of adult women with families. *Dissertation Abstracts International, 53*(02B), 0777.

Thygesen, K. H., & Esbensen, B. A. (2008). A rehabilitation trajectory for patients with lung cancer—Part II [Danish]. *Klinisk Sygepleje, 22*(2), 64–77. Abstract in English retrieved November 30, 2009, from CINAHL Plus with Full Text database.

Timmermans, O. (1999, April 7). *A practical guideline for the implementation of the Neuman Systems Model in an Institute for Mental Health Care.* Paper presented at The 7th Biennial International Neuman Systems Model Symposia, Vancouver, British Columbia, Canada.

Toot, J., Amaya, M. A., & Memmott, R. J. (1999, April 10). *Interdisciplinary applications: Neuman Systems Model as a conceptual paradigm for interdisciplinary team.* Paper presented at The 7th Biennial International Neuman Systems Model Symposia, Vancouver, British Columbia, Canada.

Trépanier, M., Dunn, S. I., & Sprague, A. E. (1995). Application of the Neuman Systems Model to perinatal nursing. In B. Neuman, *The Neuman Systems Model* (3rd ed., pp. 309–320). Stamford, CT: Appleton & Lange.

Tweed, S. A. (1999). Affective and biological responses to the inhalation of the essential oil lavender (Lavandula angustifolia, Aromatherapy). *Masters Abstracts International, 38*(04), 986. Abstract retrieved July 2, 2007, from Dissertation Abstracts Online database.

Ume-Nwagbo, P. N., DeWan, S. A., & Lowry, L. W. (2006). Using the Neuman Systems Model for best practices. *Nursing Science Quarterly, 19,* 31–35.

Vaughan, B., & Gough, P. (1995). Use of the Neuman Systems Model in England. In B. Neuman, *The Neuman Systems Model* (3rd ed., pp. 599–605). Stamford, CT: Appleton & Lange.

Verberk, F. (1995). In Holland: Application of the Neuman Model in psychiatric nursing. In B. Neuman, *The Neuman Systems Model* (3rd ed., pp. 629–636). Stamford, CT: Appleton & Lange.

Vitthuhn, K. M. (1999). Delivery of analgesics for the postoperative thoracotomy patient. *Masters Abstracts International, 37*(04), 1185. (University Microfilms No. AAG1393446)

von Bertalanffy, L. (1968). *General system theory.* New York: Braziller. [out of print]

Waddell, K. L., & Demi, A. S. (1993). Effectiveness of an intensive partial hospitalization program for treatment of anxiety disorders. *Archives of Psychiatric Nursing, 7*(1) 2–10.

Walker, P. H. (1994). Dollars and sense in health reform: Interdisciplinary practice and community nursing centers. *Nursing Administration Quarterly, 19*(1), 1–11.

Walker, P. H. (1995). Neuman-based education, practice, and research in a community nursing center. In B. Neuman, *The Neuman Systems Model* (3rd ed., pp. 415–430). Stamford, CT: Appleton & Lange.

Ware, L. A., & Shannahan, M. K. (1995). Using Neuman for a stable parent support group in neonatal intensive care. In B. Neuman, *The Neuman Systems Model* (3rd ed., pp. 321–330). Stamford, CT: Appleton & Lange.

Waters, T. (1993). Self-efficacy, change, and optimal client stability. *Addictions Nursing Network, 5*(2), 48–51.

Watson, L. A. (1991). Comparison of the effects of usual, support, and informational nursing interventions on the extent to which families of critically ill patients perceive their needs were met. *Dissertation Abstracts International, 52*(06B), 2999. (University Microfilms No. AAG9134244)

Weinberger, S. L. (1991). Analysis of a clinical situation using the Neuman Systems Model. *Rehabilitation Nursing, 16,* 278, 280–281.

Westrik, G. J. (1999, April 9). *Addiction and spiritual well being in the health perspective of the Neuman Systems Model.* Paper presented at The 7th Biennial International Neuman Systems Model Symposia, Vancouver, British Columbia, Canada.

Wilkey, S. F. (1990). The effects of an eight-hour continuing education course on the death anxiety levels of registered nurses. *Masters Abstracts International, 28*(04), 480. (University Microfilms No. AAG1340601)

Williamson, J. W. (1992). The effects of ocean sounds on sleep after coronary artery bypass graft surgery. *American Journal of Critical Care, 1*(1), 91–97.

Wright, J. G. (1996). The impact of preoperative education on health locus of control, self-efficacy, and anxiety for patients undergoing total joint replacement surgery. *Masters Abstracts International, 35*(01), 216. (University Microfilms No. AAG1382185)

Wullschleger, L. A. (1999). Fetal infant mortality in Kalamazoo (Michigan). *Masters Abstracts International, 38*(02), 422. Abstract retrieved July 2, 2007, from Dissertation Abstracts Online database.

Young, L. M. (2000). The effects of guided mental imagery on the blood pressure of clients experiencing mild to moderate essential hypertension. *Dissertation Abstracts International, 61*(02B), 787. Abstract retrieved July 2, 2007, from Dissertation Abstracts Online database.

Zavala-Onyett, N. D. (2001). The impact of a school-based health clinic on school absence. *Masters Abstracts International, 39*(04), 1134. Abstract retrieved July 2, 2007, from Dissertation Abstracts Online database.

Annotated Bibliography[*]

Barker, E., Robinson, D., & Brautigan, R. (1999). The effect of psychiatric home nurse follow-up on readmission rates of patients with depression. *Journal of the American Psychiatric Nurses Association, 5*(4), 111–116.

This study used the Neuman Systems Model as a conceptual framework to study hospital readmission rates of patients with depression in those who had home follow-up visits by psychiatric nurses and those who did not. Findings included a substantial reduction in hospital readmissions in the group that received the in-home visits, even though both groups received similar outpatient care.

Black, P., Deeny, P., & McKenna, H. (1997). Sensoristrain: An exploration of nursing interventions in the context of the Neuman systems theory. *Intensive and Critical Care Nursing, 13,* 249–258.

This paper describes the use of the Neuman Systems Model to create a framework for nursing practice using prevention-as-intervention in comfort care, knowing the patient, and therapeutic presence of the nurse to reduce sensory strain in intensive care patients. It seeks to link nursing actions with patient outcomes.

Chiverton, P., Tortoretti, D., LaForest, M., & Walker, P. H. (1999). Bridging the gap between psychiatric hospitalization and community care: Cost and quality outcomes. *Journal of the American Psychiatric Nurses Association, 5*(2), 46–53.

This study investigated quality indicators, patient satisfaction, and costs of care related to recidivism and rehospitalization in psychiatric patients who received transitional case management services and those who received traditional care. No differences in levels of depression or in mental status were found between the groups. Those who received the transitional care management expressed high levels of satisfaction had much lower readmission and emergency department visit rates. The costs of providing the transitional case management were significantly less than the costs for readmission and emergency department visits.

Gigliotti, E. (1999). Women's multiple role stress: Testing Neuman's flexible line of defense. *Nursing Science Quarterly, 12,* 36–44.

This study used the Neuman Systems Model as conceptual framework to investigate the relations between a stressor (multiple roles: maternal and student roles), flexible line of defense (perceived social support), and normal line of defense (perceived multiple role stress). Statistically significant findings included that social support helped explain multiple role stress in women aged 37 and older. This group of women broadened its social support network, including support from children, friends at school, work associates, and clergy. Support from husband was inversely associated with multiple role stress in both the younger and older groups of women.

Hanson, M. J. (1999). Cross-cultural study of beliefs about smoking among teenaged females. *Western Journal of Nursing Research, 21,* 635–651.

This study used the Neuman Systems Model as a conceptual framework to study smoking behavior in African American, Puerto Rican, and non-Hispanic White females, aged 13 to 19. Statistically significant relations between beliefs and smoking behavior in each ethnic group were found. The specific beliefs differed among the groups.

Jones, W. R. (1996). Stressors in the primary caregivers of traumatic head injured patients. *AXON, 18*(1), 9–11.

This study used the Neuman Systems Model to identify intrapersonal, interpersonal, and extrapersonal stressors in individuals who are primary caregivers for persons who have suffered a traumatic head injury. While stressors in all three categories were identified, only intrapersonal and interpersonal stressors were positively correlated with changing levels of stress.

McHolm, F. A., & Geib, K. M. (1998). Application of the Neuman Systems Model to teaching health assessment and nursing process. *Nursing Diagnosis: The Journal of Nursing Language and Classification, 9*(1), 23–33.

Faculty developed a nursing theory framework for teaching health assessment to beginning-level baccalaureate nursing students. The faculty

---

[*] Selected material published in English since 1995.

concluded that students who could make connections between the Neuman Systems Model
and NANDA nursing diagnoses within the
nursing process would be able to make better
choices about appropriate nursing diagnoses.

Marsh, V., Beard, M. T., & Adams, B. N. (1999). Job
stress and burnout: The mediational effect of
spiritual well-being and hardiness among
nurses. *Journal of Theory Construction and
Testing, 3*(1), 13–19.

An empirical test of a model developed from NSM
and Selye's stress theory. Results supported that
job stress had a direct positive effect on burnout
among nurses, while spiritual well-being had a
direct negative effect. When operating through
hardiness, spiritual well-being had an indirect
negative effect on burnout. The study supported
the inclusion of spiritual well-being in considering job burnout.

Molassiotis, A. (1997). A conceptual model of
adaptation to illness and quality of life for cancer patients treated with bone marrow transplants. *Journal of Advanced Nursing, 26,* 572–579.

The Neuman Systems Model provides the basis
for this model of adaptation to illness and the
resultant quality of life in cancer patients who
receive bone marrow transplants. The model
has five stages. The first stage begins with the
stressor or initial stimuli and the perception of
that stressor as a threat. The second stage involves the reaction to the threat producing
stressor. The third stage describes the adaptive
or maladaptive coping activities related to
dealing with the illness as a threat. The fourth
stage includes nursing care using prevention-
as-interventions. The fifth stage is the level of
adaptation—from adaptation to illness and
satisfaction with life to maladjustment and
low quality of life. Included in each of these
stages are the personal variables (physiological, psychological, social, development). It
should be noted that the spiritual variable is
not described.

Moody, N. B. (1996). Nurse faculty job satisfaction: A national survey. *Journal of Professional
Nursing, 12,* 277–288.

In a survey of nursing faculty in universities offering a doctorate of nursing, the Neuman
Systems Model was used with other theories to
construct a system's framework to investigate job satisfaction of nursing faculty.
Demographic variables were significantly
correlated with measures of job satisfaction.
The contributors to a regression model of nursing faculty job satisfaction were salary, degree
level of nursing student taught, and the length
of the annual contract for faculty.

Narsavage, G. L. (1997). Promoting function in
clients with chronic lung disease by increasing
their perception of control. *Holistic Nursing
Practice, 12*(1), 17–26.

The Neuman Systems Model provided the format
for assessing persons with chronic obstructive
pulmonary disease and developing their
perception of control as a secondary prevention-
as-intervention. Control is defined as an intrapersonal component that interacts with the
physiologic, sociocultural, developmental, and
spiritual variables to affect stability. Methods
included in the secondary prevention-as-intervention include use of assessment tools, diaries, relaxation, and other stress management
techniques.

Newman, D. M. L. (2005). A community nursing
center for the health promotion of senior citizens based on the Neuman Systems Model.
Nursing Education Perspectives, (26), 221–223.

This article described a community nursing center
in which care in based on the Neuman Systems
Model (NSM). The center was established to
meet health promotion needs for senior citizens.
Students, both undergraduate and graduate,
from two schools of nursing have experience in
the center so comprehensive documentation
was vital. Forms, based on the NSM, were designed and consistently used. Having practice
based on the NSM aided this consistency, even
with changing student populations. This project
has helped demonstrate the utility of the NSM
for education, practice, and research.

Picot, S. J., Zauszniewski, J. A., Debanne, S. M., &
Holston, E. C. (1999). Mood and blood pressure in Black female caregivers and noncaregivers. *Nursing Research, 48,* 150–161.

This study investigated the relationship between
the mood symptoms of anger, anxiety, and sadness and ambulatory daytime blood pressure
in a group of Black female caregivers of a dependent elder and in a group of noncaregivers.
The findings indicated a negative relationship
between anger and diastolic blood pressure,
leading to a recommendation for further study
of whether low anger scores represent low levels of perceived anger or suppressed anger.

Reed, K. S. (2003). Grief is more than tears. *Nursing Science Quarterly, 16,* 77–81.

This concept analysis of grief recognizes the difficulty of measuring grief due to its individual nature and vagueness about what is normal. The use of a nursing model (the Neuman Systems Model) helped to define areas of assessment and assisted in identifying appropriate outcome measures. It also assisted in creating a nursing perspective from work in other disciplines.

Sabo, C. E., & Michael, S. R. (1996). The influence of personal message with music on anxiety and side effects associated with chemotherapy. *Cancer Nursing, 19,* 283–289.

This pilot study investigated the use of a recorded message with a musical background to reduce anxiety and side effects in persons receiving chemotherapy. There was no significant difference in the severity of side effects between the experimental and control groups. Those in the experimental group did demonstrate statistically significant lower levels of state anxiety.

Skalski, C. A., DiGerolamo, L., & Gigliotti, E. (2006). Stressors in five client populations: Neuman Systems Model-based literature review. *Journal of Advanced Nursing, 56*(1), 69–78.

The Neuman Systems Model Research Institute chose stressors as the concept for its initial collaborative research project. Eighty-seven published studies, published between 1983 and February 2005, were identified through the use of the institute's bibliography developed by Jacqueline Fawcett and a CINAHL review using "Neuman systems model" and "stressors" as key words. Of these 87 studies, 13 were identified as "stressor studies." Within these studies, five client populations were identified: caregivers, cancer survivors, patients in intensive care units, recipients of care, and parents of children having day surgery. Data were most often collected using investigator developed interview guides. Evidence was found of stressors being categorized as intra-, inter- or extrapersonal. Identified stressor were burden of responsibility for the caregivers, awareness of vulnerability for the cancer survivors, being overwhelmed for the ICU patients, loss of control for the parents, and frustration with role changes for the recipients of care. The authors indicate that these findings can be the basis for nursing practice and for future collaborative research. They suggest the middle range theory of caregiver role strain could be tested empirically.

The reader is encouraged to seek information from Dissertation Abstracts International and CINAHL, either in print or online, about the multitude of thesis and dissertation reports, journal articles, and book chapters that demonstrate the use of the Neuman Systems Model in research, practice, and education. The numbers are too great to be included in this annotation.

CHAPTER 15

Other Theories from the 1970s

Julia B. George

During the 1970s additional theories were proposed. Those initially published in this period were Joan Riehl-Sisca's interaction model, Kathryn E. Barnard's Child Health Assessment Interaction Model (known then as Parent–Child Interaction Model), and Josephine G. Paterson and Loretta Zderad's Humanistic Nursing. Of these, the works of Barnard and Paterson and Zderad have continued to be developed and used by others. This chapter will focus on the Child Health Assessment Interaction Model and on Humanistic Nursing.

CHILD HEALTH ASSESSMENT INTERACTION MODEL

Kathryn E. Barnard

Kathryn E. Barnard was born in 1938 in Omaha, Nebraska. She received her bachelor's degree in nursing from the University of Nebraska, Omaha, in 1960; master's degree in nursing from Boston University, Massachusetts in 1962; and Ph.D. in early childhood development from the University of Washington, Seattle, in 1972. Her career has been in nursing education (at the University of Nebraska and the University of Washington) and research. She is Professor Emeritus of Family and Child Nursing, School of Nursing, and research affiliate, Center on Human Development and Disability, at the University of Washington (http://depts.washington.edu/chdd/mrddrc/res_aff/ barnard.html, accessed November 6, 2007). Her research has focused on infant-toddler development (Barnard, 1972; Barnard & Eyres, 1979; Kelly, Morisset, Barnard, & Patterson, 1996; Lobo, Barnard, & Coombs, 1992; Wacharasin & Barnard, 2001; Wacharasin, Barnard, & Spieker, 2003), parent–infant interaction (Barnard, 1999, 2007; Elliott, Drummond, & Barnard, 1996; Foss, Hirose, & Barnard, 1999), program models for intervention with young families (Barnard & Powell, 1972; Barnard et al., 1977; Solchany & Barnard, 2001; Thomas, Barnard, & Sumner, 1993), and postpartum depression (Jolley, Elmore, Barnard, & Carr, 2007). She is credited with developing the Feeding and Teaching Scales to assess parent–child interaction and the Nursing Child Assessment Satellite Training (NCAST) program to provide preparation in the appropriate use of the scales.

Her honors include an honorary doctorate from the University of Nebraska; the National League for Nursing Lucille Petry Leone Award for teaching (1969); induction as a fellow, American Academy of Nursing (AAN) (1975); named Maternal and Child Health Nurse of the Year by the American Nurses Association (ANA) (1984); election to the Institute of Medicine (1985); named Nurse Scientist of the Year by the ANA (1987); recipient of the T B Brazelton Lectureship Award from the American Association for the Care of Children's Health (1992); recipient of the Gustav O. Leinhard Award from the Institute of Medicine (2002); Sigma Theta Tau International's Episteme Award (2003); and named as a Living Legend by the AAN (2006). She was the first woman to deliver the Annual Faculty Lecture at the University of Washington (1985) and was the second person to be named Spence Professor of Nursing in the UW School of Nursing.

PARENT–CHILD INTERACTION   During the 1970s Barnard led the research team that conducted the federally funded Nursing Child Assessment Project and developed the NCAST program to disseminate their results (Barnard et al., 1977). Barnard's (2004) own description of her work states that her

> . . . interests have been in the primary relationship of the child and parent, usually the mother as the primary caregiver . . . we theorize that children learn through daily experiences that either there is or is not help available when they are distressed. A child, whose experience is characterized by getting the help needed when distressed, develops the trust needed to move on to further developmental challenges . . . we realize the young child's brain does not have the capacity to regulate strong negative emotions (distress). It is an important role for the caregiver to provide presence, comfort, and containment of those negative emotions since the infant cannot easily shut down the activation of the sympathetic system. Unfortunately some infants have parents with difficulty even recognizing the distress cues of the infant, let alone being able to provide the comfort the infant needs. It has been reported these unresponsive parents [sic] own cries, when they were infants, where [sic] infrequently attended causing them to repress that state; and therefore when in the role of parents themselves, they do not even hear their own child's crying. (p. 49)

CONCEPTS OF CHILD HEALTH ASSESSMENT INTERACTION MODEL   The Child Health Assessment Interaction Model (CHAIM) has four major components, as shown in Figure 15-1. They are the *child*, the *caregiver*, the *environment*, and *interaction*. The child is generally identified as no older than age three. The concepts related to child are *temperament* and *regulation*; to caregiver are *physical health, mental health, coping,* and *educational level*; to environment are *resources, inanimate,* and *animate*; and to interaction are, for the parent, *sensitivity to cues, fostering of emotional growth,* and *fostering of cognitive growth* and, for the infant, *clarity of cues given* and *responsiveness to parent.*

The *temperament* of the child includes maturity level, neurological status, activity, responsiveness to external stimuli, alertness, habituation, and irritability (Barnard & Eyres, 1979). *Regulation* refers to the child's ability to be self-calming and to evoke desired responses from caregivers. The caregiver's *physical and mental health* in the model have been essentially by self-report, *coping* involves the ability to respond to novel or stressful situations, and *educational level* has been measured by years of schooling. Educational level could be broadened to include more informal sources of education; however, Barnard and Eyres (1979) indicate that most studies of development have not supported that the mother's level of education makes a significant difference in the

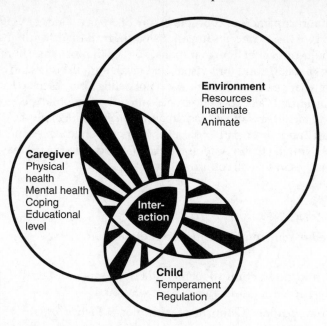

FIGURE 15-1 Child Health Assessment Interaction Model. *(From Sumner, G., & Spietz, A. (Eds). (1994). NCAST caregiver/ parent-child teaching manual (p. 3). Seattle: NCAST Publications, University of Washington School of Nursing. Used with permission.)*

child's development. The *inanimate environment* involves the nonsocial aspects that can impact the senses, such as space, materials, toys, sounds, richness, or deprivation (Barnard & Eyres, 1979); the *animate environment* represents the social aspects—in the model these aspects are most clearly represented by the caregiver portion of the interaction; *resources* in the environment represent what is available to support or hinder the relationship, including other people and finances. In interaction, *sensitivity to cues* involves the appropriateness of the caregiver's response to cues initiated by the child, and *fostering emotional growth* involves affectionate play, social interaction (such as that associated with feeding), and reinforcement of desirable social behavior, all at a developmentally appropriate level; *fostering cognitive growth* involves providing appropriate stimulation to enhance the child's understanding; in general, appropriate stimulation will involve activities just beyond the child's current level of understanding. The *clarity of the child's cues* influences the caregiver's ability to respond correctly to the child's needs. For example, consider the difference in the responses of the mother who says, "Oh, that is his hungry cry" or "That is his sleepy cry." Just as clearly different cues require different responses from the caregiver, the infant also needs to make different behavioral modifications to the differing parental responses (*responsiveness to parent*). When the hungry baby is picked up by her mother, she stops crying and begins nuzzling for food; when the tired baby is placed in her crib, she settles down to sleep.

METAPARADIGM, RESEARCH, AND PRACTICE WITH CHILD HEALTH ASSESSMENT INTERACTION   Because Barnard's goal was a model of interaction in relation to child development, she did not present her work in the framework of a nursing theory and thus did not define the four metaparadigm concepts in any one place. Fine et al. (1998) were able to identify definitions of these concepts in various works by Barnard. Nursing was defined as "the diagnosis and treatment of human responses to health problems"; humans described as having the ability "to take in auditory, visual, and tactile stimuli but also to make meaningful associations from what he takes in"; health was not defined but discussed as important; and environment as including "all experiences encountered by the child: people, objects, places, sounds, visual and tactile sensations" (as cited in Fine et al., 1998, pp. 427–428).

The CHAIM and its associated tools, the Nursing Child Assessment Teaching Scale (NCATS) and the Nursing Child Assessment Feeding Scale (NCAFS), have been involved in a number of studies in several countries:

Canada

NCATS & NCAFS:

improved parent–infant interaction (Letourneau, 1998)

NCATS:

father–child interaction (Boechler, 2000; Harrison, Magill-Evans, & Benzies, 1999; Harrison, Magill-Evans, & Sadoway, 2001)

low-income parents (Letourneau, Hungler, & Fisher, 2005)

parent–infant interaction (Harrison & Magill-Evans, 1996)

parents' childrearing history effect (Onyskiw, 1994)

program evaluation (Drummond, Weir, & Kysela, 2002)

very-low-birthweight infants (Feeley, 2001)

NCAFS:

life circumstances and interactions (St. Arnaud, 1996)

China:

NCATS: early mother–infant interaction (Zhu et al., 2007)

Japan:

NCATS:

infants with developmental disabilities (Kusaka, Ohgi, Gima, & Fujimoto, 2007)

mother–infant interaction (Loo, Ohgi, Tyler, & Hirose, 2005)

United States

CHAIM:

failure to thrive (Allen, 2005)

newborn sleep–wake cycles (Leake, 1990)

pediatric obesity (Hackie, 2006)

predicting child maltreatment (Lanik, 1993)

NCATS & NCAFS:

adolescent mothers (Free, 1988; Witt, 1984)

drug-exposed mothers/infants (Coyer, 1999)

failure to thrive (Lobo et al., 1992)

infant massage (Pardew, 1996)

mother–infant interaction (Britton, Gronwaldt & Britton, 2001)

program evaluation (Kang et al., 1995)

use by a variety of disciplines (Huber, 1991)

NCATS:

African American mothers (Lichti, 1994)

adopted children (Lucia, 1992)

bottle-feeding preterm infants (Kirvin, 1997)

children teaching toddler siblings (Hing, 1996)

chronically ill children (Lambert, 1987; Sullivan-Bolyai, 1999)

dependent-care agency of mothers and fathers (Boedecker, 1988)

drug-exposed children (Hogan, 2002; Schneider, 1993; Szwagiel, 1993)

disadvantaged/low-income/homeless mothers (Gossett, 2004; Grace, 1989; Horodynski & Gibbons, 2004; Schiffman, Omar, & McKelvey, 2003; Wacharasin, 2001; Wacharasin & Barnard, 2001)

failure to thrive (Reichard Sullivan, 1988; Stewart & Meyer, 2004)

family cohesion (Sturm, 1985)

father–infant interaction (Nakamura, Stewart, & Tatarka, 2000)

Hmong families (Boffman, Clark, & Helsel, 1997)

infant health promotion (Gaffney, Kodadek, Meuse, & Jones, 2001)

infants with developmental disabilities (Howell, 2005)

Latino families (Badr, 2001; Kolobe, 2004)

measuring caregiver–child interaction (Byrne & Keefe, 2003; Dillion, 2001)

mothers/children with HIV (Johnson, 1997; Johnson & Lobo, 2001; Klunklin & Harrigan, 2002)

Native American parents (Seideman et al., 1994)

predicting harsh discipline strategies (Gaffney, Barndt-Maglio, Myers, & Kollar, 2002)

preterm infants (Small, 1986)

program evaluation (Ellis, 1994; Horodynski & Gibbons, 2004; Huebner, 2002; Murdock, 1991; Roman et al., 1995; Sadler, Swartz, & Ryan-Krause, 2003; Schragenheim, 1996; Tineo, 2002)

teenage mothers (Diehl, 1993; Garver, 1986; Martus, 1993; Parks, 1983; Verzemnieks, 1998)

toddler–mother interaction (Tesh & Holditch-Davis, 1997)

toddler social competence (Spegman & Houck, 2005)

NCAFS:

child mental development (Foss et al., 1999)

mother–infant interaction (Huff, 1987; Robinson, 1988)

program evaluation (Arhin, 2005; Fehringer, 2003)

substance-abusing mothers (French, 1994)

The CHAIM is used in professions other than nursing. Examples include education (Dillion, 2001; Lichti, 1994), health sciences (Ananthaswamy, 2006; Szwagiel, 1993), human development (Ellis, 1994; Schneider, 1993; Small, 1986), medicine (Loo et al., 2005; Zhu et al., 2007), occupational therapy (Nakamura et al., 2000; Stewart & Meyer, 2004), physical therapy (Kolobe, 2004; Kusaka et al., 2007; Pardew, 1996), and psychology (Hogan, 2002; Howell, 2005; Letourneau, 1998; Murdock, 1991; Parks, 1983; Sturm, 1985; Tineo, 2002).

Examples of the use of the CHAIM in practice include assessment of mothering (Fowles & Horowitz, 2006; Horowitz, Logsdon, & Anderson, 2005), family nursing (Thomas et al., 1993), health visiting in the United Kingdom (Mischenko, Cheater, & Street, 2004), infant mental health (Solchany & Barnard, 2001), preterm infants (Kang et al., 1995), and rural settings (Horodynski & Gibbons, 2004; Kang, Barnard, & Oshio, 1994).

It is apparent that the CHAIM and its associated tools, the NCATS and the NCAFS, have been contagious across countries and disciplines. The model is more a model of child development than of nursing but is certainly useful in nursing. The NCAST program was initially targeted to nurses and has expanded to train observers from any discipline in which the tools may be useful. Barnard and her research team are to be congratulated on their insistence that the tools are only to be used by trained observers and on providing the mechanism for that training to occur. More information about the scales and training to use them may be found at http://www.ncast.org.

The reader of reports about use of the CHAIM must read carefully, as the acronyms NCAST, NCATS, and NCAFS are often used; at times the two scales are referred to as the NCAST scales rather than by their titles. Also, it is apparent from the brief overview of research studies presented in this chapter that use of the teaching scale has been reported much more frequently than use of the feeding scale. Part of the reason for this is that several of the studies have been longitudinal studies of development from infancy through toddlerhood and the teaching scales have been considered more appropriate to use, whether for developmental or observational reasons.

HUMANISTIC NURSING

Josephine G. Paterson and Loretta Zderad

Josephine G. Paterson was born September 1, 1924, in Freeport, New York. She received a diploma in nursing from Lenox Hill Hospital School of Nursing, New York, New York (1945); bachelor's degree in nursing education from St. John's University, Brooklyn, New York (1954); master's degree in public health with a specialty in mental health from Johns Hopkins School of Hygiene and Public Health, Baltimore, Maryland (1955); and a doctorate in nursing science with a specialty in psychiatric mental health nursing from Boston University, Massachusetts (1969) (O'Connor, 1993). She worked in public and mental health as well as psychiatric nursing as staff nurse, faculty member, consultant, educational coordinator, and clinical specialist (Paterson & Zderad, 1971). She retired in 1985 from her position as a "nursologist" at Northport Veterans Administration Hospital, Northport, New York (O'Connor, 1993).

Loretta Zderad was born June 7, 1925, in Chicago, Illinois. She received a diploma in nursing from St. Bernard's Hospital School of Nursing, Chicago (1947); bachelor's degree in nursing education from Loyola University, Chicago (1947); master's degree in nursing education with a major in psychiatric nursing from Catholic University,

Washington, D.C. (1952); and master of arts in philosophy (1960) and Ph.D. in philosophy (1968) from Georgetown University, Washington, D.C. She taught "mental health nursing at the University of Illinois, the Catholic Hospital of America, Boston University and Ohio State University" and worked as program director of psychiatric nursing for the Southern Regional Educational Board and as a clinical specialist (Paterson & Zderad, 1971). She retired in 1985 from her position as a "nursologist" at Northport Veterans Administration Hospital, Northport, New York (O'Connor, 1993).

HUMANISTIC NURSING DEFINED   Paterson and Zderad (1976/1988/2007) indicate the theory of humanistic nursing began as they cotaught a graduate seminar in 1960 in which all were encouraged to discuss, question, clarify, and be open to honest argument resulting in increased awareness, reflection, ability to struggle with rather than against differences, and being open to questions. Their book began with a course for professional nursing staff in 1972 and evolved over work with six such groups of nurses. They describe humanistic nursing practice theory as follows:

> . . . nurses consciously and deliberately approach nursing as an existential experience . . . reflect on the experience and phenomenologically describe the calls they receive, their responses, and what they come to know from their presence in the nursing situation. (p. 3)

The two major components in this description are the *existential experience* and the *phenomenological dialogue.*

The concepts related to the existential experience are *uniqueness-otherness, authenticity-experiencing, moreness-choice,* and *value-nonvalue.* Uniqueness-otherness represents the existential concept that a human being is at the same moment ("all at once") uniquely self and also like others. Each person has both uniquely individual characteristics and common characteristics shared with all others. Paterson and Zderad (1976/1988/2007) describe authenticity as "self-in-touchness" or being in touch with one's own sensations and responses. The more in touch with ourselves we are, the more we can be open to others, also known as being in presence with another or experiencing. As nurses become more aware of their individual responses and the possibilities called forth by the other, moreness occurs, and choices can be made as to whether to relate and how to relate to others. For one person to be genuinely present to another, that presence must be considered of value and as making a difference in the situation. With value, genuine presence may occur; without value (or with nonvalue), genuine presence will not occur.

Phenomenological dialogue leads us to consider *what to describe, why to describe, and how to describe phenomenologically.* "The thing itself" is described in phenomenology, and Paterson and Zderad (1976/1988/2007) identify the thing itself in humanistic nursing practice as the existentially experienced nursing situation. The nurse is asked to describe three things: the unique views and responses of the nurse, the responses of the nursed that are knowable, and the "reciprocal call and response, the between, as they occur in the nursing situation" (p. 7). Part of the "why" of description includes more knowledge and understanding of the quality of the nursing situation and of the variations in the general knowledge of human beings and the development of nursing theory and science. How to describe requires "deliberate responsible, conscious, aware, nonjudgmental existence of the nurse in the nursing situation followed by disciplined authentic reflection and description" using everyday words (p. 8).

Concepts involved in humanistic nursing include *well-being and more-being, human potential, intersubjective transaction,* and *being and doing.* Well-being is related to those aspects of nursing that deal with the quality of the other's personal survival; more-being moves beyond a view of health as the absence of disease to consider how the nurse can help the nursed become more within that person's particular life circumstances. Human potential involves all possible responses of the human being and includes both needing and helping. Paterson and Zderad (1976/1988/2007) point out these responses include both those that may be considered limiting or needing (anger, frustration, rejection, aggression) as well as those viewed as helping (caring, joy, courage, tenderness). Intersubjective transaction relates to the shared situation that occurs as the nurse and the nursed relate in a shared situation in which the nurse is nurturing, the nursed is being nurtured, and the relation or transaction is the between through which the nurturance occurs. Being and doing are described as so interrelated it is difficult, if not impossible, to truly describe one without the other. Nursing involves both being as a mode and the doing of something. Since it is easier to describe the doing, often it is the acts that are focused on. Paterson and Zderad say of being that "presence and the effect of one's presence can be known much more vividly than they can be described" (p. 14). They also discuss the importance of "being with" or "being there," in which there may be no observable doing but the nurse's attention is focused on the nursed and the nurse is open to the shared situation.

Humanistic nursing also involves *authentic commitment, choice and intersubjectivity, theory and practice,* and *the framework of the human situation.* Authentic commitment occurs when the nurse is actively present with the whole of the nurse's being both personally and professionally. It is personal because each nurse is unique and authentic commitment is a live act. It is professional when it is goal oriented. Paterson and Zderad (1976/1988/2007) recognize that it is impossible for the nurse to express authentic commitment to every patient over the course of an entire workday. However, they discuss that experienced moments of genuine presence give meaning to nursing and that humanistic nursing can occur in various degrees. They state that perhaps humanistic nursing might be considered a goal, an attitude, or a major value shaping one's practice. The process of nursing involves choices; in existential terms, a person is choices—that is, at any given moment each person is shaped by choices made in the past. Choices influence both by what is selected and what is not selected. At an intersection, choosing to turn left means you cannot pass by what is on the road straight ahead or to the right. As human beings these choices lead us to relationships with others in time and space and to the paradox of being, at the same time, a unique, independent individual and a person who is interdependent with or related to others. In this intersubjective relationship between nurse and nursed, the giving of one's self, or presence, is desired but does not occur on demand. Presence occurs only when given freely. The nurse in such intersubjective transaction seeks to encourage the making of responsible choices. Paterson and Zderad also describe theory and practice as inextricably intertwined—the practice experience leads to conceptualization about practice and examination of the values inherent in the practice situation; these evolve into humanistic nursing theory based on nurses' lived experience. Practice and theory inform each other. The framework, or human situation, for humanistic nursing is described by Paterson and Zderad as "a particular kind of human situation in which the interhuman relating is purposely directed toward nurturing the well-being or more-being of a person with perceived needs related to the health-illness quality of living . . . the elements . . . include . . . patient and nurse . . . meeting (being and becoming) in a goal directed (nurturing well-being and more-being) intersubjective transaction (being with and doing with) occurring in time and space . . . in a world of men and things" (p. 19).

Paterson and Zderad (1976/1988/2007) also describe nursing as a lived dialogue that involves *meeting, relating, presence,* and *call and response* that occur in a real world that includes *other human beings, things, time,* and *space.* The meeting of two unique individuals (nurse and nursed), each of whom has some control over how much disclosure will occur, may be expected or unexpected, is purposeful (with a goal or expectation), and thus has meaning and is experienced in light of the goal(s). Relating between nurse and nursed may be as subject to object or subject to subject; in the open lived dialogue with true presence, the relating will be subject to subject, and the unique individuality of the other will be identified with subject-to-object relating providing the "scientific" or intellectual information needed to reach goals. Presence may or may not occur; it can be invoked or evoked but does not appear on demand. Presence requires an openness or receptivity on the part of both parties in the relationship; both availability and reciprocity are involved. Call and response in the humanistic nursing situation involves the nursed's call to the nurse to be cared for or have a need met; the nurse's response relates to providing that caring or meeting the need. In turn, the nurse provides a call to the nursed, such as identifying how services may be obtained, and the nursed may respond by requesting a particular service. The call and response from both the nurse and the nursed are both sequential and simultaneous, verbal and nonverbal. While the lived dialogue in humanistic nursing is described as occurring between two individuals—nurse and nursed—there are other aspects of the real world involved. One of these is other human beings; being open to another involves also being open to that person as related to other human beings. The nursed relates to family, coworkers, and friends; the nurse will view the patient as part of a group of patients, whether others in that day's assignment or others who have been nursed. In addition the nurse is influenced by the changing role of nurses and by the nurse's own personal history. Things, such as furniture, clothing, equipment, or utensils, in the environment will also have either an inhibiting or an enhancing influence. The same things will be in the environment of both parties in the lived dialogue but will have a different degree of familiarity and utility for each of the parties. What is familiar to one may well be foreign to the other. Time should be considered both as measured in minutes or days and as lived by the nurse and patient. When both types of time are shared in a genuinely intersubjective relationship, synchronicity occurs. Space also is to be considered as measured and as experienced. Paterson and Zderad describe lived space as "large and small, far and near, long and short, high and deep, above and below, before and behind, left and right, across, all around, empty, crowded" (p. 38). Personalized space is identified as place; the hospitalized patient likely feels out of place while the nurse is comfortable in that space. Truly being with the nursed requires the nurse to know the nursed in that person's lived space.

Humanistic nursing produces, occurs in, and is influenced by *community.* Paterson and Zderad (1976/1988/2007) discuss a variety of aspects of community. A community may be defined as a group of people (family, class of students, work group), groups within a geographic area, place where people reside (from town to the world), or a profession. Persons within a community can make a difference through being open to possibilities and as-yet-unattempted choices. Each nurse can relate to others and explore personal experience to create community out of what the nurse comes to know through such exploration, recognizing that each is at once alike and different. A person's view is influenced by past experience, especially that which occurred within the nuclear family. Paterson and Zderad refer to Buber's (1958) descriptions of human relationships as "I-Thou," "I-It," and "We." In "I-Thou" relating, the human merges with another while recognizing self as also separate, with a result that each becomes more. "I-It" occurs when a person looks back at previous "I-Thou" relationships and interprets them to accrue scientific knowledge. "We" provides for community and unique contributions by an adult. Buber refers to the thinking human being as a dialogue of internalized "Thous."

Paterson and Zderad (1976/1988/2007) propose a research methodology for humanistic nursing that they call *phenomenologic nursology* (pp. 76–81). The phases of phenomenologic nursology are the following:

1. Preparation of the nurse knower for coming to know—being willing to take risks and approach the situation openly
2. Nurse knowing of the other intuitively
3. Nurse knowing the other scientifically—analyzing what is known; similar to Buber's "I-It"
4. Nurse complementarily synthesizing known others—sorting, classifying, and interpreting the information from multiple known realities.
5. Succession within the nurse from the many to the paradoxical one—pondering the multiple realities and coming to an expansion of one's view to create an ever-more-inclusive view

METAPARADIGM, RESEARCH, AND PRACTICE WITH HUMANISTIC NURSING   Paterson and Zderad (1976/1988/2007) include the four major concepts of nursing's metaparadigm in their work. The person is discussed as man or, when the recipient of nursing care, the nursed and, when the provider of nursing care, the nurse. O'Connor (1993) indicates the characteristics of *person* in humanistic nursing are freedom to choose, uniqueness, adequacy, relatedness, and having a history. Paterson and Zderad state that nursing values human potential far beyond a narrow definition of *health* as the absence of disease; their discussion of health is conducted under the rubric of well-being and more-being. The implication is that health includes both well-being and more-being, especially in situations where well-being as freedom from disease is not possible. *Environment* is not specifically defined, but Paterson and Zderad do discuss that the nurse–nursed relationship takes place in a real world that includes other human beings, things, time, and space. *Nursing* is viewed as an existential experience lived between human beings, a response to a human situation in which one person (the nursed) needs help and the other (the nurse) gives it.

Humanistic nursing has been the basis for a number of studies, in various parts of the world, as well as articles about its use in nursing practice. Examples of publications about research, practice, and education with humanistic nursing include the following:

Research
  Brazil:
    child with AIDS (de Paula & Crossetti, 2005a, 2005b; de Paula, de Mello Padoin, Vernier, & da Motta, 2003; Medeiros, & da Motta, 2008)
    families with Down syndrome child (Ramos, Caetano, Soares, & Rolim, 2006)
    hospitalized child (Cunha & Zagonel, 2008)

neonatal intensive care (Campos & Cardoso, 2004a, 2004b; Rolim, 2008; Rolim & Cardoso, 2006a, 2006b; Rolim, Pagliuca, & Cardoso, 2005)

parents of children with cancer (de Oliveira, da Costa, & da Nóbrega, 2006)

pediatric nursing (de Lourdes Castanha & Zagonel, 2005; Schaurich, Padoin, de Paula, & da Motta, 2005)

Canada:

hospital restructuring experience (Suderman, 1997)

China:

childbirth (Li, 2006)

United States:

breast cancer (Moch, 1988)

care of adolescents (Hinds, 1985; Mustain, 1999; Weissman, 1992)

contemplative spirituality (Larson, 2002)

essence of nurse practitioner–patient interaction (Kleiman, 2002)

labor and delivery (Luegenbiehl, 1986)

patient expectations (Davis, 2003, 2005)

patients with diabetes and on hemodialysis (Johnson, 2001)

psychiatric intensive care (Ward, 2003)

time (Davis, 2006)

tool development (Easter, 1999; Hines, 1991; Kostovich, 2002; Stoner, 1982)

Practice

Brazil:

critical care (Cunha & Zagonel, 2006; Mercês & Rocha, 2006; Nascimento & Trentini, 2004)

Down syndrome (Negri, Labronici & Zagonel, 2003)

theory-based practice (de Paula, Schaurich, Padoin, & Crossetti, 2004)

work-related accidents (Krug & Somavilla, 2004)

Portugal:

newborn care (Carneiro, Cardoso, Abreu, & Fernandes)

Spain:

health (Santos, Pagliuca & Fernandes, 2007)

intercultural relations (Guillaumet, 2009)

United Kingdom:

comfort (Tutton & Seers, 2003)

United States:

applicability to research and practice (McCamant, 2006)

Education:

cultural influences (Kleiman, Frederickson, & Lundy, 2004)

humanistic nursing education (Praeger, 1980)

Humanistic nursing theory is the first published nursing theory to be based in existentialism. Paterson and Zderad's (1976/1988/2007) book clearly reflects that basis and their own growth as humanistic nurses. The book is neither an easy read nor a quick guide to clinical practice. The content challenges the reader to think, reflect, and incorporate personal experience. Paterson and Zderad are to be complimented in recognizing that the time constraints and demands of clinical practice will limit the individual nurse's ability to practice humanistic nursing to its fullest and in encouraging the nurse to treasure those moments when the lived dialogue does occur.

EXPLORE PEARSON **mynursingkit**™

MyNursingKit is your one stop for online chapter review materials and resources. Prepare for success with additional NCLEX®-style practice questions, interactive assignments and activities, web links, animations and videos, and more!

Register your access code from the front of your book at
www.mynursingkit.com.

Barnard References

Allen, C. L. (2005). Prenatal care utilization as a predictor of failure to thrive. *Dissertation Abstracts International, 67*(01B), 177. Abstract retrieved August 9, 2007, from Dissertation Abstracts Online database.

Ananthaswamy, M. (2006). Measuring development of therapeutic relationships. *Dissertation Abstracts International, 68*(01B), 189. Abstract retrieved August 9, 2007, from Dissertation Abstracts Online database.

Arhin, A. O. (2005). Effect of bug-in-the-ear-feedback as an intervention to promote attachment behaviors in the adolescent mother/infant dyad. *Dissertation Abstracts International, 67*(01B), 177. Abstract retrieved August 9, 2007, from Dissertation Abstracts Online database.

Badr, L. K. (2001). Quantitative and qualitative predictors of development for low-birth weight infants and Latino background. *Applied Nursing Research, 14,* 125–135.

Barnard, K. E. (1972). The effect of stimulation on the duration and amount of sleep and wakefulness in the premature infant. *Dissertation Abstracts International, 33*(05B), 2167. Abstract retrieved February 13, 2008, from Dissertation Abstracts Online database.

Barnard, K. E. (1999). The developing family: How is it doing with nurturing young children? . . . adapted from Guest Editorial in *Canadian Journal of Nursing Research,* 1998, Vol. 30, No. 3, 7–12. *Canadian Journal of Nursing Research, 30,* 299–304.

Barnard, K. E. (2004). Guest editorial: Is there a developmental pathway leading to addictive behavior? *Journal of Addictions Nursing, 15,* 49–50.

Barnard, K. E. (2007). Ask the expert. The feeding relationship. *Zero to Three, 28*(1), 4.

Barnard, K. E., & Eyres, S. J. (Eds.). (1979). *Child health assessment, part 2: The first year of life.* Hyattsville, MD: U. S. Department of Health, Education, and Welfare.

Barnard, K. E., & Powell, M. L. (1972). *Teaching the mentally retarded child: A family care approach.* St. Louis: Mosby.

Barnard, K. E., Spietz, A. L., Snyder, C., Douglas, H. B., Eyres, S. J., & Hill, V. (1977). *The nursing child assessment satellite training study guide.* Unpublished program learning manual.

Boechler, V. L. (2000). Predictors of father–child interaction measured by the Nursing Child Assessment Teaching Scale. *Masters Abstracts International, 39*(06), 1520. Abstract retrieved August 9, 2007, from Dissertation Abstracts Online database.

Boedeker, R. J. (1988). Comparing dependent-care agency of mothers and fathers. *Masters*

Abstracts International, 28(01), 104. Abstract retrieved August 9, 2007, from Dissertation Abstracts Online database.

Boffman, J. L. H., Clark, N. J. M, & Helsel, D. (1997). Can NCAST and HOME assessment scales be used with Hmong refugees? *Pediatric Nursing, 23,* 235–244.

Britton, H. L., Gronwaldt, V., & Britton, J. R. (2001). Maternal postpartum behaviors and mother–infant relationship during the first year of life. *Journal of Pediatrics, 138,* 905–909.

Byrne, M. W., & Keefe, M. R. (2003). Comparison of two measures of parent–child interaction. *Nursing Research, 52,* 34–41.

Coyer, S. M. (1999). Vulnerability in parenting in cocaine-exposed mother/infant dyads. *Dissertation Abstracts International, 60*(5B), 2060. Abstract retrieved August 9, 2007, from Dissertation Abstracts Online database.

Diehl, P. K. (1993). Self-esteem and mother–infant interaction among teenage mothers. *Masters Abstracts International, 33*(02), 514. Abstract retrieved August 9, 2007, from Dissertation Abstracts Online database.

Dillion, P. B. (2001). The hand that rocks the cradle: A study of caregiver-child interaction. *Dissertation Abstracts International, 62*(05A), 1715. Abstract retrieved August 9, 2007, from Dissertation Abstracts Online database.

Drummond, J. E., Weir, A. E., & Kysela, G. M. (2002). Home visitation practice: Models, documentation, and evaluation. *Public Health Nursing, 19*(1), 21–29.

Elliott, M. R., Drummond, J., & Barnard, K. E. (1996). Subjective appraisal of infant crying. *Clinical Nursing Research, 5,* 237–250.

Ellis, I. J. (1994). The effect of intervention on parent–child interaction. *Masters Abstracts International, 32*(05), 1361. Abstract retrieved August 9, 2007, from Dissertation Abstracts Online database.

Feeley, N. (2001). Infant, mother and contextual factors related to mothers' interactions with their very-low-birthweight infants. *Dissertation Abstracts International, 64*(01B), 143. Abstract retrieved August 9, 2007, from Dissertation Abstracts Online database.

Fehringer, K. A. (2003). Correlates of mother–infant interaction and self-regulation in a perinatal intervention program. *Dissertation Abstracts International, 64*(12B), 6012. Abstract retrieved August 9, 2007, from Dissertation Abstracts Online database.

Fine, J. M. B., Baker, J. M., Borchers, D. A., Cochran, D. T., Kaltofen, K. G., Orcutt, N., et al. (1998). Kathryn E. Barnard: Parent–Child Interaction Model. In A. M. Tomey & M. R. Alligood (Eds.), *Nursing theorists and their work* (4th ed., pp. 423–438). St. Louis: Mosby.

Foss, L. A., Hirose, T., & Barnard, K. E. (1999). Relationship of three types of parent–child interaction in depressed and non-depressed mothers and their children's mental development at 13 months. *Nursing and Health Sciences, 1,* 211–219.

Fowles, E. R., & Horowitz, J. A. (2006). Clinical assessment of mothering during infancy. *Journal of Obstetric, Gynecologic, and Neonatal Nurses, 35,* 662–670.

Free, T. A. (1988). The relationship of family patterns to adolescent mother–infant interactions. *Dissertation Abstracts International, 50*(02B), 492. Abstract retrieved August 9, 2007, from Dissertation Abstracts Online database.

French, E. D. (1994). The effects of comforting and interactional techniques substance-abusing *mother*–infant dyads. *Dissertation Abstracts International, 55*(09B), 3814. Abstract retrieved August 9, 2007, from Dissertation Abstracts Online database.

Gaffney, K. F., Barndt-Maglio, B., Myers, S., & Kollar, S. J. (2002). Early clinical assessment for harsh child discipline strategies. *MCN: The American Journal of Maternal Child Nursing, 27*(1), 34–40.

Gaffney, K. F., Kodadek, M. P., Meuse, M. T., & Jones, G. B. (2001). Assessing infant health promotion: A cross cultural comparison. *Clinical Nursing Research, 10,* 102–116.

Garver, P. M. M. (1986). Relationships among social support dimensions, maternal age, and mother–infant interactions in adolescent mother–infant dyads. *Dissertation Abstracts International, 47*(04B), 1486. Abstract retrieved August 9, 2007, from Dissertation Abstracts Online database.

Gossett, O. M. (2004). Maternal attachment, depression, and caregiving: Relationships with child behavior in homeless mothers of toddlers. *Dissertation Abstracts International, 65*(04B), 1777. Abstract retrieved August 9, 2007, from Dissertation Abstracts Online database.

Grace, J. T. (1989). The assessment of the mother–newborn interaction. *Dissertation Abstracts International, 50*(07B), 2844. Abstract retrieved August 9, 2007, from Dissertation Abstracts Online database.

Hackie, M. (2006). Parental perception of pediatric obesity. *Masters Abstracts International, 45*(01),

283. Abstract retrieved August 9, 2007, from Dissertation Abstracts Online database.

Harrison, M. J., & Magill-Evans, J. (1996). Mother and father interactions over the first year with term and preterm infants. *Research in Nursing and Health, 19,* 451–459.

Harrison, M. J., Magill-Evans, J., & Benzies, K. (1999). Fathers' scores on the Nursing Child Assessment Teaching Scale: Are they different from those of mothers? *Journal of Pediatric Nursing, 14,* 248–254.

Harrison, M. J., Magill-Evans, J., & Sadoway, D. (2001). Scores on the Nursing Child Assessment Teaching Scale for father–toddler dyads. *Public Health Nursing, 18,* 94–100.

Hing, J. (1996). How do school age children teach their toddler age siblings? *Masters Abstracts International, 35*(01), 209. Abstract retrieved August 9, 2007, from Dissertation Abstracts Online database.

Hogan, T. M. S. (2002). Child abuse potential and mother–infant interaction among mothers of substance-exposed and nonexposed infants and toddlers. *Dissertation Abstracts International, 63*(02B), 1029. Abstract retrieved August 9, 2007, from Dissertation Abstracts Online database.

Horodynski, M. A., & Gibbons, C. (2004). Rural low-income mothers' interactions with their young children. *Pediatric Nursing, 30,* 299–306.

Horowitz, J. A., Logsdon, M. C., & Anderson, J. K. (2005). Measurement of maternal-infant interaction. *Journal of the American Psychiatric Nurses Association, 11,* 164–172.

Howell, A. (2005). Growth in the interactions of mothers and their infants with developmental disabilities. *Dissertation Abstracts International, 66* (09B), 5123. Abstract retrieved August 9, 2007, from Dissertation Abstracts Online database.

Huber, C. J. (1991). Documenting quality of parent–child interaction: Use of the NCAST scales. *Infants and Young Children: An Interdisciplinary Journal of Special Care Practices, 4*(2), 63–75.

Huebner, C. E. (2002). Evaluation of a clinic-based parent education program to reduce the risk of infant and toddler maltreatment. *Public Health Nursing, 19,* 377–389.

Huff, A. G. (1987). The predictive value of role supplementation on mother–infant interaction. *Dissertation Abstracts International, 48*(04B), 1004. Abstract retrieved August 9, 2007, from Dissertation Abstracts Online database.

Johnson, M. O. (1997). Mother–child interaction in the presence of maternal human immunodeficiency virus infection. *Dissertation Abstracts International, 58*(03B), 1213. Abstract retrieved August 9, 2007, from Dissertation Abstracts Online database.

Johnson, M. O., & Lobo, M. L. (2001). Mother–child interaction in the presence of maternal HIV infection. *JANAC: Journal of the Association of Nurses in AIDS Care, 12*(1), 40–51.

Jolley, S. N., Elmore, S., Barnard, K. E., & Carr, D. B. (2007). Dysregulation of the hypothalamic-pituitary-adrenal axis in postpartum depression. *Biological Research for Nursing, 8,* 210–222.

Kang, R., Barnard, K., Hammond, M., Oshio, S., Spencer, C., Thibodeaux, B., et al. (1995). Preterm infant follow-up project: A multi-site field experiment of hospital and home intervention programs for mothers and preterm infants. *Public Health Nursing, 12,* 171–180.

Kang, R., Barnard, K., & Oshio, S. (1994). Description of the clinical practice of advanced practice nurses in family-centered early intervention in two rural settings. *Public Health Nursing, 11,* 376–384.

Kelly, J. F., Morisset, C. E., Barnard, K. E., & Patterson, D. L. (1996). Risky beginnings: Low maternal intelligence as a risk factor for children's intellectual development. *Infants and Young Children: An Interdisciplinary Journal of Special Care Practices, 8*(3), 11–23.

Kirvin, C. F. (1997). The effect of "Keys to Caregiving" on the bottle feeding practices used with preterm neonates. *Masters Abstracts International, 35*(04), 999. Abstract retrieved August 9, 2007, from Dissertation Abstracts Online database.

Klunkin, P., & Harrigan, R. C. (2002). Child-rearing practices of primary caregivers of HIV-infected children: An integrative review of the literature. *Journal of Pediatric Nursing, 17,* 289–296.

Kolobe, T. H. A. (2004). Childrearing practices and developmental expectations for Mexican-American mothers and the developmental status of their infants. *Physical Therapy, 84,* 439–453.

Kusaka, R., Ohgi, S., Gima, H., & Fujimoto, T. (2007). Short-term effects of the Neonatal Behavioral Assessment Scale-based intervention for infants with developmental disabilities. *Journal of Physical Therapy Science, 19*(1), 1–8.

Lambert, S. A. (1987). Children with tracheotomies and the home environment. *Dissertation Abstracts International, 48*(04B), 1005. Abstract retrieved August 9, 2007, from Dissertation Abstracts Online database.

Lanik, G. E. (1993). Prediction of child maltreatment using the Family Stress Checklist and the Home Observation Scale for Measurement of the Environment (HOME) Inventory Scale. *Dissertation Abstracts International, 54*(10B), 5094. Abstract retrieved August 9, 2007, from Dissertation Abstracts Online database.

Leake, P. Y. (1990). The relationship of fetal activity patterns to newborn wake–sleep cycles. *Dissertation Abstracts International, 51*(07B), 3324. Abstract retrieved August 9, 2007, from Dissertation Abstracts Online database.

Letourneau, N. L. (1998). The effect of improved parent–infant interaction on infant development: Pilot study. *Dissertation Abstracts International, 59*(12B), 6504. Abstract retrieved August 9, 2007, from Dissertation Abstracts Online database.

Letourneau, N. L., Hungler, K. M., & Fisher, K. (2005). Low-income Canadian Aboriginal and non-Aboriginal parent–child interactions. *Child: Care, Health and Development, 31*, 545–554.

Lichti, M. O. (1994). The salience of developmental history, parenting beliefs, psychological resources, and contextual factors in determining parenting competence among high-risk African American mothers: A path model. *Dissertation Abstracts International, 55*(11A), 3417. Abstract retrieved August 9, 2007, from Dissertation Abstracts Online database.

Lobo, M. L., Barnard, K. E., & Coombs, J. B. (1992). Failure to thrive: A parent–infant interaction perspective. *Journal of Pediatric Nursing, 7*, 251–261.

Loo, K. K., Ohgi, S., Howard, J., Tyler, R., & Hirose, T. (2005). Neurobehaviors of Japanese newborns in relation to the characteristics of early mother–infant interaction. *Journal of Genetic Psychology, 166*, 264–279.

Lucia, A. E. (1992). Attachment between mothers and their adopted children. *Dissertation Abstracts International, 53*(12B), 6224. Abstract retrieved August 9, 2007, from Dissertation Abstracts Online database.

Martus, J. E. (1993). Benefits of a nurturing program: Perceptions of adolescent mothers. *Masters Abstracts International, 31*(04), 1744.

Abstract retrieved August 9, 2007, from Dissertation Abstracts Online database.

Mischenko, J., Cheater, F., & Street, J. (2004). NCAST: Tools to assess caregiver–child interaction. *Community Practitioner, 77*(2), 57–60.

Murdock, S. A. (1991). A program evaluation of the Welcome Baby Project: A primary prevention program for teenage mothers and their infants. *Dissertation Abstracts International, 52*(10B), 5543. Abstract retrieved August 9, 2007, from Dissertation Abstracts Online database.

Nakamura, W. M., Stewart, K. B., & Tatarka, M. E. (2000). Assessing father–infant interactions using the NCAST teaching scale: A pilot study. *American Journal of Occupational Therapy, 54*(1), 44–51.

Onyskiw, J. E. (1994). The relationship between parental recall of acceptance experienced in childhood, marital quality and current parent–infant interactions. *Masters Abstracts International, 35*(01), 212. Abstract retrieved August 9, 2007, from Dissertation Abstracts Online database.

Pardew, E. M. (1996). The effects of infant massage on the interactions between high risk infants and their caregivers. *Dissertation Abstracts International, 57*(06B), 3688. Abstract retrieved August 9, 2007, from Dissertation Abstracts Online database.

Parks, M. L. (1983). Maternal sensitivity to infant cues: Impact of group intervention for adolescent mothers. *Dissertation Abstracts International, 44*(11A), 3330. Abstract retrieved August 9, 2007, from Dissertation Abstracts Online database.

Reichard Sullivan, B. A. (1988). Nonorganic failure to thrive maternal-child dyads: The effect of psychoeducational interventions. *Dissertation Abstracts International, 49*(06B), 2110. Abstract retrieved August 9, 2007, from Dissertation Abstracts Online database.

Robinson, J. L. (1988). Mother–infant interaction: A description of the infant's contributions while feeding when the infant has congenital heart disease. *Masters Abstracts International, 27*(01), 102. Abstract retrieved August 9, 2007, from Dissertation Abstracts Online database.

Roman, L. A., Lindsay, J. K., Boger, R. P., DeWys, M., Beaumont, E. J., Jones, A. S., et al. (1995). Parent-to-parent support initiated in the neonatal intensive care unit. *Research in Nursing and Health, 18*, 385–394.

Sadler, L. S., Swartz, M. K., & Ryan-Krause, P. (2003). Supporting adolescent mothers and their children through a high school-based child care center and parent support program. *Journal of Pediatric Healthcare, 17*(3), 109–117.

Schiffman, R. F., Omar, M. A., & McKelvey, L. M. (2003). Mother–infant interaction in low-income families. *MCN: The American Journal of Maternal Child Nursing, 28,* 246–251.

Schneider, J. W. (1993). An investigation of focused attention in opioid-exposed toddlers. *Dissertation Abstracts International, 54*(05B), 2425. Abstract retrieved August 9, 2007, from Dissertation Abstracts Online database.

Schragenheim, K. H. (1996). Improving the interactions of mothers with their children through home intervention. Masters Abstracts International, 34(04), 1555. Abstract retrieved August 9, 2007, from Dissertation Abstracts Online database.

Seideman, R. Y., Williams, R., Burns, P., Jacobson, S., Weatherby, F., & Primeaux, M. (1994). Culture sensitivity in assessing urban Native American parenting. *Public Health Nursing, 11,* 98–103.

Small, M. C. (1986). Comparison of preterm infant development and home environments among graduates of three hospital newborn units. *Dissertation Abstracts International, 47*(10B), 4106. Abstract retrieved August 9, 2007, from Dissertation Abstracts Online database.

Solchany, J. E., & Barnard, K. E. (2001). Is mom's mind on her baby? Infant mental health in Early Head Start. *Zero to Three, 22*(1), 39–47.

Spegman, A. M., & Houck, G. M. (2005). Assessing the feeding/eating interaction as a context for the development of social competence in toddlers. *Issues in Comprehensive Pediatric Nursing, 28,* 213–236.

St. Arnaud, S. L. (1996). A comparison of life circumstances and maternal-infant feeding interactions. *Masters Abstracts International, 35*(05), 1383. Abstract retrieved August 9, 2007, from Dissertation Abstracts Online database.

Stewart, K. B., & Meyer, L. (2004). Brief report. Parent–child interactions and everyday routines in young children with failure to thrive. *American Journal of Occupational Therapy, 58,* 342–346.

Sturm, S. C. (1985). The relationship between family cohesion, mother's perception of social support and mother infant interaction. *Dissertation Abstracts International, 46*(12B), 4429. Abstract retrieved August 9, 2007, from Dissertation Abstracts Online database.

Sullivan-Bolyai, S. L. (1999). Mothers' experiences parenting the young child with Type I diabetes. *Dissertation Abstracts International, 60*(06B), 2613. Abstract retrieved August 9, 2007, from Dissertation Abstracts Online database.

Szwagiel, C. M. (1993). The association of child abuse potential with mother and infant characteristics in a group of drug-using women. *Dissertation Abstracts International, 55*(05B), 1823. Abstract retrieved August 9, 2007, from Dissertation Abstracts Online database.

Tesh, E. M., & Holditch-Davis, D. (1997). HOME Inventory and NCATS: Relation to mother and child behaviors during naturalistic observations. *Research in Nursing and Health, 20,* 295–307.

Thomas, R. B., Barnard, K. E., & Sumner, G. A. (1993). Family nursing diagnosis as a framework for family assessment. In S. L. Feetham, S. B. Meister, J. M. Bell, C. L. Gilliss (Eds.), *The nursing of families: Theory/research/education/ practice . . . selected papers from the Second International Family Nursing Conference, Portland, Oregon, 1991* (pp. 127–136). Newbury Park, CA: Sage.

Tineo, W. (2002). Impact of age-paced parenting newsletters on urban families with at-risk children. *Dissertation Abstracts International, 63*(08B), 3960. Abstract retrieved August 9, 2007, from Dissertation Abstracts Online database.

Verzemnieks, I. L. (1998). Parenting attitudes and behaviors of adolescent mothers rearing young toddlers. *Dissertation Abstracts International, 59*(09B), 4733. Abstract retrieved August 9, 2007, from Dissertation Abstracts Online database.

Wacharasin, C. (2001). Predicting child cognitive development in low-income families. *Dissertation Abstracts International, 62*(05B), 2263. Abstract retrieved August 9, 2007, from Dissertation Abstracts Online database.

Wacharasin, C., & Barnard, K. E. (2001). Predicting child cognitive development in low-income families . . . 34th Annual Communicating Nursing Research Conference/15th Annual WIN Assembly, "Health Care Challenges Beyond 2001: Mapping the Journey for Research and Practice," held April 19–21, 2001 in Seattle, Washington. *Communicating Nursing Research, 34,* 342.

Wacharasin, C., Barnard, K. E., & Spieker, S. J. (2003). Factors affecting toddler cognitive development in low-income families: Implications for practitioners. *Infants and Young Children: An Interdisciplinary Journal of Special Care Practices, 16*(2), 175–181.

Witt, S. (1984). The impact of a mother education program on the mothering skills of selected rural adolescent mothers. *Dissertation Abstracts International, 45*(09B), 2873. Abstract retrieved August 9, 2007, from Dissertation Abstracts Online database.

Zhu, H., Loo, K. H., Min, L., Yin, Q., Luo, H., & Chen, L. (2007). Relationship between neurobehaviors of Chinese neonates and early mother–infant interaction. *Journal of Reproductive and Infant Psychology, 25*(2), 106–121.

Paterson and Zderad References

Buber, M. (1958). *I and Thou* (2nd ed.) (Ronald Gregor Smith, Trans.). New York: Charles Scribner's Sons.

Campos, A. C. D., & Cardoso, M. V. L. (2004a). Application of the Paterson and Zderad theory on mothers of newborn babies under phototherapy [Portuguese]. *Texto & Contexto Enfermagem, 13*, 435–443. Abstract in English retrieved May 18, 2007, from CINAHL Plus with Full Text database.

Campos, A. C. S., & Cardoso, M. V. L. (2004b). Newborn children under phototherapy: The mother's perception [Portuguese]. *Revista Latino-Americana de Enfermagem, 12*, 606–613. Abstract in English retrieved May 18, 2007, from CINAHL Plus with Full Text database.

Carneiro, K. M., Cardoso, M. V. L., Abreu, W. J. C., & Fernandes, H. I. V. (2007). Sandwich nursing doctorate's period of training: An experience in Portugal [Portuguese]. *Revista Electrônica de Enfermagem, 9*(1), 261–274. Abstract in English retrieved November 30, 2009 from CINAHL Plus with Full Text database.

Cunha, P. J., & Zagonel, I. P. S. (2006). The lived dialogue permeating the nursing care in pediatric cardiac ICU [Portuguese]. *Revista Electronica de Enfermagem, 8*, 292–297. Abstract in English retrieved May 18, 2007, from CINAHL Plus with Full Text database.

Cunha, P. J., & Zagonel, I. P. S. (2008). The interpersonal relationships of care actions in the hospital technological environment [Portuguese]. *Acta Paulista de Enfermagem, 21*, 412–419.

Davis, L. A. (2003). A phenomenological study of patients' expectations concerning nursing care. *Dissertation Abstracts International, 64*(11B), 5448. Abstract retrieved November 6, 2007, from Dissertation Abstracts Online database.

Davis, L. A. (2005). A phenomenological study of patient expectations concerning nursing care. *Holistic Nursing Practice, 19*(3), 126–133.

Davis, L. A. (2006). The experience of time and nursing practice. *Visions: The Journal of Rogerian Nursing Science, 14*(1), 36–44.

de Lourdes Castanha, M., & Zagonel, I. P. S. (2005). Nurse's care practice according to the view of the healthcare team [Portuguese]. *Revista Brasileira de Enfermagem, 58*, 556–562. Abstract in English retrieved May 18, 2007, from CINAHL Plus with Full Text database.

de Oliveira, N. F. S., da Costa, S. F. G., & da Nóbrega, M. M. L. (2006). Lived dialogue between nurse and mothers of children with cancer [Portuguese]. *Revista Electronica de Enfermagem, 8*, 99–107. Abstract in English retrieved May 18, 2007, from CINAHL Plus with Full Text database.

de Paula, C. C., & Crossetti, M. G. O. (2005a). Happening of nursery care for the child-being who lives with AIDS: Being, knowing and shared doing [Portuguese]. *Revista Gaucha de Enfermagem, 26*, 102–114. Abstract in English retrieved May 18, 2007, from CINAHL Plus with Full Text database.

de Paula, C. C., & Crossetti, M. G. O. (2005b). The way of caring in the meeting with the child-being who lives with AIDS: Experiencing finitude and ethic [Portuguese]. *Texto & Contexto Enfermagem, 14*(2), 193–201. Abstract in English retrieved May 18, 2007, from CINAHL Plus with Full Text database.

de Paula, C. C., de Mello Padoin, S. M., Vernier, E. T. N., & da Motta, M. G. C. (2003). Reflections on the child being and on the nursing care in AIDS context [Portuguese]. *Revista Gaucha de Enfermagem, 24*, 189–195. Abstract in English retrieved May 18, 2007, from CINAHL Plus with Full Text database.

de Paula, C. C., Schaurich, D., Padoin, S. M. M., & Crossetti, M. G. O. (2004). The care as a lived and dialogued meeting in the Humanistic Nursing Theory of Paterson and Zderad [Portuguese]. *Acta Paulista de Enfermagem, 17*, 425–431.

Abstract in English retrieved May 18, 2007, from CINAHL Plus with Full Text database.

Easter, A. L. (1999). Preliminary testing of the Modes of Being Present Scale (MBPS). *Dissertation Abstracts International, 60*(09B), 4519. Abstract retrieved November 6, 2007, from Dissertation Abstracts Online database.

Guillaumet, M. (2009). Trans-cultural relationships in treatment situations [Spanish]. *Revista de Enfermería(Barcelona, Spain), 32* (7–8), 8–12. Abstract in English retrieved November 21, 2009, from PubMed database.

Hinds, P. S. (1985). An investigation of the relationships between adolescent hopefulness, caring behaviors of nurses and adolescent health care outcomes. *Dissertation Abstracts International, 46*(08B), 2623. Abstract retrieved November 6, 2007, from Dissertation Abstracts Online database.

Hines, D. R. (1991). The development of the measurement of presence scale. *Dissertation Abstracts International, 52*(08B), 4123. Abstract retrieved November 6, 2007, from Dissertation Abstracts Online database.

Johnson, R. J. (2001). The experiences of hemodialysis patients with type 2 diabetes mellitus. *Masters Abstracts International, 40*(01), 150. Abstract retrieved November 6, 2007, from Dissertation Abstracts Online database.

Kleiman, S. (2002). The essences of the lived experiences of nurse practitioners interacting with their patients. *Dissertation Abstracts International, 63*(04B), 1785. Abstract retrieved February 23, 2008, from Dissertation Abstracts Online database.

Kleiman, S., Frederickson, K., & Lundy, T. (2004). Using an eclectic model to educate students about cultural influences on the nurse–patient relationship. *Nursing Education Perspectives, 25,* 249–253.

Kostovich, C. T. (2002). Development of a scale to measure nursing presence. *Dissertation Abstracts International, 63*(01B), 178. Abstract retrieved February 23, 2008, from Dissertation Abstracts Online database.

Krug, S. B. F., & Somavilla, V. C. (2004). A reflexive analysis on professional nursing actions involving work accident victims in view of the theory of Paterson and Zderad [Portuguese]. *Revista Latino-Americana de Enfermagem, 12,* 277–279. Abstract in English retrieved May 18, 2007, from CINAHL Plus with Full Text database.

Larson, S. G. (2002). Contemplative spirituality: Towards phenomenological understanding. *Dissertation Abstracts International, 63*(05B), 2308. Abstract retrieved November 6, 2007, from Dissertation Abstracts Online database.

Li, H. (2006). Application of humanistic nursing care for parturient undergoing spontaneous delivery [Chinese]. *Chinese Nursing Research, 20*(1B), 140–141. Abstract in English retrieved May 18, 2007, from CINAHL Plus with Full Text database.

Luegenbiehl, D. L. (1986). The essence of nurse caring during labor and delivery. *Dissertation Abstracts Online, 47*(06B), 2375. Abstract retrieved November 6, 2007, from Dissertation Abstracts Online database.

McCamant, K. L. (2006). Humanistic nursing, interpersonal relations theory, and the empathy-altruism hypothesis. *Nursing Science Quarterly, 19,* 334–338.

Medeiros, H. M., & da Motta Mda G. (2008). HIV/AIDS children living in shelters under the perspective of Humanistic Nursing [Portuguese]. *Revista Gaúcha De Enfermagem, 29,* 400-407. Abstract in English retrieved November 21, 2009, from PubMed database.

Mercês, C. A. M., & Rocha, R. M. (2006). Paterson and Zderad's theory: Nursing care for critical clients sustained by the experienced dialogue [Portuguese]. *Revista Enfermagem UERJ, 14,* 470–475. Abstract in English retrieved May 18, 2007, from CINAHL Plus with Full Text database.

Moch, S. D. (1988). Health in illness: Experiences with breast cancer. *Dissertation Abstracts International, 50*(02B), 0497. Abstract retrieved February 23, 2008, from Dissertation Abstracts Online database.

Mustain, B. J. (1999). The lived experience of overweight adolescent females. *Masters Abstracts International, 37*(05), 1437. Abstract retrieved November 6, 2007, from Dissertation Abstracts Online database.

Nascimento, E. R. P., & Trentini, M. (2004). Nursing care at the intensive care unit (ICU): Going beyond objectivity [Portuguese]. *Revista Latino-Americana de Enfermagem, 12,* 250–257. Abstract in English retrieved May 18, 2007, from CINAHL Plus with Full Text database.

Negri, M. D. X., Labronici, L. M., & Zagonel, I. P. S. (2003). Inclusive nursing care for individual suffering from Down's syndrome under Paterson and Zderad's view [Portuguese].

Revista Brasileira de Enfermagem, 56, 678–682. Abstract in English retrieved May 18, 2007, from CINAHL Plus with Full Text database.

O'Connor, N. (1993). *Paterson and Zderad: Humanistic Nursing Theory.* Newbury Park, CA: Sage.

Paterson, J. G., & Zderad, L. (1971). All together thorough complementary syntheses the worlds of the many. *Journal of Nursing Scholarship, 4*(3), 13–16. Abstract retrieved February 18, 2008, from http://www.blackwell-syngery.com.

Paterson, J. G., & Zderad, L. T. (2007). *Humanistic Nursing.* Retrieved February 20, 2008, from http://www.paterson-zderad-humanistic-nursing.com (Previously published 1988 [Pub. No. 41-2218], New York: National League for Nursing; originally published 1976, New York: John Wiley & Sons)

Praeger, S. G. (1980). Humanistic nursing education: Considerations and proposals. *Dissertation Abstracts International, 41*(06B), 2122. Abstract retrieved November 6, 2007, from Dissertation Abstracts Online database.

Ramos, A. F., Caetano, J. A., Soares, E., & Rolim, K. M. (2006). The family living with Down syndrome patients in the perspective of humanistic theory [Portuguese]. *Revista Brasileira De Enfermagem, 59*, 262–268. Abstract in English retrieved November 21, 2009, from PubMed database.

Rolim, K. M. C. (2008). Humanistic nursing: Contribute for development of the nurse in the neonatal unit [Portuguese]. *Revista Eletrônica de Enfermagem, 10*(1), 251–253.

Rolim, K. M. C., & Cardoso, M. V. L. (2006). Discourse and practice of care to newborns at risk: Reflecting about humanized care [Portuguese]. *Revista Latino-Americana de Enfermagem, 14*(1), 85–92. Abstract in English retrieved May 18, 2007, from CINAHL Plus with Full Text database.

Rolim, K. M., & Cardoso, M. V. (2006b). Interaction nurse-newborn during orotracheal aspiration and blood collection [Portuguese]. *Revista da Escola de Enfermagen da U S P, 40*, 515–523.

Abstract in English retrieved November 21, 2009, from PubMed database.

Rolim, K. M. C., Pagliuca, L. M. F., & Cardoso, M. V. L. (2005). Analysis of humanistic theory and interpersonal relations of nurses in newborn care [Portuguese]. *Revista Latino-Americana de Enfermagem, 13*, 432–440. Abstract in English retrieved May 18, 2007, from CINAHL Plus with Full Text database.

Santos, M. C. L., Pagliuca, L. M. F., & Fernandes, A. F. C. (2007). Humanistic theory: Dimensional analysis of the concept of health [Spanish]. *Metas de Enfermería, 10*(4), 56–60. Abstract in English retrieved November 30, 2009, from CINAHL Plus with Full Text database.

Schaurich, D., Padoin, S. M. M., de Paula, C. C., & da Motta, M. G. C. (2005). Utilization of the humanistic theory of Paterson and Zderad as possibility of practical in pediatric nursing [Portuguese]. *Escola Anna Nery Revista de Enfermagem, 9*, 265–270. Abstract in English retrieved May 18, 2007, from CINAHL Plus with Full Text database.

Stoner, M. J. H. (1982). Hope and cancer patients. *Dissertation Abstracts International, 44*(01B), 0115. Abstract retrieved November 6, 2007, from Dissertation Abstracts Online database.

Suderman, E. M. (1997). The lived experience of nurses during a hospital restructuring. *Masters Abstracts International, 36*(02), 0517. Abstract retrieved February 23, 2008, from Dissertation Abstracts Online database.

Tutton, E., & Seers, K. (2003). An exploration of the concept of comfort. *Journal of Clinical Nursing, 12*, 689–696.

Ward, S. G. (2003). Intensive observation service: Nurses's feelings and perceptions regarding the new service. *Masters Abstracts International, 41*(05), 1423. Abstract retrieved November 6, 2007, from Dissertation Abstracts Online database.

Weissman, J. K. (1992). The adolescent's experience of being accepted by a nurse. *Masters Abstracts International, 31*(02), 0774. Abstract retrieved November 6, 2007, from Dissertation Abstracts Online database.

CHAPTER 16

Theory of Culture Care Diversity and Universality

Madeleine M. Leininger

Julia B. George

Madeleine M. Leininger was born July 13, 1925, in Sutton, Nebraska, and received her basic nursing education at St. Anthony's School of Nursing, Denver, Colorado, graduating in 1948. In 1950 she earned a bachelor of science degree in biological science from Mount St. Scholastica College (now known as Benedictine College), Atchison, Kansas; in 1954 a master of science in psychiatric-mental health nursing from The Catholic University of America, Washington, D.C.; and in 1965 a Ph.D. in cultural and social anthropology from the University of Washington, Seattle. She is a fellow in the American Academy of Nursing and holds honorary doctorates from Benedictine College; the University of Indianapolis, Indiana; and the University of Kuopio, Kuopio, Finland. In 1998 she was named a Living Legend by the American Academy of Nursing.

Dr. Leininger is the founder of transcultural nursing, the Transcultural Nursing Society, and the Journal of Transcultural Nursing. She was associate professor and director of the graduate psychiatric nursing program, College of Nursing and Health, University of Cincinnati, Ohio; professor of nursing and anthropology (the first joint appointment in nursing and another discipline in the United States), University of Colorado, Denver; dean of nursing and lecturer in anthropology, University of Washington, Seattle; dean of nursing and adjunct professor of anthropology, University of Utah, Salt Lake City; and professor of nursing, director of the Center for Health Research, and adjunct professor of anthropology, Wayne State University, Detroit, Michigan. She is Professor Emeritus, College of Nursing, Wayne State University, and adjunct professor at the University of Nebraska Medical Center College of Nursing, Omaha. She has published extensively and lectures and consults about transcultural nursing and human care theory and research worldwide. She has held visiting professorships and lectureships in Australia, Brunei, Dar es Salaam Finland, Germany, the Netherlands, Russia, Singapore, Sweden, Switzerland, Taiwan, Thailand, and the United States. Her papers are housed in the Walter Ruether Archival Center, Wayne State University. A collection of her books is housed at Madonna University, Livonia, Michigan, the location of the home office of the Transcultural Nursing Society. Her early papers are housed in the Boston Archives at Boston University, Massachusetts. More information about her activities and publications can be found on the website for the Transcultural Nursing Society at http://www.tcns.org.

In the 1940s Leininger (1991) recognized the importance of caring to nursing. Statements of appreciation for nursing care made by patients alerted her to caring values and led to her long-standing focus on care as the dominant ethos of nursing. During the mid-1950s, she experienced what she describes as cultural shock while she was working in a child guidance home in the midwestern United States. While working as a clinical nurse specialist with disturbed children and their parents, she observed recurrent behavioral differences among the children and finally concluded that these differences had a cultural base. She identified a lack of knowledge of the children's cultures as the missing link in nursing to understand the variations needed in the care of clients. This experience led her to become the first professional nurse in the world to earn a doctorate in anthropology and led to the development of the field of transcultural nursing.

Leininger first used the terms *transcultural nursing*, *ethnonursing*, and *cross-cultural nursing* in the 1960s. In 1966, at the University of Colorado, she offered the first transcultural nursing course with field experiences and has been instrumental in the development of similar courses at a number of other institutions (Leininger, 1979). In 2006, Leininger affirmed her definition of transcultural nursing as

> . . . a discipline of study and practice focused on comparative culture care differences and similarities among and between cultures in order to assist human beings to attain and maintain meaningful and therapeutic health care practices that are culturally based (2006a, p. 16)

and as

> . . . a discipline with a body of knowledge and practices to attain and maintain the goal of culturally congruent care for health and wellbeing. (2006a, p. 19)

In 2006 she defined ethnonursing as

> . . . a rigorous, systematic, and in-depth method for studying multiple cultures and care factors within familiar environments of people and to focus on the interrelationships of care and culture to arrive at the goal of culturally congruent care services. (2006a, p. 20)

The term *transcultural nursing* (rather than "cross-cultural") is used today to refer to the evolving knowledge and practices related to this field of study and practice. Leininger (1991, 1995, 2006a) stresses the importance of knowledge gained from direct experience or directly from those who have learned from experience and labels such knowledge as *emic*, or people centered. This is contrasted with *etic* knowledge, which describes the professional perspective. She contends that *emically* derived care knowledge is essential to establish nursing's epistemological and ontological base for practice.

Leininger built her theory of transcultural nursing on the premise that the peoples of each culture can not only know and define the ways in which they experience and perceive their nursing care world but also relate these experiences and perceptions to their general health beliefs and practices. Based on this premise, nursing care is derived and developed from the cultural context in which it is to be provided.

Leininger (1991, 2006a) asserts that human care is central to nursing as a discipline and as a profession. She and others have studied the phenomena of care for over five decades. They recognize and are proponents of the preservation of care as the essence of nursing. With this increasing recognition of care as essential to nursing knowledge and practice, Leininger labeled her theory *culture care*. She drew upon anthropology for the culture component and upon nursing for the care component. Her belief that cultures have both health practices that are specific to one culture and prevailing patterns that are common across cultures led to the addition of the terms *diversity* and *universality* to the title of her theory. Thus, the most current title of Leininger's theory is Culture Care or Culture Care Diversity and Universality.

LEININGER'S THEORY

In 1985, Leininger published her first presentation of her work as a theory, and in later works (1988b, 1991, 1995, 2002, 2006a) she presented further explication of her ideas. She refers to her 1991 book as the primary book for her theory and recommends it for further in-depth study of the theory (Leininger, 2006a). In the later presentations, she provided orientational definitions for the constructs of care; culture; culture care; emic and etic, including generic and professional care; cultural and social structure factors; ethnohistory; environmental context; worldview; culture care preservation, culture care accommodation, and culture care repatterning; culturally congruent care; culture care diversity; and universality. Leininger points out that these definitions are provisional guides that may be altered as a culture is studied. In addition to the definitions, she presented assumptions related to the constructs. Leininger (2002) differentiates between concept and construct as a concept dealing with a single idea and a construct including several ideas interrelated in a phenomenon.

Care as a noun is defined as those abstract and concrete phenomena related to "assistive, supportive, and enabling experiences or ideas toward others with evident or anticipated needs to ameliorate or improve a human condition or lifeway" (Leininger, 2006a, p. 12). Care is assumed to be a distinct, dominant, unifying, and central focus of nursing, and, while curing and healing cannot occur effectively without care, care may occur without cure. *Care* as a gerund is defined as "actions, activities, and practices directed to assist or help others toward healing and wellbeing" (p. 12). Assumptions related to care and caring include that they are essential for the survival of humans, as well as for their growth, health, well-being, healing, and ability to deal with handicaps and death. The expressions, patterns, and lifeways of care have different meanings in different cultural contexts. The phenomenon of care can be discovered or identified by examining the cultural group's view of the world, social structure, and language.

Culture is the "learned, shared, and transmitted . . . values, beliefs, norms, and lifeways of a particular group that guides . . . thinking, decisions, and actions in patterned ways" (Leininger, 1995, p. 60) and is often intergenerational (Leininger, 2006a). A related assumption is that the values, beliefs, and practices for culturally related care are shaped by and often embedded in "the worldview, social structure factors (e.g. religion, philosophy of life, kinship, politics, economics, education, technology, and cultural values) and the ethnohistorical and environmental context" of the culture (Leininger, 2006a, p. 19). A subculture, while closely related to the culture, is a group within the culture that differs from the main culture in its "values, beliefs, norms, moral codes, and ways of living with some distinctive features of its own" (Leininger & McFarland, 2002, p. 47).

Culture care is defined as "the synthesized and culturally constituted assistive, supportive and, facilitative, caring acts toward self or others focused on evident or anticipated needs for the client's health or well-being or to face disabilities, death, or other human conditions" (Leininger & McFarland, 2002, p. 83). A related assumption is that culture care, as a synthesis of the two major constructs of culture and care, guides the discovery and helps explain and account for the human conditions including, but not limited to, health, well-being, disabilities, and expressions of care. Another assumption is that within all facets of culture care (meanings, expressions, patterns, processes, structures), there are both commonalities and differences between and within cultures (Leininger, 2006a).

The constructs of *emic* (insider's knowledge) and *etic* (outsider or stranger's viewpoint) are also related to sources of care. Emic care, known as *generic* or *folk care*, and *caring,* is defined as "culturally learned and transmitted lay, indigenous (traditional), and largely emic folk knowledge and skills used by cultures" (Leininger & McFarland, 2002, p. 61). In 1995, Leininger identified this emic or generic care as being usually based in the home. Etic care is known as *professional care* and includes nursing care. *Professional care* is defined as "formal and explicit cognitively learned . . . knowledge and practices obtained generally through educational institutions . . . [used] to provide assistive, supportive, enabling, or facilitative acts for or to another individual or group in order to improve their health, prevent illnesses, or to help with dying or other human conditions" (Leininger, 2006a, p. 14). Table 16-1 provides a comparison of the generic and professional care systems from the consumer's view. The associated assumption is that in every culture both emic and etic practices can be discovered and used.

TABLE 16-1 Consumer's View of Generic and Professional Care

Generic (emic) View	Professional (etic) View
Orientation is humanistic	Orientation is scientific
Based in the people, uses the practical and familiar	Clients are acted upon by strangers using unfamiliar techniques
Approach is holistic and integrated; focuses on social relationships, language, and lifeways	Services are fragmented, not integrated; services focus on the physical body and mind
Primary focus is on caring	Overall focus is primarily on curing, diagnosis, and treatments
Uses folk remedies and personal relationships; essentially not technical	Primarily technological using many diagnostic tests and scientific treatments
Seeks to prevent illness, disability, and to maintain lifeways	Seeks to treat disease, disability, and pathology
Communication modes are high in context	Communication modes are low in context
Relies on folk caring and healing practices that are traditional and familiar	Relies on assessment and treatment of biophysical and emotional factors

Adapted from Leininger, M., & McFarland, M. R. (2002). *Transcultural nursing: Concepts, theories, research and practice* (3rd ed., p. 61). New York: McGraw-Hill.

Cultural and social structure factors are important considerations. While they are broad in nature, the way in which they interrelate within a given individual or group will influence the behavior of that individual or group. These factors include "religion (spirituality); kinship (social ties); politics; legal issues; education; economics; technology; political factors; philosophy of life; and cultural beliefs and values with gender and class differences" (Leininger, 2006a, p. 14).

The construct of *ethnohistory* came from anthropology but has been defined for nursing by Leininger (2006a) as those "past facts, events, instances, and experiences of human beings, groups, cultures, and institutions that occur over time in particular contexts that help explain past and current lifeways about culture care influencers of health and wellbeing or the death of people" (p. 15). "Knowledge of meanings and practices derived from world views, social structure factors, cultural values, environmental context, and language uses are essential to guide nursing decisions and actions in providing cultur[e] congruent care" (Leininger, 1988b, p. 155).

The *environmental context* in which care occurs is very important, as it, too, influences the behaviors of all who are involved in the care experience. Environmental context is "the totality of an event, situation, or particular experience that gives meaning to people's expressions, interpretations, and social interactions within particular geophysical, ecological, spiritual, sociopolitical, and technologic factors in specific cultural settings" (Leininger, 2006a, p. 15).

Worldview is the way in which people look at the world or at the universe and form a "picture or value stance" about the world and their lives (Leininger, 1995, p. 105). Information about worldview provides a broader perspective or understanding of decisions made about care and caring.

Along with the universal nature of human beings as caring beings, the cultural care values, beliefs, and practices that are specific to a given culture provide a basis for the patterns, conditions, and actions associated with human care. Knowledge of these provides the base for three *action-decision care modes*, all of which require the coparticipation of the nurse and clients. *Culture care preservation* is also known as maintenance and includes "those assistive, supportive, facilitative or enabling professional acts or decisions that help cultures to retain, preserve, or maintain beneficial care beliefs and values or to face handicaps and death" (Leininger, 2006a, p. 8). *Culture care accommodation*, also known as negotiation, includes "those assistive, accommodating, facilitative, or enabling creative provider care actions or decisions that help cultures adapt to or negotiate with others for culturally congruent, safe, and effective care for their health, wellbeing, or to deal with illness or dying" (p. 8). *Culture care repatterning*, or restructuring, includes "those assistive, supportive, facilitative, or enabling professional actions and mutual decisions that would help people to reorder, change, modify or restructure their lifeways and institutions for better (or beneficial) health care patterns, practices, or outcomes" (p. 8). Repatterning requires the creative use of an extensive knowledge of the client's culture base and must be done in a way that is sensitive to the client's lifeways while using both generic and professional knowledge. Leininger's assumption is that these three modes are unique and creative and provide a different way of offering help to human beings in diverse cultures.

Culturally congruent (nursing) care is defined as "culturally based care knowledge, acts, and decisions used in sensitive and knowledgeable ways to appropriately and meaningfully fit the cultural values, beliefs, and lifeways of clients for their health and wellbeing, or to prevent illness, disabilities, or death" (Leininger, 2006a, p. 15). Leininger (1995) asserts that nursing, as a transcultural care discipline and profession, has a central purpose to serve human beings in all areas of the world and that when culturally based nursing care is beneficial and healthy, it contributes to the well-being of the client(s)—whether individuals, groups, families, communities, or institutions—as they function within the context of their environments. Also, nursing care will be culturally congruent or beneficial only when the clients are known by the nurse and the clients' patterns, expressions, and cultural values are used in appropriate and meaningful ways by the nurse with those clients. Finally, if clients receive nursing care that is not at least reasonably culturally congruent (i.e., compatible with and respectful of the clients' lifeways, beliefs, and values), the client will demonstrate signs of stress, noncompliance, cultural conflicts, and/or ethical or moral concerns.

Cultures have both differences and similarities. In relation to care, Leininger (2006a) terms these as culture care diversity and culture care universality. *Culture care diversity* indicates "the differences or variabilities among human beings with respect to culture care meanings, patterns, values, lifeways, symbols, or other features related to providing beneficial care to clients of a designated culture" (p. 16). In contrast, *culture care universality* indicates the "commonly shared or similar culture care phenomena features of human beings or a group with recurrent meanings, patterns, values, lifeways, or symbols that serve as a guide for caregivers to provide assistive, supportive, facilitative, or enabling people care for healthy outcomes" (p. 16). It is assumed that, while human care is universal across cultures, caring may be demonstrated through diverse expressions, actions, patterns, lifestyles, and meanings. Leininger states that the purpose of the culture care theory was to explore and document these diversities and universalities between and among cultures. Her goal is "to use culture care research findings to provide specific and/or general care that would be culturally congruent, safe, and beneficial to people of diverse or similar cultures for their health, well-being, and healing, and to help people face disabilities and death" (p. 5).

Leininger also defines *nursing* as "a learned, humanistic, and scientific profession and discipline focused on human care phenomena and caring activities in order to assist, support, and facilitate or enable individuals or groups to maintain or regain their health or well-being in culturally meaningful and beneficial ways, or to help individuals face handicaps or death" (Leininger & McFarland, 2002, p. 46). *Professional nursing care (caring)* is defined as "formal and cognitively learned professional care knowledge and practice skills, obtained through educational institutions, that are expected to provide assistive, supportive, enabling or facilitative acts to or for another individual or group in order to improve a human health condition (or well-being), disability, lifeway, or to work with dying clients" (Leininger, 1995, p. 79).

Health is "a state of well-being that is culturally defined and constituted . . . a state of being to maintain and the ability to help individuals or groups to perform their daily role activities in culturally expressed beneficial care and patterned lifeways" (Leininger, 2006a, p. 10). Leininger (1995) indicates that all cultures have generic or folk health care practices, that professional practices usually vary across cultures, and that in any culture there will be cultural similarities and differences between the care receivers (generic) and the professional caregivers.

Leininger (2002) identifies the unique features of her theory as follows:

- One of the oldest theories of nursing
- Focus on the interrelationships of culture, care, well-being, health, illness, and death
- Focus on comparative culture care
- Holistic and multidimensional exploration of culturally based care meanings and practices
- Seeking to discover the cultural care diversities and universalities
- Specific nursing research method of ethnonursing
- Three action modes with both abstract and practical features
- Inclusion of both emic and etic views

Leininger named her theory *Culture Care Diversity and Universality* and depicts it in what she now terms the Sunrise Enabler (formerly known as the Sunrise Model) (see Figure 16-1). This enabler may be viewed as a cognitive map that moves from the most abstract to the least abstract. The top of the enabler is the worldview and cultural and social structure levels, which direct the study of perceptions of the world outside of the culture—the suprasystem in general system terms. Leininger (1985b) states that the world-view leads to the study of the nature, meaning, and attributes of care from three perspectives. Values and social structure could be a part of each of three perspectives. The microperspective studies individuals within a culture; these studies typically would be on a small scale. The middle perspective focuses on more complex factors in one specific culture; these studies are on a larger scale than microstudies. The macrostudies investigate phenomena across several cultures and are large in scale.

The culture care worldview flows into the cultural and social structure dimensions and the multiple factors that make up these dimensions. Aspects of these factors include their environmental context, language, and ethnohistory. The factors influence how care patterns and practices are expressed to provide holistic care in health, illness, and death. Next is knowledge about individuals, families, groups, communities, and institutions in diverse health care contexts. This knowledge provides culturally specific meanings and expressions in relation to care and health. The next focus is on the generic or folk care, professional care-cure practices, and nursing care practices. Information about these includes the characteristics and the specific care features of each. This information allows for the identification of similarities and differences or culture care universality and culture care diversity.

Next are transcultural care decisions and actions that involve culture care preservation/maintenance, culture care accommodation/negotiation, and culture care repatterning/restructuring. It is here that nursing care is delivered. Within the Sunrise Enabler, culture congruent care is developed. This care is both congruent with and valued by the members of the culture.

Leininger (Leininger & McFarland, 2002) points out that the enabler is not the theory but a depiction of the components of the theory of Culture Care Diversity and Universality. The purpose of the enabler is to aid the study of how the components of the theory influence the health status of and care provided to individuals, families, groups, communities, and institutions within a culture. She points out that one may begin at any level of the enabler but needs to explore all of its aspects. She presents cogent arguments for the use of the enabler to guide discovery research that uses qualitative and ethnographic methods of study. She speaks strongly against the use of

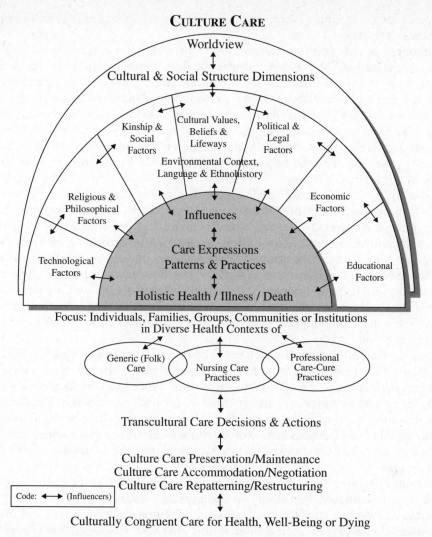

CULTURE CARE

FIGURE 16-1   Leininger's Sunrise Enabler.   *(From Leininger, M. M. (2006). Culture Care Diversity and Universality Theory and evolution of the Ethnonursing Method. In M. M. Leininger, & M. R. McFarland. Culture Care Diversity and Universality: A worldwide nursing theory (2nd ed.) (p. 25). Boston: Jones and Bartlett.)*

operational definitions and preconceived notions and the use of causal or linear perspectives in studying cultural care diversity and universality. She supports the importance of finding out what *is*, of exploring and discovering the essence and meanings of care.

LEININGER'S THEORY AND THE FOUR MAJOR CONCEPTS

Leininger defines health, nursing, and environment but does not specifically define the major concept of person. However, her view of these concepts can be derived from her conceptual definitions and assumptions. She also presents an argument for care as the central concept in nursing's metaparadigm (Leininger, 1988a, 1991, 1995; Leininger & McFarland, 2002, 2006).

Leininger is adamant that the concept of person is not culturally appropriate in many cultures; person often is not a central or dominant concept in a culture. *Human beings* are best represented in her work. Humans are believed to be caring and to be capable of being concerned about the needs, well-being, and survival of others. Human care is universal, that is, seen in all cultures. Humans have survived within cultures and through place and time because they have been able to care for infants, children, and the elderly in a variety of ways and in many different environments. Thus, humans are universally caring beings who survive in a diversity of cultures through their ability to provide the universality of care in a variety of ways according to differing cultures, needs, and settings. Leininger (1991) also indicates that nursing as a caring science should focus beyond traditional "nurse–patient interactions and dyads [to include] families, groups, communities, total cultures, and institutions" (p. 22) as well as world-wide health institutions and ways to develop international nursing care policies and practices. She points out that in many non-Western cultures, family and institutions dominate. In these cultures, person is not an important concept. Indeed, there may be no term in the language for "person." Thus, in the theory of Culture Care Diversity and Universality the focus is on human beings and not necessarily on the individual. A focus on the individual should occur only if it is appropriate to the culture in which care is being given.

Leininger defines *health*; this definition appears earlier in this chapter. She speaks of health systems, health care practices, changing health patterns, health promotion, and health maintenance. Health is an important concept in transcultural nursing. Because the emphasis is on the need for nurses to have knowledge that is specific to the culture in which nursing is being practiced, it is presumed that health is viewed as being universal across cultures but defined within each culture in a manner that reflects the beliefs, values, and practices of that particular culture. Thus, health is both universal and diverse.

Leininger speaks to social structure and worldview rather than society. She defines environment as "the totality of geophysical situations(s), or . . . the lived-in geographic and ecological settings of cultures" (Leininger 2006a, p. 10) and discusses environmental context (defined earlier in this chapter). However, society and environment, if viewed as being represented in culture, are a major theme of Leininger's theory. Leininger's (1991) definition of culture focuses on a particular group (society) and the patterning of actions, thoughts, and decisions that occurs as the result of "learned, shared, and transmitted values, beliefs, norms, and lifeways" (p. 47). This learning, sharing, transmitting, and patterning occur within a group of people who function in an identifiable setting or environment.

Nursing is defined by Leininger; this definition appears earlier in this chapter. She also discusses that nursing, as a profession, has a societal mandate to serve people and, as a discipline, is expected to discover, develop, and use knowledge distinctive to nursing's focus on human care and caring. She expresses concern that nurses do not have adequate preparation for a transcultural perspective and that they neither value nor practice from such a perspective to the fullest extent possible. She presents three types of nursing actions that are culturally based and thus congruent with the needs and values of the clients. These are culture care preservation/maintenance, culture care accommodation/negotiation, and culture care repatterning/restructuring; they have been defined earlier in this chapter. These three modes of action can lead to the delivery of nursing care that best fits with the client's culture and thus decreases cultural stress and potential for conflict between client and caregiver.

It should be noted that Leininger incorporates additional concepts as vital to nursing. These include human care, caring, and multiple cultural factors. These terms are defined elsewhere in this chapter, and their definitions will not be repeated here.

CULTURE CARE DIVERSITY AND UNIVERSALITY AND TRANSCULTURAL NURSING

After careful review of the Sunrise Enabler, it becomes apparent that there are parallels between the enabler and the nursing process. This is true, in part, because both represent a problem-solving process. The focus of the nursing process is the client who is the recipient of nursing care. The client (whether an individual, family, group, or other aggregate of human beings) is also a focus of the Sunrise Enabler, but the importance of knowledge and understanding of the client's culture is a major shaping force in the enabler. Major features of cultures are presented in Table 16-2.

Gaining knowledge and understanding of another's culture may be very time consuming for the nurse who is not familiar with that culture. Leininger (1978, 1991, 1995; Leininger & McFarland, 2002) speaks with concern about the possibility of the nurse being involved in culture shock or cultural imposition. *Culture shock* may result when an outsider attempts to comprehend or adapt effectively to a different cultural group. The outsider is likely to experience feelings of discomfort and helplessness and some degree of disorientation because of the differences in cultural values, beliefs, and practices. Culture shock may lead to anger and can be reduced by seeking knowledge of the culture before encountering that culture. *Cultural imposition* refers to efforts of the outsider, both subtle and not so subtle, to impose his or her own cultural values, beliefs, or behaviors upon an individual, family, or group from another culture. Cultural imposition has been particularly prevalent in efforts to impose Western health care practices on other cultures.

In 1995, Leininger added many other concepts related to culture to those included in her earlier discussions. *Culture values* are critical to transcultural nursing, as they

---

TABLE 16-2   Features of Cultures

- Reflect learned and shared values, ideals, and meanings that guide thoughts, decisions, and actions
- Have rules of behavior that are readily recognized (manifest) or covert and ideal (implicit)
      *care is often implicit
- Have material items or symbols that have special meaning
         *Coke or Pepsi cans in the United States; bows and arrows in New Guinea
- Have traditional ceremonial practices (religious rituals, food feasts) transmitted intergenerationally and reaffirm caring ways
- Have insider's or emic views and knowledge that are extremely important to discover and understand for meaningful care practices
- Have intercultural variations, both between and within cultures

---

Adapted from Leininger, M., & McFarland, M. R. (2002). *Transcultural nursing: Concepts, theories, research and practice* (3rd ed., pp. 48–49). New York: McGraw-Hill.

have a strong influence on behavior. They are defined as "the powerful internal and external directive forces that give meaning and order to an individual's group's thinking, decisions, and actions" (p. 63). *Cultural relativism* is the position that "cultures are unique and must be evaluated according to their own values and standards" (p. 66). *Ethnicity* relates to identity arising from language, religion, and national origins. *Ethnocentrism*, a universal phenomenon and a core concept in transcultural nursing, is "the belief that one's own ways are the best, most superior, or preferred ways to act, believe, or behave" (p. 65). In contrast, *racism* is "derived from the concept of race, and it is usually defined as a biological feature of a discrete group, whose members share distinctive genetic traits inherited from a common ancestor" (p. 70). *Prejudice* is "preconceived ideas, beliefs, or opinions about an individual, group, or culture that limit a full and accurate understanding of the individual, culture, gender, race, event, or situation" (p. 71). *Discrimination* is "the limiting of opportunities, choices, or life experiences because of prejudices about individuals, cultures, or social groups" (p. 71). *Stereotyping* is "placing people and institutions, mentally and by attitudes, into a narrow, fixed trait, rigid pattern, or with inflexible 'boxlike' characteristics" (p. 71).

> *Uniculturalism* (or monoculturalism) is "the belief that one's universe is largely constituted, centered upon and functions from a one-culture perspective and reflecting some cultural ethnocentric views" (p. 65). *Multiculturalism* is "a perspective and reality that there are many different cultures and subcultures in the world which need to be recognized, valued, and understood for their differences and similarities" (p. 65). *Cultural bias* is "a firm position or stance that one's own values and beliefs must govern the situation or decision" (p. 66). On the other hand, *cultural blindness* is "the inability of an individual to recognize one's own lifestyle, values and modes of behavior and those of another individual because of strong attitude to make them invisible due to ethnocentric tendencies" (p. 67). *Cultural pain* is "the suffering, discomfort, or unfavorable responses of an individual group towards an individual who has different beliefs or lifeways, usually reflecting the insensitivity of those inflicting the discomfort" (p. 67). *Biculturalism* is "how biological, physical, and different physical environments of diverse and similar cultures relate to care, health, illness, and disabilities" (p. 68). *Culture-bound* is "specific care, health, illness, and disease conditions that are particular, highly unique, and usually specific to a designated culture or geographical area" (p. 69). Leininger (1995) uses the terms *Western* and *non-Western* for general comparative purposes in discussing transcultural nursing. Western cultures tend to be highly industrialized and dependent on technology. Non-Western (may be identified as Eastern) cultures are much less dependent on technology, have strong philosophical ideologies, and have existed for thousands of years. *Enculturation* is "in-depth learning about a culture with its specific values, beliefs, and practices in order to prepare children and adults to function or to live effective[ly] in a particular culture" (p. 72). *Acculturation* is "the process by which an individual or group from culture A learns how to take on many of the behaviors, values, and lifeways of culture B" (p. 72). *Socialization* is "the social process whereby an individual or group from a particular culture learns how to become a part of and function within the larger society in order to know how to interact with others, vote, work, and live in a society" (p. 73).

Assimilation is "the way an individual or group from one culture selectively takes on and chooses certain features of another culture without necessarily taking on the total attributes of a particular culture" (p. 73).

Leininger and McFarland (2002) discuss concepts related to culture care:

- Culture specific care/caring—"very specific or particular ways to have care fit [the] client's needs"
- Generalized culture care—"commonly shared professional nursing care techniques, principles, and practices that are beneficial to several clients as a general and essential human care need"
- Culture care conflict—"signs of distress, concern and nonhelpful nursing care practices that fail to meet a client's cultural expectations, beliefs, values, and lifeways"
- Culture care clashes—similar to culture care conflict but are further defined as when "obvious and known situations arise that are tense and cause overt problems"
- Cultural exports—"the sending of ideas, techniques, material goods, or symbolic referents to another culture with the intention they will be valued and used to improve lifeways or to advance practices"
- Cultural imports—the "taking in or receiving [of] ideas, techniques, material goods, or other items with the position they can be useful or helpful in this culture"
- Culture time—"the dominant orientation of an individual or group to different past, present, and . . . future periods that guides one's thinking and actions"
  - Includes clock time, social time, cyclic time
- Cultural space—"the variation of cultures in the use of body, visual, territorial, and interpersonal distance to others"
  - Includes body touching
- Cultural context—"the totality of shared meanings and life experiences in particular social, cultural and physical environments that influence attitudes, thinking and patterns of living"
  - May be high (deeply involved with almost instant sharing of beliefs and values) or low (with less commonly shared meanings and more difficultly understanding strangers)
- Culture care therapy—"qualified, transcultural nurses who offer assistive, supportive, and facilitative healing reflections and practices to individuals who have experienced cultural, pain, hurts, insults, offenses, and other related concerns" (pp. 57–60)

The upper portions of the Sunrise Enabler involve the development of knowledge about cultures, people, and care systems. When appropriately used, they could help prevent culture shock, cultural imposition, and culture care conflict. These levels are similar to the *assessment* and *diagnosis* phases of the nursing process. However, in the Sunrise Enabler, knowledge of the culture could be gained before identifying a specific client who would be the focus of the nursing process. First, one is assessing or gathering knowledge and information about the social structure and worldview of the client's culture. Other information that is needed includes the language and environmental context of the client as well as the factors of technology, religion, philosophy, kinship, social structure, cultural values and beliefs, politics, legal system, economics, and education. Much of this knowledge could be gathered before the identification of a particular client and would be useful in preventing both culture shock and cultural imposition. The principles identified by Leininger as important to conducting a cultralogical assessment are presented in Table 16-3.

Worldview and social structure knowledge needs to be applied to the situation of the client, whether that client is an individual, a family, a group, a community, or a sociocultural institution. Next, it is recognized that the client exists within a health system and the values, beliefs, and behaviors of the generic (folk), professional, and nursing care portions of that health system need to be identified. Throughout this assessment process, it is important to recognize and identify those characteristics that are universal or common across cultures and those that are diverse or specific to the culture being assessed. After identifying the culture care diversities and universalities for the culture, a nursing diagnosis can be developed based on those areas in which the client is not meeting a cultural expectation of the client's culture. A short assessment guide developed by Leininger is displayed in Table 16-4. More detailed assessment guides can be found in her 1995 and 2002 (Leininger & McFarland) texts.

Once the diagnosis has been established, *planning, outcomes,* and *implementation* occur within "nursing care decisions and actions." Again, the nursing care decisions and actions need to be culturally based to best meet the needs of the client and provide culture

---

TABLE 16-3   Principles for Culturalogical Assessment

- Study the Sunrise Enabler and the Culture Care Theory first to be able to draw upon and use the different components
- Show a genuine and sincere interest in the client by listening to and learning from that client
- Give attention to gender or class differences, communication modes (including special language terms), and interpersonal space
- Remain fully aware of one's own culture, including biases and prejudices
- Be aware that the client may belong to subcultures or special groups (for example, drug users, the homeless, the deaf) and that knowledge of that subculture is needed for an accurate assessment and to avoid stereotyping
- Nurses need to know their own culture and areas of competencies as well as deficits to become culturally competent practitioners
- Clarify and explain at the outset to the client (whether an individual or a group) the focus and purpose of the assessment, including times to visit them about their health care beliefs and practices
- Seek a holistic view of the client's world within the client's environmental context using the factors in the Sunrise Enabler that influence care, illness, or well-being
- Remain an active listener and discover the client's emic and etic ways to fit client expectations and create a climate in which the client feels it is safe and beneficial to share
- Reflect on the learned "transcultural holding knowledge" about the client's culture and available research-based care and health knowledge

---

Adapted from Leininger, M., & McFarland, M. R. (2002). *Transcultural nursing: Concepts, theories, research and practice* (3rd ed., pp. 121–125). New York: McGraw-Hill.

TABLE 16-4 Leininger's Short Culturalogical Assessment Guide	

Start Here

↓

Phase I   Record observations of what you see, hear, or experience with clients (includes dress and appearance, body condition features, language, mannerisms and general behavior, attitudes, and cultural features).

↓

Phase II   Listen to and learn from the client about cultural values, beliefs, and daily (nightly) practices related to care and health in the client's environmental context. Give attention to generic (home or folk) practices and professional nursing practices.

↓

Phase III   Identify and document recurrent client patterns and narratives (stories) with client meanings of what has been seen, heard, or experienced.

↓

Phase IV   Synthesize themes and patterns of care derived from the information obtained in phases I, II, and III.

↓

Phase V   Develop a culturally based client–nurse care plan as coparticipants for decisions and actions for culturally congruent care.

Adapted from Leininger, M., & McFarland, M. R. (2002). *Transcultural nursing: Concepts, theories, research and practice* (3rd ed., p. 129). New York: McGraw-Hill.

congruent care. The three modes of action are culture care preservation/maintenance, culture care accommodation/negotiation, and culture care repatterning/restructuring. In culture care preservation/maintenance, the professional actions focus on supporting, assisting, facilitating, or enabling clients to preserve or retain favorable health, to recover from illness, or to face handicaps or death. An example would be facilitating an elderly person's access to grocery shopping so that the individual can continue to prepare healthful meals—or encouraging the sharing of those meals with another in a manner that is culturally acceptable.

Culture care accommodation/negotiation creates professional efforts to facilitate, enable, assist, or support actions that represent ways to negotiate with or adapt or adjust to the client's health and care patterns for a beneficial or satisfying health outcome. For example, in planning for prenatal classes for multigravidas in a Hispanic community, provision for child care needs to be included, as Hispanic mothers place very high value on caring for their children and do not use babysitters as freely as do many mothers in American society. The Hispanic mother's care pattern is to provide care for her child and to have the child near her. She is likely to choose to not attend the class rather than leave her child at home with a babysitter. Those who do not understand this may become involved in cultural imposition and label the mother as not caring when she does not attend meetings at which child care is not available.

Culture care repatterning/restructuring refers to professional actions that seek to help clients change meaningful health or life patterns to patterns that will be healthier for them while respecting the client's cultural values. For example, Charles Thompson, whose dietary pattern has been to eat fried and salted foods at every meal, is found to have hypertension and elevated blood cholesterol levels. Fried chicken with a salty batter is an important element in Mr. Thompson's diet—it is a food that appears on the menu at family celebrations and one that is frequently packed in the brown-bag meal he carries to work. Fortunately, the chicken itself is one of the forms of protein that is recommended in low-fat and low-cholesterol diets. The repatterning that can occur relates to the way in which the chicken is prepared. The food preparer in the Thompson family could be taught to skin the chicken (helps lower the fat and thus the cholesterol), use a coating of herbs (rather than salt to help with the hypertension), and bake in the microwave oven with no added fat rather than fry with a salty batter (helps with both cholesterol and hypertension). Such change would repattern the preparation of a favorite food into a way that could provide for the continued inclusion of this food in the diet on a regular basis. At the same time, important changes in the way in which Mr. Thompson eats would be supported. Similar repatterning could occur with other foods; for example, instead of cooking green beans with salt pork, the beans could be cooked with herbs and a little polyunsaturated or monosaturated oil.

The Sunrise Enabler does not include an area identified as *evaluation*. However, in Leininger's (1995; Leininger & McFarland, 2002) discussion of transcultural nursing, she places a great deal of importance on the need for nursing care to provide ways in which care will benefit the client and on the need to systematically study nursing care behaviors to determine which care behaviors are appropriate to the lifeways and behavioral patterns of the culture for healing, health, or well-being. Indeed, the definition of transcultural nursing speaks to comparative culture care. Such study and comparison certainly is the equivalent of evaluation. Without evaluation of the outcomes of a particular plan of care that used the nursing process or a series of such plans, the systematic study that Leininger advises cannot be completed.

Example of Transcultural Nursing

Daniel Saunders, eight years old, has been accompanied to the emergency department by his mother and grandmother. He has had acute abdominal pain for two days. The nurse notes that his mother defers questions about Daniel to him or to his grandmother and that none of the three respond immediately to questions posed or comments made by the staff or look directly at members of the staff. They sit close together but do not touch one another. The physician wants to admit Daniel for exploratory abdominal surgery. Daniel's mother will not sign the admission and surgical permission forms until his grandmother has given her approval to do so. At this point, Daniel's grandmother takes a bag of cornmeal from her pocket and begins to sprinkle it around Daniel.

The nurse who lacks transcultural knowledge, or who is unicultural, likely views this family as strange and suspicious. The lack of direct eye contact leads to questions of what they are hiding. The mother appears indecisive. The family members don't seem to care much for each other since they do not touch. And what is the deal with the cornmeal?

The transcultural nurse would recognize that this is a Navajo family and the family members are demonstrating typical characteristics as described by Phillips and Lobar (1995). The Navajo culture is a matriarchical culture whose members defer to the wisdom of elders. Thus, Daniel is accompanied by his mother and grandmother rather than by his mother and father. Also, the grandmother is viewed as the source of wisdom, so her decision and support are necessary before the permission slips are signed, even though the dominant American culture considers Daniel's mother the appropriate person to sign these permission forms. Daniel is included in responses to questions asked because a value in the Navajo culture is for the individual to speak for him- or herself. The lack of direct eye contact and pauses after questions or statements are made by another are indications of respect, not of untrustworthiness. The pauses are intended to convey both respect and a degree of thought and attention being given to the content of the message. Navajo family members demonstrate their caring for one another through being physically close but not through touching. Illness is viewed as a lack of or disturbance of one's harmony. Rituals, such as sprinkling the person with cornmeal, are important to restore harmony. The nurse needs to note that it is important to save the cornmeal to return it to the family.

After Daniel's surgery, the nurse can anticipate that he will accept pain relief. It is also likely that as many relatives as are available will want to visit—such family support is another cultural value. Finally, should Daniel be on a b.i.d. antibiotic when discharged, the timing of the administration of his medication should be tied to natural events such as sunup and sundown rather than with the clock, meals, or some other activity. The Navajo sense of time tends to be casual (as compared to the American attention to clock time) and relative, and mealtimes are likely to be flexible.

CRITIQUE OF CULTURE CARE DIVERSITY AND UNIVERSALITY

1. *What is the historical context of the theory?* Beginning with the identification of a need to understand the culture of clients, through the introduction of the terms *transcultural nursing* and *ethnonursing care,* to the presentation of the Sunrise Enabler, Madeleine Leininger developed the theory of Culture Care Diversity and Universality. Leininger began developing her ideas about culture and caring as nursing theory development in the United States was just beginning to occur, that is, in the 1950s and 1960s. While she has had multiple publications on these concepts annually since the mid-1960s, she first labeled her thinking a theory in 1985. Prior to the mid-1980s her publications tended to be about culture or about caring; since the mid-1980s the focus has been on transcultural nursing, culture care, and qualitative research. She provides an excellent discussion of the path she has taken in the development of the Sunrise Enabler and the theory of Culture Care Diversity and Universality in her 1991 book as well as in her later books (Leininger, 1995; Leininger & McFarland, 2002, 2006). Thus, her work has occurred during the same time frame as the major efforts in development of nursing theory. Her focus on caring is shared with many other theorists. She has provided the leadership in focusing on culture and its importance to the delivery of appropriate nursing care. She has also been in the forefront in advocating the use of qualitative research in nursing.

2. *What are the basic concepts and relationships presented by the theory?* Leininger developed the Sunrise Enabler to demonstrate the interrelationships of the concepts in her theory of Culture Care Diversity and Universality. The worldview and social structure portion of the model does not differ significantly from any other view of culture and its interaction with human beings, with the possible exception of the inclusion of care and health patterns. The Sunrise Enabler focuses on individuals, families, groups, communities, and sociocultural institutions, which is similar to other theories of nursing. The inclusion of the term *culture* does provide a distinguishing feature since no other nursing theory has this emphasis on culture. Health care includes generic, professional, and nursing care. The inclusion of the generic system is unique to the theory of Culture Care Diversity and Universality. Nursing care decisions and actions are identified as supporting, accommodating to, or repatterning current health and care practices. The focus of nursing care decisions and actions is shared with many other theories. The division of actions into supporting, accommodating, or repatterning is specific to this theory. The Sunrise Enabler of Culture Care Diversity and Universality in itself supports the concepts of diversity and universality. The worldview, social structure, and description of individuals, families, groups, communities, and institutions are essentially universal as they have much in common with many other theories. The identified care systems and types of nursing care actions are diverse, or more specific and unique to this particular theory. Overall, the theory of culture care was the first to focus specifically on human care from a transcultural perspective (Leininger, 1991). It provides a holistic rather than a fragmented view of people. This view includes "worldview; biophysical state; religious (or spiritual) orientation; kinship patterns; material (and nonmaterial) cultural phenomena; the political, economic, legal, educational, technological, and physical environment; language; and folk and professional care practices" (p. 23).

3. *What major phenomena of concern to nursing are presented? (These phenomena may include* but are not limited to *human beings, environment, health, interpersonal relations, caring, goal attainment, adaptation, and energy fields.*) The major phenomena of concern to nursing are culture, care, and culture care. The human being as an individual may or may not be important, depending on the cultural values. Environment is identified as environmental context and includes the multiple areas in the Sunrise Enabler. Health is also defined with the specifics of what is viewed as health, determined again by the values of the culture. Nursing is identified as a culture. Other dominant constructs include the diverse and universal aspects of culture care, the insider (emic) and stranger (etic) views, cultural and social structures, ethnohistory, three modes of care decision and action, culturally congruent care, and transcultural nursing.

4. *To whom does this theory apply? In what situations? In what ways?* Because everyone, as individuals or in groups, belongs to a culture and/or a subculture, this theory applies to anyone in any situation. For nurses, there is a special concern about being culturally appropriate in approach and in responses. Leininger particularly warns about cultural imposition and culture shock. McManus (2008) suggests that transcultural nursing can help nurse practitioners establish a practice that is friendly to lesbian, gay, bisexual, and transgender individuals.

5. *By what method or methods can this theory be tested?* The theory of Culture Care Diversity and Universality is based on and calls for qualitative rather than quantitative research. The development of hypotheses is characteristic of positivistic, quantitative research. The development of research questions and of relational statements is characteristic of qualitative research. Leininger (1991) states that nursing science should be defined "as the creative study of nursing phenomena which reflects the systematization of knowledge using rigorous and explicit research methods within either the qualitative or quantitative paradigm in order to establish a new or to advance nursing's discipline knowledge" (p. 30). Leininger developed a qualitative method for studying culture and care known as the ethnonursing research method; she indicates that the qualitative methodology is the most appropriate for studying the emic views and beliefs of people. The principles that guide the ethnonursing research method are the following:

- Maintain an open discovery, active listening, and a genuine learning attitude in working with informants in the total context in which the study is conducted.
- Maintain an active and curious posture about the "why" of whatever is seen, heard, or experienced, and with appreciation of whatever informants share with you.
- Record whatever is shared by informants in a careful and conscientious way for full meanings, explanations, or interpretations to preserve informant ideas.
- Seek a mentor who has experience with the ethnonursing research method to act as a guide.
- Clarify the purposes of additional qualitative research methods if they are combined with the ethnonursing method, such as combining life histories, ethnography, phenomenology, or ethnoscience. (Leininger, 1991, pp. 106–109)

In addition to the Sunrise Enabler, Leininger has developed the following enablers to aid in conducting ethnonursing studies: the Observation-Participation-Reflection Enabler; the Researcher's Domain of Inquiry, Stranger to Trusted Friend Enabler; the Ethnodemographic Enabler; and the Acculturation Enabler (Leininger & McFarland, 2002, 2006). Nearly 75 cultures or subcultures have been studied using this research method. McFarland (2002) and Leininger (2006a, 2006b) provide information on selected findings from such studies. Leininger (2007) indicates that more diversities than universalities about care phenomena have been identified but that the most universal care construct is respect for and about cultures. The major source of information about this method, its tools, and studies conducted using it is the *Journal of Transcultural Nursing*. Other information may be found through the Transcultural Nursing Society.

6. *Does this theory direct nursing actions that lead to satisfactory outcomes?* The theory of Culture Care Diversity and Universality does not give specific direction for nursing actions such as "ambulate three times a day." However, it does provide direction on how to learn about the culture of another and how to exhibit caring in relation to another's cultural values, especially in relation to health. Leininger emphasizes that culturally congruent care is vital for lasting satisfactory outcomes.

7. *How contagious is this theory?* This theory is very contagious in that it is universally applicable and widely presented. Not only has Leininger spoken and consulted worldwide, but many international students have come to the United States to study transcultural nursing with her. The theory has been used to guide research, education, and nursing practice about and with a wide variety of cultures and subcultures. Clarke, McFarland, Andrews, and Leininger (2009) present additional information on the worldwide impact of this theory.

Research has been reported about cultures and subcultures including African American women and prenatal care (Morgan, 1996); African American elders (Sanchez-Jones, 2006); adolescents (Rosenbaum & Carty, 1996); American Indian community health (Tyree, 2007); Arab childbearing women (El-Adham, 2005); American gypsies (Bodnar & Leininger, 1992, 1995); American Hare Krishnas and pregnancy (Morgan, 1992); American hospital nurses (Leininger, 1995); Anglo and African American elders in long-term care (McFarland, 1997); Anglo American males in the rural Midwest (Sellers, Poduska, Propp & White, 1999); Anglo American and Philippine American nurses (Spangler, 1991);

Baganda women as AIDS caregivers (MacNeil, 1994, 1996); care needs of African American male juvenile offenders (Canty-Mitchell, 1996); childbirth experiences of European American women (Finn, 1994); Civil War nurse-caring (Urban Cordeau, 2004); culture and pain (Villarruel, 1995); Czech-Americans (Miller, 1997a, 1997b); diabetes education in a Hispanic community (Garcia, 1996); dying patients (Gates, 1988, 1991); elderly Anglo-Canadian caregivers (Cameron, 1990); elderly Polish Americans (McFarland, 1995); ethnicity and immunizations (Spitznagle, 1999); the evolution of transcultural nursing (Husting, 1991); Finnish birthing practices (Lamp, 1998); the Gadsup of New Guinea (Leininger, 1991, 1995); the goal of culturally sensitive care (Kirkham, 1998); Greek Canadian widows (Rosenbaum, 1990, 1991); health experiences of Athabascans in Galena, Alaska (Paul, 1991); health as viewed by Vietnamese immigrants in central New York State (Dean-Kelly, 1997); home care in a Jewish community (Racine, 1996); the homeless (Drury, 1995); hospitalized Muslim women in Nebraska (Rashidi, 2005); Iranian immigrants in New South Wales, Australia (Omeri, 1997); Japanese children with congenital heart disease (Masumori, 1997); Lebanese Muslims in the United States (Luna, 1994); Lithuanian Americans (Gelazis, 1994); male nurses in Brazil (Nobrega, Lopes Neto, Dantas, & Perez, 1996); midwifery practice in South Africa (Maputle & Jali, 2006); the mentally ill (George, 1998); midwestern U.S. spiritual care meanings (Sellers, 2001); Morroccan immigrant families in Spain (Gentil García, 2008); the Muckleshoots (Horn, 1995); Muscogee Creek Indians (Wing & Thompson, 1996); native Hawaiians (Kinney, 1985); nurse anesthesia (Horton, 1998); nurses and caring (Enns, 2002; Ingle, 1988; Miers, 1993; Schweiger, 1992); nurses confidence in culturally diverse care (Lowe-Nurse, 2001); nursing and medicine in America (Leininger, 1995); Old Order Amish (Wenger, 1991, 1995); perceptions of caring by Pakistanis in the United Kingdom (Cortis, 2000); Philippine Americans (Leininger, 1995); Portuguese chemotherapy patients (Soares, Klering, & Schwartz, 2009); postpartum depression in Jordanian Australian women (Nahas & Amasheh, 1999); prenatal care in Tunisia (Lazure, 2000); Puerto Rican infant feeding practices in New York (Higgins, 1995); psychiatric care values in Finland (Nikkonen, 1994); quality of life (Leininger, 1994); students who study in countries other than their native country (Martsolf, 1991); The Farm and midwifery services to the Amish (Finn, 1995); transitions to caregiver in middle age (Kuhns-Hastings, 2000); trends in transcultural research (Leininger, 1997b); Tunisian hospital nurses (Lazure, Vissandjee, Pepin, & Kerouac, 1997); types of health practitioners and cultural imposition (Leininger, 1995); Ukrainian American mothers (Bohay, 1991); urban Mexican Americans (Stasiak, 1991); and viligance as a caring expression (Carr, 1998). Studies are not limited to nursing; for example, Rizvi's (2000) master's thesis is in occupational therapy.

Discussions about the use of Culture Care Diversity and Universality in education include comparing the transcultural practices of RNs and baccalaureate students (Baldonado et al., 1998), English-as-second-language nursing students (Taggar, 1998), graduate curriculum in mental health nursing (Redmond, 1988), impact on nursing curricula in the United States (Andrews, 1995; Campinha-Bacote, Yahle, & Langenkamp, 1996), inclusion of African American diversity in in-service education (Dowe, 1990), incorporation in basic nursing texts in Canada (Morse & English, 1986), key references for staff development and nursing in-service (Mahon, 1997), metaphor use (Weitzel, 2003), nursing curriculum in South Africa (de Villiers & van der Wal, 1995), simulation games (Talabere, 1996), retention of minority nursing students (McManemy, 2002), undergraduate and graduate education (Haylock, 1992; Leininger, 1995), use as a context for considering education and health care in India (Basuray, 1997), use in an associate degree program (Jeffreys & O'Donnell, 1997), and use in a transcultural, transnational setting (Baker & Burkhalter, 1996). Unfortunately, Kardong-Edgren and Campinha-Bacote (2008) found that students who graduated from bachelor of science nursing programs all tested as only culturally aware regardless of whether they had had a cultural emphasis in their program.

Reports of transcultural nursing practice include the cultures and subcultures of adolescent homosexuals (Dootson, 2000); advocacy and diversity (Kavanagh, 1993); African Americans (Morgan, 1995); Anglo-Americans in the United States (Leininger, 1995); Aotearoa, New Zealand (Smith, 1997); Arab Muslims (Luna, 1995); Ayurveda medicine (Larson-Presswalla, 1994); breast cancer screening for elderly Black women in the United States (Brown & Williams, 1994); care of hospitalized children in Australia (Alsop-Shields & Nixon, 1997); care of the wounded in Brazil (da Silva & Mocelin, 2007); caregivers of children with cancer in Taiwan (Laing, 2002); childbirth in Brazil (Santos, Prado, & Boehs, 2000); children with muscular dystrophy in Japan (Komura, 2006); Chinese, Korean, and Vietnamese (Leininger, 1995); dialysis care in Brazil (Dias, Arujo, & Barroso, 2001); community assessment in a Hispanic community (Ludwig-Beymer, Blankemeier, Casas-Byots, & Suarez-Baleazar, 1996); comparison and contrast with Sartre (Rajan, 1995); culturally sensitive care in the United Kingdom (McGee, 1994); the deaf (Stebnicki & Coeling, 1999); developing of a caring culture practice model in hospitals in Canada (MacDonald & Miller-Grolla, 1995); ethical, moral, and legal aspects (Leininger, 1995; Zoucha & Husted, 2000); Greek culture (Larson, 2003); the Hausa of northwestern Africa (Chmielarczyk, 1991); health values in China (Finn & Lee, 1996); home health care in the United States (Hahn, 1997; Narayan, 1997); impact on practice (Leininger, 1996, 1997a, 1999); interaction with American families in relation to child rearing (Campinha-Bacote & Ferguson, 1991); Japanese Americans (Leininger, 1995); Jewish Americans (Leininger, 1995); Lithuanian Americans (Gelazis, 1995); mental health nursing (Leininger, 1995); Mexican Americans (Villarruel & Leininger, 1995); Navajo child health beliefs (Phillips & Lobar, 1995); nursing administration (Leininger, 1991); nursing in Japan (Inaoka, 1997), Saudi Arabia (Luna, 1998), South Africa (Mashaba, 1995), Switzerland (Rohrbach-Viadas, 1997), and Germany (Brouns, 1993; Kollak & Kupper, 1998; Leininger & Gstottner, 1998); self-perception of cultural competence of nurses (Alexander, 1996); and terminal patients (Piqué & del Pozo Flórez, 1999).

STRENGTHS AND LIMITATIONS

A major strength of Leininger's theory is the recognition of the importance of culture and its influence on everything that involves the recipients and providers of nursing care. The development of this theory over a number of years has allowed its concepts and constructs to be tested by a number of people in a variety of settings and cultures. The Sunrise Enabler provides guidance for the areas in which information needs to be collected.

Some limitations, as identified by Leininger in 1991 and still appropriate, include the limited number of graduate nurses who are academically prepared to conduct the investigations needed to provide transcultural nursing care. An associated concern is that too few nursing programs include courses and planned learning experiences that provide a knowledge base for transcultural nursing practice. While there has been some increase in the number of nurses prepared in transcultural nursing, it is important to note the danger of cultural biases and cultural imposition occurring with nurses' personal cultural values. There is also a need for research funds to support continued study of caring practices—both those that are universal and those that are particular to a culture. Leininger (1997b) identifies that the three greatest continuing needs are for education of nurses to practice transcultural nursing, to use the existing findings from transcultural nursing research, and to continue research to develop new knowledge and reaffirm credible findings in a continually changing world.

It is interesting to note that in spite of Leininger's emphasis on the importance of avoiding cultural imposition and cultural shock, Domenig (1999) expresses concern that Leininger does not make interaction the main object of her theory and that nurses need to be encouraged to analyze their own cultural backgrounds. It would be difficult to identify how Leininger could have put greater emphasis on the importance of these aspects.

The change of the label of what is now known as the Sunrise Enabler from that of Sunrise Model is a bit awkward. It is understandable that Leininger may have wanted to emphasize the use of the Sunrise Enabler, along with her other enablers, to enhance ethnonursing research. However, the Sunrise Enabler is pictorial and has long been known and even discussed by Leininger as a model.

The complexity of the Sunrise Enabler can be viewed as both strength and a limitation. The complexity is a strength in that it emphasizes the importance of the inclusion of anthropological and cultural concepts in nursing education and practice. On the other hand, the complexity can lead to misinterpretation or rejection, both of which are limitations.

Summary

Madeleine Leininger has been working since the 1950s on the development of her theory of Culture Care Diversity and Universality. In the 1960s, she first began to use the terms *transcultural nursing* and *ethnonursing*. While she has slightly different definitions of these terms, she has used them interchangeably, an action that can be confusing to the reader. She defines each of her concepts and presents assumptions that she considers to be relevant. The concepts and their interrelationships provide the basis for the Sunrise Enabler of this theory. The Sunrise Enabler presents a cognitive model that, when viewed from the top down, moves from the cultural and social structure dimensions through individuals, families, groups, communities, and institutions in generic, professional, and nursing care to nursing care decisions and actions that are cultural care preserving, accommodating, and repatterning to culturally congruent care. The Sunrise Enabler also indicates the need to move from knowledge generation through substantive knowledge to application of the knowledge. In discussing the Sunrise Enabler, Leininger (1991) presents the idea that care patterns and processes may be universal or diverse. Universal care indicates care patterns, values, and behaviors that are common across cultures. Care diversities represent those patterns and processes that are unique or specific to an individual, family, or cultural group. Leininger (2006) indicates and lists 175 care constructs, identified in studies of 58 cultures. As ethnonursing research studies continue, the list is likely to grow.

The theory of Culture Care Diversity and Universality is of significance in a society that is becoming more and more aware of the cultural diversity within its boundaries. While this theory does not provide specific directions for nursing care, it does provide guidelines for the gathering of knowledge and a framework for the making of decisions about what care is needed or would be of the greatest benefit to the client. Leininger has clearly identified what has been a major deficit in our provision of nursing care and provided a road map to begin to fill the gaps created by that deficit.

Thought Questions

1. Discuss how you might use the Sunshine Enabler to develop an assessment tool for use in your clinical practice.
2. How would the use of Leininger's theory alter your approach to caring for someone from a culture other than your own?
3. How would the use of Leininger's theory alter your approach to caring for someone from your own culture?

4. Select a culture other than your own and identify two examples of possible care for each of the three modes of culture care actions appropriate to that culture.

PEARSON

EXPLORE mynursingkit™

MyNursingKit is your one stop for online chapter review materials and resources. Prepare for success with additional NCLEX®-style practice questions, interactive assignments and activities, web links, animations and videos, and more!

Register your access code from the front of your book at
www.mynursingkit.com.

References

Alexander, B. J. (1996). Self-perceived cultural competence of Delaware nurses. *Dissertation Abstracts International, 58*(06B), 2954. Abstract retrieved April 1, 2008, from Dissertation Abstracts Online database.

Alsop-Shields, L., & Nixon, J. (1997). Transcultural nursing and its use in the care of children in hospital. *Australian Paediatric Nurse, 6*(2), 2–5.

Andrews, M. (1995). Transcultural nursing: Transforming the curriculum. *Journal of Transcultural Nursing, 6*(2), 4–9.

Baker, S. S., & Burkhalter, N. C. (1996). Teaching transcultural nursing in a transcultural setting. *Journal of Transcultural Nursing, 7*(2), 10–13.

Baldonado, A., Beymer, P. L., Barnes, K., Starsiak, D., Nemivant, E. B., & Anonas-Ternate, A. (1998). Transcultural nursing practice described by registered nurses and baccalaureate nursing students. *Journal of Transcultural Nursing, 9*(2), 15–25.

Basuray, J. (1997). Nurse Miss Sahib: Colonial culture-bound education in India and transcultural nursing. *Journal of Transcultural Nursing, 9*(1), 14–19.

Bodnar, A., & Leininger, M. (1992). Transcultural nursing care values, beliefs, and practices of American (USA) Gypsies. *Journal of Transcultural Nursing, 4*(1), 17–28.

Bodnar, A., & Leininger, M. (1995). Transcultural nursing care of American Gypsies. In M. Leininger, *Transcultural nursing: Concepts, theories, research and practices* (2nd ed., pp. 445–470). New York: McGraw-Hill.

Bohay, I. Z. (1991). Culture care meanings and experiences of pregnancy and childbirth of Ukrainians. In M. M. Leininger (Ed.), *Culture care diversity and universality: A theory of nursing* (pp. 203–229) (Pub. No. 15-2402). New York: National League for Nursing Press.

Brouns, G. (1993). Leininger's theory of cultural nursing diversity and universality [German]. *Pflege, 6*, 191–196.

Brown, L. W., & Williams, R. D. (1994). Culturally sensitive breast cancer screening programs for older black women. *Nurse Practitioner, 19*(3), 21, 25–26, 31.

Cameron, C. F. (1990). An ethnonursing study of the influence of extended caregiving on the health status of elderly Anglo-Canadian wives caring for physically disabled husbands. *Dissertation Abstracts International, 52(02B)*, 746.

Campinha-Bacote, J., & Ferguson, S. (1991). Cultural considerations in child-rearing practices: A transcultural perspective. *Journal of National Black Nurses' Association, 5*(1), 11–17.

Campinha-Bacote, J., Yahle, T., & Langenkamp, M. (1996). The challenge of cultural diversity for nurse educators. *Journal of Continuing Education in Nursing, 2*(2), 59–64.

Canty-Mitchell, J. (1996). The caring needs of African American male juvenile offenders. *Journal of Transcultural Nursing, 8*(1), 3–12.

Carr, J. M. (1998). Vigilance as a caring expression and Leininger's theory of cultural care diversity and universality. *Nursing Science Quarterly, 11*, 74–78.

Chmielarczyk, V. (1991). Transcultural nursing: Providing culturally congruent care to the Hausa of Northwest Africa. *Journal of Transcultural Nursing, 3*(1), 15–19.

Clarke, P. N., McFarland, M. R., Andrews, M. M., & Leininger, M. (2009). Caring: Some reflections on the impact of the culture care theory by McFarland & Andrews and a conversation with Leininger. *Nursing Science Quarterly, 22*, 233–239.

Cortis, J. D. (2000). Caring as experienced by minority ethnic patients. *International Nursing Review, 47*(1), 53–62.

da Silva, D. M., & Mocelin, K. R. (2007). The nurse care to wounds bearers under the view of transcultural care [Portuguese]. *Revista Nursing, 9*(105), 81–88. Abstract in English retrieved April 1, 2008, from CINAHL Plus with Full Text database.

Dean-Kelly, L. A. (1997). Concept and process of attaining and maintaining health for a selected Vietnamese immigrant population. *Dissertation Abstracts International, 58(07B)*, 3554.

de Villiers, L., & van der Wal, D. (1995). Putting Leininger's nursing theory "Culture Care Diversity and Universality" into operation in the curriculum—Part I. *Curationis, 18*(4), 56–60.

Dias, M. S. A., Araujo, T. L., & Barroso, M. G. T. (2001). Developing the care proposed by Leininger with a person in dialysis treatment [Portuguese]. *Revista da Escola de Enfermagem da USP, 35*, 354–360. Abstract in English retrieved April 1, 2008, from CINAHL Plus with Full Text database.

Domenig, D. (1999). The mediation of transcultural nursing care in the clinical context: A tightrope walk [German]. *Pflege, 12*, 362–369.

Dootson, L. G. (2000). Adolescent homosexuality and culturally competent nursing. *Nursing Forum, 35*(3), 13–20.

Dowe, D. S. (1990). African-American diversity in nursing inservice programs. *Masters Abstracts International, 29-02*, 261.

Drury, L. J. (1995). Lifeways of homeless chronically mentally ill individuals in a community housing program. *Dissertation Abstracts International, 56*(03B), 1345. Abstract retrieved April 4, 2008, from Dissertation Abstracts Online database.

El-Adham, A. F. M. (2005). Childbirth pain experience recall of United States Arab immigrant women: A cross cultural comparison. *Dissertation Abstracts International, 66*(02B), 827. Abstract retrieved April 1, 2008, from Dissertation Abstracts Online database.

Enns, C. L. (2002). Expressions of caring by contemporary surgical nurses: A phenomenological study. *Masters Abstracts International, 41*(05), 1418. Abstract retrieved April 1, 2008, from Dissertation Abstracts Online database.

Finn, J. M. (1994). Culture care of Euro-American women during childbirth: Using Leininger's theory. *Journal of Transcultural Nursing, 5*(2), 25–37.

Finn, J. M. (1995). Leininger's model for discoveries at The Farm and midwifery services to the Amish. *Journal of Transcultural Nursing, 7*(1), 28–35.

Finn, J. M., & Lee, M. (1996). Transcultural nurses reflect on discoveries in China using Leininger's Sunrise model. *Journal of Transcultural Nursing, 7*(2), 21–27.

Garcia, C. M. (1996). Diabetes education in the Hispanic community. *Masters Abstracts International, 35-02*, 517.

Gates, M. F. G. (1988). Care and cure meanings, experiences and orientations of persons who are dying in hospital and hospice settings. *Dissertation Abstracts International, 50-02B*, 493.

Gates, M. F. (1991). Culture care theory for study of dying patients in hospital and hospice contexts. In M. M. Leininger (Ed.), *Culture care diversity and universality: A theory of nursing* (pp. 281–304) (Pub. No. 15-2402). New York: National League for Nursing Press.

Gelazis, R. (1994). Humor, care, and well-being of Lithuanian Americans: An ethnonursing study using Leininger's theory of Culture Care

Diversity and Universality. *Dissertation Abstracts International, 55(04B)*, 1377.

Gelazis, R. (1995). Lithuanian Americans and culture care. In M. Leininger, *Transcultural nursing: Concepts, theories, research and practices* (2nd ed., pp. 427–444). New York: McGraw-Hill.

Gentil Garciá, I. (2008). Education for health in Moroccan immigrant families [Spanish]. *Cultura de los Cuidados, 12*(24), 114–119. Abstract in English retrieved November 30, 2009, from CINAHL Plus with Full Text database.

George, T. B. (1998). Meanings, expressions, and experiences of care of chronically mentally ill in a day treatment center using Leininger's culture care theory. *Dissertation Abstracts International, 59(12B)*, 6262.

Hahn, J. A. (1997). Transcultural nursing in home health care: Learning to be culturally sensitive. *Home Health Care Management and Practice, 10*(1), 66–71.

Haylock, P. J. (1992). Commentary on "Teaching cultural content: A nursing education imperative" [original article by C. F. Capers in *Holistic Nursing Practice, 6*(3), 19–28]. *ONS Nursing Scan in Oncology, 1*(3), 20.

Higgins, B. J. (1995). Puerto Rican cultural beliefs: Influence on infant feeding practices in western New York. *Dissertation Abstracts International, 56*(10B), 5417. Abstract retrieved April 1, 2008, from Dissertation Abstracts Online database.

Horn, B. (1995). Transcultural nursing and child-rearing of the Muckleshoots. In M. Leininger, *Transcultural nursing: Concepts, theories, research and practices* (2nd ed., pp. 501–515). New York: McGraw-Hill.

Horton, B. J. (1998). Nurse anesthesia as a subculture of nursing in the United States. *Dissertation Abstracts International, 59(11B)*, 5786.

Husting, P. M. (1991). An oral history of transcultural nursing. *Dissertation Abstracts International, 52(07A)*, 2608.

Inaoka, F. (1997). Leininger's theory of nursing: Its meaning for nursing in Japan [Japanese]. *Kango Kenkyu, 30*(2), 3–6.

Ingle, J. R. (1988). The business of caring: The perspective of men in nursing. *Dissertation Abstracts International, 50*(02B), 0495. Abstract retrieved April 4, 2008, from Dissertation Abstracts Online database.

Jeffreys, M. R., & O'Donnell, M. (1997). Cultural discovery: An innovative philosophy for

creative learning activities. *Journal of Transcultural Nursing, 8*(2), 17–22.

Kardong-Edgren, S., & Campinha-Bacote, J. (2008). Cultural competency of graduating US Bachelor of Science nursing students. *Contemporary Nurse: A Journal for the Australian Nursing Profession, 28*(1-2), 37–44.

Kavanagh, K. H. (1993). Transcultural nursing: Facing the challenges of advocacy and diversity/universality. *Journal of Transcultural Nursing, 5*(1), 4–13.

Kinney, G. L. (1985). Caring values and caring practices of native Hawaiians in a Hawaiian home lands community. *Dissertation Abstracts International, 47*(09B), 3706.

Kirkham, S. R. (1998). Nurses' descriptions of caring for culturally diverse clients. *Clinical Nursing Research, 7*, 125–146.

Kollak, I., & Kupper, H. (1998). Culturally sensitive care as an extension of Leininger's nursing theory [German]. *Pflege Aktuell, 52*, 226–228.

Komura, H. (2006). Progressive muscular dystrophy: Nurses' interaction and awareness of children's feeling and wishes [Japanese]. *Journal of Japan Academy of Nursing Science, 26*(2), 31–38. Abstract in English retrieved June 6, 2007, from CINAHL Plus with Full Text database.

Kuhns-Hastings, J. J. (2000). Middle-aged daughters' transitions from non-caregiver to caregiver for elderly dependent parents. *Dissertation Abstracts International, 61*(03B), 1324. Abstract retrieved April 1, 2008, from Dissertation Abstracts Online database.

Lamp, J. K. (1998). Generic and professional culture care meanings and practices of Finnish women in birth within Leininger's theory of Culture Care Diversity and Universality. *Dissertation Abstracts International, 60*(01B), 0131. Abstract retrieved November 6, 2007, from Dissertation Abstracts Online database.

Larson, M. (2003). The Greek-connection: Discovering cultural and social structure dimensions of the Greek culture using Leininger's Sunrise Model. *ICUs and Nursing Web Journal, 15*. Abstract retrieved June 6, 2007, from CINAHL Plus with Full Text database.

Larson-Presswalla, J. (1994). Insights into eastern health care: Some transcultural nursing perspectives. *Journal of Transcultural Nursing, 5*(2), 21–24.

Lazure, G. (2000). Le soin generique et le soin professionel a la periode prenatale: L'experience de femmes de la region du sud de la Tunisie [French text]. *Dissertation Abstracts International, 61*(07B), 3509. Abstract retrieved April 4, 2008, from Dissertation Abstracts Online database.

Lazure, G., Vissandjee, B., Pepin, J., & Kerouac, S. (1997). Transcultural nursing and a care management partnership project. *Nursing Inquiry, 4,* 160–166.

Leininger, M. (1978). *Transcultural nursing: Concepts, theories, and practices.* New York: Wiley. [out of print]

Leininger, M. (1979). *Transcultural nursing.* New York: Masson. [out of print]

Leininger, M. M. (1985). Transcultural care diversity and universality: A theory of nursing. *Nursing and Health Care, 6,* 209–212.

Leininger, M. M. (1988a). *Care: Discovery and uses in clinical and community nursing.* Detroit: Wayne State University Press.

Leininger, M. M. (1988b). Leininger's theory of nursing: Cultural Care Diversity and Universality. *Nursing Science Quarterly, 1,* 152–160.

Leininger, M. M. (Ed.). (1991). *Culture Care Diversity and Universality: A theory of nursing* (Pub. No. 15-2402). New York: National League for Nursing Press.

Leininger, M. (1994). Quality of life from a transcultural nursing perspective. *Nursing Science Quarterly, 7,* 22–28.

Leininger, M. (1995). *Transcultural nursing: Concepts, theories, research and practices* (2nd ed.). New York: McGraw-Hill.

Leininger, M. (1996). Culture care theory, research, and practice. *Nursing Science Quarterly, 9,* 71–78.

Leininger, M. M. (1997a). Transcultural nursing as a global care humanizer, diversifier, and unifier. *Hoitotiede, 9,* 219–225.

Leininger, M. (1997b). Transcultural nursing research to transform nursing education and practice: 40 years. *Image, Journal of Nursing Scholarship, 29,* 341–347.

Leininger, M. M. (1999). Transcultural nursing: An imperative for nursing practice. *Imprint, 46*(5), 50–52.

Leininger, M. (2002). Culture care theory: A major contribution to advance transcultural nursing knowledge and practices. *Journal of Transcultural Nursing, 13,* 189–192.

Leininger, M. M. (2006a). Culture Care Diversity and Universality theory and evolution of the ethnonursing method. In M. M. Leininger & M. R. McFarland (Eds.), *Culture Care Diversity and Universality: A worldwide nursing theory* (2nd ed., pp. 1–42). Boston: Jones and Bartlett.

Leininger, M. M. (2006b). Selected culture care findings of diverse cultures using culture care theory and ethnomethods [Revised Reprint]. In M. M. Leininger & M. R. McFarland (Eds.), *Culture Care Diversity and Universality: A worldwide nursing theory* (2nd ed., pp. 281–306). Boston: Jones and Bartlett.

Leininger, M. M. (2007). Theoretical questions and concerns: Response from the theory of Culture Care Diversity and Universality perspective. *Nursing Science Quarterly, 20,* 9–15.

Leininger, M., & Gstottner, E. (1998). Cultural dimensions of humane care—The Sunrise Model [German]. *Osterr Krankenpflegez, 51*(12), 26–29.

Leininger, M., & McFarland, M. R. (2002). *Transcultural nursing: Concepts, theories, research and practice.* New York: McGraw-Hill.

Leininger, M. M., & McFarland, M. R. (2006). *Culture Care Diversity and Universality: A worldwide nursing theory* (2nd ed.). Boston: Jones and Bartlett.

Liang, H. (2002). Understanding culture care practices of caregivers of children with cancer in Taiwan. *Journal of Pediatric Oncology Nursing, 19,* 205–217. Abstract retrieved June 6, 2007, from CINAHL Plus with Full Text database.

Lowe-Nurse, D. D. (2001). Assessment of nurses' confidence levels when caring for culturally diverse patients. *Masters Abstracts International, 39*(04), 1128. Abstract retrieved April 1, 2008, from Dissertation Abstracts Online database.

Ludwig-Beymer, P., Blankemeier, J. R., Casas-Byots, C., & Suarez-Balcazar, Y. (1996). Community assessment in a suburban Hispanic community: A description of method. *Journal of Transcultural Nursing, 8*(1), 19–27.

Luna, L. (1994). Care and cultural context of Lebanese Muslim immigrants: Using Leininger's theory. *Journal of Transcultural Nursing, 5*(2), 12–20.

Luna, L. J. (1995). Arab Muslims and culture care. In M. Leininger, *Transcultural nursing: Concepts, theories, research and practices* (2nd ed., pp. 317–333). New York: McGraw-Hill.

Luna, L. J. (1998). Culturally competent health care: A challenge for nurses in Saudi Arabia. *Journal of Transcultural Nursing, 9*(2), 1–14.

MacDonald, M. R., & Miller-Grolla, L. (1995). Developing a collective future: Creating a culture specific nurse caring practice model for hospitals. *Canadian Journal of Nursing Administration, 8,* 78–95.

MacNeil, J. M. (1994). Culture care: Meanings, patterns and expressions for Baganda women as AIDS caregivers within Leininger's theory. *Dissertation Abstracts International, 56-02B,* 743.

MacNeil, J. M. (1996). Use of culture care theory with Baganda women as AIDS caregivers. *Journal of Transcultural Nursing, 7*(2), 14–20.

Mahon, P. Y. (1997). Transcultural nursing: A source guide. *Journal of Nursing Staff Development, 13,* 218–222.

Martsolf, D. S. (1991). The relationship between adjustment, health, and perception of care in two groups of cross-cultural students migrants. *Dissertation Abstracts International, 53(02B),* 770.

Mashaba, G. (1995). Culturally-based health-illness patterns in South Africa and humanistic nursing care practices. In M. Leininger, *Transcultural nursing: Concepts, theories, research and practices* (2nd ed., pp. 591–602). New York: McGraw-Hill.

Masumori, K. (1997). A study of children's experiences with congenital heart disease: Using Leininger's ethnonursing method [Japanese]. *Kango Kenkyu, 30,* 233–244.

McFarland, M. (1995). Culture care theory and elderly Polish Americans. In M. Leininger, *Transcultural nursing: Concepts, theories, research and practices* (2nd ed., pp. 401–426). New York: McGraw-Hill.

McFarland, M. R. (1997). Use of culture care theory with Anglo- and African American elders in a long-term care setting. *Nursing Science Quarterly, 10,* 186–192.

McFarland, M. R. (2002). Part II: Selected research findings from the culture care theory. In M. Leininger & M. R. McFarland (Ed.), *Transcultural nursing: Concepts, theories, research, and practices* (3rd ed., pp. 99–116). New York: McGraw-Hill.

McGee, P. (1994). Culturally sensitive and culturally comprehensive care . . . including commentary by Shomaker, D. *British Journal of Nursing, 3,* 789–793.

McManus, A. J. (2008). Creating an LGBT-friendly practice: Practical implications for NPs. *American Journal for Nurse Practitioners, 12*(4), 29–32, 35–38.

Maputle, M. S., & Jali, M. N. (2006). Dealing with diversity: Incorporating cultural sensitivity into midwifery practice in the tertiary hospital of Capricorn district, Limpopo province. *Curatonis, 29*(4), 61–69.

McManemy, J. C. (2002). Caring behaviors and cultural influences: Retention strategies for minority nursing students. *Dissertation Abstracts International, 63*(04B), 1785. Abstract retrieved April 1, 2008, from Dissertation Abstracts Online database.

Miers, L. J. (1993). The meaning of professional nurse caring: The experience of family members of critically ill patients. *Dissertation Abstracts International, 55*(02B), 0369. Abstract retrieved April 4, 2008, from Dissertation Abstracts Online database.

Miller, J. E. (1997a). Politics and care: A study of Czech Americans within Leininger's theory of Culture care diversity and universality. *Dissertation Abstracts International, 58-03B,* 1216.

Miller, J. E. (1997b). Politics and care: A study of Czech Americans within Leininger's theory of Culture Care Diversity and Universality. *Journal of Transcultural Nursing, 9*(1), 3–13.

Morgan, M. (1992). Pregnancy and childbirth beliefs and practices of American Hare Kirshna devotees within transcultural nursing. *Journal of Transcultural Nursing, 4*(1), 5–10.

Morgan, M. (1995). African Americans and cultural care. In M. Leininger, *Transcultural nursing: Concepts, theories, research and practices* (2nd ed., pp. 383–400). New York: McGraw-Hill.

Morgan, M. (1996). Prenatal care of African American women in selected USA urban and rural cultural contexts. *Journal of Transcultural Nursing, 7*(2), 3–9.

Morse, J. M., & English, J. (1986). The incorporation of cultural concepts into basic nursing texts. *Nursing Papers: Perspectives in Nursing, 18,* 69–76.

Nahas, V., & Amasheh, N. (1999). Culture care meanings and experiences of postpartum depression among Jordanian Australian women: A transcultural study. *Journal of Transcultural Nursing, 10*(1), 37–45.

Narayan, M. C. (1997). Cultural assessment in home healthcare. *Home Healthcare Nursing, 15,* 663–670.

Nikkonen, M. (1994). Changes in psychiatric caring values in Finland. *Journal of Transcultural Nursing, 6*(1), 12–17.

Nobrega, M., Lopes Neto, D., Dantas, H. F., & Perez, V. L. (1996). Being a nurse in a transcultural context [Portuguese]. *Rev Bras Enferm, 49,* 399–408.

Omeri, A. (1997). Culture care of Iranian immigrants in New South Wales, Australia: Sharing transcultural nursing knowledge. *Journal of Transcultural Nursing, 8*(2), 5–16.

Paul, D. M. (1991). Description of the health experience of Athabascans living in Galena: A modified ethnographic approach. *Masters Abstracts International, 30-02*, 301.

Phillips, S., & Lobar, S. (1995). Navajo child health beliefs and rearing practices within a transcultural nursing framework: Literature review. In M. Leininger, *Transcultural nursing: Concepts, theories, research and practices* (2nd ed., pp. 485–500). New York: McGraw-Hill.

Piqué Prado, E., & del Pozo Flórez, J. A. (1999). Nursing and the terminal patient: Anthropological perspective [Spanish]. *Metas de Enfermeria, 2*(18), 47–51. Abstract in English retrieved April 1, 2008, from CINAHL Plus with Full Text database.

Racine, L. (1996). Etude des perceptions culturelles d'un groupe d'ai nees et d'ai nes de la communaute juive et d'un groupe d'infirmieres sur les soins infirmiers de maintien a domicile du clsc cote-ds-neiges [French text]. *Masters Abstracts International, 35*(05), 1381. Abstract retrieved April 4, 2008, from Dissertation Abstracts Online database.

Rajan, M. J. (1995). Transcultural nursing: A perspective derived from Jean-Paul Sartre. *Journal of Advanced Nursing, 22*, 450–455.

Rashidi, A. (2005). Experience of practicing Muslim women in hospitals in Omaha, Nebraska from January, 1988 to October, 2004. *Dissertation Abstracts International, 66*(02B), 850. Abstract retrieved April 1, 2008, from Dissertation Abstracts Online database.

Redmond, G. T. (1988). An examination of the influence of transcultural nursing on graduate curriculum in mental health nursing. *Dissertation Abstracts International, 49*(12A), 3608.

Rizvi, Z. B. A. (2000). Phenomenological perspectives on a culturally diverse client-therapist relationship in occupational therapy. *Masters Abstracts International, 38*(04), 1008. Abstract retrieved April 1, 2008, from Dissertation Abstracts Online database.

Rohrbach-Viadas, C. (1997). Visit by Madeleine Leininger, June 1997. "In Switzerland transcultural nursing is indispensable" [French]. *Krankenpfl Soins Infirm, 90*(9), 65–66.

Rosenbaum, J. (1990). Cultural care of older Greek Canadian widows within Leininger's theory of culture care. *Journal of Transcultural Nursing, 2*(1), 37–47.

Rosenbaum, J. (1991). Culture care theory and Greek Canadian widows. In M. M. Leininger (Ed.), *Culture Care Diversity and Universality: A theory of nursing* (pp. 305–339) (Pub. No. 15-2402). New York: National League for Nursing Press.

Rosenbaum, J. N., & Carty, L. (1996). The subculture of adolescence: Beliefs and care, health and individuation with Leininger's theory. *Journal of Advanced Nursing, 23*, 741–746.

Sanchez-Jones, T. R. (2006). A qualitative analysis of health promotion among older African Americans. *Dissertation Abstracts International, 67*(04B), 1920. Abstract retrieved April 1, 2008, from Dissertation Abstracts Online database.

Santos, V. S. C., Prado, M. L., & Boehs, A. E. (2000). Nurse performance next to the couple/newborn in the parturition process founded on Madeleine Leininger's theory [Portuguese]. *Texto & Contexto Enfermagem, 9*(2, part 1), 375–387. Abstract in English retrieved June 6, 2007, from CINAHL Plus with Full Text database.

Schweiger, J. L. (1992). Commitment to clinical nursing: A case study. *Dissertation Abstracts International, 53*(11B), 5648. Abstract retrieved April 4, 2008, from Dissertation Abstracts Online database.

Sellers, S. C. (2001). The spiritual care meanings of adults residing in the Midwest. *Nursing Science Quarterly, 14*, 239–248.

Sellers, S. C., Poduska, M. D., Propp, L. H., & White, S. I. (1999). The health care meanings, values, and practices of Anglo-American males in the rural Midwest. *Journal of Transcultural Nursing, 10*(4), 320–330.

Smith, M. (1997). False assumptions, ethnocentrism and cultural imposition . . . Madeleine Leininger's theory of culture care and its place in Aotearoa. *Nurs Prax NZ, 12*(1), 13–16.

Soares, L. C., Klering, S. T., & Schwartz, E. (2009). Transcultural care to oncology patients in chemotherapy treatement and their relatives [Portuguese]. *Ciencia, Cuidado e Saude, 81*(1), 101–108.

Spangler, Z. D. L. (1991). Nursing care values and caregiving practices of Anglo-American and Philippine-American nurses conceptualized within Leininger's theory. *Dissertation Abstracts International, 52-04B*, 1960.

Spitznagle, C. L. (1999). Ethnicity and immunization compliance. *Masters Abstracts International, 37*(04), 1184. Abstract retrieved April 1, 2008, from Dissertation Abstracts Online database.

Stasiak, D. B. (1991). Culture care theory with Mexican Americans in an urban context. In M. M. Leininger (Ed.), *Culture Care Diversity and Universality: A theory of nursing* (pp. 179–201) (Pub. No. 15-2402). New York: National League for Nursing Press.

Stebnicki, J. A. M., & Coeling, H. V. (1999). The culture of the deaf. *Journal of Transcultural Nursing, 10*, 350–357.

Taggar, R. K. (1998). Nursing faculty perceptions of teaching practices which help English as a second language nursing students. *Masters Abstracts International, 36*(05), 1320. Abstract retrieved April 4, 2008, from Dissertation Abstracts Online database.

Talabere, L. R. (1996). Meeting the challenge of culture care in nursing: Diversity, sensitivity, competence, and congruence. *Journal of Cultural Diversity, 3*(2), 53–61.

Tyree, E. M. (2007). Culture care values, beliefs and practices observed in empowerment of American Indian community health representatives. *Dissertation Abstracts International, 68*(04B), 2259. Abstract retrieved April 1, 2008, from Dissertation Abstracts Online database.

Urban Cordeau, M. A. (2004). Acts of caring: A history of the lived experience of nurse-caring by northern women during the American Civil War. *Dissertation Abstracts International, 65*(03B), 1253. Abstract retrieved April 1, 2008, from Dissertation Abstracts Online database.

Villarruel, A. (1995). Cultural perspectives of pain. In M. Leininger, *Transcultural nursing: Concepts, theories, research and practices* (2nd ed., pp. 263–277). New York: McGraw-Hill.

Villarruel, A., & Leininger, M. (1995). Culture care of Mexican Americans. In M. Leininger, *Transcultural nursing: Concepts, theories, research and practices* (2nd ed., pp. 365–382). New York: McGraw-Hill.

Watson, J. (1988). *Nursing: Human science and human care.* (Pub. No. 15-2236). New York: National League for Nursing.

Weitzel, M. L. (2003). The use of metaphors only versus metaphors with elaborations in nursing education instruction for Asian and majority culture students. *Dissertation Abstracts International, 64*(01A), 51. Abstract retrieved April 4, 2008, from Dissertation Abstracts Online database.

Wenger, A. F. (1991). The culture care theory and the Old Order Amish. In M. M. Leininger (Ed.), *Culture care diversity and universality: A theory of nursing* (pp. 147–178) (Pub. No. 15-2402). New York: National League for Nursing Press.

Wenger, A. F. (1995). Cultural context, health and health care decision making 1994. *Journal of Transcultural Nursing, 7*(1), 3–14.

Wing, D. M., & Thompson, T. (1996). The meaning of alcohol to traditional Muscogee Creek Indians. *Nursing Science Quarterly, 9*, 175–180.

Zoucha, R., & Husted, G. L. (2000). The ethical dimensions of delivering culturally congruent nursing and health care. *Issues in Mental Health Nursing, 21*, 325–340.

Selected Annotated Bibliography

Baker, S. S., & Burkhalter, N. C. (1996). Teaching transcultural nursing in a transcultural setting. *Journal of Transcultural Nursing, 7*(2), 10–13.

The authors present a cultural encounter between the faculty and students in a baccalaureate nursing program and the nurse–patient–community system found in the Texas–Mexico border town of Laredo. This transnational, transcultural setting provided a challenging environment for assessing the effectiveness of the theory of Culture Care Diversity and Universality and its three modes of nursing action.

Baldonado, A., Beymer, P. L., Barnes, K., Starsiak, D., Nemivant, E. B., and Anonas-Ternate, A. (1998). Transcultural nursing practice described by registered nurses and baccalaureate nursing students. *Journal of Transcultural Nursing, 9*(2), 15–25.

This study of 767 registered nurses and senior baccalaureate nursing students found that neither group was confident about providing care to culturally diverse patients. The registered nurses did report a higher degree of use of cultural assessment data to modify care than did the students. Both groups identified an overwhelming need for transcultural nursing care and reported they seek to respond to cultural challenges through modifications of care. Care modifications were based on communication, language, perception of pain and pain relief, aspects of religious and spiritual beliefs, gender, family roles, and identified cultural values. Respondents did not identify the use of a conceptual framework to conduct these assessments and to plan the modifications of care.

Bodner, A., & Leininger, M. (1992). Transcultural nursing care values, beliefs, and practices of American (USA) gypsies. *Journal of Transcultural Nursing, 4*(1), 17–28.
This study was based on the theory of Culture Care Diversity and Universality and used the ethnonursing research method. Findings substantiated the importance of culture to Gypsies. Care meanings identified include protective ingroup caring, watching over and guarding against Gadje (outsiders), facilitating care rituals, respecting the values of the Gypsy culture, alleviating Gadje harassment, remaining suspicious of Gadje, and dealing with moral codes and rules related to purity and impurity.

Cameron, C. F. (1990). An ethnonursing study of the influence of extended caregiving on the health status of elderly Anglo-Canadian wives caring for physically disabled husbands. *Dissertation Abstracts International, 52*(02B), 746.
This qualitative study investigated the care experiences and health status of elderly Anglo-Canadian wives as they provided care for their physically disabled spouses over an extended period of time. These women were of English, Scottish, and Irish descent. The major commonalities found included that culture care patterns of caregiving influenced the health status of the spouse; the meanings and experiences of the caregivers reflected cultural care values, social structure, and environmental context; female caregiving was culturally transmitted as caring for others throughout the life cycle; and caring activity patterns helped maintain the health of the caregivers and of others. Diversity was found in the potential for neglect, acceptance of caregiving by strangers, and culture-specific planning for care in the future. Several generic care constructs were identified. These included concern for both affectionate and spiritual love, attention, and duty. Obligation and care concepts included commitment to care, continuous caring, care enculturation, other care, and care appreciation.

Canty-Mitchell, J. (1996). The caring needs of African American male juvenile offenders. *Journal of Transcultural Nursing, 8*(1), 3–12.
This ethnonursing study investigated the social and cultural needs of male African American juvenile offenders. Five juveniles, aged 12 to 15 years old, living in a southeastern U.S. inner city participated in the interviews. A general theme was found to be survival in the face of loss. Domains of loss were family, social, and self-identity, and the categories of loss in each domain were loss of caring, loss of protection, loss of discipline, and loss of support, with the threat to survival dominant in each type of loss. Culturally congruent nursing actions were identified.

Cortis, J. D. (2000). Caring as experienced by minority ethnic patients. *International Nursing Review, 47*(1), 53–62.
This qualitative study reports the results of indepth interviews with Pakistanis (20 males and 18 females) from Bradford, West Yorkshire, United Kingdom, about their perceptions of caring. In general, findings indicated a lack of congruence between the respondents' expectations of caring and their experiences of caring received from nurses.

Garcia, C. M. (1996). Diabetes education in the Hispanic community. *Masters Abstracts International, 35-02*, 517.
This master's thesis examined the effects of a community based, culturally congruent educational program on diabetes self-efficacy and hemoglobin A1C measurements in a Hispanic community. A pretest–posttest design was used with a sample of 32 subjects. The difference in diabetes self-efficacy was found to be statistically significant, while a statistically significant difference in A1C was not found.

Gelazis, R. (1994). Humor, care, and well-being of Lithuanian Americans: An ethnonursing study using Leininger's theory of Culture Care Diversity and Universality. *Dissertation Abstracts International, 55*(04B), 1377.
This ethnonursing research study investigated the cultural implications of humor in Lithuanian Americans. The findings indicated that cultural humor assists in bearing life's burdens, diffusing potential confrontations, and supporting and enhancing well-being through

supporting a positive outlook on life; serves a survival function; is subtle and abstract and expressed in daily life events; and has a caring function to increase a sense of closeness and well-being. Care themes indicate that care is a basic orientation with an attitude of concern for others, expressed as a community, and means protection with protective care modalities. Well-being themes indicated that well-being is broadly defined as a positive state of mind about self and the world and is holistic (including spiritual, emotional, physical, social, and economic aspects in balance) and that the history of their culture strongly influenced identity and commitment to survival of the culture, which led to a sense of well-being. The two constructs of cultural humor and culture care humor were identified.

Horton, B. J. (1998). Nurse anesthesia as a subculture of nursing in the United States. *Dissertation Abstracts International, 59(11B)*, 5786.

Horton sought to demonstrate that nurse anesthesia is a subculture of nursing through this ethnonursing study of 55 registered nurse and certified registered nurse anesthetists. The five identified themes were that nurse anesthetists have a common worldview of the cultural values of nurse anesthesia; are committed to and show responsibility for the patients they serve; remain active and vigilant to defend and maintain their professional practice rights; reflect a subculture distinctly different from, while having commonalities with, the culture of nursing; and have rituals and symbols that provide patient benefits and reinforce solidarity within nurse anesthesia. The findings support nurse anesthesia as a subculture of nursing.

Morgan, M. (1996). Prenatal care of African American women in selected USA urban and rural cultural contexts. *Journal of Transcultural Nursing, 7(2)*, 3–9.

This ethnonursing study investigated prenatal care of African American women within their familiar cultural contexts. The impetus for the study arose from studies that connected lack of prenatal care in African American women with low birth weights and high infant mortality rates. Four major themes were identified. Cultural care meant protection, presence, and sharing. Health and well-being were influenced by such social structural factors as spirituality, kinship factors, and economics. While professional prenatal care was seen as necessary, even

essential, barriers, including distrust of noncaring professionals, inhibited the receipt of such care. African American women reported wide use of folk health beliefs and practices as well as indigenous health care providers.

Redmond, G. T. (1988). An examination of the influence of transcultural nursing on graduate curriculum in mental health nursing. *Dissertation Abstracts International, 49(12A)*, 3608.

The data for this study were derived from telephone interviews with Leininger and National League for Nursing Self Study reports from the "Top Twenty" schools of nursing in the United States. Findings indicated very few cultural and transcultural elements in the curricular documents studied. Data supported that faculty influence the cultural and transcultural content in graduate mental health nursing programs. Also, the philosophical foundations and curricular components of the programs studied demonstrated discontinuities, and qualitative research methods were seldom taught. In contrast, quantitative research methods were universally included in the programs. Finally, those curricula that included more cultural or transcultural elements also included more content on implementation of civil rights laws.

Sellers, S. C. (2001). The spiritual care meanings of adults residing in the Midwest. *Nursing Science Quarterly, 14*, 239–248.

This ethnonursing study interviewed six key and 12 general informants in the midwestern United States to discover their perceptions of spiritual nursing care. Five themes were developed from the data analysis: defining spirituality as a motivating force; spirituality as a dynamic, lifelong search; spirituality as unique in expression and practice; spirituality as influenced by environmental context; and how nurses can enhance spirituality. Sadly, both key and general informants perceived nurses as ineffective in addressing client spirituality. The author recommends both further research and careful examination of nursing service and education practices.

Spangler, Z. D. L. (1991). Nursing care values and caregiving practices of Anglo-American and Philippine-American nurses conceptualized within Leininger's theory. *Dissertation Abstracts International, 52(04B)*, 1960.

This ethnonursing study sought to identify the cultural care diversities and universalities in relation to nursing care values and caregiving practices of Anglo-American and Philippine-American nurses in hospital practice. The identified diversity themes were that the care of Anglo-American nurses was characterized by promotion of autonomy (self-care), assertiveness, and situation control. The care of Philippine-American nurses was characterized by an obligation to care based on the care values of conscience, physical comfort, respect, and patience. Nurse-to-nurse conflicts were generated by cultural conflicts. Philippine-American nurses sought cultural care congruence through use of the three modes of nursing action. Two universal themes were also identified. These were the concerns associated with the nursing shortage (increased workload, frustration, inability to provide total patient care) and the influence of institutional norms, standards, and regulations on nursing practice. Implications of this study include the need to reexamine the expectation that foreign-educated nurses should adopt American nursing care values, rather than American and foreign-educated nurses learning from each other.

CHAPTER 17

Health as Expanding Consciousness
Margaret A. Newman

Julia B. George

Margaret Ann Newman (b. 1933) received a B.S.H.E. in home economics and English from Baylor University, Waco, Texas, in 1954; a B.S. in nursing from the University of Tennessee, Memphis, in 1962; an M.S. in nursing from the University of California, San Francisco, in 1964; and a Ph.D. in nursing science and rehabilitation nursing from New York University, New York, in 1971. She relates that she resisted the feeling that she should become a nurse as she completed her first bachelor's degree and during the next eight years while she served as the primary caregiver during her mother's struggle with amyotrophic lateral sclerosis. Her mother died just as Newman had prayed that she was willing to become a nurse. Within two weeks of her mother's death, Newman was a nursing major at the University of Tennessee and quickly decided that nursing was right for her.

Newman has held faculty positions at the University of Tennessee, Memphis; New York University; and Pennsylvania State University, University Park. She retired as professor in the School of Nursing at the University of Minnesota in 1996. In addition to these faculty positions, she has served as director of nursing for the University of Tennessee Clinical Research Center, acting director of nursing for the Ph.D. program in nursing science at New York University, and professor-in-charge of the graduate program in nursing at Pennsylvania State University.

She is an active scholar and the recipient of many honors. She has served or is serving on the editorial boards of many scholarly nursing journals, including Advances in Nursing Science, Journal of Professional Nursing, Nursing and Health Care, Nursing Research, Nursing Science Quarterly, *and* Western Journal of Nursing Research. *She is a fellow in the American Academy of Nursing and is, listed in Who's Who in American Women and in Who's Who in America and the recipient of the Outstanding Alumnus Award from the University of Tennessee College of Nursing and the Distinguished Alumnus Award and Distinguished Scholar in Nursing from the New York University Division of Nursing. She has also received the Sigma Theta Tau International Founders Award for Excellence in Nursing Research and the E. Louise*

Grant Award for Nursing Excellence from the University of Minnesota. The Zeta Chapter of Sigma Theta Tau International offers the Margaret Newman Scholar Award to support doctoral students whose work extends Newman's theory. She has been a Latin American Teaching fellow and an American Journal of Nursing scholar. She has conducted workshops and conferences and served as a consultant around the world, including Australia, Brazil, Canada, Czechoslovakia, France, Finland, Germany, Japan, New Zealand, Poland, and the United Kingdom, in addition to the United States.

Margaret Newman states that during her doctoral study she was interested in theory in nursing (Wallace & Coberg, 1990). More specifically, as a result of her experiences during her mother's illness, she was interested in the relationships between movement, time, and space, for she describes her mother as having been immobilized in time and space. Newman states that she did not intentionally begin to develop a theory but, rather, "slid" into theory development. Her preparations to speak at a conference in 1978 marked the beginning of her defined intention to explicate the temporal and spatial patterns of health. She says that at this time she was moving toward a theory of health. She chose health as a focus because she saw disease as a meaningful aspect of health and believed health needed better definition.

In developing her theory, Newman (1994a, 2005) was influenced by Martha Rogers (1970), Bentov (1978), Bohm (1980, 1981, 1992), Moss (1981), Prigogine (1976), and Young (1976a, 1976b). From Rogers she drew upon the concepts of pattern and the unitary nature of human beings, with particular emphasis on the importance of the basic assumption of pattern. The unitary human being is open and in interaction with its environment. There are no real boundaries between human and environment; pattern is an identification of the wholeness of the person. Newman identified disease as a manifestation of pattern (Newman, 2005; Wallace & Coberg, 1990). Bentov's view of consciousness as evolving and being coextensive with the universe supported Newman's concept of health as expanding consciousness. Bohm's discussion of implicate and explicate order supported the idea of health as a pattern of the whole with a normal progression toward higher levels of organization. Moss's presentation of love as the highest level of consciousness was affirming of Newman's views of the nature of health and nursing. Prigogine's theory of dissipative structures supported the idea that seemingly negative events are part of the process of expanding consciousness (Newman, 1997a). Young's discussion of the importance of insight, pattern recognition, and choice provided the impetus for the integration of the concepts of movement, time, and space into a dynamic theory of health.

HEALTH AS EXPANDING CONSCIOUSNESS

Concepts and Assumptions

Newman (2003) describes a discussion with Martha Rogers that led to the view of health as a unitary concept. In discussing health and illness with Rogers, Newman spoke of them as opposite ends of the spectrum, to which Rogers simply replied, "No." The next description, as opposite sides of the same coin, drew the same response from Rogers. Finally, Newman indicates that "Martha understood that opposites create boundaries and that there were no boundaries between health and illness. I had to give up my way of viewing things as opposites." Giving up her view of opposites led to the creation of the theory of Health as Expanding Consciousness (HEC).

HEC is summarized by Jones (2006, p. 331) as

. . . reflected in pattern. A person's wholeness is identified by *pattern* and is a reflection of the dynamic person-environment interaction. Through pattern recognition, meaningful people and events are discussed as the lived experience is uncovered. During periods of disorganization (Prigogine, 1976) such as illness, opportunities for new life choices may become more easily identified. In a caring relationship with the nurse, the person can recognize opportunities for action and direction. When new choices are made, opportunities for increased freedom and connectedness, as well as for relationships, are possible through a new awareness of the human potential. (Newman, 2005)

Concepts in HEC include consciousness and expanding consciousness, person-environment interaction, pattern, pattern recognition, transformation, and disorganization.

Consciousness is "the *information* of the system; the capacity of the system to interact with the environment" (Newman, 1994a, p. 33). In humans this "informational capacity includes not only all the things we normally associate with consciousness, such as thinking and feeling, but also all the information embedded in the nervous system, the endocrine system, the immune system, the genetic code and so on" (p. 33). As human beings develop, consciousness grows, or expands. As consciousness expands, the more it coexists with the universe. Consciousness is the essence of all matter; persons do not *possess* consciousness, they *are* consciousness. The direction of life is ever toward higher levels of consciousness.

Pattern depicts the whole and is characterized by movement, diversity, and rhythm. Movement is constant and rhythmic, and the parts are diverse. Pattern is relatedness; the process of patterning occurs as human energy fields penetrate one another and transformation occurs. As more information is obtained, pattern evolves unidirectionally and becomes more highly organized.

Pattern recognition occurs within the observer. Although we may predict the next event in a sequence, on the basis of knowledge of the sequence to date, we cannot make such predictions *with certainty* because additional information that indicates a change in the sequence has not happened (Bateson, 1979). Thus, if given a sequence of 3, 6, 9, 12, we are likely to predict that the next number would be 15 when in reality the sequence is 3, 6, 9, 12, 16, 20, 24, 28, 33, 38, and so on. It may not be possible to see the pattern all at once. We need to remind ourselves that the piece of reality that is known to us is only a portion of the total reality. Newman (1994a) suggests that more of the pattern is revealed as the time frame is expanded. We follow this concept of increased knowledge of pattern with increased time when we need three elevated blood pressure readings taken at different times to identify an individual as hypertensive. It is also important to note that each pattern is embedded in another pattern. The pattern in the individual is embedded in the pattern of the family, and of the family in the pattern of the community, and so on. The more we comprehend the whole, the more knowledge of the parts becomes meaningful. Paradoxically, the whole may be seen in the parts. A change in the way an individual walks may communicate an overall mood of sadness or glee. Pattern recognition helps find meaning and understanding and in doing so speeds up the evolution of consciousness (Newman, 1997a).

Disorganization is drawn from the work of Prigogine and relates to change in pattern. Patterns tend to become more highly organized as information increases. However, at times the new information, such as illness, does not fit into the existing pattern, and the pattern becomes less orderly, disorganized, or even chaotic. Such times of disorganization provide an indication that change is necessary; Newman (1994a) terms this as a choice point. The disorganization and associated choices may lead to transformation. *Transformation* is change that occurs all at once rather than in a gradual and linear fashion.

Health as the Whole

Newman (1994a) provides a new view of *health*. The old view of health as the absence of disease has been associated with a tendency to view those without health as inferior. She proposes that Hegel's dialectical fusion of opposites to form a synthesized new could fuse disease and nondisease to form a new concept of health. She adds Jantsch's (1980) idea that such fusion may transcend synthesis and, indeed, opposites come to include each other. Bohm (1981) states that when such synthesis is followed to its logical conclusion the opposites pass into each other, reflect each other, and are recognized as identical to each other. From these viewpoints, disease becomes "a meaningful reflection of the whole [of health]" (Newman, 1994a, p. 7). Newman states that Rogers (1970) eliminated the view of health and disease as dichotomies when she proposed persons as unitary human beings. Within such a view, health and disease are not separate entities but *"are each reflections of the larger whole"* (Newman, 1994a, p. 9). Again drawing on Bohm, Newman uses the example of the two views of the same scene provided by cameras that photograph that scene from different angles. Just as the pictures from each camera provide different pictures of the same whole, disease and nondisease provide different views of health.

Newman states that health, disease, and the pattern of the whole are consistent with Bohm's (1980) theory of implicate and explicate order. Implicate order is that "unseen, multidimensional pattern that is the ground, or basis, for all things" (Newman, 1994a, p. 10). Explicate order arises out of the implicate order and includes the tangibles—those things we can identify with our senses—of the world. Because we can see, touch, hear, and feel the tangibles, we tend to identify them as primary, which is contrary to Bohm's statement that implicate order is primary. In this sense, *"manifest health, encompassing disease and non-disease, can be regarded as the explication of the underlying pattern of person-environment"* (Newman, 1994a, p. 11). The explicate is a manifestation of the implicate (Newman, 1997a, p. 22).

Newman proposes that those fluctuations in patterns identified as sickness can provide the disturbance needed to reorganize the relationships of a pattern more harmoniously. Illness may achieve what people have wanted but have been unable to acknowledge; it can provide or represent the disequilibrium needed to maintain the vital active exchange with the environment. We grow or evolve through experiencing disequilibrium and learning how to attain a new sense of balance. Thus, disease may be seen as both emergent pattern and expanding consciousness. It is important to remember that although an individual may exhibit the emergent pattern labeled disease, that individual's pattern relates to and affects the patterns of others—family, friends, community. As open energy systems in constant interaction, humans influence one another's patterns and evolve together.

Newman (1994a) cites Ferguson's (1980) discussion of the paradigm shift occurring in the view of health. She describes it as a shift from an instrumental to a relational view. The shift includes searching for *patterns* instead of treating symptoms, perceiving pain and disease as *information* instead of seeing them as totally negative, viewing the body as a *dynamic field of energy* that is continuous with a larger field instead of as a machine in various states of repair or disrepair, and seeing disease as a *process* rather than an entity. The new paradigm of health, in its embrace of a unitary pattern of changing relationships, is essential to nursing. Within this paradigm the task is not to seek to change the pattern of another but to recognize that pattern as information that represents the whole and to seek to relate to the pattern as it unfolds. The relational paradigm of health incorporates and transforms the old instrumental paradigm. The characteristics of the instrumental paradigm—linear, causal, predictive, rational, controlling, dichotomous—need to be seen as special cases of the new relational paradigm. The characteristics of the new paradigm are pattern, emerging, unpredictable, unitary, intuitive, and innovative.

When health is seen as a pattern of the whole, disease becomes an emergent pattern that can be understood in terms of a pattern of energy (Newman, 1994a). Seeing disease as a manifestation of pattern can help people become aware of their pattern of person–environment interaction. The insight that is gained can be transforming, both for the person and for the family. Newman draws on Young's (1976b) discussion of the acceleration of the evolution of consciousness to explain such transformation. Young emphasizes the process of interaction both among individuals and between people and society in reaching the goal of a higher level of development. He describes seven stages in this evolution. The first is potential freedom, which moves into the second stage, or binding. In binding, the collective is primary, the individual is not important, everything is regulated, and initiative is not needed. In the third stage, centering, individual identity, self-consciousness, and self-determination develop as the person breaks with authority. The fourth stage, choice, is the turning point in which the individual learns the "law." The emphasis in choice is on science and a search for laws with a new awareness of self-limitation. When the law is learned, the fifth stage, or decentering, begins and the emphasis shifts away from self-development to something greater than the individual. Energy is a dominant feature and one's works develop a life of their own; the experience is one of unlimited growth. The sixth stage, unbinding, involves increasing freedom from time, and the seventh stage represents complete freedom and unrestricted choice. Newman (1994a) says that most of us do not experience stages 6 and beyond. She does state that Young's conception of evolution and her own model of health as expanding consciousness are corollaries:

> We come into being from a state of potential consciousness, are bound in time, find our identity in space, and through movement we learn the "law" of the way things work and make choices that ultimately take us beyond space and time to a state of absolute consciousness. (p. 46)

It is from Young that Newman derived her emphasis on the importance of a choice point. A choice point occurs when the old ways of doing things no longer work and new answers must be sought. The experience is one of disconnectedness—the familiar does not function in the expected way; things are falling apart. This sense of disorder is a predecessor of a transformation to a higher level of consciousness. Such transformation is characterized by the knowledge that the old rules no longer apply and by the willingness to tolerate some degree of uncertainty and ambiguity until the emerging pattern becomes clearer.

Newman (1994a) says that disease is not necessary for evolution to higher levels of consciousness. She cites Bentov (1978) and Moss (1981) in discussing that the degree of flexibility one uses in responding to stress helps to determine how disabling that stress will be. The more open and flexible one is, the more energy can flow through and the less negative effects result from the stress. Newman recommends that "we accept the experience as *our* experience regardless of how contrary it is to what we might have wished would happen" (p. 29).

> In the model of health as expanding consciousness it does not matter where one is in the spectrum. There is no basis for rejecting any experience as irrelevant. The important factor is to be fully present in the moment and know that whatever the experience, it is a manifestation of the process of evolving to higher consciousness. (p. 68)

New Paradigm

Newman, Sime, and Corcoran-Perry (1991) proposed a perspective for nursing that they call the unitary–transformative paradigm. The unitary–transformative paradigm views "the human being as a unitary phenomenon unfolding in an undivided universe" (Newman, 1994a, p. 82). Phenomena are identified by pattern and by interaction with the larger whole. Change is unidirectional, unpredictable, and transformative. Change occurs as systems move through periods or stages of organization and disorganization (choice points) to become more complex. Disruptive processes are seen as phases of reorganization. Health is seen as the evolving pattern of the whole, which illustrates the unfolding implicate order. The person is seen as unitary *and* continuous with the undivided wholeness of the universe. As either person or universe transforms, the other transforms and there are no identifiable boundaries. Characteristics of this paradigm are shown in Table 17-1.

The appropriate methodology for studying this paradigm is a hermenutic, dialectic approach (Newman, 1994, 1997a). Hermenutic represents the search for meaning and dialectic represents the process and content aspects, with each revealing the other—process as content and content as process. Newman supports research as praxis (Newman, 1990a, 1994a). She uses Wheeler and Chinn's (1984) definition of praxis as "thoughtful reflection and action that occur in synchrony, in the direction of transforming the world" (p. 2). Newman indicates that both the participants and the researchers

TABLE 17-1   The Unitary–Transformative Paradigm

Moving From	To Unitary–Transformative
Attention to other as object	Attention to the "we" in relationship
Fixing things	Attending to the meaning of the whole
Hierarchical one-way interventions	Mutual process partnering
Focus on power, manipulation, and control	Reflective compassionate consciousness
Seeking cause (the past) and prediction (the future)	Process (the present) "relaxing into the uncertainty and unpredictability of this process"

Adapted from Newman, M. M. (1997). *Experiencing the whole.* Advances in Nursing Science, 20(1), 34–49.

experience growth as her interactive research methodology is carried out. She believes that research must focus on practice realities and not be limited to outcomes. It is important that the nursing research help practitioners understand and act in their unique situations. The content of the research is the process of the nursing, seeking pattern recognition. The theory of expanding consciousness is used as *a priori* theory to inform and illuminate the experiences of the participants in the research. In 2005, she refers to praxis as TheoryPracticeResearch.

HEALTH AS EXPANDING CONSCIOUSNESS AND THE FOUR MAJOR CONCEPTS

Newman (1994a) deals with all of the concepts in nursing's metaparadigm. *Human beings* are unitary with the *environment*. There are no boundaries. Human beings are identified by their patterns. The patterns of individuals are embedded in those of their family and, in turn, these are embedded in the patterns of the community and society. Humans are moving toward ever-increasing organization and are capable of making their own decisions. Progression to a higher level of organization often occurs after a period of disorganization, or choice point, when the older ways no longer work. Movement is a pivotal choice point in evolving consciousness and is the expression of consciousness. Restriction of movement forces one beyond space–time. Marchione (1993) states that Newman's implicit assumptions are that humans have the following characteristics:

- Open energy systems
- In continual interconnectedness with a universe of open systems (environment)
- Continuously active in evolving their own pattern of the whole (health)
- Intuitive as well as affective and cognitive beings
- Capable of abstract thinking as well as sensation
- More than the sum of their parts (p. 6)

Health is expanding consciousness: "the evolving pattern of the whole, the explication of the unfolding implicate order" (Newman, 1994a, pp. 82–83). Health is a synthesis of disease and nondisease. Newman's theory is about health; further discussion of health can be found in the presentation of the theory in this chapter.

Newman (1994a) discusses *nursing* as a profession, presenting three stages in the growth of the profession. The first stage is formative. In this stage nursing was in the process of becoming, of establishing its identity, and individual practitioners were responsible for their own practice. In the second or normative stage, nursing lost some of its authority and was more competitive and persuasive in relation to the environment. During this stage, nursing moved primarily into the hospital setting and nurses became employees. The third stage is the integrative stage. Newman thinks that nursing is moving into the third stage but has not yet completed the process. In the integrative stage nursing will relate to other health care providers and to clients as partners, in a cooperative, mutual manner. Newman (1990b) suggests that three nursing roles are essential to the integrative model. The professional nursing role is the primary integrative role; Newman refers to this role as nursing clinician/case manager. The other two roles are that of nursing team leader and staff nurse. The nursing clinician/case manager embraces the whole of the nursing paradigm, the staff nurse functions primarily from the medical or disease-oriented paradigm, and the nursing team leader serves as a liaison between the two to integrate and coordinate all into individualized care for every client. Notice that these three roles demonstrate the incorporation of the old (disease-oriented paradigm) within the new (nursing paradigm), with the old becoming part of the whole rather than the primary focus of activity.

Newman (1994a) defines nursing as *"caring in the human health experience"* (p. 139). She believes that caring is a moral imperative for nursing. On the basis of Moss's (1981) statement on love, she says that caring is something that transforms all of us and all that we do, rather than something that we do. Caring reflects the whole of the person. Caring requires that we be open. Being open is being vulnerable. Being vulnerable may lead to suffering, which we tend to avoid. Avoiding suffering can impede our efforts to move to higher levels of consciousness. "The need is to let go, embrace our experience, and allow the expansion of consciousness to unfold" (Newman, 1994a, p. 142). Without caring, nursing does not occur.

HEALTH AS EXPANDING CONSCIOUSNESS AND THE NURSING PROCESS

When health is conceptualized as the expansion of consciousness in a universe of undivided wholeness, intervention aimed at producing a particular result becomes a problem. To intervene with a particular solution in mind is to say we know what form the pattern of expanding consciousness will take, and we don't. Moss (1981), who declares himself a *former* general practitioner of medicine, asks where is the world going anyway, except around in circles. Somehow this bigger picture makes it easier to relax and enjoy an authentic involvement/evolvement with another person. (Newman, 1994a, p. 97)

In the relational paradigm described by Newman (1994a), the focus is not on the professional identifying what is wrong (*assessment* and *diagnosis*) or on planning and taking steps to correct the problem (*outcomes, planning, implementation, evaluation*). Rather, the professional enters into partnership with the client. The situation that brings the client to the attention of the nurse is often one of chaos and, at the minimum, involves circumstances that the client does not know how to handle. The client is at a choice point and is seeking a partner to participate in an authentic relationship. The nurse and client trust that, through the process of the unfolding of the relationship, both will emerge at a higher level of consciousness. The nurse is with the client throughout the process.

The intent of the nurse is to "enter into the process with the client to be present with it, attend to it and live it, even if it appears in the form of disharmony, catastrophe, or disease" (Newman, 1994a, p. 99). To accomplish this, the nurse must give up the compulsion to fix things, to shape the world in a previous image of what health is or should be. Newman believes that the joy of nursing is in being present with clients through disorganization and disharmony with "an unconditional acceptance of the unpredictable, paradoxical nature of life" (p. 103). Such acceptance does not mean doing nothing. Action becomes apparent as pattern becomes apparent. In the client situations Newman presents as examples, she identifies the nurse as "doing" many of the things that would be done within the old framework—providing support and information, for example. It is the intent with which these things are done that differs. In the unitary–transformative paradigm, the nurse's actions are part of the process of being with another as both nurse and client seek expanded consciousness. The actions are not oriented toward achieving a preestablished goal determined by the nurse. Newman describes successful outcomes as "a shift from concentration on self to a broader perspective that extends beyond self, a kind of universal perspective . . . manifest in congruence between inner and outer experience and a greater capacity for love and relatedness in the world. The health professional's awareness of being, rather than doing, is the primary mechanism" (p. 103).

Newman describes this nurse–client relationship as similar to the events that occur after two pebbles are thrown into a pool of water. From the entry point of each pebble ripples begin to emanate. These ripples continue to radiate, meet, interact, and develop an interference pattern. The interference pattern spreads and is part of the whole of each of the original patterns. If we substitute two people for the pebbles and the waves of each of their patterns for the ripples in the water, we have an interaction pattern similar to that shown in Figure 17-1. To be in touch with another, one needs to be in touch with one's own pattern. The more we know ourselves, the clearer we can be in expressing our patterns to others and in coming to know them. There are no separate parts; the pattern is to be sensed as a whole, as a continuous flow of movement with relationships that continue to merge and move apart. "The nurse–client relationship is a rhythmic coming together and moving apart of the client and the nurse" (Newman, 1994, p. 112).

The five-step nursing process does not apply to Newman's theory. The implication of the five-step process that predictive goals can be set and that outcomes should be measured against these goals is not compatible with Newman's statements that we cannot make predictions with certainty and that we do not know what form expanding consciousness will take. For Newman, the process of nursing is one of coming together as partners during a time of chaos when the client is at a choice point. The nurse is there to be with the client and to accept the unpredictable nature of life. Accepting the circumstances decreases the stress in responding to those circumstances. Although the nurse may share knowledge, provide support, or be an organizing force in the relationship, the primary function for the nurse in this caring relationship is awareness of being. Attending to silence is at least as crucial as attending to utterances and movements. When the client is ready, the nurse and

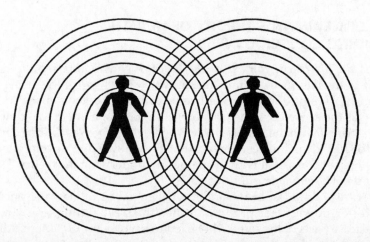

FIGURE 17-1 Interaction pattern of two persons: A holographic model of intervention. (*Used by permission from Newman, M. A. (1994). Health as expanding consciousness (2nd ed.). New York: National League for Nursing Press. Used with permission of National League for Nursing, New York, NY.*)

client will again move apart. It is hoped that each will have reached a higher level of consciousness through the experience.

An example of a Newman-based nurse–client experience is demonstrated in Michaels's (2000) story, "About Marie":

> I visited Marie, who was living with severe chronic obstructive pulmonary disease. Being on continuous oxygen and many medications for heart and lung disease, Marie's goal was to discontinue all the prescribed medications and shift to herbs. She was an avid shopper in health food stores and had considerable knowledge about the desired effects of herbs and other nonprescribed medications. Marie felt vulnerable and expended much of her energy taking care of herself. She was easily frightened. For example, Marie would startle when the phone rang. In dialogue with her about her life situation, Marie decided she wanted to learn to relax. She found in her closet a hand-held biofeedback device intended for a family member. She used that device continuously for more than a month and finally reached a point where she was able to relax no matter what was happening to her. Several months later she had to undergo a cholecystectomy. Her physicians wondered whether she would survive the surgery or be able to get off the ventilator. She did survive the surgery and came off the ventilator effortlessly. She attributed her success to the biofeedback device. Marie was never able to attribute success to herself alone. She relied on and gave credit to external agents for success—her medication, or herbs, or the hand-held biofeedback device. She used the hand-held biofeedback device to change her response to environmental stimuli and life events. In her efforts, Marie began to discern her pattern and meaning. She remained steadfast in believing that it was only something outside of herself that would help her. With a strong faith, Marie was not afraid of death, but she did fear dying alone. Several months later, Marie contracted pneumonia, was hospitalized, and died. (Michaels, 2000, p. 29)

CRITIQUE OF NEWMAN'S THEORY OF HEALTH AS EXPANDING CONSCIOUSNESS

1. *What is the historical context of the theory?* Newman began the development of her theory in the late 1970s, a time during which much work was being done in the development of nursing theories. She began using the deterministic, positivist approach that was the accepted mode of knowledge development at that time. She found she was not satisfied with the results she was achieving; she was finding some evidence of support for her ideas but recognized that the knowledge development methods being used were not consistent with the paradigm underlying the theory. Therefore, the findings could not adequately guide practice.

For over three decades, Newman has challenged us to view the phenomenon of health in a different way. Her proposal of health as expanding consciousness, with health and disease parts of the same whole, led to a new view of pattern. Although concepts are present within her work, they are not primary to understanding the unitary–transformative paradigm. She indicates that she has moved beyond the interrelationship of concepts to the interrelationship of human beings.

2. *What are the basic concepts and relationships presented by the theory?* The basic concepts are health, expanding consciousness, the whole or unitary person, choice points, pattern, pattern recognition, disorganization, and transformation. Newman recognizes that there are movement–time–space dimensions in the unitary evolving patterns of consciousness (Newman, 1997a, p. 25). The major relationship is that health is expanding consciousness.

3. *What major phenomena of concern to nursing are presented? (These phenomena may include* but are not limited to *human beings, environment, health, interpersonal relations, caring goal attainment, adaptation, and energy fields.)* Human beings and environment are unitary, thus inseparable. Health is a major focus of the theory. Nursing and caring are also major phenomena of concern.

4. *To whom does it apply? In what situations? In what ways?* Newman's theory of Health as Expanding Consciousness is not limited by person or setting. It is generalizable to anybody, anywhere. Her presentation of nursing within this theory is limited to those situations in which caring occurs. She states that without caring, nursing is not present.

5. *By what method or methods can this theory be tested?* Newman supports the use of the theory of health as expanding consciousness as *a priori* in research. However, she does not support the positivistic view of hypothesis development and testing. In her research methodology, the patterns that are identified through interviews with research participants are tested against the theory. Thus, the theory of health as expanding consciousness can be used in research and in testing. The hermeneutic dialectic methodology to be used does not include hypotheses, which represent a view of the world that is incongruent with the theory.

Research has been conducted by using Newman's theory. Newman has conducted studies on the needs of hospitalized patients (1966), time and movement (1972, 1976), subjective time (1982; Newman & Guadiano, 1984), and patterns in persons with coronary artery disease (Newman & Moch, 1991). These studies have both added to the general body of nursing knowledge and served to refine and develop her theory. Fryback's (1993) and Moch's (1988, 1990) studies supported Newman's thesis that disease is a part of health and that the emergence of disease allows health to unfold. Schorr, Farnham, and Ervin (1991) also report support for Newman's theory, whereas Mentzer and Schorr (1986) found that perceived duration of time was not related to age. Newman says that Engle's (1984, 1986) conclusion that the faster one moves, the healthier one is, is based on a paradigm other than Newman's even though Engle used the methodology that Newman had identified at that time. It is important to note that in the mid-1980s Newman had not yet explicated her hermeneutic dialectic methodology for the unitary–transformative paradigm.

6. *Does this theory direct nursing actions that lead to favorable outcomes?* Since the focus is on process and not on fixing what is wrong, it is difficult to define favorable outcomes in light of the theory of Health as Expanding Consciousness. The theory is not intended to be measured by outcomes.

7. *How contagious is this theory?* As identified in the biographical sketch at the beginning of this chapter, Newman has made worldwide presentations of her work. In her writings she has focused primarily on theory development, research, and practice. This is reflected in the areas of focus of publications about her work as there has been little mention of the use of this theory in education. Two examples found are Vandemark's (2006) and Picard and Mariolis's (2002) discussion of the use of nursing theory in the preparation of psychiatric nurses.

Newman's (1994a) discussion of research as praxis makes it clear that her intention and belief is that theory must be derived from practice, reflect the realities of practice, and inform practice. She has also proposed a model for practice that is derived from the theory (Newman, 1990b). Bramlett, Gueldner, and Sowell (1990) discussed consumer-centric advocacy as accomplished through the nurse–client interpersonal relationship and supported by Newman's indication of client freedom to be the decision maker. Others have spoken of the utility of Newman's work in guiding and improving practice. Areas of discussion have included parish nursing (Gustafson, 1990), caring for high-risk pregnant women (Kalb, 1990), caring for women with rheumatoid arthritis (Neill, 2002b), parternership in practice (Jonsdottir, Litchfield, & Pharris, 2003), pattern recognition as the essence of practice (M. C. Smith, 1990), practicing in a professional manner (Nelson, 1991), praxis (Pharris & Endo, 2007), and relating (Newman, 1999). The use of the theory at Carondelet St. Mary's has also been described (Ethridge, 1991; Michaels, 1992; Newman, Lamb, & Michaels, 1991). Other publications about practice include case examples (Capasso, 1998), case management (Newman, Lamb, & Michaels, 1991); community nursing (Bunkers, Michaels, & Ethridge, 1997), death (Zust, 2006), an integrative model (Newman, 1990c), and partnering of researcher and practicing nurses (Endo, Miyahara, Suzuki, & Ohmasa, 2005).

Areas of reported research include adults with cancer (Barron, 2000); binge/purge behaviors (Muscari, 1992); cancer survivors (DeMarco, Picard, & Agretelis, 2004; Karian, Jankowski, & Beal, 1998; Picard, Agretelis, & DeMarco, 2004); caregiving couples (Brown & Alligood, 2004; Brown, Chen, Mitchell, & Province, 2007; Schmitt, 1991); chronic pain and music (Schorr, 1993); chronic skin wounds (Rosa, 2006); community pattern recognition (Pharris, 2002); cultural diversity (Butrin, 1992); experience with breast cancer (Moch, 1988, 1990; Roux, 1993); families, in Canada and Japan, dealing with mental illness (Yamashita, 1998a, 1998b, 1999); family with death of a child (Picard, 2002); family health (Litchfield, 1997); families with children with health care needs (Falkenstern, 2003; Tommet, 1997, 2003); guided imagery (Gross, 1995); health behavior change life patterns (Berry, 2002); health in older adults (Engle, 1984; Kelley, 1990; Noveletsky-Rosenthal, 1996; Schorr, Farnham & Ervin, 1991); high-risk pregnancy (Schroeder, 1993); HIV/AIDS as expanding consciousness (Kendall, 1996; Lamendola & Newman, 1994); Japanese women with ovarian cancer and their families (Endo, 1996, 1998; Endo et al., 2000); middle adolescent females (Shanahan, 1993); menopause (Musker, 2008); midlife women (Picard, 1998, 2000); movement and time (Schorr & Schroeder, 1991); Native American women with breast cancer (Kiser Larson, 1999); pattern recognition (Batty, 1999; Hayes & Jones, 2007); peer support groups (Bruce-Barrett, 1998); perceptions of control and time duration (Mentzer & Schorr, 1986); persons with chronic illnesses (Brauer, 2001; Dingley, Bush & Roux, 2001; Jonsdottir, 1994, 1998; Neill, 2002a, 2005; Newman & Moch, 1991; Predeger & Mumma, 2004; Schlotzhauer & Farnham, 1997); preadmission nursing practice (Flanagan, 2002); pre-surgery practice (Flanagan, 2009); professional identity (Brenner, 1986); rural Black families (C. T. Smith, 1989); synchrony (Krejci, 1992); and victimizing sexualization (S. K. Smith, 1997a, 1997b). Publications about research and theory development include Connor (1998), Endo (2004), Holmes (1993), Newman (1987, 1990a, 1990b, 1992,

1994b, 1997b), Solari-Twadell, Bunkers, Wang, and Snyder (1995), Wade (1998), Wendler (1996), and Yamashita and Tall (1998).

STRENGTHS AND LIMITATIONS

Strengths of Newman's work include that it is a work in progress, one that is evolving through the use of an identified research method. Also, Newman's presentation is logical. She presents the material from which she derived her ideas as needed and discusses with clarity those works that support her theory.

Her statement that health is expanding consciousness, seen in the evolving pattern of the whole, is relatively simple. Her ideas represent a paradigm shift in our view of health and of nursing and may be complex to those who do not comprehend the paradigm. This is true for any paradigm shift and should not be seen as a limitation of this theory.

There are some areas of potential confusion in her work. For example, she describes disease as disequilibrium or disruption and discusses the role played by disequilibrium in growth or the expansion of consciousness. At another point, she states that disease is not necessary and may not occur if human beings can be open to and accepting of the turn of events in their lives. She also describes humans and their environment as an undivided whole and speaks eloquently to the importance of viewing them in this way. Again, in another discussion, she indicates that the whole can be seen in its parts. She does discuss the fact that the smaller the piece being viewed is, the fuzzier the picture of the whole will be.

For those who seek structure and direction in providing nursing care, a limitation of this theory is its focus on the process in the present. For those to whom relationships are more important than products, this focus will be beneficial and a strength.

Summary

Newman developed a theory of health as expanding consciousness in which disease and nondisease are synthesized to form a new view of health. Health is seen as the explication of the underlying pattern of person–environment. Humans are unitary beings moving in space–time and unfolding in an undivided universe toward increasing organization. Humans are ever changing in a unidirectional, unpredictable, and transformative (all-at-once) manner. Change is associated with periods of organization and disorganization. During disorganization, when old ways no longer are effective, humans face choice points. It is during such times that clients and nurses come together. Nursing is "caring in the human health experience" (Newman, 1994a, p. 139). In the unitary–transformative paradigm, caring involves the whole of the nurse and the whole of the client. Nurse and client become partners in living through the period of disharmony and emerging at a higher level of consciousness. Newman proposes a hermeneutic dialectic approach to research and states that research is praxis. Both the participants and the researchers grow and learn in the interactive process of conducting the research. The experience of the participant and researcher is not unlike that of the client and nurse. Newman has provided a new view of the world of health in a logical manner. Her theory of health as expanding consciousness can be applied in any setting, and can be used in research and practice. Continued research is needed as this theory evolves.

Thought Questions

1. Describe an example of expanding consciousness in your own life.
2. According to Newman, what is the importance of a crisis point?
3. Describe the role of the nurse, according to Newman, when encountering some one who is at a crisis point.

4. Consider a clinical situation in which you were not satisfied with the outcome; -- describe how using Health as Expaning Consciousness might have made a difference in that outcome.

PEARSON

EXPLORE mynursingkit™

MyNursingKit is your one stop for online chapter review materials and resources. Prepare for success with additional NCLEX®-style practice questions, interactive assignments and activities, web links, animations and videos, and more!

Register your access code from the front of your book at
www.mynursingkit.com.

References

Barron, A. (2000). Life meanings and the experience of cancer: Application of Newman's research method and phenomenological analysis. *Dissertation Abstracts International, 62*(03B), 1313. Abstract retrieved April 7, 2008, from Dissertation Abstracts Online database.

Bateson, G. (1979). *Mind and nature: A necessary unity.* Toronto: Bantam.

Batty, M. L. E. (1999). Pattern identification and expanding consciousness during the transition of "low-risk" pregnancy. *Masters Abstracts International, 39*(03), 826. Abstract retrieved April 7, 2008, from Dissertation Abstracts Online database.

Bentov, I. (1978). *Stalking the wild pendulum.* New York: E. P. Dutton.

Berry, D. C. (2002). Newman's theory of Health as Expanding Consciousness in women maintaining weight loss. *Dissertation Abstracts International, 63*(05B), 2300. Abstract retrieved June 6, 2007, from Dissertation Abstracts Online database.

Bohm, D. (1980). *Wholeness and the implicate order.* London: Routledge & Kegan Paul.

Bohm, D. (1981). The physicist and the mystic—Is a dialogue between them possible? A conversation with David Bohm conducted by Renee Weber. *Re-Vision, 4*(1), 22–35.

Bohm, D. (1992). On dialogue. *Noetic Sciences Review, 23,* 16–18.

Bramlett, M. H., Gueldner, S. H., & Sowell, R. L. (1990). Consumer-centric advocacy: Its connection to nursing frameworks. *Nursing Science Quarterly, 3,* 156–161.

Brauer, D. J. (2001). Common patterns of person-environment interaction in persons with rheumatoid arthritis. *Western Journal of Nursing Research, 23,* 414–430.

Brenner, P. S. (1986). Temporal perspective, professional identity, and perceived well-being. *Dissertation Abstracts International, 47*(12B), 4821.

Brown, J. W., & Alligood, M. R. (2004). Realizing wrongness: Stories of older wife caregivers. *Journal of Applied Gerontology, 23*(2), 104–119.

Brown, J. W., Chen, S., Mitchell, C., & Province, A. (2007). Help-seeking by older husbands caring for wives with dementia. *Journal of Advanced Nursing, 59,* 353–360.

Bruce-Barrett, C. A. (1998). Patterns of health and healing: Peer support and prostate cancer. *Masters Abstracts International, 37-01,* 233.

Bunkers, S. L., Michaels, C., & Ethridge, P. (1997). Advanced practice nursing in community: Nursing's opportunity. *Advanced Practice Nursing Quarterly, 2,* 79–84.

Butrin, J. E. (1992). Cultural diversity in the nurse–client encounter. *Clinical Nursing Research, 1,* 238–251.

Capasso, V. A. (1998). The theory is the practice: An exemplar. *Clinical Nurse Specialist, 12,* 226–229.

Connor, M. J. (1998). Expanding the dialogue on praxis in nursing research and practice. *Nursing Science Quarterly, 11,* 51–55.

DeMarco, R. F., Picard, C., & Agretelis, J. (2004). Nurse experiences as cancer survivors: Part I—Personal. *Oncology Nursing Forum, 31,* 523–530.

Dingley, C. E., Bush, H. A., & Roux, G. (2001). Inner strength in women recovering from coronary artery disease: A grounded theory. *Journal of Theory Construction and Testing, 5*(2), 45–52.

Endo, E. (1996). Pattern recognition as a nursing intervention with adults with cancer. *Dissertation Abstracts International, 57*(06B), 3653.

Endo, E. (1998). Pattern recognition as a nursing intervention with Japanese women with ovarian cancer. *Advances in Nursing Science, 20*(4), 49–61.

Endo, E. (2004). Nursing praxis within Margaret Newman's theory of Health as Expanding Consciousness. *Nursing Science Quarterly, 17,* 110–115.

Endo, E., Miyahara, T., Suzuki, S., & Ohmasa, T. (2005). Partnering of researcher and practicing nurses for transformative nursing. *Nursing Science Quarterly, 18,* 138–145.

Endo, E., Nitta, N., Inayoshi, M., Saito, R., Takemura, K., Minegishi, H., et al. (2000). Pattern recognition as a caring partnership in families with cancer. *Journal of Advanced Nursing, 32,* 603–610.

Engle, V. F. (1984). Newman's conceptual framework and the measurement of older adults' health. *Advances in Nursing Science, 7*(1), 24–36.

Engle, V. F. (1986). The relationship of movement and time to older adults' functional health. *Research in Nursing and Health, 9,* 123–129.

Ethridge, P. (1991). A nursing HMO: Carondelet St. Mary's experience. *Nursing Management, 22*(7), 22–27.

Falkenstern, S. K. (2003). Nursing facilitation of health as expanding consciousness in families who have a child with special health care needs. *Dissertation Abstracts International, 64*(07B), 3186. Abstract retrieved April 7, 2008, from Dissertation Abstracts Online database.

Ferguson, M. (1980). *The aquarian conspiracy: Personal and social transformation in the 1980s.* Los Angeles: J. P. Tarcher.

Flanagan, J. M. (2002). Nurse and patient perceptions of the Pre-Admission Nursing Practice Model: Linking theory to practice. *Dissertation Abstracts International, 63*(05B), 2304. Abstract retrieved June 6, 2007, from Dissertation Abstracts Online database.

Flanagan, J. M. (2009). Patient and nurse experience of theory-based care. *Nursing Science Quarterly, 22,I* 160–172.

Fryback, P. B. (1993). Health for people with a terminal diagnosis. *Nursing Science Quarterly, 6,* 147–159.

Gross, S. W. (1995). The impact of a nursing intervention of relaxation with guided imagery on breast cancer patients' stress and health as expanded consciousness. *Dissertation Abstracts International, 56*(10B), 5416.

Gustafson, W. (1990). Application of Newman's theory of health: Pattern recognition as nursing practice. In M. E. Parker (Ed.), *Nursing theories in practice* (pp. 141–161) (Pub. No. 15-2350). New York: National League for Nursing.

Hayes, M. O., & Jones, D. (2007). Health as expanding consciousness: Pattern recognition and incarcerated mothers, a transforming experience. *Journal of Forensic Nursing, 3*(2), 61–66.

Holmes, C. A. (1993). Praxis: A case study in the depoliticization of methods in nursing research...including commentary by Thompson, J. L. *Scholarly Inquiry for Nursing Practice, 3*(1), 3–15.

Jantsch, E. (1980). *The self-organizing universe.* New York: Pergamon.

Jones, D. A. (2006). Newman's Health as Expanding Consciousness. *Nursing Science Quarterly, 19,* 330–332.

Jonsdottir, H. (1994). Life patterns of people with chronic obstructive pulmonary disease: Isolation and being closed in. *Dissertation Abstracts International, 56*(03B), 1346.

Jonsdottir, H. (1998). Life patterns of people with chronic obstructive pulmonary disease: Isolation and being closed in. *Nursing Science Quarterly, 11,* 160–166.

Jonsdottir, H., Litchfield, M., & Pharris, M. D. (2003). Partnership in practice. *Research and Theory for Nursing Practice, 17*(1), 51–63.

Kalb, K. A. (1990). The gift: Applying Newman's theory of health in nursing practice. In M. E. Parker (Ed.), *Nursing theories in practice* (pp. 163–186) (Pub. No. 15-2350). New York: National League for Nursing.

Karian, V. E., Jankowski, S. M., & Beal, J. A. (1998). Exploring the lived-experience of childhood cancer survivors. *Journal of Pediatric Oncology Nursing, 15,* 153–162.

Kelley, F. J. (1990). Spatial–temporal experiences and self-assessed health in the older adult. *Dissertation Abstracts International, 51,* 1194B.

Kendall, J. (1996). Human association as a factor influencing wellness in homosexual men with human immunodeficiency virus disease. *Applied Nursing Research, 9,* 195–203.

Kiser Larson, N. K. (1999). Life patterns of Native American women experiencing breast cancer. *Dissertation Abstracts International, 60(05B),* 2062.

Krejci, J. W. (1992). An exploration of synchrony in nursing. *Dissertation Abstracts International, 53,* 2247.

Lamendola, F. P., & Newman, M. A. (1994). The paradox of HIV/AIDS as expanding consciousness. *Advances in Nursing Science, 16(3),* 13–21.

Litchfield, M. (1997). The process of nursing partnership in family health. *Dissertation Abstracts International, 58(04B),* 1802.

Marchione, J. (1993). *Margaret Newman: Health as expanding consciousness.* Newbury Park, CA: Sage.

Mentzer, C. A., & Schorr, J. A. (1986). Perceived situational control and perceived duration of time: Expressions of life patterns. *Advances in Nursing Science, 9(1),* 12–20.

Michaels, C. (1992). Carondelet St. Mary's nursing enterprise. *Nursing Clinics of North America, 27,* 77–85.

Michaels, C. (2000). Becoming a bard: A journey to self. *Nursing Science Quarterly, 13,* 28–30.

Moch, S. D. (1988). Health in illness: Experiences with breast cancer. *Dissertation Abstracts International, 50(02B),* 497.

Moch, S. D. (1990). Health within the experience of breast cancer. *Journal of Advanced Nursing, 15,* 1426–1435.

Moss, R. (1981). *The I that is we.* Millbrae, CA: Celestial Arts.

Muscari, M. E. (1992). Binge/purge behaviors and attitudes as manifestations of relational pattern-ings in a woman with bulimia nervosa. *Dissertation Abstracts International, 53(11B),* 5647.

Musker, K. M. (2008). Life patterns of women transitioning through menopause: A Newman research study. *Nursing Science Quarterly, 21,* 330–342.

Neill, J. (2002a). From practice to caring praxis through Newman's theory of Health as Expanding Consciousness: A personal journey. *International Journal for Human Caring, 6(2),* 48–54.

Neill, J. (2002b). Transcendence and transformation in the life patterns of women living with rheumatoid arthritis. *Advances in Nursing Science, 24(4),* 27–47.

Neill, J. (2005). Health as Expanding Consciousness: Seven women living with multiple sclerosis or rheumatoid arthritis. *Nursing Science Quarterly, 18,* 334–343.

Nelson, J. I. (1991). A crab or a dolphin: A new paradigm for nursing practice. *Nursing Outlook, 39,* 136–137.

Newman, M. A. (1966). Identifying and meeting patients' needs in short-span nurse–patient relationships. *Nursing Forum, 5(1),* 76–86.

Newman, M. A. (1972). Time estimation in relation to gait tempo. *Perceptual and Motor Skills, 34,* 359–366.

Newman, M. A. (1976). Movement tempo and the experience of time. *Nursing Research, 25,* 273–279.

Newman, M. A. (1979). *Theory development in nursing.* Philadelphia: F. A. Davis.

Newman, M. A. (1982). Time as an index of expanding consciousness with age. *Nursing Research, 31,* 290–293.

Newman, M. A. (1987). Aging as increasing complexity. *Journal of Gerontological Nursing, 13(9),* 16–18.

Newman, M. A. (1990a). Newman's theory of health as praxis. *Nursing Science Quarterly, 3,* 37–41.

Newman, M. A. (1990b). Shifting to higher consciousness. In M. Parker (Ed.), *Nursing theories in practice* (pp. 129–139) (Pub. No. 15-2350). New York: National League for Nursing.

Newman, M. A. (1990c). Toward an integrative model of professional practice. *Journal of Professional Nursing, 6,* 167–173.

Newman, M. A. (1992). Prevailing paradigms in nursing. *Nursing Outlook, 40,* 10–13, 32.

Newman, M. A. (1994a). *Health as expanding consciousness* (2nd ed.) (Pub. No. 14-2626). New York: National League for Nursing Press.

Newman, M. A. (1994b). Theory for nursing practice. *Nursing Science Quarterly, 7,* 153–157.

Newman, M. A. (1997a). Evolution of the theory of Health as Expanding Consciousness. *Nursing Science Quarterly, 10,* 22–25.

Newman, M. A. (1997b). Experiencing the whole. *Advances in Nursing Science, 20*(1), 34–49.

Newman, M. A. (1999). The rhythm of relating in a paradigm of wholeness. *Image: Journal of Nursing Scholarship, 31,* 227–230.

Newman, M. A. (2003). A world of no boundaries. *Advances in Nursing Science, 26,* 240–245.

Newman, M. A. (2005). Caring in the human health experience. In C. Picard & D. Jones (Eds.), *Giving voice to what we know: Margaret Newman's theory of Health as Expanding Consciousness in nursing practice, research, and education* (pp. 3–10). Boston: Jones and Bartlett.

Newman, M. A., & Guadiano, J. K. (1984). Depression as an explanation for decreased subjective time in the elderly. *Nursing Research, 33,* 137–139.

Newman, M. A., Lamb, G. S., & Michaels, C. (1991). Nursing case management: The coming together of theory and practice. *Nursing and Health Care, 12,* 404–408.

Newman, M. A., & Moch, S. D. (1991). Life patterns of persons with coronary artery disease. *Nursing Science Quarterly, 4,* 161–167.

Newman, M. A., Sime, A. M., & Corcoran-Perry, S. A. (1991). The focus of the discipline of nursing. *Advances in Nursing Science, 14*(1), 1–6.

Noveletsky-Rosenthal, H. T. (1996). Pattern recognition in older adults living with chronic illness. *Dissertation Abstracts International, 57(10B),* 6180.

Pharris, M. D. (2002). Coming to know ourselves as community through a nursing partnership with adolescents convicted of murder. *Advances in Nursing Science, 24*(3), 21–42.

Pharris, M. D., & Endo, E. (2007). Flying free: The evolving nature of nursing practice guided by the theory of Health as Expanding Consciousness. *Nursing Science Quarterly, 20,* 136–143.

Picard, C. A. (1998). Uncovering pattern of expanding consciousness in mid-life women: Creative movement and the narrative as modes of expression. *Dissertation Abstracts International, 59(03B),* 1049.

Picard, C. (2000). Pattern of expanding consciousness in midlife women: Creative movement and the narrative as modes of expression. *Nursing Science Quarterly, 13,* 150–157.

Picard, C. (2002). Family reflections on living through sudden death of a child. *Nursing Science Quarterly, 15,* 242–250.

Picard, C., Agretellis, J., & DeMarco, R. F. (2004). Nurse experiences as cancer survivors: Part II—Professional. *Oncology Nursing Forum, 31,* 537–542.

Picard, C., & Mariolis, T. (2002). Praxis as a mirroring process: Teaching psychiatric nursing grounded in Newman's theory of Health as Expanding Consciousness. *Nursing Science Quarterly, 15,* 118–122.

Predeger, E. & Mumma, C. (2004). Connectedness in chronic illness: Women's journeys. *International Journal for Human Caring, 8*(1), 13–19.

Prigogine, I. (1976). Order through fluctuations: Self-organization and social systems. In E. Jantsch & C. H. Waddington (Eds.), *Evolution and consciousness: Human systems in transition* (pp. 93–133). Reading, MA: Addison-Wesley.

Rogers, M. (1970). *An introduction to the theoretical basis of nursing.* Philadelphia: F. A. Davis.

Rosa, K. C. (2006). A process model of healing and personal transformation in persons with chronic skin wounds. *Nursing Science Quarterly, 19,* 349–358.

Roux, G. M. (1993). Phenomenologic study: Inner strength in women with breast cancer. *Dissertation Abstracts International, 55(02B),* 370.

Schlotzhauer, M., & Farnham, R. (1997). Newman's theory and insulin dependent diabetes mellitus in adolescence. *Journal of School Nursing, 13*(3), 20–23.

Schmitt, N. A. (1991). Caregiving couples: The experience of giving and receiving social support. *Dissertation Abstracts International, 52(11B),* 5761.

Schorr, J. A. (1993). Music and pattern change in chronic pain. *Advances in Nursing Science, 15*(4), 27–36.

Schorr, J. A., Farnham, R. C., & Ervin, S. M. (1991). Health patterns in aging women as expanding consciousness. *Advances in Nursing Science, 13*(4), 52–63.

Schorr, J. A., & Schroeder, C. A. (1991). Movement and time: Exertion and perceived duration. *Nursing Science Quarterly, 4,* 104–112.

Schroeder, C. A. (1993). Perceived duration of time and bed rest in high risk pregnancy: An exploration of the Newman model. *Dissertation Abstracts International, 54(04B),* 1894.

Shanahan, S. M. (1993). The lived experience of life-time passing in middle adolescent females. *Masters Abstracts International, 32-05,* 1376.

Smith, C. T. (1989). The lived experience of staying healthy in rural black families. *Dissertation Abstracts International, 50(09B),* 3925.

Smith, M. C. (1990). Pattern in nursing practice. *Nursing Science Quarterly, 3,* 57–59.

Smith, S. K. (1997a). Women's experience of victimizing sexualization, part I: Responses related to abuse and home and family environment. *Issues in Mental Health Nursing, 18,* 395–416.

Smith, S. K. (1997b). Women's experience of victimizing sexualization, part II: Community and longer term personal impacts. *Issues in Mental Health Nursing, 18,* 417–432.

Solari-Twadell, P. A., Bunkers, S. S., Wang, C. E., & Snyder, D. (1995). The Pinwheel Model of Bereavement. *Image: Journal of Nursing Scholarship, 27,* 323–326.

Tommet, P. A. (1997). Nurse–parent dialogue: Illuminating the pattern of families with children who are medically fragile. *Dissertation Abstracts International, 58(05B),* 2359.

Tommet, P. A. (2003). Nurse-parent dialogue: Illuminating the evolving pattern of families with children who are medically fragile. *Nursing Science Quarterly, 16,* 239–246.

Vandemark, L. M. (2006). Awareness of self and expanding consciousness: Using nursing theories to prepare nurse-therapists. *Issues in Mental Health Nursing, 27,* 605–615.

Wade, G. H. (1998). A concept analysis of personal transformation. *Journal of Advanced Nursing, 28,* 713–719.

Wallace, D. (Producer), & Coberg, T. (Director). (1990). *Margaret Newman—The nurse theorists: Portraits of excellence* [Videotape]. Oakland, CA: Studio Three Production, Samuel Merritt College of Nursing.

Wendler, M. C. (1996). Understanding healing: A conceptual analysis. *Journal of Advanced Nursing, 24,* 836–842.

Wheeler, C. E., & Chinn, P. L. (1984). *Peace and power: A handbook of feminist process.* Buffalo: Margaret-daughters.

Yamashita, M. (1998a). Family coping with mental illness: A comparative study. *Journal of Psychiatric Mental Health Nursing, 5,* 515–523.

Yamashita, M. (1998b). Newman's theory of Health as Expanding Consciousness: Research on family caregiving in mental illness in Japan. *Nursing Science Quarterly, 11,* 110–115.

Yamashita, M. (1999). Newman's theory of health applied in family caregiving in Canada. *Nursing Science Quarterly, 12,* 73–79.

Yamashita, M., & Tall, F. D. (1998). A commentary on Newman's theory of health as expanding consciousness. *Advances in Nursing Science, 21,* 65–75.

Young, A. M. (1976a). *The geometry of meaning.* San Francisco: Robert Briggs.

Young, A. M. (1976b). *The reflective universe: Evolution of consciousness.* San Francisco: Robert Briggs.

Zust, B. L. (2006). Death as a transformation of wholeness: An "Aha" experience of Health as Expanding Consciousness. *Nursing Science Quarterly 19,* 57–60.

Selected Annotated Bibliography

Bruce-Barrett, C. A. (1998). Patterns of health and healing: Peer support and prostate cancer. *Masters Abstracts International, 37-01,* 233.

This study used Newman's hermeneutic dialectic research methodology to explore the meaning and pattern of health experiences of five men diagnosed with prostate cancer. The diagnosis of cancer was identified as a choice point and the resulting expansion of consciousness included attuning to one's personal pattern, developing more authentic relationships, and transcending limitations imposed by the disease, its treatment, and lack of knowledge.

Jonsdottir, H. (1994). Life patterns of people with chronic obstructive pulmonary disease: Isolation and being closed in. *Nursing Science Quarterly, 11,* 160–166.

This hermeneutic dialectic study involved 10 persons with chronic obstructive pulmonary disease. Findings included describing the life pattern as resignation, unsuccessful solution to traumatic events, and difficulties expressing oneself and relating to others. None of the participants described having experienced a choice point.

Newman, M. A. (1995). *A developing discipline: Selected works of Margaret Newman*

(Pub. No. 14-2671). New York: National League for Nursing Press.

This is a helpful volume for the student of Newman's work. Gathered in this one work are 22 previously published articles authored or coauthored by Margaret Newman. They are divided into the categories of the emerging structure of the discipline; identifying the pattern of the whole; transforming the meaning of health and practice; integrating theory, education, and practice; retrospective; and prospective.

Schmitt, N. A. (1991). Caregiving couples: The experience of giving and receiving social support. *Dissertation Abstracts International, 52(11B)*, 5761. This study investigated the experience of giving and receiving social support among spouses and spouse caregivers. Twenty older adult couples participated in the study. Results included that helping involved a readjustment of roles; the most valuable help was that keyed to what was most important to the recipient; all agreed they would rather help than be helped and saw helping as a normal part of marriage and identified the helper as a good person. Possibly the most important aspect of this study is its demonstration that the couple or family can be the unit of analysis and family patterns can be identified.

Tommet, P. A. (1997). Nurse–parent dialogue: Illuminating the pattern of families with children who are medically fragile. *Dissertation Abstracts International, 58(05B)*, 2359. This study used the hermeneutic dialectic method to investigate the pattern of families in the process of choosing an elementary school for a medically fragile child. The process of the study helped the parents identify their patterns. A major theme with these families was that of uncertainty and the families identified having moved from disruption and disorganization to reorganization in which instead of seeking to control uncertainty, they were learning to live with uncertainty. The family patterns included being isolated from other family and friends; having evolving relationships with health care providers; developing mutually supportive relationships; experiencing changes in space, time, and movement; interacting with bureaucracy; identifying personal growth and strengths; and making decisions. Developing new ways of relating within and without the family was identified as expanding consciousness.

CHAPTER **18**

Theory of Transpersonal Caring
Jean Watson

Brenda P. Johnson and Jane H. Kelley

Jean Watson was born in 1940 in West Virginia, earned a diploma from Lewis Gale Hospital School of Nursing in Roanoke, Virginia; a baccalaureate degree in nursing from the University of Colorado, Boulder, in 1964; a master's degree in psychiatric–mental health nursing from the University of Colorado, Denver, in 1966; and a Ph.D. in educational psychology and counseling from the University of Colorado, Boulder, in 1973. She has held faculty and administrative positions at the University of Colorado Health Sciences Center, including deanship of the School of Nursing from 1983 to 1990 and founding director of the Center for Human Caring. In 1992, Dr. Watson was named Distinguished Professor at the University of Colorado, the highest honor accorded University of Colorado faculty for scholarly work. She is a widely published author and recipient of numerous awards and honors, including an international Kellogg Fellowship in Australia, a Fulbright Research Award in Sweden, and six honorary doctoral degrees, including three international doctorates (Sweden, United Kingdom, and Quebec, Canada) as well as membership in the American Academy of Nursing and the National League for Nursing's Martha E. Rogers Award for nursing scholarship in 1993. In 1999 Dr. Watson assumed the University of Colorado School of Nursing Murchinson-Scoville Chair in Caring Science, the nation's first endowed chair in caring science. Her latest books range from empirical measurements of caring to philosophies of caring and healing. Theoretical constructs from Dr. Watson's theory have been used to guide academic programs and new models of care in diverse settings around the globe. For additional information about Dr. Jean Watson, the theory of human caring, and programs of study in the caring sciences, you may refer to Dr. Watson's website at the University of Colorado Health Sciences Center School of Nursing (http://www2.uchsc.edu/son/caring/content/default.asp).

The essence of Watson's theory is caring for the purpose of promoting healing, preserving dignity, and respecting the wholeness and interconnectedness of humanity. Her work characterizes nursing as a healing art and science dedicated to the pursuit of harmonious and sacred relationships. It challenges nursing to rediscover its healing traditions while expanding its mission for caring relationships at the societal and planetary level.

The tenets of Watson's theory harken back to Nightingale's concept of nursing as a calling. Just as Nightingale answered the call to transform the profession and the institutions within which nurses learn and practice, Watson's theory has been used extensively as a model by schools and hospitals for putting the human element back into the study and practice of nursing. In the tradition of Florence Nightingale, Jean Watson advocates for a strong liberal arts education with its emphasis on philosophy and values.

Although Watson's theory of human care has been adopted worldwide as a model for the delivery of nursing care, Watson has often stated that the original intent of her work was not to be prescriptive but rather to serve as more of a worldview or ethic by which nursing could explore and understand its traditions and purpose in caring and healing. Since the initial publication of her theory in 1979, Watson has attempted to serve as a bridge by which nursing could transition from a biomedical/natural science model to a postmodern/human science perspective. Aligning nursing with caring was both an attempt by Watson to honor nursing's traditions in herbal and natural healing modalities as well as to make it distinct from medicine with its emphasis on diagnosing and curing disease. Watson believes that language is essential to this endeavor. Watson's theory is constantly evolving as a reflection of her own life journey as well as the availability of words with which to express her beliefs. For example, Watson's original 1979 work was organized around 10 "carative factors." While the basic tenets of these factors have not changed, Watson's current version refers to them as "clinical caritas processes." Although "caritas" and "carative" are similar, the word "caritas" comes "from the Latin word meaning to cherish, to appreciate, to give special attention, if not loving attention to . . ." (http://www2.uchsc.edu/son/caring/content/evolution.asp, accessed January 1, 2008). The shift in terminology reflects Watson's growing emphasis on the metaphysical and spiritual dimensions, the ultimate expression of which Watson views as love. Increasingly, Watson posits "love as an ethic" and ontology as the starting point for nursing's existence, broad societal mission and the basis for caring–healing practices (Watson, 2005a, 2005b). This terminology is also more congruent with a postmodern paradigm. Watson (1999) delineates the basic tenets of postmodernism as follows:

- no one Truth, but multiple truths;
- no one universally known reality that is defined by physical-material world;
- multiple, constructed realities, . . . attention to valuing multiple meanings;
- acknowledgement of physical and non-physical reality and phenomena;
- non-linearity of thinking and acting, introduces relativity of time and space;
- open to ideas that include context, critiques, challenges, multiple interpretations, stories, narratives, text and search for meaning and wholeness;
- utilizes emerging metaphors of art, artistry, creativity, harmony, beauty, spirit-metaphysical, and a holographic nature for exploring and understanding life and the meaning of life and human existence. (p. 289)

Postmodernism is a critique of cultural norms and common notions of truth and reality. It is transdisciplinary and is evident in fields ranging from physics to ecofeminism. Postmodernism uses a deconstructive process to question dominant patterns of thought and governance, which have led to the modernist paternalistic system of hierarchy, followed by a reconstructive process to envision more holistic and egalitarian patterns of thought and being. Watson situates nursing within a postmodern worldview, which acknowledges the holistic and interconnected nature of the universe and the importance of subjectivity. The human science paradigm, thus, is the creation of postmodernism and contrasts with the traditional science paradigm espoused by predominant beliefs of the 19th and 20th centuries and known as the modern age.

There are fundamental differences in ways of being (ontology), knowing (epistemology), and doing (praxis) within the traditional versus the human science paradigm (see Table 18-1). The purpose of traditional science is identification and prediction. Human science is predominantly concerned with the meaning of the lived experience. Thus, different approaches to knowledge development are espoused by the contrasting paradigms. Whenever nursing aligns itself within a biomedical model, key elements of a traditional science paradigm are description of symptoms, variables, and physiological or behavioral outcomes. A human science paradigm would envision the key elements to knowledge formation to be understanding of the human–environment, person–life spirit, or human–human interaction. Methodological ways by which knowledge is acquired also differ. Traditional science recognizes only the legitimacy of verifiable, objective data. This has been interpreted to mean observation of variables in controlled conditions for the purpose of identifying and determining causes of various symptoms, behaviors, and physiological manifestations. A human science approach accepts the legitimacy of multiple ways of knowing or imagining (e.g., phenomenological or aesthetic methods) in order to understand the lived experience or how human–environmental energy patterns are transformed within specific contexts.

Nursing actions (praxis) differ greatly within contrasting paradigms also. Professional nursing within a traditional science and biomedical model is focused on "doing" by controlling and manipulating physical and behavioral parameters through specific actions and environments that maintain physiological or behavioral homeostasis. Within a human science paradigm, the emphasis is on "being" and the cocreation of nurse–patient interactions on human–environmental energy patterns that restore harmony and a sense of well-being.

Watson, through the theory of caring, seeks to give nursing the epistemological and ontological structure by which to pursue a return to the sacredness and mystery of living

TABLE 18-1   A Contrast of Traditional Science and Human Science

	Traditional Science Paradigm	Human Science Paradigm
Ontology	Identify Predict Human as mind/body	Meaning of the experience as lived by a person Human as embodied spirit
Epistemology	Describe outcomes in terms of physical indicators or as behaviors	Knowing about interaction of human–environment, person–life spirit, or human–human
Methodology	Structured studies relying on control of conditions and seeking to establish cause and effect	Multiple approaches seeking to understand lived experience in identified contexts
Praxis	Focus/goal is homeostasis and stability	Seeks harmony and well-being

in relationship rather than the pursuit of domination and self-determination in a health care system that mimics a society that has become fragmented and spiritually bereft.

WATSON'S THEORY OF TRANSPERSONAL CARING

Philosophical Background

Watson's work reflects a blend of Eastern and Western philosophical beliefs. In her early works, transcendental phenomenology was a strong influence on her focus on the metaphysical and spiritual nature of being human. Philosophical beliefs of several philosophers, such as Whitehead (1953), Kierkegaard (1941), and deChardin (1959), influenced her concepts of self and ontological caring. The interpersonal nature of caring was influenced by the psychological teachings of Carl Rogers (1961). Nurse theorists and philosophers who were especially influential in shaping Watson's beliefs about health, culture, environment, dignity, and caring were Nightingale (1859/1957), Henderson (1966), Leininger (1980, 1981), Martha Rogers (1970), and Gadow (1980). Eastern views on the importance of mind/body harmony as can be achieved through meditation and ritual, and metaphysics, and the noetic sciences (Harman, 1991) have influenced Watson's more recent emphasis on the power of intentionality and consciousness on health and healing. Watson acknowledges the influence of the views of Danish philosopher Knud Logstrup (1997) and French philosopher Emmanuel Levinas (1969) on the unity of holiness to life and the moral foundations of humanity on her theory. The similarities of ancient wisdoms espoused by mystics and tribal cultures and more recent beliefs of a holographic science provide the basis for "the emerging/converging paradigm," which has led to Watson's current interest in a caring–healing consciousness that transcends time and space. Watson (2005a) envisions a universal energy field to which all belong and that serves as a healing life force. Watson expresses the hope that such a relational ontology can heal not only individuals but unhealthy health care, sociopolitical, and cultural institutions as well.

Contents of the Theory

In a review of her theory, Watson (1996) presents the major conceptual elements of the original theory along with elements that have evolved over time. The major conceptual elements of Watson's original theory were *transpersonal caring relationship, the 10 carative factors*, and *caring occasion/caring moment*. Current dimensions of Watson's theory (1996, p. 151; 2005a) that have evolved and emerged from these original tenets are the following:

- Expanded views of self and person; transpersonal mind/body/spirit oneness; embodied spirit
- Importance of caring–healing consciousness within the human–environment energy field
- Consciousness as energy; forgiveness and surrender as highest level of consciousness.
- Phenomenal field/unitary consciousness: unbroken wholeness and connectedness of all (subject-object-person-environment-nature-universe-all living things)
- Advanced caring–healing modalities/nursing arts that involve not only the mind and hands, but also the human heart and soul
- Ultimate form of healing and transcendence is love
- Nurse as sacred healing environment

Transpersonal Caring Relationship

Originally defined as a human-to-human connectedness occurring in a nurse–patient encounter wherein "each is touched by the human center of the other" (1989, p. 131; quoted in Watson, 1996, p. 151), the transpersonal caring relationship has always been the key element of Watson's theory.

By 1985/1988 and continuing in her 1996 work, Watson provided a list of specifications on which a transpersonal caring relationship depends:

- The moral commitment, intentionality, and consciousness needed to protect, enhance, promote, and potentiate human dignity, wholeness, and healing, wherein a person creates or cocreates his or her own meaning for existence, healing, wholeness, and caring.
- Orientation of the nurse's intent, will, and consciousness toward affirming the subjective/intersubjective significance of the person. . . .
- The nurse's ability to realize, accurately detect, and connect with the inner condition (spirit) of another. . . .
- The nurse's ability to assess and realize another's condition of being-in-the-world and to feel a union with the other. . . .
- The caring–healing modalities potentiate harmony, wholeness, and comfort, and promote inner healing by releasing some of the disharmony and blocked energy that interfere with the natural healing processes.
- The nurse's own life history and previous experiences. . . . To some degree, the necessary knowledge and sensitivity can be gained through work with other cultures, study of the humanities (art, drama, and literature), and exploration of one's own values, beliefs, and relationship with self . . . personal growth experiences such as psychotherapy, meditation, bioenergetics work, and spiritual awakening. . . . (Watson, 1996, pp. 153–154)

Watson has always stated that the ability to care for others is dependent upon one's ability to care for self. Watson has recently (2005a) expanded the nature of self-care to the ability and readiness for forgiveness of self and others, gratitude for life and all its blessings, and to surrender, to let go of ego and to accept our experiences without resistance or the constant need to control. Watson suggests that forgiveness, gratitude, and surrender are gifts of the universe that place the nurse in "right relation"—a spiritual state that makes the nurse ready to care for others in a way that brings healing and meaning to those who are vulnerable, suffering, or in despair.

Ten Carative Factors to Clinical Caritas Processes

Ten carative factors were identified by Watson (1979, 1985/1988, 1996) as characterizing a caring relationship based upon the nurse's conscious, moral commitment to each person in such a way that facilitates healing and dignity, and that conveys a spiritual dimension influenced by the caring consciousness of the nurse. Watson's intent was not for them to be used as a checklist but rather as a philosophical and conceptual guide for nursing. Indeed, they have served as guiding principles for theory-guided practice models and research around the world. The evolving nature of Watson's theory has led to the redefining and renaming of the original factors to *clinical caritas processes* (see Table 18-2). The caritas processes are intended to be instrumental in reintegrating a

TABLE 18-2   Carative Factor to Clinical Caritas Processes

Carative Factor (Watson, 1996)	Clinical Caritas Processes[1]
Forming a humanistic-altruistic system of values	Practice of loving-kindness and equanimity within context of caring consciousness
Enabling and sustaining faith-hope	Being authentically present and enabling and sustaining the deep belief system and subjective life world of self and one-being-cared-for
Being sensitive to self and others	Cultivation of one's own spiritual practice and transpersonal self, going beyond ego self
Developing a helping-trusting, caring relationship (seeking transpersonal connections)	Developing and sustaining helping-trusting, authentic caring relationship
Promoting and accepting the expression of positive and negative feelings and emotions	Being present to, and supportive of, the expression of positive and negative feelings as a connection with deeper spirit of self and the one-being-cared-for
Engaging in creative, individualized, problem-solving caring processes	Creative use of self and all ways of knowing a part of the caring process, to engage in artistry of caring–healing practices
Promoting transpersonal teaching-learning	Engaging in genuine teaching-learning experience that attends to unity of being and meaning, attempting to stay within other's frame of reference
Attending to supportive, protective, and/or corrective mental, physical, societal, and spiritual environments	Creating healing environment at all levels, (physical as well as nonphysical, subtle environment of energy and consciousness, whereby wholeness, beauty, comfort, dignity, and peace are potentiated
Assisting with gratification of basic human needs while preserving human dignity and wholeness	Assisting with basic needs, with an intentional caring consciousness, administering "human care essentials," which potentiate alignment of mind/body/spirit, wholeness, and unity of being in all aspects of care; tending to both embodied spirit and evolving spiritual emergence
Allowing for, and being open to, existential-phenomenological and spiritual dimensions of caring and healing that cannot be fully explained scientifically through modern Western medicine	Opening and attending to spiritual-mysterious and existential dimensions of one's own life-death; soul care for self and the one-being-cared-for

[1](http://www2.uchsc.edu/son/caring/content/evolution.asp)

sense of harmony and dignity into sociopolitical and environmental relationships as well as interpersonal ones.

Caring Occasion/Caring Moment

A *caring occasion/caring moment* occurs whenever nurse and other(s) come together with their unique life histories and phenomenal field in a human-to-human transaction and is "a focal point in space and time . . . has a field of its own that is greater than the occasion itself . . . arise[s] from aspects of itself that become part of the life history of each person, as well as part of some larger, deeper, complex pattern of life" (Watson, 1985/1988, p. 59).

Once again, language limits Watson's ability to explain the concept of "caring moment." While described as a moment, Watson believes that connecting of human spirits in a caring, loving interaction exists in a timeless field of cosmic energy. As such, the "caring occasion" is manifested as a discrete moment but also exists in a dimension not bound by space or time. When spirits connect in this way, both the nurse and the one being cared for have the potential for transcendence, which can be manifested as healing, wholeness, harmony, and diversity. Watson (2005a) also believes that every caring occasion has the potential for collectively expanding the field of interconnected consciousness of the universe in a way that expands the universal field of harmony and wholeness.

WATSON'S THEORY AND NURSING'S METAPARADIGM

Watson's earlier works address the metaparadigm concepts of person (human being), health, environment, and nursing as somewhat more discrete concepts than do her later works. As Watson has been inspired by quantum physics and has integrated varied ways of knowing and being and doing, her descriptions of the metaparadigm concepts have been modified. The concepts are dealt with as nondiscrete, intertwined, and discontinuous.

Person (Human Being)

In 1996, Watson elaborated on this transcendent nature of being human. She uses a quote of de Chardin (1967):

> *We are not human beings having a spiritual experience.*
> *We are spiritual beings having a human experience.* (as quoted in Watson, 1996, p. 148)

Of the basic premises identified by Watson (1985/1988, pp. 50–51) on which her caring model is based, five relate to person:

1. A person's mind and emotions are windows to the soul . . .
2. A person's body is confined in time and space, but the mind and soul are not confined to the physical universe . . .
3. A nurse may have access to a person's mind, emotions, and inner self indirectly through any sphere—mind, body or soul—provided the physical body is not perceived or treated as separate from the mind and emotions and higher sense of self (soul) . . .
4. The spirit, inner self, or soul (geist) of a person exists in and for itself . . .
5. People need each other in a caring, loving way . . .

In her recent works (1996, 2005a), Watson's focus shifts more to the connectedness of all of existence. She further develops the concept of the "unity of mindbodyspirit/nature, and of a field of connectedness between and among persons and environments at all levels, into infinity and into the universal or cosmic level of existence" (1996, p. 147). There is an "unbroken wholeness and connectedness of all (subject-object-person-environment-nature-universe-all living things)" (1996, p. 151).Watson increasingly emphasizes how the human consciousness and body are interconnected with the planet and even the universe. Using Emoto's (2002) scientific and aesthetic work with water crystals, Watson (2005a) discusses how the individual and collective human consciousness is inseparable from the environment in which we live.

Health and Illness

Watson considers *illness* to be a perceived state rather than presence of disease. Illness is defined as

> subjective turmoil or disharmony within a person's inner self or soul at some level or disharmony within the spheres of the person, for example, in the mind, body, and soul, either consciously or unconsciously. . . . Illness connotes a felt incongruence within the person such as an incongruence between the self as perceived and the self as experienced. (Watson, 1985/1988, p. 48)

Watson notes that illness can result from a troubled inner soul, and illness can lead to disease, but the two concepts do not fall on a continuum and can exist apart from one another.

"Health refers to unity and harmony within the mind, body, and soul" (Watson, 1985/1988, p. 48). Within such a context, human beings are in a near perpetual state of healing. Feeling gratitude for life's gifts, surrendering to life's challenges, and giving and receiving love are at the center of healing and health (Watson, 2005a). From this perspective, a person can experience a healthy state in the absence or presence of physical disease. In fact, Watson believes that it is often the times "when we are most alone, despairing, suffering, longing, and hurting; at the same time, most grateful for when we experience joy, hope, and healing insights that come after or during the midst of pain and darkness" (Watson, 2005a, p. 82).

Environment

Watson focuses on the healing environment and nurse *as* healing environment. "I now invite us to *consider the practitioner and their* [sic] *evolved caring consciousness, presence, intentionality, heart-centered foci, and so forth, as the environment!*" (Watson, 2005a, p. 94). Whether it be at the personal, interpersonal, societal, planetary, or universal level, harmonious relationships are associated with healing and transcendence; fragmented, broken, and disharmonious relationships are associated with suffering and illness. Disharmony can take the form of individuals resisting their own physical pain or disability. In such a situation, through meditation individuals may learn how to channel their energy to redirect the pain in such a way that the suffering is diminished. Ever increasingly, Watson cries out for the need for healing at the societal and planetary level. As interconnected beings with the cosmos, the health of the planet and the harmony of human existence with natural rhythms of the planet are fundamental to health and healing: ". . . we learn that what we perceive as suffering, at one level, is our own congealing and freezing of the divine flow of life energy; in other words, not being in flow with natural laws of nature and natural timeless rhythm of all things in the universe . . ." (Watson, 2005a, p. 137).

In much of her recent work, Watson addresses the importance of institutional value systems, policies, and administrative practices, which can be considered part of the environment. Tools such as the Caring Factor Scale (Nelson, Watson, & INOVA Health System, 2006) have been designed for measuring institutional caring from a theory of human care perspective.

Nursing as Profession and Praxis

In her own words, Watson (1985/1988) defined *nurse* to be both a noun and a verb and nursing to consist

> of knowledge, thought, values, philosophy, commitment, and action, with some degree of passion . . . related to human care transactions and intersubjective personal human contact with the lived world of the experiencing person. (p. 53)

The verb "to nurse" is carried out through human care and caring, which Watson views as the moral ideal of nursing, and

> consists of transpersonal human-to-human attempts to protect, enhance, and preserve humanity by helping a person find meaning in illness, suffering, pain, and existence; to help another gain self-knowledge, control, and self-healing wherein a sense of inner harmony is restored regardless of the external circumstances. (p. 54)

Human care nursing involves a reciprocal relationship between the nurse and others as coparticipants in a pattern of subjectivity–intersubjectivity evidenced in "consciousness; intentionality; perceptions and lived experiences related to caring, healing, and health-illness conditions in a given 'caring moment'; and experiences or meanings that transcend the moment and go beyond the actual experience" (Watson, 1996, p. 148).

Watson (1996) determines nursing to be both scientific and artistic, based on caring–healing knowledge and practices drawn from the arts and humanities as well as from traditional and emerging sciences (p. 142). As a profession, nursing "exists in order to sustain caring, healing, and health where, and when, they are threatened biologically, institutionally, environmentally, or politically, by local, national, or global influences" (p. 146).

The practice of nursing based on Watson's theoretical and philosophical concepts differs substantially from biomedical/natural-science-based practice. The physical body is cared for, but the care is never separated from the context of the unity of mind/body/spirit/nature.

Nursing Interventions

Effective nursing interventions are related to the goals being sought through the interventions. The goals of Watson's theory of transpersonal caring relate to "mental-spiritual growth for self and others, finding meaning in one's own existence and experiences, discovering inner power and control, and potentiating instances of transcendence and self-healing" (Watson, 1985/1988, p. 74). In such a theoretical context, the nurse intervenes through "a way of being" rather than through use of a set of behaviors. The nurse serves as a coparticipant with the patient, who is the agent of change.

Interventions, or the human care processes, within the human care context require a wide scope of knowledge:

- of human behavior and human responses to actual or potential health problems . . .
- of individual needs . . .

- of how to respond to others' needs . . .
- of our strengths and limitation . . .
- of who the other person is . . . strengths and limitations, the meaning of the situation for him or her . . .
- of how to comfort, offer compassion and empathy. (Watson, 1985/1988, p. 74)

All interventions within a human care context presuppose a knowledge base and clinical competence and, in addition, require an intention, a will, a relationship, and actions. Watson describes this interaction as a "heart-centered awareness" and "loving/caring consciousness." Thus, it is not only actions in the form of voice, touch, hands, and healing modalities such as massage but also the nurse's "being" and "presence" that are instruments of healing.

CASE STUDY   Applying Watson's theory of transpersonal caring entails first and foremost a belief in the value and dignity of each human being. The nurse must honor and respect the power of intention inherent in the caring moment. Thus, the intent with which the nurse engages in another's life force is as important as the specific interventions and will, in fact, guide the actions taken. Using the clinical caritas processes as a guide to nursing interventions is intended to encourage creativity and inspiration for restoring harmony and unity within an individual's environment and personhood rather than provide a prescriptive rubric.

SITUATION   Mr. W., 82 years old, has recently left his home of 43 years to move in with his son and daughter-in-law. Mr. W.'s wife died of cancer 13 months ago, and his son and family have become increasingly concerned over the past few months about Mr. W.'s safety and well-being. His health has been gradually failing to the point that he is now very unsteady when walking, unable to hear the telephone, and eating very little. The family has also noticed that Mr. W. has not been keeping up with the routine maintenance on his house (e.g., basic cleaning and yard work). Mr. W. has become very suspicious of family and friends and frequently says they are trying to "take advantage" of him.

The approach to nursing care in this situation is guided by the paradigmatic perspective from which it is viewed. If it is viewed within a totality, particularistic paradigm and the nursing process is applied, the initial step of *assessment* is undertaken for the purpose of identifying problems. In Mr. W.'s case, the assessment identifies functional deficits in the realms of mobility, socialization, and nutrition with an identified risk to Mr. W.'s physical safety and emotional well-being. Nursing *diagnoses* could include risk for social isolation r/t suspiciousness; risk for injury r/t unsteady ambulation; altered nutrition: less than body requirements r/t decreased appetite and interest in food preparation; and risk for dysfunctional grieving r/t recent death of spouse and evidence of possible depression. *Goals and outcomes* would relate to physical safety and psychological well-being. *Nursing interventions* would focus on coordinating services for Mr. W. for the purpose of arranging a safer environment that allows for the highest level of independent function. Nursing actions, thus, might include teaching Mr. W to use a cane or walker and referral for an audiological exam to determine if hearing aids would improve his hearing and thereby possibly diminish the paranoid behaviors he is exhibiting. Teaching interventions may include education for the family and client as to the possibility of a dementia. If a psychiatric referral is made, an assessment for depression may be undertaken, and a possible diagnosis may be followed by treatment. In this case, such a diagnosis would be labeled a "pseudodementia" since depression in the elderly frequently results in cognitive changes and behavioral changes that may appear to be a type of dementia. If antidepressant therapy is prescribed for Mr. W., another nursing intervention may be to monitor for and to teach about the possible side effects of antidepressant medication. *Evaluation* would focus on data to indicate improvements in the identified areas of functional deficit.

Nursing care that is derived from a unitary–transformative paradigm and a perspective of Watson's theory of transpersonal caring would be primarily concerned with the way in which Mr. W.'s situation is affecting the relationships and activities that give meaning to his everyday life. The first step would be a *mutual engagement* of the nurse and Mr. W. in order to reflect on that which makes Mr. W.'s life meaningful. This process reflects the clinical caritas process of *being authentically present and enabling and sustaining the deep belief system and subjective lifeworld of self and one-being-cared-for*. In Mr. W.'s situation, the nurse learns that Mr. W. had always taken special pride in his home. This had included doing all of his own home repairs and a hobby of woodworking and furniture making. In the last few years, however, Mr. W. had not been doing much woodworking because he had become the primary caregiver for his ailing wife. Mr. W. tells the nurse that since his wife died, he sees very little purpose to "struggling alone" and reluctantly agreed to move in with his son and family only because they "left me little choice" and because he was afraid that his house would soon be in such bad need of repairs that it would sell for "next to nothing." From this very basic and somewhat cursory understanding of Mr. W.'s perspective, the nurse engages the family in a discussion of some of the ways in which Mr. W.'s move may be expected to be a struggle and present hardships, as well as the possible enriching and fulfilling aspects to the situation. This *discussion* reflects the clinical caritas process of *being present to and supportive of the expression of positive and negative feelings as a connection with deeper spirit of self and the one-being-cared-for*. Referrals to an audiologist and physical therapist are made for Mr. W. The nurse, however, also discusses with Mr. W. and the family possible ways to enhance the nonverbal aspect of communication in order to compensate for Mr. W.'s hearing loss. The son and daughter-in-law also suggest that Mr. W. use a part of the garage to set up a small workshop of his own—one that will be on the same level as his bedroom and to which he will have safe and ready access. The family decides that Mr. W. could possibly relieve an older son and daughter-in-law of some of the yard work (reflecting the clinical caritas process of *creative use of self and all ways of knowing a part of the caring process, to engage in artistry of caring–healing practices*). Mr. W. decides that he would like to have breakfast and lunch in his room but will plan to eat dinner with the family. It is hoped that such a plan will improve his nutritional intake.

In Mr. W.'s case, the purpose of nursing care derived from the perspective of Watson's theory is to promote dignity and harmony of mind/body/spirit. This entails a process of mutual reflection on the possibilities for growth and fulfillment in the situation rather than mere maintenance of function. Thus, Mr. W.'s frailty and greater dependency are seen as an opportunity for the family to give and receive love and concern rather than merely as a greater burden and imposition (reflecting the clinical caritas process of *opening and attending to spiritual-mysterious, and existential dimensions of one's own life-death; soul care for self and the one-being-cared-for*). Refer to Table 18-3 for a summary of the approaches to nursing care for Mr. W.

TABLE 18-3   Paradigmatic Approaches to Nursing Care for Mr. W.

	Totality/Particularistic Paradigm	Holographic/Simultaneity Paradigm
Ontology (values; mission)	Identifying problems and functional deficits—mobility, socialization, and nutrition	Engagement with patient and family for purpose of identifying potential meaningful aspects of the situation—pride in his home, struggle with change
Epistemology (framework for approach)	Nursing process; nursing diagnosis—risk for social isolation r/t suspiciousness; risk for injury r/t unsteady ambulation; altered nutrition: less than body requirements r/t decreased appetite and interest in food preparation; risk for dysfunctional grieving r/t recent death of spouse and evidence of possible depression	Carative factors—faith–hope; expressing positive and negative feelings; and transpersonal teaching/learning
Praxis (knowledgeable actions and interventions)	Coordinating services Teaching Referrals	Engagement and caring occasion Teaching Referrals
Goal (purpose)	Promotion of highest level of independent function and prevention of injury	Promotion of dignity, harmony of mind/body/spirit, and enhancing possibility for growth and fulfillment

CRITIQUE OF WATSON'S THEORY OF TRANSPERSONAL CARING

1. *What is the historical context of the theory?*   A theory should be judged in light of the historical context within which it was created and the purpose for which it was intended. Jean Watson has stated that the purpose of the theory of transpersonal caring is to "help others to see, to view phenomena in a new or different way, perhaps to develop or to attempt a new starting point, to use a new lens when focusing on the phenomena of human behavior in health and illness" (Watson, 1985/1988, p. 1). Watson's theory was never designed to be a theory with specific testable constructs in the natural science tradition. It began as a philosophy and with delineation of the carative factors and explication of the constructs. In Watson's 1985/1988 version, it became more of a theory at the grand or middle range level. Watson's theory attempts to move nursing from the modernist view of the human body as machine and reality as discrete, elemental, and concrete into a world of the metaphysical where the interdependent and nondiscrete nature of a world and the spiritual nature of humans is of paramount importance. Watson's theory is based on the Nightingale concept of a healing environment. Watson believes not only that interpersonal and environmental factors affect healing but also that healing and a sense of well-being can occur in the presence as well as in the absence of disease. Thus, a core concept of Watson's theory is that caring is independent of curing.

2. *What are the basic concepts and relationships presented by the theory?* Watson's theory defines health and illness as harmony/disharmony of the mind/body/spirit. Eastern philosophies regarding the nature of the spirit and consciousness in health and healing greatly influenced Watson's original conceptualization of caring in the human health experience. The influence of chaos theory (Kellert, 1993), quantum physics, and quantum mechanics (Pelletier, 1985) on later 20th-century ideas about a universal consciousness and energy fields is seen in Watson's most recent thoughts on nursing as a caring ontology and the transpersonal occasion as an exchange of energy and consciousness with the capability to facilitate healing.

A common criticism of Watson's work is that by separating the person into mind, body, and spirit, Watson contradicts the core of her theory, which is that the essence of being human is wholeness and interconnectedness. This clearly is an invalid criticism, as it is not Watson's conceptualization that is flawed but rather that the language used to express these concepts is limited. Watson has frequently stated that metaphor and poetry portray the lived experience in a much richer and more meaningful way than does the language of traditional science adopted by the medical and clinical professions. For this reason, Watson's writings are uniquely elegant as she intersperses everyday language with metaphors and images of classical literature and poetry. Often such writings are used not only to describe the ontological aspect of her theory but also to argue for an expansion of the epistemology of nursing to include aesthetic and creative methods of discovering knowledge beyond the more traditional prescriptive methods of laboratory and social sciences.

Watson's conceptualization of the human form as an open, transforming system capable of growth and transcendence has roots in the concept of the unitary person developed by Martha Rogers (1970) as well as in existentialism. Her belief that "the body resides in a field of consciousness, rather than consciousness residing in the body" (Watson, 1999, p. 169) is based on ancient writings such as those of the 12th-century mystic Hildegard of Bingen (1985) as well as 20th-century artists such as Alex Grey (1990) and postmodern thinkers who write about the universal consciousness and the body as soul (Campbell, 1972; Wilber, 1982; Zukav, 1990). The embeddedness of body in soul is a complex concept and can be confusing in a culture that envisions the body as separate from the mind—as a mechanistic system of parts capable of replacement (consider the widespread notion of organ transplantation as a viable cure for disease and potential hope of the future for extending life). Therefore, while Watson has never excluded the "body physical" in her writings, many readers focus on the relational (e.g., transpersonal occasion) aspect of her theory instead of the connection between body and soul. In her earlier works, Watson refers to the skills and techniques of nursing as the "trim." Although she recognized the importance of the nurse to be "confident and competent in delivery of care" (Watson, 1985/1988, p. xvi), she clearly emphasized the carative factors as the core of nursing (p. xvii). Watson's recent theoretical writings emphasize to a much greater degree the human as "embodied spirit" and, thus, can no longer be misinterpreted as diminishing the importance of the body at the expense of the concepts of mind and spirit.

3. *What major phenomena of concern to nursing are presented?* (These phenomena may include but are not limited to *human beings, environment, health, interpersonal relations, caring, goal attainment, adaptation, and energy fields.*)** Caring is the essence of Watson's theory. Caring, however, is not unique to nursing knowledge or practice. It is, rather, the pattern of the concepts and the way in which caring is defined in terms of specific human actions as well as the context within which it occurs that makes it unique to nursing. Worldviews reflecting ideas on energy fields, wholeness, processes, and patterns have been the basis on which theories in nursing have been built (Boykin & Schoenhofer, 1993). Regardless of whether caring is conceptualized as a human trait, a moral imperative, an affect, an interpersonal interaction, or an intervention, it is about a unique way of living and caring in the world (Morse, Solberg, Neander, Bottorff, & Johnson, 1990). The focus of Watson's theory, thus, is not outcome driven. Rather, the focus of Watson's theory is about the "lived experience" of caring for oneself, one's fellow human beings, and one's environment. Watson refers to this as "ontological caring" and believes that nurses have a moral commitment to care (Watson, 2005a, 2005b). Thus, while Watson uses everyday language to express the concepts of caring, the philosophical underpinnings are anything but simplistic.

Watson's theory is based on a cosmology of consciousness and possibility rather than one of matter and predictability. She posits nursing to be "metaphor for the sacred feminine archetypal energy, now critical to the healing needed in modern Western nursing and medicine" (Watson, 1999, p. 11). This cosmology is grounded in a moral ontology of caring, an epistemology open to multiple ways of being, knowing, and doing, and a postmodern quantum reality of nonlinear, complex, holographic systems. All of reality exists between the real and the possible and intentionality as consciousness and energy have the power to heal. Within this framework, the transpersonal caring occasion is not just an affect or emotion expressed between two people, but is energy with the potential for transforming and creating a new order or reality.

Thus, Watson articulates each of the metaparadigm concepts of human, health, environment, and nursing within an expanded worldview. The Nightingale emphasis on fresh air and clean water is broadened to include the healing power of the higher-frequency energy transmitted by loving, caring intentions and actions. Human beings are envisioned not only as a system of cells, tissues, and organs but also as energy manifested in the ancient Hindu chakra system and the concept of the extrasensory. Energy and its balance play a role in health and healing. Within this worldview, the ontological state of the nurse is as essential to the caring–healing act as is any technological competency.

4. To whom does this theory apply? In what situations? In what ways? The values and constructs of Watson's theory are applicable in any situation or setting where the integrity, wholeness, and "soul" of humanity is of concern. Within nursing, the theory of transpersonal caring has been applied in both educational programs as well as practice settings. Numerous universities use nursing education models based on ontologically congruent caring philosophies. This list includes an extensive international community represented by countries such as Sweden, Finland, Norway, Japan, Thailand, and South America. There are also models of practice being used worldwide in clinics, hospitals, and home-based and community health programs that are based on a caring science and the constructs of Watson's theory (http://www2.uchsc.edu/son/caring/content/CaritasPractice.asp).

Although practice models based upon Watson's theory now circle the globe and vary greatly across cultures and settings, one of the first clinical models, The Caring Center, provided an early example of a practice model. The Caring Center (DNPHC) was opened in 1988 as a totally nurse-directed center for clients with HIV/AIDS (Neil, 1990, 1994). Its mission was to facilitate high-quality health care for HIV-positive clients and their lovers, friends, and families. The Center believed that the healing process is fostered by the understanding, love, and concern of those who care. Each client was linked to a particular nurse who had a responsibility to be the patient's advocate. Clients had the opportunity to change nurses at their request. The Center was a model for research as praxis in that focus group meetings of staff and clients cocreated understanding and insights into the personal experience as well as the way in which the Center was operated. Programmatic decisions were based on the insights that developed out of these group meetings. Watson's theory provided the framework for the Center from the outset. In order to keep the caring theory alive and to facilitate greater consistency in applying the theory, every six months chart audits were done in which the narratives were analyzed for the way in which the carative factors had been applied in specific nurse–patient situations. In keeping with Watson's view of nursing as human science, aesthetic methods of inquiry, such as photography, were incorporated into the programmatic evaluation. The DNPHC is an excellent exemplar of how a clinical model of care uses a theory of nursing to design its purpose, organization, and program of evaluation.

5. *By what method or methods can this theory be tested?* Smith (2004) reviewed 40 studies that were based on Watson's theory of caring and published between 1988 and 2003. A broad range of designs and methods were utilized in these studies—phenomenology, quantitative descriptive surveys, and quasi-experimental designs using standardized scales and physiological measurement (p. 13). In addition to qualitative designs, Watson's (2002) text describes measurement issues and available instruments for quantifying caring behaviors. Smith (2004) notes that a paucity of studies address the more unitary-transformative nature of Dr. Watson's recent work. Such research would need to identify the indicators and qualities of healing relationships and healing environments. One example of an attempt at measuring the attributes of a healing environment is the Caring Factor Scale (Nelson et al., 2006). Watson's view of caring–healing relationships mandates that evidence/knowledge be studied within the context of personal meaning, wholeness, and understanding of life processes. Thus, designs that integrate multiple perspectives and ways of knowing (including aesthetics and metaphysical) are clearly those that are most congruent with the philosophy and values of the theory of transpersonal caring.

6. *Does this theory direct nursing actions that lead to favorable outcomes?* Three eras, corresponding to three paradigms that have affected nursing's progress and maturity, have been identified by nursing leaders and are discussed by Watson (1999, p. 98). Dossey (1991) described these paradigms as eras of medical science and treatment models: Era I (particulate–deterministic), Era II (integrative–interactive), and Era III (unitary–transformative). Until health care systems are congruent with the worldview identified by Era III, there is no systematic way by which the outcomes of Watson's theory may be judged.

In order to maximize the impact of Watson's theory on nursing practice, the philosophy and environment within which the nurse acts must be congruent with the cosmology that undergirds the constructs and principles of Watson's theory. In general, schools of thought that allow for linear, mechanistic models of thought, such as nursing diagnosis and critical thinking, are barriers to the enactment of Watson's theory. However, incongruency between a worldview that values highly rational thought and a unitary–transformative worldview that values multiple ways of knowing may exist mainly because of the inability of the individual to embrace both views.

Smith (2004) attempts to explain the seeming incongruence between "medico-technological competence" and the transpersonal dimension of caring reflected in studies that ask patients and nurses to rank the importance of nurse caring behaviors. "Incompetent practice cannot be perceived as caring in any situation. On the other hand, the highest levels of medico-technological competence do not necessarily reflect transpersonal caring" (p. 15). Smith asserts that the context of the situation is a key factor in how nursing behaviors are ranked. In life-threatening situations, technical skills may be given a higher priority by patients. Nurses, on the other hand, assume the presence of competence and "describe something more and different as caring" (p. 15). Nurses know, also, that the type and degree of technical skills vary by setting and role. This is congruent with Watson's view of technical knowledge and competence, which is that the dimensions of transpersonal caring do not negate technical competence but rather assume that it is present in any professional nursing setting or role in which it is necessary.

In a meta-analysis of 130 studies published between 1980 and 1996 pertaining to Watson's theory, Swanson (1999) described reported outcomes as including positive outcomes for both the patient and the nurse. Positive outcomes for patients ranged from enhanced healing to positive emotional-spiritual outcomes such as enhanced coping, self-esteem, and trust. Nurses reported positive satisfaction with nursing, a sense of accomplishment, and enhanced relationships with patients.

The American Nurses Credentialing Center's Magnet hospital designation has been credited with newfound interest in theory-guided practice in hospitals (Foster, 2006; Watson, 2006). Positive outcomes for both patients and nurses have resulted from innovative models of care based upon Watson's theory (see http://www2.uchsc.edu/son/caring/content/connections.asp for descriptions of models and reported outcomes).

As has been previously discussed, Watson intended for her work to inform of another dimension—one that "goes beyond clinical views of medical illness and pathology and enters into a deeper subjective human dimension related to self-knowledge, self-control, self-caring, and even self-healing potential" (Watson, 2007, p. 13). There are numerous examples of ways by which the documentation of nursing care (Neil, 1994; Rosenberg, 2006) and specific nursing behaviors (Baldursdottier & Jonsdottir, 2002; Cronin & Harrison, 1988; Gleeson & Higgins, 2009; Gray, 1993; Marini, 1999; Mullins, 1996) may be made congruent with a key construct of Watson's (1979) early work, the carative factors. Manifesting and communicating the more recent aspects of Watson's theory as they relate to such concepts as energy fields, embodied spirit, cardio-energetics, and heart-centered living (Watson, 2005a) present a greater challenge. Verbal and written language are often too limiting, and thus Watson relies frequently on metaphors and aesthetics (Emoto, 2002) for communicating her beliefs, thoughts, and visions. A growing body of work is developing that supports the integration of art and literature as nursing interventions that facilitate health and healing (Chinn & Watson, 1994; Walder, 2001).

7. *How contagious is this theory?* Watson's (1979) theory of human caring, introduced over 25 years ago, has informed and inspired across cultures and disciplines those interested in the caring sciences for the purpose of bringing "soulful," meaningful practice into a modern health care system that is all too often influenced to a great degree by theories of safety, finance, and organizational development from a corporate perspective (Foster, 2006).

Clinical nurses and academic programs throughout the world use Watson's published works on the philosophy and theory of human caring and the art and science of nursing. Watson's caring philosophy is used to guide new models of caring and healing practices in diverse settings and in several different countries. Research, educational, and practice projects can be found in Canada, Denmark, Hong Kong, Ireland, Japan, Korea, Portugal, Taiwan, and across the United States (see, e.g., http://www.caritas consortium.org/research.html, accessed January 24, 2008). Favero, Meier, Lacerda, Mazza, and Kalinowski (2009) conducted a systematic review of the inclusion of Watson's theory in Brazilian studies over a 10-year period and found 34 publications. Examples of master's theses and doctoral dissertations using Watson's work can be found in the references at the end of this chapter. Publications in relation to practice relate to caring in Brazil (Medeiros & Leite, 2008), critical care in Brazil (Mathias, Zagonel, & Lacerda, 2006; Nascimento & Erdmann, 2006), care during pregnancy (Pessoa, Pagliuca, & Damasceno, 2006), creating a profile of the caring nurse (Persky, Nelson, Watson, & Bent, 2008), holistic nursing (McKern, 2004), home care in Spain (Porcel, 2007), mindful leadership (Pipe & Bortz, 2009), persons with rheumatoid arthritis (Nyman & Lutzen, 1999), reflective practice in Canada (Cara & O'Reilly, 2008), role modeling excellence in practice in Canada (Perry, 2009) touch in mental health nursing (Gleeson & Higgins, 2009), transforming practice (Watson & Foster, 2003), and trust in nursing practice in Italy and China (Masera, 2009; Wu & Wu, 2007).

STRENGTHS AND LIMITATIONS OF WATSON'S THEORY

Watson's work has been criticized by many who do not operate from the same Era III paradigm that serves as context for the theory. The lack of emphasis on physical as a separate entity on which to focus care disturbs those still practicing from the mechanistic medical model. Watson's "embodied spirit" does not satisfy those who perceive the world from that model.

Watson's work is transformative at all levels and realms of nursing. Her theory directs the focus back onto the person and mandates that technology be used selectively for the betterment of humankind rather than as the sole guiding factor in health care. Watson attempts to rekindle the passion of nursing for the sacredness of being human and the sacred traditions of health and healing. In Watson's theory limitations are not to be found in the validity of her work but rather in the barriers to enacting these principles created by a bureaucratic health care system guided by an entirely different set of values and beliefs. The future of Watson's theory will be determined largely by the degree to which the public and the, as yet, minority of professional healers and clinicians can transform "sickness treatment systems" into the "healing/health care centers" of a caring, holographic cosmology.

Summary

Jean Watson has played a major role in reorienting nursing from a biomedical, mechanistic model to one of caring as a transpersonal, interactive process. While never intending to exclude the physical body from the mind/body/spirit, Watson does diminish the importance of the physical. The body is conceived to be inside consciousness. The self and person are viewed as transpersonal mind/body/spirit oneness, part of an unbroken wholeness of subject–object–person–environment–nature–universe–all living things. The role of body is best conceived as embodied spirit.

For the nurse, as coparticipant with the client as change agent, nursing care is a "way of being" rather than doing. However, all of transpersonal caring–healing is expected to take place in a context of a broad knowledge base, including physical and skill-based knowledge. It is the definitions of health and illness and the goals of caring–healing that differ and reorient nursing care. Health as unity and harmony within body, mind, and soul and the degree of convergence between self as perceived and self as experienced, determining health or illness, drive the goals of care in Watson's theory. The goals of mental and spiritual growth for self and others, finding meaning in one's existence and experiences, discovering inner power and control, and potentiating instances of transcendence and self-healing reflect a caring–healing consciousness that transcends time and space. Dr. Watson believes that the caring healing consciousness of a caring occasion or caring moment opens up a higher energy field with potential for healing beyond body and self, with potential movement toward greater harmony, wholeness, health, and spiritual evolution.

Thought Questions

1. How is Watson's concept of caring different from the concept of caring in everyday life?
2. Describe a modification that Jean Watson has made to her theory since its inception in 1979. What were the influences for this change?
3. Find an aesthetic mode or object (art, music, object from nature) that is symbolic of a meaningful aspect of your life and identify why it is symbolic.
4. How are Nightingale's concept of environment and Watson's concept of environment similar? How are they different? In your current practice, what are ways by which you could facilitate a caring–healing environment?
5. Think of a specific situation from your practice that exemplifies one or more of Watson's clinical caritas processes. What were the manifestations of the "caring moment"?

References

Baldursdottier, G., & Jonsdottier, H. (2002). The importance of nurse caring behaviors as perceived by patients receiving care at an emergency department. *Heart and Lung, 31*, 67–75.

Bingen, H. (1985). *Illuminations of Hildegard of Bingen* (Text by Hildegard of Bingen, commentary by M. Fox). Santa Fe, NM: Bear Publications.

Boykin, A., & Schoenhofer, S. (1993). *Nursing as caring: A model for transforming practice* (Pub. No. 15-2549). New York: National League for Nursing Press.

Campbell, J. (1972). *Myths to live by*. New York: Viking Press.

Cara, C., & O'Reilly, L. (2008). Embracing Jean Watson's theory of Human Caring through a reflective [*sic*] practice within a clinical situation [French]. *Recherche en Soins Infirmiers, 95*, 37–45. Abstract in English retrieved November 30, 2009, from CINAHL Plus with Full Text database.

Chinn, P. L., & Watson, J. (Eds.). (1994). *Art and aesthetics in nursing*. New York: National League for Nursing Press.

Cronin, S. N., & Harrison, B. (1988). Importance of nurse caring behaviors as perceived by patients after myocardial infarction. *Heart and Lung, 17*, 374–380.

de Chardin, P. (1967). *On love*. New York: Harper & Row.

Dossey, L. (1991). *Meaning and medicine*. New York: Bantam.

Emoto, M. (2002). *Messages from water*. Tokyo, Japan: Hado Publ. Taito-su, © I.H.M Co., Ltd.; http://www.hado.net;book@hado.net.

Favero, L., Meier, M. J., Lacerda, M. R., Mazza, V. A., & Kalinowski, L. C. (2009). Jean Watson's Theory of Human Caring: A decade of Brazilian publication [Portuguese]. *Acta Paulista de Enfermagem, 22*, 213–218. Abstract in English retrieved November 30, 2009, from CINAHL Plus with Full Text database.

Foster, R. (2006). A perspective on Watson's theory of human caring. *Nursing Science Quarterly, 19*, 332–333.

Gadow, S. (1980). Existential advocacy: Philosophical foundation of nursing. In S. Spicker & S. Gadow (Eds.), *Nursing images and ideals* (pp. 86–101). New York: Springer.

Gleeson, M., & Higgins, A. (2009). Touch in mental health nursing: An exploratory study of nurses' views and perceptions. *Journal of Psychiatric and Mental Health Nursing, 16*, 382–389.

Gray, P. (1993). Perioperative nurse caring behaviors: Perceptions of surgical patients. *AORN, 57*, 1106–1114.

Grey, A. (1990). *Sacred mirrors: The visionary art of Alex Grey*. Rochester, NY: Inner Traditions International.

Harman, W. (1991). *A re-examination of the metaphysical foundation of modern science*. Sausalito, CA: Institute of Noetic Sciences.

Henderson, V. (1966). *The nature of nursing: A definition and its implications for practice, research, and education*. New York: Macmillan.

Kellert, S. (1993). *In the wake of chaos*. Chicago: University of Chicago Press.

Kierkegaard, S. (1941). *Concluding: Unscientific postscript* (D. S. Swenson & W. Lowrie, Trans.). Princeton, NJ: Princeton University Press.

Leininger, M. (1980). Caring: A central focus of nursing and health care. *Nursing and Health Care, 1*(3), 135–143.

Leininger, M. (Ed.). (1981). *Caring: An essential human need*. Thorofare, NJ: Charles B. Slack.

Levinas, E. (1969). *Totality and infinity*. Pittsburgh, PA: Duquesne University.

Logstrup, K. (1997). *The ethical demand*. Notre Dame, IN: University of Notre Dame Press.

Marini, B. (1999). Institutionalized older adults' perceptions of nurse caring behaviors. *Journal of Gerontological Nursing, 25*(5), 10–16.

Masera, G. (2009). The feeling of trust in nursing practice: Some interpretations [Italian]. *International Nursing Perspectives, 9*(1), 17–20. Abstract in English retrieved November 30, 2009, from CINAHL Plus with Full Text database.

Mathias, J. J. S., Zagonel, I. P. S., & Lacerda, M. R. (2006). Human caring processes: Direction for nursing care [Portuguese]. *Acta Paulista de Enfermagem, 19*, 332–337. Abstract in English retrieved April 14, 2007, from CINAHL Plus with Full Text database.

McKern, B. (2004). Gathering the threads: Reweaving the soul of nursing. *International Journal for Human Caring, 8*(3), 47–52.

Medeiros, F. A. L., & Leite, K. A. O. (2008). The act of taking care in the perspective of Programa Saude da Familia (PSF) [Portuguese]. *Revista Nursing, 11*(126), 518–523. Abstract in English retrieved November 30, 2009, from CINAHL Plus with Full Text database.

Morse, J., Solberg, S., Neander, W., Bottorff, J., & Johnson, J. (1990). Concepts of caring and caring as a concept. *Advances in Nursing Science, 13*(1), 1–14.

Mullins, I. (1996). Nurse caring behaviors for persons with acquired immunodeficiency syndrome/human immunodeficiency virus. *Applied Nursing Research, 9*(1), 18–23.

Nascimento, K. C., & Erdmann, A. L. (2006). Transpersonal nursing care to human beings in a critical care unit [Portuguese]. *Revista Enfermagem, 14*, 333–341. Abstract in English retrieved April 14, 2007, from CINAHL Plus with Full Text database.

Neil, R. (1990). Watson's theory of caring in nursing: The rainbow of and for people living with AIDS. In M. Parker (Ed.), *Nursing theories in practice* (pp. 289–301). New York: National League for Nursing Press.

Neil, R. (1994). Authentic caring: The sensible answer for clients and staff dealing with HIV/AIDS. *Nursing Administration Quarterly, 18*(2), 36–40.

Nelson, J. , Watson, J., & INOVA Health System (2006). *Caring Factor Scale*. Available online at http://www2.uchsc.edu/son/caring/content/Articles/CaringFactorScale.pdf.

Nightingale, F. (1957). *Notes on nursing: What it is, and what it is not* (Com. ed.). Philadelphia: Lippincott. (Original work published 1859)

Nyman, C., & Lutzen, K. (1999). Caring needs of patients with rheumatoid arthritis. *Nursing Science Quarterly, 12*(2), 164–169.

Pelletier, K. (1985). *Toward a science of consciousness*. Berkeley, CA: Celestial Arts.

Perry, R. N. B. (2009). Role modeling excellence in clinical nursing practice. *Nurse Education in Practice, 9*(1), 36–44.

Persky, G. J., Nelson, J. W., Watson, J., & Bent, K. (2008). Creating a profile of a nurse effective in caring. *Nursing Administration Quarterly, 32*(1), 15–20.

Pessoa, S. M. F., Pagliuca, L. M. F., & Damasceno, M. M. C. (2006). The theory of human care: Critical analysis and possible applications for women with pregnancy [Portuguese]. *Revista Enfermagem, 14*, 463–469. Abstract in English retrieved April 14, 2007, from CINAHL Plus with Full Text database.

Pipe, T. B., & Bortz, J. J. (2009). Mindful leadership as healing practice: Nurturing self to serve others. *International Journal for Human Caring, 13*(2), 34–38.

Porcel, M. A. (2007). Nursing care adopted for use in homes for the elderly based on Watson model [Spanish]. *Gerokomos, 18*(4), 18–22. Abstract in English retrieved November 30, 2009, from CINAHL Plus with Full Text database.

Rogers, C. R. (1961). *On becoming a person: A therapist's view of psychology*. Boston: Houghton Mifflin.

Rogers, M. (1970). *An introduction to the theoretical basis of nursing*. Philadelphia: F. A. Davis.

Rosenberg, S. (2006). Utilizing the language of Jean Watson's caring theory within a computerized clinical documentation system. *CIN: Computers, Informatics, Nursing, 24*(1), 53–56.

Smith, M. (2004). Review of research related to Watson's theory of caring. *Nursing Science Quarterly, 17*, 13–25.

Swanson, K. (1999). What is known about caring in nursing science. In A. S. Hinshaw, S. Fleetham, & J. Shaver (Eds.), *Handbook of clinical nursing research* (pp. 31–60). Thousand Oaks, CA: Sage.

Walder, D. W. (2001). Unfolding transpersonal caring–healing through story. *International Journal of Human Caring, 6*(1), 18–24.

Watson, J. (1979). *Nursing: The philosophy and science of caring*. Boston: Little, Brown.

Watson, J. (1988). *Nursing: Human science and human care: A theory of nursing*. New York: National League for Nursing. (Original work published 1985, Appleton-Century-Crofts)

Watson, J. (1989). Keynote address: Caring theory. *Journal of Japan Academy of Nursing Science, 9*(2), 29–37.

Watson, [M.] J. (1996). Watson's theory of transpersonal caring. In P. H. Walker & B. Neuman (Eds.), *Blueprint for use of nursing models: Education, research, practice and administration* (pp. 141–184) (Pub. No. 14-2696). New York: National League for Nursing Press.

Watson, J. (1999). *Postmodern nursing and beyond*. New York: Harcourt, Brace.

Watson, J. (2002). *Instruments for assessing and measuring caring in nursing and health sciences*. New York: Springer.

Watson, J. (2005a). *Caring science as sacred science*. Philadelphia: F. A. Davis.

Watson, J. (2005b). Caring science: Belonging before being as ethical cosmology. *Nursing Science Quarterly, 18*, 304–305.

Watson, J. (2006).Caring theory as ethical guide to administrative and clinical practices. *Journal of Nursing Administration, 8*(1), 87–93. [Reprinted from NAQ. (2000). *30*(1), 48–55]

Watson, J. (2007). Theoretical questions and concerns: Response from a caring science framework. *Nursing Science Quarterly, 20*, 13–15.

Watson, J., & Foster, R. (2003). The Attending Nurse Caring Model®: Integrating theory, evidence and advanced caring–healing therapeutics for transforming professional practice. *Journal of Clinical Nursing, 12*, 360–365.

Whitehead, A. N. (1953). *Science and the modern world*. Cambridge, England: Cambridge University Press.

Wilber, K. (Ed.). (1982). *The holographic paradigm and other paradoxes*. Boston: New Science Library.

Wu, S., & Wu, P. (2007). The experience of nursing an AIDS patient whose secret was divulged to his family [Chinese]. *Journal of Nursing, 54*(3), 98–102. Abstract in English retrieved November 30, 2009, from CINAHL Plus with Full Text database.

Zukav, G. (1990). *The seat of the soul*. New York: Fireside (Simon & Schuster).

Master's Theses

Blais, J. (1999). Le caring comme indicateur en evaluation de la qualite des soins infirmiers en sante communautaire. *Masters Abstracts International, 37*(06), 1815. Abstract retrieved December 17, 2007, from Dissertation Abstracts Online database.

Braun, M. L. (2009). Incidence of acute depressive episode up to one year post surgical experience. *Masters Abstracts International, 47*(05), 2829. Abstract retrieved December 1, 2009, from Dissertation Abstracts Online database.

Calladine, M. L. (1997). A descriptive study of nurses' perceptions of caring and codependency within nursing. *Masters Abstracts International, 37*(04), 0997. Abstract retrieved December 17, 2007, from Dissertation Abstracts Online database.

Cormier, G. (2005). La pratique des soins lies a l'hydratation chez les personnes agees vivant en foyer do soins. *Masters Abstracts International, 44*(03), 1333. Abstract retrieved December 17, 2007, from Dissertation Abstracts Online database.

Francoeur, N. (2006). Une description de l'attirance vers le cannabis de la personne atteinte de schizophrenie. *Masters Abstracts International, 45*(01), 281. Abstract retrieved December 17, 2007, from Dissertation Abstracts Online database.

Harrison, B. P. (1988). Development of the Caring Behaviors Assessment based on Watson's theory of caring. *Masters Abstracts International, 27*(01), 0095. Abstract retrieved December 17, 2007, from Dissertation Abstracts Online database.

Hill, S. A. (2000). A descriptive study of the caring behaviors of intensive care unit nurses. *Masters Abstracts International, 38*(06), 1584. Abstract retrieved December 17, 2007, from Dissertation Abstracts Online database.

Martin, N. A. (1995). A phenomenological study of faith-hope in wives caring for husbands who have recently experienced myocardial infarction. *Masters Abstracts International, 34*(03), 1150. Abstract retrieved December 17, 2007, from Dissertation Abstracts Online database.

Mullins, I. C. (1993). Watson's carative factors in relation to care needs indicated by AIDS patients. *Masters Abstracts International, 32*(01), 0229. Abstract retrieved December 17, 2007, from Dissertation Abstracts Online database.

Narasi, B. H. (1992). Hospice, humor, and Watson. *Masters Abstracts International, 31*(01), 0279. Abstract retrieved December 17, 2007, from Dissertation Abstracts Online database.

Oburo, F. I. (2008). Caring at the end of life: A phenomenological study. *Masters Abstracts International, 47*(01), 328. Abstract retrieved December 1, 2009, from Dissertation Abstracts Online database.

O'Keefe, C. S. (2000). A descriptive study of the caring behaviors of nurses practicing in long-term care facilities. *Masters Abstracts International, 38*(04), 982. Abstract retrieved December 17, 2007, from Dissertation Abstracts Online database.

Schindel Martin, L. J. (1990). A phenomenological study of faith-hope in aging clients undergoing long-term hemodialysis. *Masters Abstracts International, 28*(04), 0583. Abstract retrieved December 17, 2007, from Dissertation Abstracts Online database.

Sitzman, K. L. (2001). Effective ergonomic teaching for positive client outcomes. *Masters Abstracts International, 39*(03), 830. Abstract retrieved December 17, 2007, from Dissertation Abstracts Online database.

Stobie, M. M. (1994). The experience of nurses caring for the primary caregivers of persons living with AIDS. *Masters Abstracts International, 33*(02), 0519. Abstract retrieved December 17, 2007, from Dissertation Abstracts Online database.

Willson, B. E. (1997). The relationship of trust between the gynecological patient experiencing radiation therapy and the nurse. *Masters Abstracts International, 35*(04), 1003. Abstract retrieved December 17, 2007, from Dissertation Abstracts Online database.

Doctoral Dissertations

Baird, K. S. (1996). A comparative study of differences in caring ability and the role of social support in associate degree nursing and dental hygiene students. *Dissertation Abstracts International, 57*(07B), 4292. Abstract retrieved December 17, 2007, from Dissertation Abstracts Online database.

Carson, E. M. (2002). A comparison of evidence of Watson's carative factors in performance appraisals for medical surgical registered nurses in the state of Illinois. *Dissertation Abstracts International, 63*(09B), 4117. Abstract retrieved December 17, 2007, from Dissertation Abstracts Online database.

Clark, C. M. (2006). Incivility in nursing education: Student perceptions of uncivil faculty behavior in the academic environment. *Dissertation Abstracts International, 67*(05A), 1663. Abstract retrieved December 17, 2007, from Dissertation Abstracts Online database.

Clark, C. S. (2004). Human caring theory: Expansion and explication. *Dissertation Abstracts International, 65*(12B), 6288. Abstract retrieved December 17, 2007, from Dissertation Abstracts Online database.

Donohue, M. A. T. (1991). The lived experience of stigma in individuals with AIDS: A phenomenological investigation. *Dissertation Abstracts International, 53*(01B), 0200. Abstract retrieved December 17, 2007, from Dissertation Abstracts Online database.

Flanagan, J. M. (2002). Nurse and patient perceptions of the pre-admission nursing practice model: Linking theory to practice. *Dissertation Abstracts International, 63*(05B), 2304. Abstract retrieved December 17, 2007, from Dissertation Abstracts Online database.

Gauna, M. C. (1998). An exploration of the carative beliefs and behavior of female emergency room nurses: A study of caring in theory and practice. *Dissertation Abstracts International, 59*(06B), 2679. Abstract retrieved December 17, 2007, from Dissertation Abstracts Online database.

Gibson, M. H. (1995). The quality of life of adult hemodialysis patients. *Dissertation Abstracts International, 56*(10B), 5416. Abstract retrieved December 17, 2007, from Dissertation Abstracts Online database.

Gramling, K. L. (1999). The art of nursing: Portraits from the critically-ill. *Dissertation Abstracts International, 60*(08B), 3851. Abstract retrieved December 17, 2007, from Dissertation Abstracts Online database.

Mouton, C. (2007). The development of a measuring instrument to determine the educational focus of students at a nursing college. *Dissertation Abstracts International, 68*(06B), 3694. Abstract retrieved December 1, 2009, from Dissertation Abstracts Online database.

O'Reilly, L. (2007). La signification de l'experience d' "etre avec" la personne soignée et sa contribution a la readaptation: La perception d'infirmieres. *Dissertation Abstracts International, 68*(12B), 7933. Abstract retrieved December 1, 2009, from Dissertation Abstracts Online database.

Osborne, M. E. (1995). Dimensions of understanding in cross-cultural nurse–client relationships: A qualitative nursing study. *Dissertation Abstracts International, 56*(06B), 3129. Abstract retrieved December 17, 2007, from Dissertation Abstracts Online database.

Perkins, J. B. (2004). A cosmology of compassion for nursing explicated via dialogue with self, science and spirit. *Dissertation Abstracts International, 65*(07B), 3386. Abstract retrieved December 17, 2007, from Dissertation Abstracts Online database.

Simonson, C. L. S. (1990). A lived experience of caring in an educational environment. *Dissertation Abstracts International, 52*(02B), 0751. Abstract retrieved December 17, 2007, from Dissertation Abstracts Online database.

Smith, J. S. (1989). Implications for values education in health care systems: An exploratory study of nurses in practice. *Dissertation Abstracts International, 50*(11A), 3449. Abstract retrieved December 17, 2007, from Dissertation Abstracts Online database.

Stanfield, M. H. (1991). Watson's caring theory and instrument development. *Dissertation Abstracts International, 52*(08B), 4128. Abstract retrieved December 17, 2007, from Dissertation Abstracts Online database.

Annotated Bibliography

Chinn, P., & Watson, J. (1994). Introduction: Art and aesthetics as passage between centuries. In P. Chinn & J. Watson (Eds.), *Art and aesthetics in nursing*. New York: National League for Nursing Press.

The authors propose that the lost art of nursing is now being reclaimed and restored. They assert that art conspires with the spirit to emancipate humans and allows us to locate ourselves in another space and place, to change our perceptions and points of view. They propose to move nursing beyond the 20th century, during which spirituality has been separated from art, and art from science. A reintegrating paradigm of caring–healing arts, with new visions, new vocabulary, and new traditions, is being developed. The themes that emerge are art as asking and knowing, art as learning, art as practice, and art as reflective experience.

Clark, J. S. (2004). An aging population with chronic disease compels new delivery systems focused on new structures and practices. *Nursing Administration Quarterly, 28*(2), 105–115.

Describes a clinical leadership role for nurses (patient care facilitator) within a smaller area of patient responsibility (12 beds) for the purpose of providing caring professional nursing practice and one guided by Watson's theoretical constructs.

Mullaney, J. A. Barnes. (2000). The lived experience of using Watson's actual caring occasion to treat depressed women. *Journal of Holistic Nursing, 18*(2), 129–142.

Describes the ways by which Watson's "caring occasion" and the "transpersonal caring relationship" are manifested in the therapy sessions of 11 depressed women. Five essential themes emerged from data analysis of 110 pages of therapeutic notes. The findings support Watson's theoretical constructs with depressed women for their ability to persist in therapy and to adopt health-seeking behaviors.

Neil, R. (1994). Authentic caring: The sensible answer for clients and staff dealing with HIV/AIDS. *Nursing Administration Quarterly, 18*(2), 36–40.

An overview of the theory and operation of the Denver Nursing Project in Human Caring is provided. The nurse-managed outpatient community center provides integrated care and services to persons living with HIV/AIDS, their family members, and friends. Care theories of Parse and Watson are examined for areas of agreement and differences. Major tenets of existential phenomenology are described along with each theory's anchoring motifs, concepts, and principles. The theories are applied to a case study.

Schroeder, C., & Maeve, M. K. (1992). Nursing care partnerships at the Denver Nursing Project in Human Caring: An application and extension of caring theory in practice. *Advances in Nursing Science, 15*(2), 25–38.

Describes the development of nursing care partnerships as a new model of nursing practice using Watson's theory as the framework in this nurse-managed center for people living with HIV/AIDS. Includes narrative accounts from both nurses and clients to describe the relationships that are formed in this journey.

Sitzman, K. (2002). Interbeing and mindfulness: A bridge to understanding Jean Watson's theory of human caring. *Nursing Education Perspectives, 23*(3), 118–123.

The practice of mindfulness in the tradition of Thich Naht Hanh's concept of interbeing is described as a means of teaching Jean Watson's theory of human caring to nursing students. Simple mindfulness practices, such as nonjudgmental attention to thoughts, imagery, and awareness of breath, are proposed as a starting point.

Smith, M. (2004). Review of research related to Watson's theory of caring. *Nursing Science Quarterly, 17*, 13–25.

Provides a critical review of 40 studies, covering the period of time from 1988 to 2003, that were based on Watson's theory of caring. Four major categories of research were represented by these studies: (a) nature of nurse caring, (b) nurse caring behaviors, (c) human experiences and caring needs, and (d) outcomes of caring in nursing practices and education. Results and methodologies are discussed as well as implications for future research.

Wade, G. H., & Karper, N. (2006). Nursing students' perceptions of instructor caring: An instrument based on Watson's theory of transpersonal caring. *Journal of Nursing Education, 45*(5), 162–168.

An instrument based on Watson's theory for measuring students' perceptions of instructor caring was developed and tested with baccalaureate nursing students; 69 original statements were reduced to 31 statements that use a 6-point Likert scale. The instrument was found to have internal consistency and validity.

Watson, J. (1988). New dimensions of human caring theory. *Nursing Science Quarterly, 1,* 175–181.

Watson redefines contemporary nursing based on a caring–healing consciousness embedded in an ethic of caring as a moral ideal. She describes human caring and healing as transpersonal and intersubjective and opening up a "higher energy field-consciousness that has metaphysical, transcendent potentialities" (p. 181). A new metaparadigm for nursing is presented, consistent with holographic views of science.

Watson, J. (1990). The moral failure of the patriarchy. *Nursing Outlook, 38*(2), 62–66.

The moral failure of the patriarchal worldview in health care, in which caring is viewed as women's work and is not valued or is considered less important than men's work, is asserted. Suggestions for overcoming the patriarchy are offered.

Watson, J. (1994). Poeticizing as truth through language. In P. Chinn & J. Watson (Eds.), *Art and aesthetics in nursing*. New York: National League for Nursing Press.

Because we are humans, our truths are cocreated through a process of values and meaning-making via language. Discussed are concepts of truth and the relationship of poetry and truth, and ways of knowing. When our values become human values of caring for self, others, and all living things and when the meaning making of truth involves humans and cocreation of meaning via language, then a different scenario is revealed, one of the possibilities of poeticizing as truth. This is a way of inverting the paradigm and understanding human experiences from the inside out. This shift to a new dynamic of understanding human experience also shifts nursing's subject matter to a more authentic and poetic expression of the postmodern perspective.

Watson, J. (1995). Nursing's caring–healing paradigm as exemplar for alternative medicine? *Alternative Therapies, 1*(3), 64–69.

Provides an overview of the crisis in modern (biomedical) and postmodern (human) science

and method. The evolving of nursing's caring and healing system within a unitary–transformative context is presented as an exemplar for alternative medicine.

Watson, J. (1996). United States of America: Can nursing theory and practice survive? *International Journal of Nursing Practice, 2,* 241–247.

Watson argues that the concept of caring and caring theory take on new meaning in the most contemporary discourse about theory and practice. If caring as value, ethic, concept, and theory is reconsidered, it offers a metanarrative for placing professional practice and knowledge within the distinct context of nursing. She proposes that caring theory—with its explicit philosophy and ethic of caring, context, and meaning, along with its set of embedded values toward person, unity of mind/body/spirit, healing, wholeness, relation, and so on—could serve as an overarching ideal for nursing, its critique of knowledge, and its application to science and practice. She calls for international models of caring–healing excellence, with communities of researchers in multiple sites sharing assessment tools, protocols, and outcome data.

Watson, J. (1997). The theory of human caring: Retrospective and prospective. *Nursing Science Quarterly, 10*(1), 49–52.

Watson provides an overview of her original work and a description of the contemporary status of her caring theory. She offers projections for the future of the theory's use. She notes that use of the theory requires new ways of thinking, being, and acting that converge and requires a personal, social, moral, and spiritual engagement of self. She invites users of the theory to participate as cocreators of the theory's further emergence.

Watson, J. (1999). *Postmodern nursing and beyond.* Edinburgh: Churchill Livingstone.

This work expounds and expands on Watson's philosophical concepts. She proposes that the shift from traditional, modern, Western thought to what is emerging goes beyond a paradigm shift toward an ontological shift. The elements of this ontological shift are reflected in the following paths (p. xv):

Path of awareness, of awakening to the sacred feminine archetype/cosmology . . . ;

Path of cultivation of higher/deeper self and a higher consciousness: transpersonal self;

Path of honoring the sacred within and without . . . ;

Path of acknowledging the metaphysical/spiritual level . . . ;

Path of acknowledging quantum concepts and phenomena such as caring–healing energy, intentionality and consciousness . . . toward . . . the evolving human consciousness;

Path of honoring the connectedness of all . . . ;

Path of honoring the unity of mindbodyspirit . . . ;

Path of reintegrating the caring–healing arts, as an artistry of being, into healing practices . . . ;

Path of creating healing space . . . ;

Path of a relational ontology . . . ;

Path of moving beyond the modern–postmodern into the open, transpersonal space and the new thinking required for the next millennium.

Watson notes that this work is grounded in nursing but paradoxically and simultaneously transcends nursing. The proposed ontological shift is inviting and requiring a reconstruction and revision of all medical and professional health education and practice.

Watson, J. (2005). *Caring science as sacred science.* Philadelphia: F. A. Davis.

This work is both a visionary and personal treatise on health, healing, consciousness, and the cosmos. Dr. Watson posits caring science as sacred science and, in so doing, describes not so much a specific theory but rather an ever-expanding paradigm. The hope is that these expanded thoughts on healing may inspire healing for a society and a world fragmented and chaotic and in great need of peace, harmony, and a respect for ancient mysteries and truth.

CHAPTER 19

Human Becoming School of Thought

Rosemarie Rizzo Parse

Janet S. Hickman

Rosemarie Rizzo Parse earned her B.S. degree in nursing from Duquesne University, Pittsburgh, and her master's degree in nursing and Ph.D. from the University of Pittsburgh, Pennsylvania. She holds the Marcella Niehoff Chair at Loyola University in Chicago and is a fellow of the American Academy of Nursing. Previous positions include faculty at the University of Pittsburgh; dean of the Nursing School at Duquesne University, Pittsburgh; and professor and coordinator of the Center for Nursing Research at Hunter College, City University of New York. She has been visiting professor at the University of Cincinnati, Ohio; University of South Carolina, Columbia; Wright State University, Dayton, Ohio; University of Western Sydney, Australia; and Florida Atlantic University, Boca Raton (as the first Christine E. Lynn Eminent Scholar in Nursing). In 2001, the Unitary Research Section of the Midwest Nursing Research Society recognized Dr. Parse's contributions to the discipline of nursing by presenting her with a Lifetime Achievement Award.

Parse initiated and currently chairs the nursing theory-guided practice expert panel of the American Academy of Nursing. She is the founding editor of Nursing Science Quarterly, *a journal that focuses on theory development and research in nursing science. She is also president of Discovery International, Inc., a firm that sponsors international theory conferences, and the founder of the Institute of Human Becoming, where she teaches the ontology, epistemology, and methodology of the human becoming school of thought. Recent works include* Community: A Human Becoming Perspective (2003) *and* Qualitative Inquiry: The Path of Sciencing *(2001). Previous major works include* Man-Living-Health: A Theory of Nursing *(1981),* Nursing Science: Major Paradigms, Theories, and Critiques *(1987),* Nursing Research: Qualitative Methods *(Parse, Coyne, & Smith, 1985),* The Human Becoming School of Thought: A Perspective for Nurses and Other Health Care Providers *(1998), and* Hope: An International Human Becoming Perspective *(1999).*

Parse's theory supports clinical nursing practice in a variety of settings in Canada, Finland, and Sweden as well as the United States. Her research methodology has influenced the work of nurse scholars in Australia, Canada, Denmark, Finland, Greece, Italy, Japan, South Korea, Sweden, the United Kingdom, and the United States.

In 1981, Parse presented a unique theory of nursing titled "Man–Living–Health," which synthesized principles and concepts from Rogers (1970, 1984) and concepts and tenets from existential phenomenology. Parse (1981, 1992b) said that *man* refers to *Homo sapiens,* a generic term for all human beings. She stated that her purpose was to posit an idea of nursing rooted in the human sciences as an alternative to ideas of nursing grounded in the natural sciences. She defined natural-science-based nursing as having to do with the quantification of man and illness rather than the qualification of man's total experience with health.

In 1987, Parse refined this discussion by presenting two paradigms, or worldviews, of nursing. The first discussed is the totality paradigm, in which man is posited as a total summative being whose nature is a combination of bio-, psycho-, social, and spiritual aspects. The environment is viewed as the external and internal stimuli surrounding man. Man interacts and adapts with his environment to maintain equilibrium and to achieve goals. This is a refined definition of the natural, or medical, science approach to nursing. Parse states that the works of Peplau (1952/1988), Henderson (1991), Hall (1965), Orlando (1961), Levine (1989, 1990), Johnson (1980), Roy (1984; Andrews & Roy, 1986; Roy & Andrews, 1991), Orem (1991), and King (1981, 1989) are representative of the totality paradigm.

The second worldview that Parse (1987) discusses is the simultaneity paradigm, which views man as "more than and different from the sum of the parts . . . an open being free to choose in mutual rhythmical interchange with the environment . . . gives meaning to situations and is responsible for choices in moving beyond what is . . . experiencing the what was, is, and will be, all at once . . ." (p. 136). This is a refined definition of the human science approach to nursing. Parse states that her own work and that of Rogers (1970, 1992) are representative of the simultaneity paradigm.

Parse (1998) further differentiates the paradigms by stating that the totality paradigm views nursing as an *applied* science, drawing knowledge from all other sciences, while the simultaneity paradigm views nursing as a *basic* science with its own body of distinct knowledge. Consequently, totality-paradigm-based nursing practice focuses on diagnosis and treatment in curing, controlling, and preventing disease. In contrast, simultaneity-paradigm-based nursing practice focuses on the optimal well-being of unitary human beings (Rogers, 1970, 1992) and quality of life (Parse, 1981, 1992b, 1995, 1997, 1998).

In the spring of 1992, Parse (1992b) changed the name of her theory of Man–Living-Health to the theory of Human Becoming. She reworded the assumptions accordingly. No other aspects of the theory were changed. The revision was made as a response to a change in the dictionary definition of the term *man.* The current dictionary definition is gender-based as opposed to the previous use of the word *man* to identify humankind.

In the preface to the 1998 revision of her work, Parse describes ". . . a global move toward more concern for the perspective of the person and family to satisfy the concerns of the public for more humane treatment, yet at the same time there is a growing trend toward diminishing services, with the blurring of disciplinary boundaries and cross-education of health care providers to lower the cost of health care" (1998, p. ix).

Parse (1998) describes her original 1981 work as a theory of nursing, which has over time evolved into a *school of thought*. She defines a school of thought as "a theoretical view held by a community of scholars. . . . It is a knowledge tradition, including a specific ontology (assumptions and principles), a specified epistemology (focus of inquiry), and congruent methodologies (approaches to research and practice)" (p. ix). Parse writes that the term *theory* refers to the principles of human becoming.

Parse (2007b) specified that *human becoming* and *humanuniverse* be written as one word each in order to make the idea of indivisibility more explicit. By joining the words to create one concept, she believes that the idea of indivisible cocreation is more explicit. She has also chosen to elaborate certain truths embedded in the conceptualizations of the ontology. These changes will be presented in the next section.

SUMMARY OF PARSE'S HUMAN BECOMING SCHOOL OF THOUGHT

Parse's school of thought makes assumptions about humans and health and deduces from them the principles, concepts, and theoretical structures of human becoming. These assumptions are based on Rogers's principles and concepts and the works of Heidegger (1962, 1972), Sartre (1963, 1964, 1966), and Merleau-Ponty (1973, 1974) on existential-phenomenological thought. Parse uses Rogers's three major principles of helicy, complementarity (now called integrality), and resonancy and her four major concepts of energy field, openness, pattern and organization, and four-dimensionality (now called pandimensionality) as part of the theoretical basis for her own assumptions about man and health. Parse synthesizes these principles and concepts with the following tenets and concepts of existential-phenomenological thought: intentionality, human subjectivity, coconstitution, coexistence, and situated freedom. It is important to remember that the process of synthesis is, by definition, the combining of elements to create something new and different. Therefore, as will be demonstrated in the discussion of Parse's assumptions, the products of her synthesis are new and different from the original principles, tenets, and concepts on which they are based.

Parse's human becoming school of thought is a human science system of interrelated concepts describing the humanuniverse's process of becoming. The school of thought has its roots in the human sciences, which posit methodologies directed toward uncovering the meaning of phenomena as humanly experienced. The methods of inquiry lead to the creation of theories about the meaning of lived experiences. A fundamental tenet to the ontology of human becoming is the individual's (or humanuniverse's) participation in health (Parse, 1998).

The human becoming school of thought posits quality of life from each person's own perspective as the goal of nursing practice (Parse, 2006a). Cody (n.d.) states that nurses whose practice is "guided by the Human Becoming Theory live the processes of the Parse practice methodology by illuminating meaning, synchronizing rhythms, and mobilizing transcendence. . . . Research guided by the Human Becoming Theory explores the meaning of universal humanly lived experiences such as hope, taking life day-by-day, grieving, suffering, and time passing" (Cody, n.d., ¶5).

ASSUMPTIONS

As language of this theory/school of thought has changed over time, it is helpful to look at the assumptions as they were originally stated. In Parse's 1981 book *Man-Living-Health: A Theory of Nursing*, she posited nine assumptions, each of which was based on three of the 12 previously identified principles, tenets, and concepts from Rogers's theory and on existential-phenomenological thought. Phillips (1987) points out that for six of the nine assumptions, two of the three concepts used as the basis for each assumption come from Rogers, leaving three assumptions for which two of the three concepts come from existential phenomenology. Quantitatively, Phillips implies a greater grounding of the assumptions in Rogers's theory than in existential phenomenology. In contrast, Winkler (1983) states that Parse's assumptions come primarily from philosophical sources and secondarily from Rogers's theory.

Parse's (1981) original nine assumptions are the following:

1. Man is coexisting while coconstituting rhythmical patterns with the environment (based on *pattern and organization, coconstitution,* and *coexistence*).
2. Man is an open being, freely choosing meaning in situation, bearing responsibility for decisions (based on *energy field, openness,* and *situated freedom*).
3. Man is a living unity continuously coconstituting patterns of relating (based on *energy field, pattern and organization,* and *coconstitution*).
4. Man is transcending multidimensionally with the possibles (based on *openness, four-dimensionality,* and *situated freedom*).
5. Health is an open process of becoming, experienced by man (based on *openness, coconstitution,* and *situated freedom*).
6. Health is a rhythmically coconstituting process of the man–environment interrelationship (based on *pattern and organization, four dimensionality,* and *coconstitution*).
7. Health is man's pattern of relating value priorities (based on *openness, pattern and organization,* and *situated freedom*).
8. Health is an intersubjective process of transcending with the possibles (based on *openness, coexistence,* and *situated freedom*).
9. Health is unitary man's negentropic unfolding (based on *energy field, four-dimensionality,* and *coexistence*). (pp. 25–36)

In Parse's 1998 revision, each assumption is a synthesis of postulates with concepts in unique three-way combinations. Each of the postulates and concepts (energy field, openness, pattern, pandimensionality, coconstitution, coexistence, and situated freedom), is connected at least once with the assumptions in which they appear. The assumptions about the human becoming school of thought are the following:

- The human is coexisting while coconstituting rhythmical patterns with the universe.
- The human is open, freely choosing meaning in situation, bearing responsibility for decisions.
- The human is unitary, continuously coconstituting patterns of relating.
- The human is transcending multidimensionally with the possibles.
- Becoming is unitary human-living-health.
- Becoming is a rhythmically coconstituting process of the human–universe process.
- Becoming is the human's pattern of relating value priorities.
- Becoming is an intersubjective process of transcending with the possibles.
- Becoming is unitary human's emerging. (pp. 19–20)

ASSUMPTION ONE (The human is coexisting while coconstituting rhythmical patterns with the universe.)   The first assumption means that the human lives with others mutually evolving with the universe. The human pattern and the universe pattern are unique and distinct but are rhythmical and together coexist. Parse's (2007b) language would change this assumption to *The humanuniverse is coconstituting rhythmical patterns.*

ASSUMPTION TWO (The human is open, freely choosing meaning in situation, bearing responsibility for decisions.)   The second assumption means ". . . that the human, in open process with the universe, chooses ways of becoming in situation and is account-able for these choices" (Parse 1998, p. 21). In choosing the meanings of situations, the human gives up other choices and is therefore both enabled and limited by the choices made. The human remains responsible for all the outcomes of choices made, even though these outcomes may be unknown at the time of the original choice. Using Parse's (2007b) language this assumption would change to *The humanuniverse is open, freely choosing meaning in situation, bearing responsibility for decisions.*

ASSUMPTION THREE (The human is unitary, continuously coconstituting patterns of re-lating.)   This assumption means that the human is unitary and cannot be divided into parts. It also means that "Coconstituted patterns of relating are . . . illuminated through speech, words, symbols, silence, gesture, movement, gaze, posture, and touch" (Parse, 1998, p. 22). Using Parse's (2007b) language, this assumption would change to *The humanuniverse is continuously coconstituting patterns of relating.*

ASSUMPTION FOUR (The human is transcending multidimensionally with the possibles.)   This assumption means that the human, in conjunction with the human–universe mutual process, chooses to move beyond the actual, the contextual sit-uation, with possibilities. This movement is unidirectional; it is not repeatable or re-versible. A human moves beyond who one is via the mutual human–universe process in imaging possibilities. The human transcends the possibles by experiencing events in context. This experiencing opens or illuminates other possibilities that the human reaches toward while continually becoming through choosing. Using Parse's (2007b) language, this assumption would change to *The humanuniverse is transcending illimit-lessly with the possibles.*

ASSUMPTION FIVE (Becoming is unitary human-living-health.)   This assumption means that there is continuous movement that both enables and limits becoming in the human–universe mutual process. The human's view of the options or choices one makes is based on personal history as that human knows it. An experience of a situa-tion, though cocreated, belongs to only one person. "Choosing some options eliminates others so that possibilities are cocreated and experienced perspectively in the process of becoming—living health. . . . The unique perspective of each human being's experienc-ing the human-universe mutual process is health" (Parse, 1998, p. 23). Using Parse's (2007b) language, this assumption would change to *Becoming is humanuniverse health.*

ASSUMPTION SIX (Becoming is a rhythmically coconstituting process of the human–uni-verse process.)   This assumption means that human becoming is the rhythmical process of changing through the mutual connecting-separating of human with uni-verse. In each connecting, there is also separating, and with each separating, there is also connecting. This is paradoxical and it coconstitutes the emergence of health as a rel-ative present. Using Parse's (2007b) language, this assumption is *Becoming is a rhythmi-cally coconstituting process of the humanuniverse.*

ASSUMPTION SEVEN (Becoming is the human's pattern of relating value priorities.)   "This assumption means that becoming is the human's style of living chosen cherished ideals, which are values—prized beliefs. Value priorities are the preferred prized beliefs. Becoming or health is a synthesis of the human's values selected from multidimensional experiences cocreated in mutual process with the universe" (Parse, 1998, p. 24). Using Parse's (2007b) language, this assumption would change to *Becoming is the humanuniverse's pattern of relating value priorities*.

ASSUMPTION EIGHT (Becoming is an intersubjective process of transcending with the possibles.)   This assumption means that becoming is moving beyond with the possibles through a subject-to-subject mutual human–universe process. "Moving beyond with possibles" means experiencing the familiar while at the same time struggling with the unfamiliar of an imaged not-yet. Parse's (2007b) language change does not alter the wording of this assumption.

ASSUMPTION NINE (Becoming is unitary human's emerging.)   This assumption means that becoming is the human's multidimensional changing in process with the universe. The human's coexisting multidimensional experience with the universe powers the creation of individual patterns of relating that arise as rhythms of human becoming. Therefore, human health is continually changing in diverse ways. Using Parse's (2007b) language, this assumption would change to *Becoming is the humanuniverse's emerging*.

The original nine assumptions are further synthesized into three assumptions on human becoming (updated from Parse, 1992b, p. 38):

- Human becoming is freely choosing personal meaning in situations in the intersubjective process of relating value priorities.
- Human becoming is cocreating rhythmical patterns of relating in open interchange with the universe.
- Human becoming is cotranscending multidimensionally with the unfolding possibilities. (Parse, 1998, pp. 28–29)

The first assumption states that human becoming is a subject–subject or subject–universe interchange where the meaning assigned to the experience reflects one's personal values. This is a synthesis of numbers 2, 5, and 7 of her original nine, which are based on the concepts of energy field, openness, situated freedom, coconstitution, and pattern and organization.

The second assumption states that human becoming is an open interchange with the universe while *together* the human being and the environment create rhythmical patterns. This assumption appears to be a synthesis of original assumptions 1, 3, and 6, which are based on the concepts of energy fields, openness, situated freedom, pattern and organization, and coconstitution. Using Parse's (2007b) language, this would change to *Human becoming is the humanuniverse cocreating rhythmical patterns of relating*.

The third assumption states that human becoming is moving beyond the self at all levels of the universe as dreams become realities. Cotranscending is moving beyond with others and the universe multidimensionally. Multidimensionally refers to the various levels of the universe that humans experience "all at once" and choose possibles from in various situations. This is a synthesis of original assumptions 4, 8, and 9, which are based on the concepts of openness, four-dimensionality, situated freedom, coexistence, and energy field. It is important to note that Parse is viewing humans as being multidimensional, not four-dimensional. Parse (2007b) replaces the term *multidimensionality* with *limitlessness,* and *self* with *humanuniverse.* Thus, this assumption would change to *Human becoming is the humanuniverse transcending limitlessly.*

Parse (1987) cites the following distinctives of her theory:

1. The belief that humans (now humanuniverse) are more and different than the sum of their parts.
2. Human beings evolve mutually with the environment. Parse (2007b) states the humanuniverse is indivisible.
3. Human beings (now humanuniverse) cocreate personal health by choosing meaning in situations.
4. Human beings (now humanuniverse) convey meanings that are personal values that reflect their dreams and hopes.

Parse (2007b) elaborated certain truths embedded in the conceptualizations of the ontology. With this elaboration, some of the wording of her principles has changed without changing their actual intent. She states that it is important to note that cocreating reality as a seamless symphony of becoming (Parse, 1996), a central foundational thought to the ontology, occurs with the four postulates of illimitability, paradox, freedom, and mystery. "Thus, reality as a seamless symphony of becoming, a central thought of the ontology, is cocreated illimitably with living paradox in the contextually construed freedom of the impenetrable mystery of humanuniverse" (2007b, p. 309). Parse states that these four postulates permeate all three of her principles, although they are not explicitly stated in them:

- *Illimitability* is the indivisible unbounded knowing extended to infinity, the all-at-once remembering and prospecting with the moment. The word illimitability expresses indivisible, unpredictable, everchanging much more clearly than *multidimensionality* [the term previously used]. . . .
- *Paradox* is an intricate rhythm expressed as a pattern preference. Paradoxes are not opposites to be reconciled or dilemmas to be overcome but, rather, are lived rhythms. . . .
- *Freedom* is contextually construed liberation. . . . The contextual construction is humanuniverse.
- *Mystery* is the unexplainable . . . a puzzlement . . . the unfathomable with the . . . humanuniverse. (pp. 308–309)

PRINCIPLES

Three main themes can be identified in Parse's (1998) assumptions: meaning, rhythmicity, and transcendence. "Meaning refers to the linguistic and imagined content of something and the interpretation that one gives to something. It arises with the human-universe process and refers to ultimate meaning or purpose in life and the meaning moments of everyday living"(p. 29). Cody (n.d.) states that this principle means that "people coparticipate in creating what is real for them and through self-expression in living their values in a chosen way" (¶ 2).

Rhythmicity refers to the paced, paradoxical patterning of the human–universe mutual process. This can be visualized as the ebb and flow of waves coming into shore.

Rhythmical patterns moving in one direction are shown and hidden all-at-once as a flowing process as cadence changes with new experiences (Parse, 1998). Cody (n.d.) states that this principle means that "in living moment-to-moment, one shows and does not show self as opportunities and limitations emerge in moving with and apart from others" (¶ 3).

Transcedence is described as reaching beyond with possibles—the hopes and dreams as seen in multidimensional experiences. The possibles are options from which to choose personal ways of becoming (Parse, 1998). Cody (n.d.) states that this principle means that "moving beyond the 'now' moment is forging a unique personal path for oneself in the midst of ambiguity and continuous change" (¶ 4).

Each of Parse's themes leads to a principle of human becoming (see Table 19-1).

TABLE 19-1   The Human Becoming School of Thought—Ontology

Assumptions About the Human and Becoming	Assumptions About Human Becoming (Themes)	Principles of Human Becoming
The human is coexisting while coconstituting rhythmical patterns with the universe.	Human becoming is freely choosing personal meaning in situation in the intersubjective process of living value priorities. (Meaning)	*Structuring meaning multidimensionally* is cocreating reality through the languaging of valuing and imaging.
The human is open, freely choosing meaning in situation, bearing responsibility for decisions.	Human becoming is cocreating rhythmical patterns of relating in mutual process with the universe. (Rhythmicity)	*Cocreating rhythmical patterns of relating* is living the paradoxical unity of revealing–concealing and enabling–limiting while connecting–separating.
The human is unitary, continuously coconstituting patterns of relating.	Human becoming is cotranscending multidimensionally with emerging possibles. (Transcendence)	*Cotranscending with the possibles* is powering unique ways of originating in the process of transforming.
The human is transcending multidimensionally with the possibles.		
Becoming is unitary human-living-health.		
Becoming is a rhythmically coconstituting human–universe process.		
Becoming is the human's patterns of relating value priorities.		
Becoming is an intersubjective process of transcending with the possibles.		
Becoming is unitary human's emerging.		

Adapted from Parse, R. R. (1998). *The Human Becoming School of Thought.* Thousand Oaks, CA: Sage; and http://www.discoveryinternationalonline.com/site/ontology.html.

PRINCIPLE I *Structuring meaning multidimensionally is cocreating reality through the languaging of valuing and imaging* was changed in 2007b *Structuring meaning is the imaging and valuing of languaging.*

Parse's (1992b) first principle interrelates the concepts of *imaging, valuing,* and *languaging.* This principle indicates that human beings structure meaning to reality that is based on lived experiences. The meaning changes or is stretched to different possibilities based on limitless lived experiences. It arises with inherent freedom in the mystery of being human. Cocreating in this principle refers to the humanuniverse participation in the creation of the pattern. Languaging reflects images and values through speaking and movement or being silent and being still. Valuing is the process of living cherished beliefs while adding to one's personal worldview. Imaging refers to knowing and includes both explicit and tacit knowledge.

From this principle, Parse has identified a nursing practice dimension and a process (see Table 19-2). The practice dimension is illuminating meaning through discussion. This happens by explicating or making clear what is appearing now through telling about the meaning (the process). Nurses guide individuals and families to relate the meaning of a situation by making the meaning more explicit.

PRINCIPLE II *Cocreating rhythmical patterns of relating is living the paradoxical unity of revealing–concealing, and enabling–limiting, while connecting–separating* was changed in 2007b to *Configuring rhythmical patterns of relating is the revealing–concealing and enabling–limiting of connecting–separating.*

The second principle interrelates the concepts of *revealing–concealing, enabling–limiting,* and *connecting–separating.* This principle speaks to humanuniverse's configuring rhythmical patterns of relating in cocreating reality illimitably with paradoxical rhythms. Patterns of relating arise with inherent freedom in the mystery of being human. Human beings, in configuring patterns of relating, live humanuniverse rhythms (2007b).

The paradoxes identified are revealing–concealing, enabling–limiting, and connecting–separating. Parse (1981, 1998) states that these rhythmical patterns are not opposites; they are two aspects of the same rhythm and exist simultaneously—one in the foreground and the other in the background. In interpersonal relationships, one reveals part of the self but also conceals other parts; in revealing joy, sorrow is

TABLE 19-2   Human Becoming Practice Methodology

Dimensions

Illuminating meaning is explicating what was, is, and will be.
Synchronizing rhythms is dwelling with the pitch, yaw, and roll of the human–universe process.
Mobilizing transcendence is moving beyond the meaning moment with what is not-yet.

Processes

Explicating is making clear what is appearing now through languaging.
Dwelling with is immersing with the flow of connecting-separating.
Moving beyond is propelling with envisioned possibles of transforming.

From Parse, R. R. (1987). *Nursing science: Major paradigms, theories, and critiques* (p. 167). Philadelphia: Saunders. Used with permission.

concealed. Making choices or decisions enables an individual in some ways but limits in others; choosing to stay at home on New Year's Eve enables one to be with family but limits one from attending the party at a friend's house. Connecting–separating is a rhythmical process of moving together and moving apart.

The practice dimension Parse (1987) describes for this principle is the synchronizing of rhythms, which happens in dwelling with the pitch, yaw, and roll of the humanuniverse cadence. She likens dwelling-with (the process) as moving with the flow of the individual/family, leading them to recognize the harmony that exists within its own lived context. The nurse would not try to calm or balance rhythms or attempt to help the family adapt.

PRINCIPLE III   *Cotranscending with the possibles is powering unique ways of originating in the process of transforming* changed in 2007b *Cotranscending with possibles is the powering and originating of transforming.*

The third principle of the theory of human becoming interrelates the concepts of *powering, originating,* and *transforming.* Powering is an energizing force, the rhythm of which is the pushing–resisting of inter-human encounters (Parse, 1981). Originating is "inventing new ways of conforming-not conforming in the certainty-uncertainty of living" (Parse, 1998, p. 98). It is creating ways of distinguishing personal uniqueness by living out the paradoxical rhythms all-at-once. Transforming is defined as the changing of change and is recognized by increasing diversity (Parse, 1981). The principle means that humanuniverses cotranscend with possibles in cocreating reality illimitably with paradoxical rhythms of pushing–resisting, affirming–not-affirming, being–nonbeing of powering, certainty–uncertainty and conformity–nonconformity of originating, and the familiar–unfamiliar of transforming. The possibles arise with inherent freedom in the mystery of being humanuniverse (2007b).

The practice dimension identified by Parse (1987) for this principle is mobilizing transcendence, which happens in moving beyond the meaning of the moment with what is not yet. The process she identifies is moving beyond or "propelling toward the possibles in transforming" (p. 167). Here the nurse would guide individuals and/or families to plan for the changing of lived health patterns.

THEORETICAL STRUCTURES

The theoretical structures of the human becoming school of thought are noncausal in nature and consistent with the assumptions and principles. They are designed to guide research and practice (see Figure 19-1). To operationalize the structures for research and practice, practice propositions must be derived. Three theoretical structures are identified: (1) powering emerges with the revealing–concealing of imaging, (2) originating emerges with the enabling–limiting of valuing, and (3) transforming emerges with the languaging of connecting–separating (Parse, 1998, p. 56).

In her 1987 book, Parse restates her theoretical structures at a less abstract level in order for them to be used to guide nursing practice. She explains that *powering emerges with the revealing–concealing of imaging,* and "can be stated as *struggling to live goals discloses the significance of the situation*" (p. 170). The nursing practice focus "is on illuminating the process of revealing–concealing unique ways a person or family can mobilize transcendence in considering new dreams, to image new possibles" (p. 170). Parse describes a nurse–family situation in which members share their thoughts and feelings

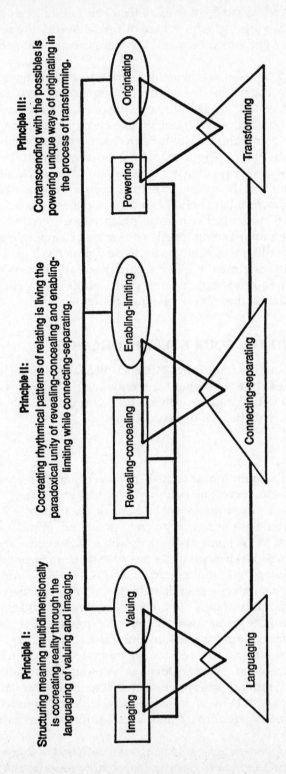

Principle I:

Structuring meaning multidimensionally is cocreating reality through the languaging of valuing and imaging.

Principle II:

Cocreating rhythmical patterns of relating is living the paradoxical unity of revealing-concealing and enabling-limiting while connecting-separating.

Principle III:

Cotranscending with the possibles is powering unique ways of originating in the process of transforming.

Relationship of the concepts in the *squares*:
Relationship of the concepts in the *ovals*:
Relationship of the concepts in the *triangles*:

Powering **is a way of** *revealing and concealing imaging.*
Originating **is a manifestation of** *enabling and limiting values.*
Transforming **unfolds in the** *languaging of connecting and separating.*

FIGURE 19-1 Principles, concepts, and theoretical structures of human becoming. (*From Parse, R. R. (1998). The Human Becoming School of Thought (p. 56). Thousand Oaks, CA: Sage. Reprinted by permission of Sage Publications, Inc.*)

about a situation, which both reveals and conceals all they know about their struggle to meet personal goals. In disclosing the significance of the situation, the meaning of the situation changes for the family members and therefore the meaning changes for the family.

According to Parse (1987), the second theoretical structure, *originating emerges with the enabling–limiting of valuing,* can be restated as *"creating anew shows one's cherished beliefs and leads in a directional movement"* (p. 170). The nursing practice focus with a person or family would be on "illuminating ways of being alike and different from others in changing values" (p. 170). By synchronizing rhythms, the members discover opportunities and limitations created by the decisions made in choosing ways to be together. Parse states that the choices of new ways of being together mobilize transcendence.

As a restatement of the third theoretical structure, *transforming emerges with the languaging of connecting–separating,* Parse (1987) suggests *"changing views emerge in speaking and moving with others"* (p. 170). The nursing practice focus would be "on illuminating meaning of relating ways of being together as various changing perspectives shed different light on the familiar, which gives rise to new possibles" (p. 170). Parse suggests that in synchronizing rhythms in a nurse–family situation, members relate their values through speech and movement. In so doing, their views change, and, through mobilizing transcendence, the ways of relating change.

HUMAN BECOMING AND THE FOUR MAJOR CONCEPTS

Human becoming will be discussed in terms of Parse's beliefs about humanuniverse, health, and nursing. Parse (1987, 1998) identifies her theory, and that of Rogers, as being representative of the simultaneity paradigm. Hence, her assumptions about the four major concepts are congruent with those of this paradigm.

Humanuniverse

Parse's (1992b, 1998) first four assumptions specify the human being as an open being in mutual process with the universe, cocreating patterns of relating with others. She states that the human being "lives at multidimensional realms of the universe all at once, freely choosing ways of becoming as meaning is given to situations" (1992b, p. 37).

Human beings are central to the human becoming school of thought. Parse's views about human beings are evident in all elements of her theory—assumptions, principles, theoretical structures, practice dimensions, and research methods. Her 2007 work changes the language, now viewing humanuniverse as inseparable in the creation of the experience of living. It is not possible or appropriate to define human beings or universe alone, for together they create a lived experience greater than and different from each seen separately.

The concept of relationships (society) is assumed under the larger view of humanuniverse. She states that what humans choose from the multiple possibles unfolds and surfaces in relationships with others and the universe. Although humanuniverse is described as having unique rhythmical patterns, it is difficult to interpret if Parse identifies a difference in the actual pattern between individuals and the humanuniverse interchange. If one assumes that "others" are a part of the human's universe, the interpretation becomes clearer.

Parse's view of humanuniverse is generally consistent with that of Rogers's (1984) presentation of the person–environment as inseparable, complementary, and evolving together. Parse's language revisions, however, delete general system terminology that is still evident in Rogers's work. Parse's view of humanuniverse is indivisible rather than complementary. It is also consistent with the existentialist view of a person being in the world all-at-once and together and the phenomenological belief that the universe is made up of everything shown to the person in the lived experience (Husserl, 1931/1962; Idie, 1967).

Winkler (1983) notes that although Parse states that all lived experiences are relevant, the omission of any references to biological manifestations of the person in his or her becoming limits Parse's theory. Phillips (1987) rejects this criticism and states that the lived experience deals with the wholeness of the person. Cody and Mitchell (1992) also reject this criticism, stating that Parse does not ignore "biological manifestations" but subsumes them within the experience of the person, which is the focus of the inquiry and practice guided by her theory.

Health

Parse (1998) describes unitary human's health as a synthesis of values, a way of living. It is not the opposite of disease or a state that a human has but rather a continuously changing process that the human cocreates in mutual process through the humanuniverse experience and is incarnated as patterns of relating value priorities. Parse proposes that health is a personal commitment and that humanuniverses are the creative authors of their own unfolding (health). She emphasizes that this unfolding cannot be prescribed or described by societal norms; it can only be lived by the person. Health is viewed by Parse as a process of changing life's meanings, a personal power emerging from the individual's collective relationships with others and the universe (Parse, 1990).

The concept of situated freedom is evident in Parse's perspective of health. Individuals choose various ways of unfolding and have personal responsibility for their choices. Phillips (1987) describes Parse's theory as a way of dealing with experience, a coming to know, rather than a product orientation. He states that the fundamental tenet of Parse's theory is that man participates in health.

Parse's theory speaks to health as humanuniverse's lived experience as it unfolds. This is a very different conceptualization of health from that of the totality paradigm theorists. From the totality worldview, health is a state of balance or well-being to which a person can aspire. The totality worldview infers a norm or standard of health that individuals and their health care providers aspire to attain. These two different worldviews have very different nursing practice methodologies that are presented in the next section.

Nursing

Parse (1992a, 1998) defines nursing as a basic science, the practice of which is a performing art. She places nursing in the company of drama, music, and dance, where, in each, the artist creates something unique. The knowledge base of the discipline is the science of the art, and the performance is the art creatively lived. Parse states,

> So too, the nurse, an artist like the dancer, unfolds the meaning of the moment with a person or family consistent with personal knowledge and cherished beliefs. The nurse artist creatively lives knowledge about the human–universe–health connectedness (nursing's phenomenon of concern),

which incarnates personal cherished beliefs. The knowledge and beliefs are *there* in the way the nurse approaches the person, the way the nurse talks and listens to the person, what the nurse is most concerned about, and how the nurse moves with the flow of the person. When the nurse artist is guided by a particular nursing theory or framework, the art form reflects that theory or framework, which represents a school of thought in nursing. (Parse, 1992a, p. 147)

Parse (1981) states that nursing's responsibility to society is the guiding of individuals and families in choosing possibilities in changing the health process, which is accomplished by intersubjective participation with people. She further states that nursing practice involves innovation and creativity, which are not encumbered by prescriptive rules.

This theorist contends that the goals of nursing focus on the quality of life from the person's perspective. Nursing is practiced with all individuals and families, regardless of societal designations of health/illness status. Parse's (1987, 1992b, 1998, 2006a) human becoming school of thought guides practice that focuses on illuminating meaning and moving beyond with the person/family relative to changing health patterns. An important aspect in regard to Parse's view of nursing is that the client, not the nurse, is the authority figure and prime decision maker in the relationship. The client, in true presence with the nurse, determines the activities for changing health patterns. Nursing, according to this theory, is "loving, true presence with the other to promote health and the quality of life" (1987, p. 169). The practice of nursing is not a prescriptive approach based on medical or nursing diagnoses, nor is it the offering of professional advice and opinions that stem from the personal value system of the nurse.

Parse (1987) has presented a practice methodology for human becoming that includes dimensions and processes (see Figure 19-1). The dimensions are *illuminating meaning, synchronizing rhythms*, and *mobilizing transcendence*. The processes are the empirical activities of *explicating, dwelling with,* and *moving beyond*. There is a clear flow of these dimensions and processes from her assumptions and principles.

In Parse's school of thought the nurse is an interpersonal guide who acts in true presence. Nursing is an active, energetic way of being with others. Authority, responsibility, and the consequences of decisions are accorded to the client. The traditional nursing roles of caregiver, advocate, counselor, and leader are not congruent with Parse's view of nursing. Teaching, however, is reflected in the dimension of illuminating meaning by explicating. The nurse as a change agent is reflected in the dimension of mobilizing transcendence by moving beyond the meaning to what is not yet.

In an editorial in *Nursing Science Quarterly*, Parse (1989) proposes a "set of fundamentals essential for fully practicing the art of nursing." These include the following:

- Know and use nursing frameworks and theories
- Be available to others
- Value the other as a human presence
- Respect differences in view
- Own what you believe and be accountable for your actions
- Move on to the new and untested
- Connect with others
- Take pride in self

- Like what you do
- Recognize the moments of joy in the struggles of living
- Appreciate mystery and be open to new discoveries
- Be competent in your chosen area
- Rest and begin anew (p. 111)

Parse (1998) defines the contextual situations of nursing practice as being nurse–person or nurse–group/community participation. She does not define specific practice settings as being more or less appropriate for practice application of the human becoming school of thought. She does, however, advise the nurse to approach the client as a nurturing gardener, not as a fix-it mechanic.

PARSE'S HUMAN BECOMING SCHOOL OF THOUGHT AND NURSING PRACTICE

The Nursing Process

Parse (1987) states that the nursing process "evolves from the discipline of philosophy and does not flow from an ontological base in the discipline of nursing" (p. 166). She further states that the steps of the nursing process are the steps of the problem-solving method and are not unique to nursing. The assumptions underlying the nursing process, that the nurse is the authority on health and that the person adapts or can be "fixed," are not congruent with the human becoming school of thought. Parse posits that as practice is the empirical life of a theory, the practice of one theory would be different from the practice of another.

Parse's Practice Methodology

Parse (1998) describes nursing practice as the art of living human becoming. The art of nursing is described as using nursing's body of knowledge in service to people with the goal of quality of life from the person's perspective. The practice methodology of human becoming includes dimensions and processes that were presented earlier in this chapter (see Table 19-2).

The human becoming nurse lives in true presence with others in the processes of illuminating meaning, synchronizing rhythms, and mobilizing transcendence. True presence is described as a special way of "being with" another person. True presence is a free-flowing attentiveness that is different from trying to attend to another—as the *trying to* distracts one from the focus. Parse states that preparation and attention are essential for true presence. "*Preparation* involves an emptying to be available . . . to the . . . other(s), . . . being flexible, . . . gracefully present, . . . and open to another. *Attention* is focus. To attend to, is to focus on the moment at hand" (Parse, 1998, p. 71). Persons share with the nurse only what they choose to disclose. The nurse in true presence joins the reality of others at all realms of experience without judging or labeling.

Parse (1998) states that "the nurse is with the other(s) in true presence through face-to-face discussions, silent immersions, and lingering presence. . . . In face-to-face discussions the nurse and person or group engage in dialogue" (p. 72). The conversation may be expressed through oral discussion, poetry, music, art, movement, photographs, and other expressions. The person/group always leads the discussion, the nurse goes with the group . A second way of being-with is silent immersion. This situation is "true presence without words, just 'being-with' through immediate engaging in the presence of another or through imagination with . . . the intention to bear witness to the other's becoming" (p. 73). Lingering presence, the third way of being-with another, is "living the remembered . . . recalling . . . a lingering presence that arises after the immediate engagement" (p. 73). It is a reflective recollection.

Parse (1998) states that in true presence with the nurse, people may change their health patterns when they change their value priorities. Through *creative imaging*, one pictures what a situation might be if lived a different way. This is a safe trying-on of a might-be. It enables a person to imagine the not-yet, and it is a way of changing meaning, thus changing health. Through *affirming personal becoming*, critically thinking about the person one is becoming, one can uncover personal patterns of preference. Living these patterns of preference confirms the values by which the person is known. An attitude of "I can" or "I will" toward a given desire for change affirms it in a new way and changes health. Through *glimpsing the paradoxical*, one looks at the incongruence in a situation as the apparent opposites emerge. This is a way of moving beyond the moment in changing patterns of health.

Parse (1998) stresses that "for nursing practice, being in true presence with another means that all realms of the universe of the nurse and the person(s) are interconnecting"(p. 76) or cocreating becoming. It is a way of being present that values "the others' human dignity and freedom to choose within situations, and it is fundamental to living the art of human becoming, the focus of which is the quality of life from the person's or group's perspective" (p. 76).

Two examples of practice applications of the human becoming school of thought will be presented.

Martin, Forchuk, Santopinto, and Butcher (1992) describe how the nurse, guided by the human becoming school of thought, relates to Mrs. W., a terminally ill cancer client:
Emergent Patterns of Health for Mrs. W.

1. Mrs. W. says she does not want to discuss her situation with her family, yet she makes plans to broach the subject with them.
2. Mrs. W. says that this is the worst time of her life, yet she says that she has never enjoyed the natural world so much as now.

Mrs. W.–Nurse Activities

1. Be truly present with Mrs. W. as she imagines familiar and unfamiliar ways of engaging with and withdrawing from family during the coming days and weeks. Through presence, seek deeper levels of meaning as she describes her hopes and dreams for the days ahead. Be with her as she shares how she intends to make these hopes come to pass and what meaning these hopes hold for her. Be present with Mrs. W. as she imagines new ways of being close to her family. Invite her to describe how her relationships are changing for her.
2. Be with Mrs. W. while she imagines aspects of nature which have special meaning for her. Invite her to describe how she can come to enjoy these aspects in her current situation. Be with her as she creates words, images and movements which bring her in touch with nature. (p. 84)

Mitchell (1986) describes the application of the human becoming school of thought to Mrs. M., an elderly woman in a long-term care facility. In true presence with Mrs. M., Mitchell is able to tease out the multiple and complex realities the client experiences. The client transcends time and space to be all-at-once a child, a mother, and a lonely elder. All the realities lived and valued by Mrs. M. continue to be lived despite the passage of time (Illuminating meaning).

In order to understand the meaning of Mrs. M.'s languaging, the nurse dwells with her. The nurse does not try to bring Mrs. M. back to reality or to control or alter Mrs. M.'s experience. The nurse goes with the flow to assist the client in finding meaning. In doing so, the nurse has the opportunity to validate feelings with the client. Mrs. M. states that she felt joy when her mother met her after school. The nurse then states, "You feel good when your mother is waiting for you." Mrs. M. responds by saying, "Yes, she's waiting for me now too. I'm waiting to go home" (Synchronizing rhythms).

This statement helps the nurse to understand that Mrs. M. perceives her present environment to be a temporary waiting area, that the client's detached behavior has occurred because she attaches little meaning to her current surroundings. Two nursing interventions are selected to guide Mrs. M.'s care. First, the nurse continues to facilitate the expression of Mrs. M.'s meaning in the present situation. Second, the nurse provides Mrs. M. with information and the freedom to make choices such as participation or detachment from unit activities (Mobilizing transcendence).

Parse's approach to practice is clearly one of nurses *in true presence with* people rather than doing for people. Articles detailing Parse's practice applications are presented in the professional literature as case studies.

HUMAN BECOMING AND THEORY CRITIQUE QUESTIONS

1. *What is the historical context of the theory?* Parse published the theory of Man-Living-Health in 1981. This theory is based on the work of a nurse scientist, Martha Rogers (1970), and existential phenomenology. Parse created new ways of looking at man, health, environment, and nursing. In synthesizing Rogers's principles of helicy, complementarity (now called integrality), and resonancy and her four concepts of openness, energy field, pattern and organization, and four-dimensionality (now called pandimensionality) with the tenets of existential-phenomemological thought, Parse created a new vision of nursing science.

Parse's theory/school of thought of nursing is rooted in the human sciences and has the goal of quality of life from the perspective of the person. The theory was first presented in 1981 and was radical thinking at that time. From this view, the health–illness continuum was rendered irrelevant, as were care plans based on health problems. Using this approach to nursing care, the authority, the responsibility, and the consequences of decision making reside with the person, not with the nurse. This thinking was revolutionary at its inception, and now, more than two decades later, this school of thought is well supported by research findings.

In 1987, Parse differentiated the totality and simultaneity paradigms in nursing. Her work is clearly representative of the simultaneity paradigm.

Parse's human becoming school of thought describes a logical sequence of events. Parse (1981) presents Rogers's principles and concepts as well as tenets and concepts from existential-phenomenological thought. She then synthesizes these tenets, principles, and concepts to create her nine assumptions. The principles of the theory of human becoming are derived from the assumptions, with each principle relating three concepts to each other (see Figure 19-1).

Parse then derived three theoretical structures, each of which uses three concepts, one from each principle (see Figure 19-1). She defines theoretical structure as a statement that interrelates concepts in a way that can be verified (Parse, 1992b). Phillips (1987) points out that the stem of each theoretical structure is taken from the third principle. He speculates that greater importance might be attached to this principle but qualifies this thought by saying that Parse makes it clear that other theoretical structures may be generated from her principles.

Levine (1988), Phillips (1987), and Winkler (1983) speak to the difficulty of Parse's terminology for those unfamiliar with existential phenomenology. They concur, however, that there is consistency in meaning at each level of discourse.

2. *What are the basic concepts and relationships presented by the theory?* The human becoming school of thought is grounded in the belief that humans coauthor their own health or becoming in mutual process with the universe, cocreating distinguishable patterns that specify the uniqueness of the humanuniverse (Parse, 1995, 2007b). Parse's concepts, postulates, themes, and theoretical structures are all clearly defined and used in a consistent manner. The relationships are clear and flow with logical precision from the assumptions, to the principles, to the theoretical structures, to the practice dimensions, and to the research methodology. Concepts and relationships become more clear to the reader as one's familiarity with the terminology increases.

3. *What major phenomena of concern to nursing are presented? (These phenomena may include* but are not limited to *human beings, environment, health, interpersonal relations, caring, goal attainment, adaptation, and energy fields.)* For Parse, the central phenomenon of nursing science is the *human–universe–health process*, or the humanuniverse and health interrelationship. *Humanuniverse* is viewed as the experience of living (Parse, 2007b). *Health* is viewed as the quality of life as experienced by the person (Parse, 1992b). Mitchell states that most nursing theories describe nursing, while human becoming describes human becoming and then presents what nursing art looks like when humanity is viewed in a particular way.

4. *To whom does this theory apply? In what situations? In what ways?* Parse's human becoming school of thought focuses on the lived experiences of unitary human beings and therefore is applicable to all individuals, families, and communities at all times and in all contexts.

5. *By what method or methods can this theory be tested?* As Parse's school of thought is rooted in the human sciences rather than the natural sciences, qualitative rather than quantitative research methodologies are used to expand it. Since the early 1980s, studies about Parse's theory have been conducted using research methods borrowed from the social sciences (descriptive), psychology (van Kaam and Giorgi modifications), and anthropology (ethnography). The studies have been of two types—basic and applied. *Basic* research is conducted with the goal of uncovering the structure of lived experiences to expand knowledge of the science or may be an interpretive hermeneutic process that specifies the meaning of texts from a human becoming perspective. *Applied* research, on the other hand, has the goal of evaluating human becoming as a guide to practice (Parse, 1998 see Table 19-3).

Parse (1987) describes the human becoming research methodology, which includes the identification of major entities for study, the scientific processes of investigation, and the details of the processes appropriate for inquiry. She states that the two aspects

TABLE 19-3   Research Guided by Human becoming

<table>
<tr><th colspan="4" align="center">Modes of Inquiry</th></tr>
<tr><th colspan="3">Basic Research</th><th>Applied Research</th></tr>
<tr><td>**Purpose:**</td><td colspan="2">To advance the science of human becoming.</td><td>To understand what happens when human becoming is lived in the nurse–person/family/ community process.</td></tr>
<tr><td>**Methods:**</td><td>**Parse Method**</td><td>**Human Becoming Hermeneutic Method**</td><td>**Qualitative Descriptive Preproject-Process-Postproject Method**</td></tr>
<tr><td>**Phenomena:**</td><td>Lived experiences (descriptions from participants)</td><td>Lived experiences (descriptions from published texts and art forms)</td><td>Changing patterns (descriptions from participants and documents)</td></tr>
<tr><td>**Processes:**</td><td>Dialogical engagement
Extraction and synthesis
Heuristic interpretation</td><td>Discoursing with penetrating engaging
Interpreting with quiescent beholding
Understanding with inspiring envisaging</td><td>Preproject information gathering by evaluator
Teaching/learning on human becoming with health professionals or living human becoming with individuals or groups
Midway information gathering by evaluator
Teaching/learning on human becoming with health professionals or living human becoming with individuals or groups
Postproject information gathering by evaluator
Analysis/synthesis of themes from each information source
Synthesis of themes from all information sources</td></tr>
<tr><td>**Discover:**</td><td>The structure of the experience (the paradoxical living of the remembered, the now moment, and the not-yet all-at-once)</td><td>Emergent meanings of human experiences</td><td>Thematic conceptualizations</td></tr>
<tr><td>**Contributions:**</td><td colspan="2">Knowledge and understanding of humanly lived experiences</td><td>Knowledge about what happens when human becoming is lived in the nurse–person/family/community process.</td></tr>
</table>

Adapted from http://www.discoveryinternationalonline.com/site/research.html; Parse, R. R. (1998). *The Human Becoming School of Thought*. Thousand Oaks, CA: Sage; and Parse, R. R. (2001). *Qualitative Inquiry: The Path of Sciencing*. Sudbury, MA: Jones & Bartlett.

of lived experience to consider in selecting an entity for study are nature and structure. The aspect of nature refers to common lived experiences that surface in the humanuniverse and are health related; examples include "being-becoming, value priorities, negentropic unfolding, and quality of life" (p. 174). Parse cites the example of "waiting" as being consistent with her definition of a common lived experience.

The second aspect of the lived experience to consider in selecting an entity for study is structure. Parse (1987) defines structure as "the paradoxical living of the remembered, the now moment and the not-yet all at once" (p. 175). Thus, the research question would be "What is the structure of the lived experience of waiting?" (p. 175). The researcher would then proceed to uncover the structure of this lived experience.

The Parse (1998) basic research methodology was constructed in congruence with the principles of human becoming. The methodology has four principles, five assumptions, and a three-step process. Parse states that her methodology "is a phenomenological-hermeneutic method in that the universal experiences [are] described by participants who lived them . . . and participants' descriptions are interpreted in light of the Human Becoming Theory" (p. 63). The phenomena for study are lived experiences of health, such as hope, loss, happiness, laughter, sorrow, and pain. Participants are persons who can describe the meaning of the lived experience under study through words, symbols, music, metaphors, poetry, photographs, drawings, or movements.

The first process of the method is *dialogical engagement.* This is a discussion between the researcher and the participant, in true presence, that focuses on the participant's description of the lived experience under study. These dialogues are recorded, preferably on videotape. After securing the participant's signed consent, the researcher opens the dialogue by requesting that the participant describe his or her experience with the lived experience under study. The researcher does not ask specific questions but may encourage the participant to elaborate about the lived experience.

The second process is *extraction-synthesis,* which is a sorting of the essences or patterns of the dialogue using the language of the participant. These essences are then conceptualized in the language of science to form a structure of the experience. Parse relates that this process occurs through dwelling with the transcribed dialogues in order to elicit the meaning of the experience as described by the participant. The structure, which Parse describes as "the paradoxical living of the remembered, the now moment, and the not-yet-all-at-once" (1998, p. 65), arising from this process is the answer to the research question.

The third step of the process is *heuristic interpretation,* which "weaves the structure with the principles of human becoming and beyond to enhance the knowledge base and create ideas for further research (Parse, 1987, 1992b, 1995, 1997). Structural transposition and conceptual integration are the processes of heuristic interpretation that move the discourse of the structure to the language of the theory" (Parse, 1998, p. 65).

The findings from studies conducted using the Parse methodology contribute new knowledge and understanding about human experiences and add to the knowledge base of nursing science. Recent studies using the Parse research methodology include feeling respected/not respected (Bournes & Milton, 2006), having faith (Doucet, 2006), sacrificing something important (Florczak, 2006), feeling unsure (Morrow, 2006), feeling respected (Parse, 2006b), feeling confident (Mitchell, Bunkers, & Bournes, 2006), suffering (Pilkington & Kilpatrick, 2006), doing the right thing (Smith, 2006), and feeling unsure (Bunkers, 2007).

A second Parse (1998) basic research methodology is called the human becoming hermeneutic method, which is a mode of inquiry focusing on interpretation and understanding. Parse describes this as a dialogical process between the researcher and the text, uncovering meaning interpreted through a particular perspective. The interpretation itself is the meaning given to the text from the frame of reference of the researcher; thus, the understanding of the text incarnates that frame of reference. Cody (1995) used this method in interpreting selected poems by Whitman using Parse's human becoming theory. In his study he identified three processes of hermeneutics: discoursing, interpreting, and understanding. Parse states that when a researcher is conducting a hermeneutic study from the human becoming perspective, a literary work or other text will be interpreted using the language of the principles of human becoming. More recent studies using this method include Ortiz's study on lingering presence (2003), Cody's study of Tennessee Williams's *Cat on a Hot Tin Roof* (2001), and Parse's study of hope (2007a).

A third methodology is the applied research method. The preproject-process-post-project descriptive qualitative method (QDPPP) is appropriate for evaluating the human becoming school of thought in practice. The purpose is to identify changes that occur as a result of using the school of thought in practice. Data are gathered prior to use of the school of thought, midway through the project, and at the end point of the project. Data sources include direct observation of nurse's documentation; written and taped interviews with participants regarding their beliefs about human beings, health, and nursing; and interviews with recipients of nursing care.

A review of the research related to Parse's theory of human becoming was published in *Nursing Science Quarterly* (Doucet & Bournes, 2007). Ninety-three research studies were included in the review, 63 of which used the Parse research method, five used the human becoming hermeneutic method, and five used the QDPPP method.

Frik and Polluck (1993) report the use of Parse's theory by graduate students practicing in a chronic illness setting, a community mental health setting, and an emergency department. The theory was used in promoting compliance in adults with diabetes, implementing hypertensive screening in the emergency room, promoting effective coping skills related to drug abuse, and improving the nutrition of neurologically impaired adults.

Mitchell (1991) reports successful use of Parse's theory on an acute medical-surgical unit. Cody and Mitchell (1992) report successful use of this theory by Jonas (1989) in an outpatient setting, and by Santopinto (1989) in a long-term care setting. Cody and Mitchell report that nurses in all of these studies identified initial difficulties in changing their approach to being with persons and giving up the urge to apply the nursing process in the traditional manner. However, increased professional satisfaction convinced them of the validity of the new approach.

Mitchell, Bournes, and Hollett (2006) describe a 24-month study in a large teaching hospital in Canada. The research project evaluated the outcome of providing nurses 20% of their time for learning and self-development. Half of the teaching/learning was aligned with the commitment of the organization to advance patient-centered care and in particular patient-centered care guided by the nursing theory of human becoming. The other half was self-directed by nurse participants according to their interests and priorities. The findings included increased patient satisfaction and increased nurse satisfaction.

Other evaluative studies that have been conducted about the theory of human becoming include Jonas (1995), Mitchell (1995), Santopinto and Smith (1995), and Northup and Cody (1998). Findings continue to support use of the human becoming school of thought in nursing practice.

6. *Does this theory direct nursing actions that lead to favorable outcomes?* The nurse, in true presence with the person, invites a discussion of the meaning of a situation.

The process of explicating, in the presence of the nurse, sheds new light on, or illuminates, meaning connected with the moment. The nurse goes with the flow of the person's rhythms as she or he moves beyond the moment, reaching for hopes and dreams that have been illuminated through the process of being with the nurse. As persons, families, and communities move beyond the moment, reaching for hopes and dreams that have been illuminated through the process of being with the nurse, transcendence is mobilized.

Parse's theory does not direct nursing actions in the traditional sense. Human becoming is a being-with, in true presence, nursing relationship with another person, family, or community. The person, family, or community in true presence with the nurse determines what would be (or would not be) beneficial to their quality of life. The value system of the person, not the value system of the nurse, directs the outcome(s).

In a review of Canadian evaluation studies of Parse's theory in practice (in a variety of health care settings from 1988 to 1994), Mitchell (1995) reports that findings indicate three main areas of change. First, with Parse's theory, nurses in all studies changed their views of human beings from seeing clients as problems to seeing them as unique human beings in relationship with others. Second, nurses reported having a different respect for persons, for the meaning they gave life and for their relationships and choices. Nurses described a new appreciation for thinking about the person's perspective of what is important for his or her own health and quality of life. The third area of change was that nurses reported an increased morale and understanding of professional, autonomous practice. A review of the comments of persons cared for by nurses living Parse's theory indicated that they felt important, cared about, and involved in decisions.

Evaluation studies of human becoming have been conducted in various clinical settings to investigate what happens when the theory is used to guide nursing practice. The published studies include Jonas (1989, 1995), Mitchell (1995, 1998), Santopinto and Smith (1995), Bournes (2002, 2006), Legault and Ferguson-Pare (1999), Mitchell, Closson, Coulis, Flint, and Gray (2000), and Mitchell, Bournes, and Hollett (2006). The findings from all of these studies have demonstrated that when this theory guides nursing practice, patients, families, and nurses feel greater satisfaction with nursing care.

Northup and Cody (1998) report findings of a descriptive evaluative study of human becoming theory in practice in the acute psychiatric setting. Findings supported prior studies regarding nurses' enhanced respect for and concern with people as self-determining human beings who create their chosen way of being with the world. One different theme, *altered job satisfaction*, demonstrated mixed findings. Although some nurses reported enhanced job satisfaction and meaningfulness in practice, others rejected Parse's practice methodology and spoke of it as inadequate to guide practice with clients who they felt were incapable of making decisions.

7. How contagious is this theory? A short answer to this question is—very contagious!   In 1998, the South Dakota State Board of Nursing adopted a regulatory decisioning model based on Parse's theory. This model integrates the values of the Board of Nursing—vision, integrity, commitment, courage, flexibility, and collaboration—with the three principles of human becoming theory and the tenets and values of public policymaking (the best interests of the practitioner, the health care institutions, and the population). This is a landmark event, as it is the first regulatory adoption of nursing-theory-guided professional nursing practice (Daamgard & Bunkers, 1998).

Since 1981, Parse's Man-Living-Health theory/human becoming school of thought has generated many articles and research studies, both published and unpublished. Parse

(2006a) reports there are currently over 300 subscribers to Parse-L on the Internet, and many more access the Parse home page for information.

More than 100 persons from many countries belong to the International Consortium of Parse Scholars. The Consortium conducts an immersion weekend each fall, offering members an opportunity to explore issues directly with Parse and to clarify ideas regarding the theory in research and practice. Opportunities are also available to have one's own original work regarding the theory critiqued. The Consortium has produced a videotape on true presence with persons in various settings and a set of teaching modules for those interested in incorporating the theory as a guide to practice (Parse, 2006a). The Web address for the Consortium is http://www.human becoming.org.

In 1992, the Institute of Human Becoming was created to offer summer sessions given by Parse on the theory and its research and practice methodologies. These sessions attract international participants. The Institute of Human Becoming website address is http://www.discoveryinternationalonline.com.

Since 1994, Parse has hosted the International Colloquium in Qualitative Research related to human becoming theory at Loyola University in Chicago. This event features doctoral students, nurse scholars, and international visiting nurse scholars who present their research.

A process model of teaching/learning is supported by Parse's human becoming school of thought, which Bunkers (1999) describes as "an all at once process of engaging with others in coming to know" (p. 227). She describes eight teaching/learning processes that emphasize the idea that teaching/learning is a dynamic interactive human encounter with ideas, places, people, and events. These processes include "expanding the imaginal margins, naming the new, going with content-process shifts, abiding with paradox, giving meaning, inviting dialogue, noticing the now and growing story" (p. 227). Recently, Aquino-Russell, Maillard Struby, and Revicsky (2007) describe using living attentive presence with a Web-based nursing theory course.

STRENGTHS AND WEAKNESSES

A strength of Parse's theory is the logical flow from construction of her assumptions to the deductive derivation of principles, theoretical structures, practice dimensions, and research processes. Another strength of the human becoming school of thought is that it focuses on all individuals, not only those defined by societal norms as being ill. The individual in the nurse–person relationship uncovers the meaning of his or her lived experience. The nurse is in true presence with the client and together they illuminate meaning, synchronize rhythms, and mobilize transcendence. This occurs as individuals/families/communities interrelate with the nurse limitlessly.

Parse is a prolific theorist and researcher. She has developed and nurtured the human becoming school of thought with great care and precision, refining it as needed since its original presentation in 1981. *Nursing Science Quarterly*, the Parse home page, and Parse-L have provided the profession with excellent and ready access to cutting-edge information, discussion, and research about the theory. The International Consortium of Parse Scholars and the Institute of Human Becoming provide both education and resources for nurses to learn more about the theory.

In 1987, Phillips suggested that Parse's theory of human becoming would speed a transformation from the mechanistic approach to health care to one that has a unitary perspective of the health care of humans. Unfortunately, the current health system (or nonsystem) is focusing on cost containment and rationing of care rather than meeting human needs. Research in nursing science, however, does demonstrate the identification of common elements and themes in lived experiences that are enhancing the knowledge base of nursing science. As these common elements and themes are validated further, they will give additional direction to a perspective of the health care of humanuniverses.

Another strength of this theory is the assumption about humans freely choosing personal meaning in the process of relating value priorities. Coupled with this assumption is the thinking that the authority and responsibility of choices resides with the person or client, not the nurse. This is an opposing stance to the tradition of paternalistic health care, where physicians make decisions and nurses and patients accept them without question. It is a contemporary stance. Consumers *do* in fact question health care professionals, seek other opinions and alternative treatment modalities, and resort to the legal system for redress of their perceived damages.

A limitation of the human becoming school of thought is its lack of articulation with the body of knowledge and psychomotor skills that most nurses and society generally attribute to the practice of professional nursing. It is an entirely new conceptualization of nursing practice and is not congruent with the "assess, diagnose, and treat" language of current nurse practice acts. The South Dakota Board of Nursing led the nation in recognizing the simultaneity paradigm and Parse's theory of human becoming a base for professional nursing practice (Daamgard & Bunkers, 1998).

A question posed to this author by graduate students in nursing is whether you have to be a nurse to practice the theory of human becoming. Many students felt that true presence could be achieved by physicians, social workers, therapists, and members of the clergy. Parse (personal communication, 1994) responded to this idea by noting that as the knowledge base is different in each discipline, what occurs in true presence with the client will be different. She also noted that other disciplines have different goals. Different goals will affect and direct a professional's ability to be in true presence with the client.

Parse's 1998 book is titled *The Human Becoming School of Thought: A Perspective for Nurses and Other Health Care Professionals*. She states in the preface that the book ". . . is intended for professional nurses and other health care providers . . . concerned with quality of life from the perspective of the people they serve" (p. x). Phillips (1999) applauds this expansion of Parse's school of thought to other health professionals. He states that ". . . a school of thought that includes a diversity of persons transcends the current struggle in interdisciplinary and collaborative endeavors. . . . Imagine the possible advancement in knowledge and science when people in the sciences and arts and humanities use nursing's schools of thought" (p. 87). Expansion of this school of thought to other health care professionals can only be seen as an added strength of Parse's work.

Parse's theory has been criticized in the past for its exclusion of the discussion of the role of the natural sciences in nursing practice. While Parse does not address this specifically in relation to her theory, she does advocate a pre-professional core curriculum that would be appropriate for the professions of law, medicine, theology, and nursing. This undergraduate pre-professional core assumes professional education to occur at the graduate level. Parse's proposed pre-professional core contains a strong natural science and liberal arts base.

Parse has clearly been successful in creating a new paradigm or worldview of nursing. Her human becoming school of thought has gained considerable support both in the United States and internationally. Current definitions of nursing science (see Chapter 1) are reflective of the simultaneity paradigm, and a wealth of both basic and applied research supports the theory of human becoming.

Thought Questions

1. Discuss Parse's description of nursing as a basic science, the practice of which is a performing art. How is it a basic science and how is it a performing art?
2. Consider Parse's concept of true presence. In what ways is this different from a traditional view of the nurse's role? In what ways is it the same?
3. Discuss Parse's definition of health. What would (or should) the nurse's role be if she believes that the patient is demonstrating unhealthy practices or behaviors?
4. Describe the nurse's role in illuminating meaning.
5. Discuss how Parse's human becoming school of thought can be used to direct nursing practice.
6. Describe a clinical scenario and compare assessment using a totality paradigm theory with assessment using Parse's theory.

PEARSON

EXPLORE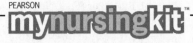

MyNursingKit is your one stop for online chapter review materials and resources. Prepare for success with additional NCLEX®-style practice questions, interactive assignments and activities, web links, animations and videos, and more!

Register your access code from the front of your book at
www.mynursingkit.com.

References

Andrews, H. A., & Roy, C. (1986). *Essentials of the Roy Adaptation Model.* Norwalk, CT: Appleton & Lange.

Aquino-Russell, C., Maillard Struby, F. V., & Revicsky, K. (2007). Living attentive presence and changing perspectives with a web-based nursing theory course. *Nursing Science Quarterly, 20,* 128–134.

Bournes, D. A. (2002). Research evaluating human becoming in practice. *Nursing Science Quarterly 15,* 190–195.

Bournes, D. A. (2006). Human becoming-guided practice. *Nursing Science Quarterly 19,* 329–330.

Bournes, D. A., & Milton, C. L. (2009). Nurses experiences of feeling respected—Not respected. *Nursing Science Quarterly, 22,* 47–56.

Bunkers, S. S. (1999). The teaching-learning process and the theory of human becoming. *Nursing Science Quarterly, 12,* 227–232.

Bunkers, S. S. (2007). The experience of feeling unsure for women at end-of-life. *Nursing Science Quarterly 20,* 56–63.

Cody, W. K. (1995). Of life immense in passion, pulse, and power: Dialoguing with Whitman and Parse—A hermeneutic study. In R. R. Parse (Ed.), *Illuminations: The human becoming theory in practice and research* (pp. 269–307). New York: National League for Nursing Press.

Cody, W. K. (2001). Mendacity as the refusal to bear witness: A human becoming hermeneutic study of a theme from Tennessee Williams' *Cat on a Hot Tin Roof.* In R. R. Parse (Ed.), *Qualitative inquiry: The path to sciencing* (pp. 205–220). Sudbury, MA: Jones & Bartlett.

Cody, W. K. (n.d.). *Parse's theory of human becoming, a brief introduction.* Retrieved June 7, 2007, from http://www.human becoming.org/site/theory.html.

Cody, W. K., & Mitchell, G. J. (1992). Parse's theory as a model for practice: The cutting edge. *Advances in Nursing Science, 15,* 52–65.

Daamgard, G., & Bunkers, S. S. (1998). Nursing science-guided practice and education: A state board of nursing perspective. *Nursing Science Quarterly, 11,* 142–144.

Doucet, T. J. (2006). *The lived experience of having faith: A Parse method study.* Unpublished doctoral dissertation, Loyola University, Chicago, IL.

Doucet, T. J., & Bournes, D. A. (2007). Review of research related to Parse's theory of human becoming. *Nursing Science Quarterly 20,* 16–32.

Edle, J. M. (1967). Transcendental phenomenology and existentialism. In J. J. Kockelmans (Ed.), *Phenomenology* (p. 247). New York: Doubleday.

Florczak, K. L. (2006). The lived experience of sacrificing something important. *Nursing Science Quarterly 19,* 133–141.

Frik, S. M., & Polluck, S. E. (1993). Preparation for advanced nursing practice. *Nursing and Health Care, 14,* 190–195.

Hall, L. (1965). *Another view of nursing care and quality.* Address given at Catholic University Workshop, Washington, DC.

Heidegger, M. (1962). *Being and time.* New York: Harper & Row.

Heidegger, M. (1972). *On time and being.* New York: Harper & Row.

Henderson, V. (1991). *The nature of nursing— Reflections after 25 years.* New York: National League for Nursing.

Husserl, E. (1962). *Ideas: General introduction to pure phenomenology.* New York: Collier-Macmillan. (Original work published 1931)

Johnson, D. E. (1980). The behavioral system model for nursing. In J. P. Riehl, & C. Roy (Eds.), *Conceptual models for nursing practice* (2nd ed., pp. 207–216). New York: Appleton-Century-Crofts. [out of print]

Jonas, C. C. (1995). Evaluation of the human becoming theory in family practice. In R. R. Parse (Ed.), *Illuminations: The human becoming theory in practice and research* (pp. 347–366). New York: National League for Nursing Press.

Jonas, C. M. (1989). *Practicing Parse's theory with groups of individuals in the community.* Paper presented at The Queen Elizabeth Hospital, Toronto, Ontario, Canada.

King, I. M. (1981). *A theory for nursing: Systems, concepts, process.* New York: Wiley. [out of print]

King, I. M. (1989). King's general systems framework and theory. In J. Riehl-Sisca (Ed.), *Conceptual models for nursing practice* (3rd ed., pp. 149–158). Norwalk, CT: Appleton & Lange.

Legault, F., & Ferguson-Pare, M. (1999). Advancing nursing practice: An evaluation study of Parse's theory of human becoming. *Canadian Journal of Nursing Leadership, 12*(1), 30–35.

Levine, M. E. (1988). [Review of the book *Nursing science*]. *Nursing Science Quarterly, 1,* 184–185.

Levine, M. E. (1989). The conservation principles of nursing: Twenty years later. In J. Riehl-Sisca (Ed.), *Conceptual models for nursing practice* (3rd ed., pp. 325–337). Norwalk, CT: Appleton & Lange.

Levine, M. E. (1990). Conservation and integrity. In M. E. Parker (Ed.), *Nursing theories in practice* (pp. 189–201) (Pub. No. 15-2350). New York: National League for Nursing.

Martin, M. L., Forchuk, C., Santopinto, M., & Butcher, H. K. (1992). Alternative approaches to nursing practice: Application of Peplau, Rogers, and Parse. *Nursing Science Quarterly, 5,* 80–85.

Merleau-Ponty, M. (1973). *The prose of the world.* Evanston, IL: Northwestern University Press.

Merleau-Ponty, M. (1974). *Phenomenology of perception* (C. Smith, Trans.). New York: Humanities Press.

Mitchell, G. J. (1986). Utilizing Parse's theory of man–living–health in Mrs. M's neighborhood. *Perspectives, 10*(4), 5–7.

Mitchell, G. J. (1991). Distinguishing practice with Parse's theory. In I. E. Goertzen (Ed.), *Differentiating nursing practice: Into the 21st century.* Kansas City, MO: American Academy of Nursing.

Mitchell, G. J. (1995). Evaluation of the human becoming theory in practice in an acute care setting. In R. R. Parse (Ed.), *Illuminations: The human becoming theory in practice and research* (pp. 367–399). New York: National League for Nursing Press.

Mitchell, G. J. (1998). Standards of nursing and the winds of change. *Nursing Science Quarterly, 11,* 97–98.

Mitchell, G. J., Bournes, D. A., & Hollett, J. (2006). Human becoming-guided patient centered care: A new model transforms nursing practice. *Nursing Science Quarterly, 19,* 218–224.

Mitchell, G. J., Bunkers, S. S., & Bournes, D. (2006). Part two: Applications of Parse's human becoming school of thought. In M. E. Parker,

Nursing theories and nursing practice (2nd ed., pp. 194–216). Philadelphia: F. A. Davis.

Mitchell, G. J., Closson, T., Coulis, N., Flint, F., & Gray, B. (2000). Patient-focused care and human becoming thought: Connecting the right stuff. *Nursing Science Quarterly, 13,* 121–125.

Morrow, M. R. (2006). *Feeling unsure: A universal lived experience.* Unpublished doctoral dissertation, Loyola University, Chicago, IL.

Northup, D. T., & Cody, W. K. (1998). Evaluation of human becoming in practice in an acute psychiatric setting. *Nursing Science Quarterly, 11,* 23–30.

Orem, D. E. (1991). *Nursing: Concepts of practice* (4th ed.). St. Louis: Mosby.

Orlando, I. J. (1961). *The dynamic nurse–patient relationship: Function, process and principles.* New York: Putnam's.

Ortiz, M. R. (2003). Lingering presence: A study using the human becoming hermeneutic method. *Nursing Science Quarterly, 16,* 146–154.

Parse, R. R. (1981). *Man-living-health: A theory of nursing.* New York: Wiley.

Parse, R. R. (1987). *Nursing science—Major paradigms, theories, and critiques.* Philadelphia: Saunders.

Parse, R. R. (1989). Essentials for practicing the art of nursing. *Nursing Science Quarterly, 2,* 111.

Parse, R. R. (1990). Health: A personal commitment. *Nursing Science Quarterly, 3,* 136–140.

Parse, R. R. (1992a). Editorial: The performing art of nursing. *Nursing Science Quarterly, 5,* 147.

Parse, R. R. (1992b). Human becoming: Parse's theory of nursing. *Nursing Science Quarterly, 5,* 35–42.

Parse, R. R. (1995). *Illuminations: The human becoming theory in practice and research.* New York: National League for Nursing Press.

Parse, R. R. (1997). Human becoming theory: The was, is, and will be. *Nursing Science Quarterly, 10,* 32–38.

Parse, R. R. (1998). *The human becoming school of thought.* Thousand Oaks, CA: Sage.

Parse, R. R. (1999). *Hope: An international perspective.* Boston: Jones & Bartlett.

Parse, R. R. (2001). *Qualitative inquiry: The path of sciencing.* Sudbury. MA: Jones & Bartlett.

Parse, R. R. (2003). *Community: A human becoming perspective.* Sudbury, MA: Jones & Bartlett .

Parse, R. R. (2006a). Part one: Rosemarie Rizzo Parse's human becoming school of thought. In M. E. Parker (Ed.), *Nursing theories and nursing*

practice (2nd ed., pp.187–194). Philadelphia: F. A. Davis.

Parse, R. R. (2006b) Feeling respected: A Parse method study. *Nursing Science Quarterly, 19,* 51–56.

Parse, R. R. (2007a). Hope in *Rita Hayworth* and *Shawshank Redemption*: A human becoming hermeneutic study. *Nursing Science Quarterly, 20,* 148–154.

Parse, R. R. (2007b). A human becoming perspective on quality of life. *Nursing Science Quarterly, 20,* 308–311.

Parse, R. R., Coyne, A. B., & Smith, M. J. (1985). *Nursing research: Qualitative methods.* Bowie, MD: Brady.

Peplau, H. E. (1988). *Interpersonal relations in nursing.* New York: Springer. (Original work published 1952, New York: Putnam's)

Phillips, J. R. (1987). A critique of Parse's man-living-health theory. In R. R. Parse (Ed.), *Nursing science: Major paradigms, theories, and critiques* (pp. 181–204). Philadelphia: Saunders.

Phillips, J. R. (1999). [Review of the book *The human becoming school of thought*]. *Nursing Science Quarterly, 12,* 87–89.

Pilkington, F. B., & Kilpatrick, D. (2008). *The lived experience of suffering:* A Parse research method study. *Nursing Science Quarterly, 21,* 228–237.

Rogers, M. E. (1970). *The theoretical basis of nursing.* Philadelphia: F. A. Davis. [out of print]

Rogers, M. E. (1984). *Science of unitary human beings: A paradigm for nursing.* Paper presented at International Nurse Theorist Conference, Edmonton, Alberta, Canada.

Rogers, M. E. (1992). Nursing science and the space age. *Nursing Science Quarterly, 5,* 27–34.

Roy, C. (1984). *Introduction to nursing: An adaptation model* (2nd ed.). Englewood Cliffs, NJ: Prentice Hall.

Roy, C., & Andrews, H. A. (1991). *The Roy Adaptation Model: The definitive statement.* Norwalk, CT: Appleton & Lange.

Santopinto, M. D. A. (1989). *An evaluation of Parse's practice methodology in a chronic care setting.* Paper presented at the 19th Quadrennial Congress of the International Council of Nurses, Seoul, South Korea.

Santopinto, M. D. A., & Smith, M. C. (1995). Evaluation of the human becoming theory in practice with adults and children. In R. R. Parse (Ed.), *Illuminations: The human becoming theory in practice and research* (pp. 309–346)

(Pub. No. 15-2670). New York: National League for Nursing Press.

Sartre, J. P. (1963). *Search for a method*. New York: Alfred A. Knopf.

Sartre, J. P. (1964). *Nausea*. New York: New Dimensions.

Sartre, J. P. (1966). *Being and nothingness*. New York: Washington Square Press.

Smith, S.M. (2006). *Doing the right thing*. Unpublished doctoral dissertation, Loyola University, Chicago, IL.

Winkler, S. J. (1983). Parse's theory of nursing. In J. J. Fitzpatrick & A. L. Whall (Eds.), *Conceptual models of nursing—Analysis and application* (pp. 275–294). Bowie, MD: Brady.

Bibliography (since 1997)

Aquino-Russell, C. (2005). Practice possibilities for nurses choosing true presence with persons who live with a different sense of hearing. *Nursing Science Quarterly, 17*, 32–36.

Aquino-Russell, C., Struby, F. V. M., & Reviczky, K. (2007). Living attentive presence and changing perspectives with a web-based nursing theory course. *Nursing Science Quarterly, 20*, 128–134.

Baumann, S. L. (1997a). Contrasting two approaches in a community-based nursing practice with older adults: The medical model and Parse's nursing theory. *Nursing Science Quarterly, 10*, 124–130.

Baumann, S. L. (1997b). Qualitative research with children as participants. *Nursing Science Quarterly, 10*, 68–69.

Baumann, S. L. (2004). Similarities and differences in experiences of hope. *Nursing Science Quarterly, 17*, 339–344.

Baumann, S. L. (2005). Exploring being: An international dialogue. *Nursing Science Quarterly, 18*, 171–175.

Baumann, S. L., & Carroll, K. (2001). Human becoming practice with children. *Nursing Science Quarterly, 14*, 120–125.

Baumann, S. L., & Englert, R. (2003). A comparison of three views of spirituality in oncology nursing. *Nursing Science Quarterly, 16*, 52–59.

Bournes, D. A. (2006). Human becoming-guided practice. *Nursing Science Quarterly, 19*, 329–330.

Bournes, D. A., Bunkers, S. S., & Welch, A. J. (2004). Human becoming: Scope and challenges. *Nursing Science Quarterly, 16*, 227–232.

Bournes, D. A., & Naef, R. (2006). Human becoming practice around the globe: Exploring the art of true presence. *Nursing Science Quarterly, 19*, 109–115.

Bunkers, S. S. (1998). A nursing theory-guided model of health ministry: Human becoming in parish nursing. *Nursing Science Quarterly, 11*, 7–8.

Bunkers, S. S. (2000). Dialogue: A process of structuring meaning. *Nursing Science Quarterly, 13*, 210–213.

Bunkers, S. S. (2002a). Lifelong learning: A human becoming perspective. *Nursing Science Quarterly, 15*, 294–300.

Bunkers, S. S. (2002b). Nursing science as human science: The new world. *Nursing Science Quarterly, 15*, 25–30.

Bunkers, S. S. (2003a). Comparison of three Parse method studies on feeling very tired. *Nursing Science Quarterly, 16*, 341–344.

Bunkers, S. S. (2003b). Understanding the stranger. *Nursing Science Quarterly, 16*, 305–309.

Bunkers, S. S. (2004a). The classroom for a learning community. *Nursing Science Quarterly, 17*, 121.

Bunkers, S. S. (2004b). The lived experience of feeling cared for: A human becoming perspective. *Nursing Science Quarterly, 17*, 36–41.

Bunkers, S. S. (2004c). Socrates' questions: A focus for nursing. *Nursing Science Quarterly, 17*, 212–218.

Bunkers, S. S. (2006). What stories and fables can teach us. *Nursing Science Quarterly, 19*, 104–107.

Carroll, K. A. (2002) *Attentive presence: A lived experience of human becoming*. Doctoral dissertation, Loyola University, Chicago, IL.

Carroll, K. (2004). Mentoring: A human becoming perspective. *Nursing Science Quarterly, 17*, 318–322.

Cody, W. K. (1997). The many faces of change: Discomfort with the new. *Nursing Science Quarterly, 10,* 65–67.

Cody, W. K. (2000). Parse's human becoming school of thought and families. *Nursing Science Quarterly, 13,* 281–284.

Cody, W. K. (2003). Diversity and becoming: Implications of human existence as coexistence. *Nursing Science Quarterly, 16,* 195–200.

Cody, W. K., Mitchell, G. J., Jonas-Simpson, C., & Maillard Strüby, F. V. (2004). Human becoming: Scope and challenges continued. *Nursing Science Quarterly, 17,* 324–329.

Dobratz, M. C., & Pilkington, F. B. (2004). A dialogue about two nursing science traditions: The Roy Adaptation Model and the human becoming theory. *Nursing Science Quarterly, 17,* 301–307.

Fawcett, J. (2001). The nurse theorists: 21st century updates—Rosemarie Rizzo Parse. *Nursing Science Quarterly, 14,* 126–131.

Fawcett, J. (2004). Theory of human becoming in action: Continuation of the dialogue. *Nursing Science Quarterly, 17,* 323.

Hansen-Ketchum, P. (2004). Parse's theory in practice: An interpretive analysis. *Journal of Holistic Nursing, 22,* 57–72.

Jonas-Simpson, C. (1997a). Living the art of the human becoming theory. *Nursing Science Quarterly, 10,* 175–179.

Jonas-Simpson, C. (1997b). The Parse research method through music. *Nursing Science Quarterly, 10,* 112–114.

Jonas-Simpson, C. (2004a). Community: A unitary perspective posited by Rosemarie Rizzo Parse. *Nursing Science Quarterly, 17,* 176.

Jonas-Simpson, C. (2004b). Musical expressions of life: A look at the 18th and 19th century from a human becoming perspective. *Nursing Science Quarterly, 17,* 330–334.

Jonas-Simpson, C. (2006). The possibility of changing meaning in light and place. *Nursing Science Quarterly, 19,* 89–94.

Jonas-Simpson, C., & McMahon, E. (2005). The language of loss when a baby dies prior to birth: Cocreating human experience. *Nursing Science Quarterly, 18,* 124–130.

Josephson, D., & Bunkers, S. S. (2004). *Eighth Street Bridge*: A dream of human becoming. *Nursing Science Quarterly, 17,* 122–127.

Karnick, P. M. (2005). Human becoming theory with children. *Nursing Science Quarterly, 18,* 221–226.

Kim, M. S., Shin, K. R., & Shin, S. R. (1998). Korean adolescents experience of smoking cessation: A prelude to research with the human becoming perspective. *Nursing Science Quarterly, 11,* 105–109.

Lee, M., Lee, M. & Baumann, S. K. (2005). Challenges in coming of age in Korea. *Nursing Science Quarterly, 18,* 71–74.

Lee, O. J., & Pilkington, F. B. (1999). Practice with persons living their dying: A human becoming perspective. *Nursing Science Quarterly, 12,* 324–328.

Letcher, D. C., & Yancey, N. R. (2004). Witnessing change with aspiring nurses: A human becoming teaching-learning process in nursing education. *Nursing Science Quarterly, 17,* 36–41.

Malinski, V. (2004). Nursing theory-based research: Parse's theory. *Nursing Science Quarterly, 17,* 201.

Malinski, V. (2005). Research issues: Emerging research methods. *Nursing Science Quarterly, 18,* 293.

Malinski, V. (2006). Research in cyberspace. *Nursing Science Quarterly, 19,* 95.

Menke, E. M. (2005). Children's experiences of being without a place to call home: What the research tells us. *Nursing Science Quarterly, 18,* 59–65.

Milton, C. L. (2003a). A graduate curriculum guided by human becoming: Journeying with the possible. *Nursing Science Quarterly, 16,* 214–218.

Milton, C. L. (2003b). Structuring meaning through new languaging: Going beyond the ethics of caring. *Nursing Science Quarterly, 16,* 21–24.

Mitchell, G. J. (2002). Human science practice models: Developing art of nursing science. *Nursing Science Quarterly, 15,* 31.

Mitchell, G. J. (2003). Abstractions and particulars: Learning theory for practice. *Nursing Science Quarterly, 16,* 310–314.

Mitchell, G. J. (2004). An emerging framework for human becoming criticism. *Nursing Science Quarterly, 17,* 103–109.

Mitchell G. J. (2006a). Human becoming criticism—A critique of Florczak's study on the lived experience of sacrificing something important. *Nursing Science Quarterly, 19,* 142–146.

Mitchell, G. J. (2006b). Views in a mirror: Illustrations of human becoming practice. *Nursing Science Quarterly, 19,* 108.

Mitchell, G. J. (2007). Picturing the nurse-person/family/community process in the year 2050. *Nursing Science Quarterly, 20,* 43–50.

Mitchell, G. J., & Cody, W. K. (1999). Human becoming theory: A complement to medical science. *Nursing Science Quarterly, 12*, 304–310.

Mitchell, G. J., & Halifax, N. D. (2005). Feeling respected-not respected: The embedded artist in Parse method research. *Nursing Science Quarterly, 18*, 105–112.

Noh, C. H. (2004). Meaning of the quality of life for persons living with serious mental illness: Human becoming practice with groups. *Nursing Science Quarterly, 17*, 220–225.

Paille, M., & Pilkington, F. B. (2002). The global content of nursing: A human becoming perspective. *Nursing Science Quarterly, 15*, 165–170.

Papendeck, J. K. (2002). A human science practice model for long-term care. *Nursing Science Quarterly, 15*, 35–37.

Parse, R. R. (1997a). Concept inventing: Unitary creations. *Nursing Science Quarterly, 10*, 63–64.

Parse, R. R. (1997b). The language of nursing knowledge: Saying what we mean. In I. M. King & J. Fawcett (Eds.), *The language of nursing theory and metatheory* (pp. 73–77). Indianapolis: Center for Nursing Press.

Parse, R. R. (1997c). Leadership: The essentials. *Nursing Science Quarterly, 10*, 109.

Parse, R. R. (1997d). New beginnings in a quiet revolution. *Nursing Science Quarterly, 10*, 1.

Parse, R. R. (1997e). Transforming research and practice within the human becoming theory. *Nursing Science Quarterly, 10*, 171–174.

Parse, R. R. (1998a). The art of criticism. *Nursing Science Quarterly, 11*, 43.

Parse, R. R. (1998b). Moving on. *Nursing Science Quarterly, 11*, 135.

Parse, R. R. (1998c). Will nursing exist tomorrow? A reprise. *Nursing Science Quarterly, 11*, 1.

Parse, R. R. (1999a). Expanding the vision: Tilling the field of nursing knowledge. *Nursing Science Quarterly, 12*, 3.

Parse, R. R. (1999b). Nursing: The discipline and the profession. *Nursing Science Quarterly, 12*, 275.

Parse, R. R. (2000a). Into the new millennium. *Nursing Science Quarterly, 13*, 3.

Parse, R. R. (2000b). Language: Words reflect and cocreate meaning. *Nursing Science Quarterly, 13*, 187.

Parse, R. R. (2000c). Obfuscating: The persistent practice of misnaming. *Nursing Science Quarterly, 13*, 91.

Parse, R. R. (2000d). Paradigms: A reprise. *Nursing Science Quarterly, 13*, 275.

Parse, R. R. (2002). Transforming health care with a unitary view of the human. *Nursing Science Quarterly, 15*, 46–50.

Parse, R. R. (2004a). A human becoming teaching-learning model. *Nursing Science Quarterly, 17*, 33–35.

Parse, R. R. (2004b). Another look at vigilance. *Illuminations, 13*(2), 1.

Parse, R. R. (2004c). The ubiquitous nature of unitary: Major change in human becoming language. *Illuminations, 13*(1), 1.

Parse, R. R. (2005a). Community of scholars. *Nursing Science Quarterly, 18*, 119.

Parse. R. R. (2005b). Parse's criteria for evaluation of theory with comparisons to Fawcett's. *Nursing Science Quarterly, 18*, 135–137.

Parse, R. R. (2005c). Research issues. The human becoming modes of inquiry: Emerging sciencing. *Nursing Science Quarterly, 18*, 297–300.

Parse, R. R. (2006a). Research findings evince benefits of nursing theory-guided practice. *Nursing Science Quarterly, 19*, 87.

Parse, R. R. (2006b). Research issues. The human becoming modes of inquiry: Emerging sciencing. *Nursing Science Quarterly, 19*, 297–300.

Parse, R. R. (2007). A human becoming perspective on quality of life. *Nursing Science Quarterly, 20*, 217.

Parse, R . R., & Bunkers, S. S. (2005). Teaching-learning processes: Community of scholars. *Nursing Science Quarterly, 18*, 119.

Parse, R. R., & Fawcett, J. (2005). Scholarly dialogue. Parse's criteria of evaluation of theory with a comparison of Fawcett's and Parse's approaches. *Nursing Science Quarterly, 18*, 135–137.

Parse, R. R., & Kelley, L. S. (1999). Hope as lived by Native Americans. In R. R. Parse (Ed.), *Hope: An international human becoming perspective* (pp. 251–272). Sudbury, MA: Jones & Bartlett.

Pilkington, F. B. (1997). Knowledge and evidence: Do they change patterns of health? *Nursing Science Quarterly, 10*, 156–157.

Pilkington, F. B. (2005a). The concept of intentionality in human science nursing theories. *Nursing Science Quarterly, 18*, 98–104.

Pilkington, F. B. (2005b). Myth and symbol in nursing theories. *Nursing Science Quarterly, 18*, 198–203.

Pilkington, F. B. (2006a). Developing nursing knowledge on grieving: A human becoming perspective. *Nursing Science Quarterly, 19,* 299–303.

Pilkington. F. B. (2006b). Exploring the ontology of space, place, and meaning, *Nursing Science Quarterly, 19,* 88.

Pilkington, F. B. (2006c). On joy-sorrow: A paradoxical pattern of human becoming. *Nursing Science Quarterly, 19,* 290–295.

Ramey, S. L., & Bunkers, S. S. (2006). Teaching the abyss: Living the art-science of nursing. *Nursing Science Quarterly, 19,* 311–315.

Smith, M. K. (2002). Human becoming and women living with violence: The art of practice. *Nursing Science Quarterly, 15,* 302–307.

Vander Woude, D., Damgaard, G., Hegge, M. J., Soholt, D., & Bunkers, S. S. (2003). The unfolding: Scenario planning in nursing. *Nursing Science Quarterly, 16,* 27–35.

Vander Woude, D. L., & Letcher, D. (2005). Becoming a living-learning organization. *Nursing Science Quarterly, 18,* 24–30.

Walker, K. M. (2000). Situated immersion: An experience of dialogue. *Nursing Science Quarterly, 13,* 214–215.

Wang, C. H. (1997). Quality of life and health for persons with leprosy. *Nursing Science Quarterly, 10,* 144–145.

Wang, C. H. (2000). Developing a concept of hope from a human science perspective. *Nursing Science Quarterly, 13,* 248–251.

Welch, A. J. (2004). The researcher's reflections on the research process. *Nursing Science Quarterly, 17,* 201–207.

Willman, A. (1999). Hope: The lived experience for Swedish elders. In R. R. Parse (Ed.), *Hope: An international perspective* (pp. 129–142). Sudbury, MA: Jones & Bartlett.

Yancy, N. R. (2005). The experience of the novice nurse: A human becoming perspective. Nursing *Science Quarterly, 18,* 215–220.

Annotated Research Bibliography (since 1997)

Allchin-Petardi, L. (1998). Weathering the storm: Persevering through a difficult time. *Nursing Science Quarterly, 11,* 172–177.
Parse's theory and research methodology were used to uncover the structure of the lived experience of persevering through a difficult time for eight women with ovarian cancer. Three core concepts surfaced: deliberately persisting, significant engagements, and shifting life patterns. The first concept was supported in the literature on perseverance, the second concept was further clarified, and the third concept represents new knowledge to the discipline of nursing.

Allchin-Petardi, L. (1999). Hope for American women with children. In R. R. Parse (Ed.), *Hope: An international perspective* (pp. 273–286). Boston: Jones & Bartlett.
This study found that the lived experience of hope for women with children is contemplating potentials with tenacious abiding amid arduous diversity.

Aquino-Russell, C. E. (2006). A phenomenological study: The lived experience of persons having a different sense of hearing. *Nursing Science Quarterly, 19,* 339–348.
Living with a different sense of hearing, including loss of hearing, is a worldwide phenomenon, known to be a condition that can change persons' patterns of relating and divest effective ways of giving and receiving messages of sound. This research describes the meaning of this experience for seven participants. The researcher followed Giorgi's descriptive phenomenological method for analysis/synthesis to arrive at a general structural description of the experience. Parse's theory of human becoming framed the researcher's theoretical perspective. Findings build on Parse's theory and may enhance nurses' understanding, in turn altering the way nurses approach persons having a different sense of hearing.

Baumann, S. L. (1999). The lived experience of hope: Children in families struggling to make a home. In R. R. Parse (Ed.), *Hope: An international perspective* (pp. 191–210). Boston: Jones & Bartlett.
This study found that the structure of the lived experience of hope for children in families struggling to make a home is the envisioning of nurturing engagements while inventing possibilities.

Baumann, S. L. (2000). The lived experience of feeling loved. *Nursing Science Quarterly, 13,* 332–338.

The purpose of this study was to uncover the meaning of the lived experience of *feeling loved.* The site of this study was a shelter-based parolee program. The framework that guided the study was Parse's human becoming theory, and the method was Parse's research methodology. The finding of this study is that the lived experience of *feeling loved* is an unshakable presence arising with moments of uplifting delight amid bewildering trepidation. The findings integrated into the human becoming theory show the paradoxical and dialectic nature of *feeling loved. Feeling loved* is linked to living freedom, trust, and hope.

Baumann, S. L. (2003). The lived experience of feeling very tired: A study of adolescent girls. *Nursing Science Quarterly, 16,* 326–333.

This study was part of a multisite study on feeling very tired using the human becoming theory and the Parse research method. The purpose of study was to explore the meaning of feeling very tired as described by a group of high school girls. The finding of this study is the following structure: *Feeling very tired is struggling with being attentively present as calming contentment emerges aid discomforting discordance.* The conclusion of this study is that feeling very tired is a complex paradoxical rhythm.

Baumann, S. L., Carroll, K. A., Damgaard, G. A., Miller, B., & Welch, A. J. (2001). An international human becoming hermeneutic study of Tom Hegg's *A cup of Christmas tea. Nursing Science Quarterly, 14,* 316–321.

This article reports a human becoming hermeneutic study of Thomas Hegg's *A Cup of Christmas Tea.* The human becoming hermeneutic method was used to discover emergent meanings about human experiences. The authors discovered three emergent meanings: honoring the cherished; communing with the was, is, and will be; and triumphing with new vision. The conclusion for families and nurses is that by remaining open to all possibilities that exist in each now, moments of serendipitous togetherness can transform human trepidation and negative views of later life.

Baumann, S. L., Dyches, T. T., & Braddick, M. (2005). Being a sibling. *Nursing Science Quarterly, 18,* 51–58.

The purpose of this descriptive study was to explore the meaning of being a sibling using Parse's theory. The finding of this study is the descriptive statement: being a sibling is an arduous charge to champion others amid restricting-enhancing commitments while new endeavors give rise to new possibilities.

Bournes, D. A. (2002a). Having courage: A lived experience of human becoming. *Nursing Science Quarterly, 15,* 220–229.

The purposes of this research were to discover the structure of the *experience* of *having courage* and to contribute to knowledge about human becoming. Participants were 10 persons with spinal cord injuries. The Parse research method was used to answer the research question, What is the structure of the *lived experience* of *having courage?* The central finding of this study is the following structure: The *lived experience* of *having courage* is a fortifying tenacity arising with triumph amid the burdensome, while guarded confidence emerges with the treasured. The findings are discussed in relation to human becoming, relevant literature, and future research.

Bournes, D. A. (2002b). Research evaluating human becoming in practice. *Nursing Science Quarterly, 13,* 190–195.

The author discusses the findings of six studies conducted to examine what happens for nurses and patients when human becoming is the guide for practice. In all of the studies, nurse participants' descriptions led to three main themes: transforming intent, unburdening joy, and struggling with change. Patient and family participants' descriptions of nursing care guided by human becoming are also summarized. This article concludes with a presentation of the universal and overarching values for knowledge development in nursing that emerged with the synthesis of the findings that have the potential to ensure personalized, meaningful, and dignified nursing service delivery.

Bournes, D. A. (2007). Human becoming and 80/20: An innovative professional development model for nurses. *Nursing Science Quarterly, 20,* 237–253.

This study evaluated the implementation of a professional development model in which nurses spend 80% of their salaried time in direct patient care and 20% of their salaried time on professional development. The findings show that on the study unit overtime hours decreased significantly, the education hours were sustained throughout the study period, workload hours per patient day increased significantly, sick time stayed low, patient satisfaction scores increased, and staff satisfaction scores were significantly higher than for comparison groups.

Bournes, D. A., & Ferguson-Pare, M. (2005). Persevering through a difficult time during the SARS outbreak in Toronto. *Nursing Science Quarterly, 18*, 324–333.

The purpose of this study was to describe the experience of *persevering through* a *difficult* time for patients, family members of patients, nurses, and allied health professionals during the severe acute respiratory syndrome outbreak. Van Kaam's phenomenological research method, with the human becoming theory as the theoretical perspective, was used to gather and analyze data from 63 participants who agreed to describe a situation that illuminated their experience of *persevering through* a *difficult* time (either online or using a voice-mail system). Data gathering occurred in early April 2003 in the midst of the severe acute respiratory syndrome outbreak in Toronto, Canada. The finding was the structural definition, *persevering through* a *difficult time* is dispiriting trepidation arising with witnessing suffering. It is a smothering connectedness with sequestering protection as unsettling contentment emerges amid unburdening hope. It sheds light on what is important for preparing for possible future outbreaks of this and other infectious diseases.

Bournes, D. A., & Mitchell, G. J. (2002). Waiting: The experience of persons in a critical care waiting room. *Research in Nursing and Health, 25*, 58–67.

The purposes of this phenomenological study were to discover the essences of the experience of waiting for 12 persons who have family members or friends in a critical care unit, to provide new knowledge about what it is like to wait that can be used as a guide in research and practice, and to contribute to knowledge about human becoming—the nursing perspective underpinning this study.

The central finding of this study was this structure: The lived experience of waiting is a vigilant attentiveness surfacing amid an ambiguous turbulent lull as contentment emerges with uplifting engagements.

Bunkers, S. S. (1998). Considering tomorrow: Parse's theory-guided research. *Nursing Science Quarterly, 11*, 56–63.

This study investigated the meaning of tomorrow for homeless females. Findings expand Parse's theory in relation to considering tomorrow, health, and quality of life. The structure of considering tomorrow is contemplating desired endeavors in longing for the cherished, while intimate alliances with isolating distance emerge as resilient endurance surfaces amid disturbing unsureness.

Bunkers, S. S. (1999). The lived experience of hope for those working with homeless persons. In R. R. Parse (Ed.), *Hope: An international perspective* (pp. 227–250). Boston: Jones & Bartlett.

This study found that the structure of the lived experience of hope for those working with homeless persons is envisioning possibilities amid disheartenment, as close alliances with isolating turmoil surface in inventive endeavoring.

Bunkers. S. S. (2004). The lived experience of feeling cared for: A human becoming perspective. *Nursing Science Quarterly, 17*, 63–71.

The purpose of this study was to answer the research question, What is the structure of the lived experience of feeling cared for? The major finding of this study is the following structure: *Feeling cared for is contentment with intimate affiliations arising with salutary endeavors, while honoring uniqueness amid adversity.*

Bunkers, S. S. (2007). The experience of feeling unsure for women at end-of-life. *Nursing Science Quarterly, 20*, 56–63.

The purpose of this study was to answer the research question, What is the structure of the lived experience of feeling unsure? The participants were nine women in the end-of-life stage. The Parse research method was used, and through the process of extraction/synthesis, three core concepts were identified: disquieting apprehensiveness, pressing on, and ultimate sorrows. For these nine women the lived experience of feeling unsure is disquieting apprehensiveness arising while pressing on with intimate sorrows.

Bunkers, S. S., & Daly, J. (1999). The lived experience of hope for Australian families living with coronary disease. In R. R. Parse (Ed.), *Hope: An international perspective* (pp. 45–61). Boston: Jones & Bartlett.

The lived experience of hope for Australian families living with coronary disease is anticipating possibilities amid anguish while enduring with vitality in intimate affiliations.

Cody, W. K. (1995). Of life immense in passion, pulse, and power: Dialoguing with Whitman and Parse—A hermeneutic study. In R. R. Parse (Ed.), *Illuminations: The human becoming theory in practice and research* (pp. 269–308). New York: National League for Nursing Press.

This study led to the following interpretation, which answers the research question, What does it mean to be human? To be human means to be *oneself*, embodied and sensual yet "not contained between my hat and boots." The self is one's interrelationship with the "kosmos," free and unbounded by space and time; the self includes all that is in one's universe.

Cody, W. K., & Filler, J. E. (1999). The lived experience of hope for women residing in a shelter. In R. R. Parse (Ed.), *Hope: An international perspective* (pp. 211–226). Boston: Jones & Bartlett.

This study found that the structure of the lived experience of women residing in a shelter is picturing attainment in persisting amid the arduous, while trusting in potentiality.

Florczak, K. L. (2006). The lived experience of sacrificing something important. *Nursing Science Quarterly, 19*, 133–141.

The purposes of this research, using the Parse method, were to discover the structure of sacrificing something important and to expand the theory of human becoming. The core concepts were discovered during the process of extraction/synthesis using synapse of dialogues for 10 church parishioners. The structure *sacrificing something important is relinquishing the cherished while shifting preferred options amid fortifying affiliations* is the central finding of this study,

Gates, K. M. (2000). The experience of caring for a loved one: A phenomenological study. *Nursing Science Quarterly, 13*, 54–59.

The purpose of this research was to uncover the meaning of caring for an elderly relative. Nine middle-aged and elderly people volunteered to take part in audio-recorded interviews to describe their experience of caring for a loved one. The following structural definition emerged from the study: The meaning of caring for an elderly relative is surfacing poignant remembering while doggedly continuing with nurturant giving and confirmatory receiving, as swells of enjoyment merge with tides of sorrow amid uplifting togetherness and valleys of aloneness. Parse's theory of human becoming and van Kaam's operations for phenomenological analysis are applied. Implications for practice and research are discussed.

Huch, M. H., & Bournes, D. A. (2003). Community dwellers' perspectives on the experience of feeling very tired. *Nursing Science Quarterly, 16*, 334–339.

The concept of feeling very tired was explored with 10 community dwelling individuals who had no expressed health concerns. The central finding of this study is the structure: *The lived experience of feeling very tired is dissipated vigor arising with monotonous disquietude amid spirited cherished engagements*. This structure was conceptually integrated with the human becoming theory as *feeling very tired is powering the languaging of valuing connecting-separating*.

Jonas-Simpson, C. (2001). Feeling understood: A melody of human becoming. *Nursing Science Quarterly, 14*, 222–230.

The study was conducted with 10 women living with an enduring health situation who discussed feeling understood and to create a musical expression of this phenemonon. The major finding of this study is the following structure: *Feeling understood is an unburdening quietude with triumphant bliss arising with the attentive reverence of nurturing engagements, while fortifying integrity emerges amid potential disregard*.

Jonas-Simpson, C. (2003). The experience of being listened to: A human becoming study with music. *Nursing Science Quarterly, 16*, 232–238.

The purpose of this study was to discover the structure of the lived experience of being listened to from the perspectives of 10 older women receiving inpatient rehabilitation. The Parse research method was used to guide this study where music was used in the dialogical engagement process. The findings include three core concepts—an *acknowledging engagement, gratifying contentment,* and an *unburdening respite*. Findings extend the theory of human becoming, enhance understanding of the experience of being listened to, and affirm its value.

Jonas-Simpson, C. (2006). The experience of being listened to: A qualitative study of older adults in long-term care settings. *Journal of Gerontological Nursing, 32*(1), 46–53.

The experience of being listened to for older adults living in long-term care facilities was explored using a qualitative descriptive method, with the human becoming theory as the theoretical framework. The themes that emerged from this study were nurturing, contentment, vital genuine connections, and deference triumphs mediocrity. The themes affirmed the experience of being listened to as fundamental to the participants' quality of life.

Kelley, L. S. (1999). Hope as lived by Native Americans. In R. R. Parse (Ed.), *Hope: An international perspective* (pp. 251–272). Boston: Jones & Bartlett.

The structure of the lived experience of hope for Native Americans is a transfiguring enlightenment arising with engaging affiliations as encircling the legendary surfaces with fortification.

Kruse, B. G. (1999). The lived experience of serenity, *Nursing Science Quarterly, 12,* 143–150.

Parse's research method was used to investigate the meaning of serenity for cancer survivors. Ten survivors told their stories of the meaning of serenity as they had lived it in their lives. Descriptions were aided by photographs chosen by each participant to represent the meaning of serenity for them. The structure of serenity was generated through the extraction/ synthesis process. Four main concepts—steering yielding with the flow, savoring remembered visions of engaging surroundings, abiding with aloneness-togetherness, and attesting to a loving presence—emerged and led to a theoretical structure of serenity from the human becoming perspective. Findings confirm serenity as a multidimensional process.

Legault, F., & Ferguson-Pare, M. (1999). Advancing nursing practice: An evaluation study of Parse's theory of human becoming. *Canadian Journal of Nursing Leadership, 12,* 30–35.

The purpose of this study was to evaluate the changes in nursing practice and the patient/ family perspectives of nursing care when Parse's theory of human becoming was used as a guide for nursing practice in an acute care surgical setting. The patterns of transition in nursing practice were understanding the unique contribution of nursing from a theoretical perspective, living value priorities to enhance quality of care for patients and families, shifting the focus of care from problems to the nurse–person relationship, finding meaning in nursing through reflection on self and others, supporting colleagues to move towards patient-centered care, persisting with new ways while facing resistance to change, and

enhancing personal and professional growth. It is evident from the positive patterns of change in nursing practice and patient and family experiences of *nursing* care that Parse's theory of human becoming is congruent with and supports patient-centered nursing practice.

Liu, S. (2004). What caring means to geriatric nurses. *Journal of Nursing Research, 12*(2), 143–152.

Using Parse's method, the finding of this study was the meaning of caring for nurses engaged in caring for the elderly: "Through the initiative deliberation from sincerity, the nurse is to dedication by the empathy and tolerance." The core concepts of caring were: deliberation, initiative, sincerity, tolerance, empathy, and dedication.

Mitchell, G. J., Bournes, D. A., & Hollett, J. (2006). Human becoming-guided patient-centered care: A new model transforms nursing practice. *Nursing Science Quarterly, 19,* 218–224.

A report of a 24-month research project in a large teaching hospital in Canada to evaluate what happens when nurses are provided 20% of time for the purpose of learning and self-development.

Mitchell, G. J., Bunkers, S. S., & Bournes, D. A. (2006). Feeling confident. In M. E. Parker (Ed.), *Nursing theories and nursing practice* (pp. 200–204). Philadelphia: F. A. Davis..

A study of the lived experience of feeling confident of people living with a spinal cord injury. Participants included three women and seven men between the ages of 22 and 42 years. Three core concepts were extracted/synthesized: *buoyant assuredness amid unsureness, sustaining engagements,* and *persistently pursuing the cherished.* These core concepts led to the structure of *feeling confident is a buoyant assuredness amid unsureness that arises with sustaining engagements while persistently pursuing the cherished.*

Mitchell, G. J., Pilkington, F. B., Aiken, F., Carson, M.G., Fisher, A., & Lyon, P. (2005). Exploring the lived experience of waiting for persons in long-term care. *Nursing Science Quarterly, 18*(3), 162–170.

This study describes the meaning of waiting for persons who reside in long-term care settings. Parse's theory of human becoming provided the nursing perspective and a qualitative descriptive-exploratory design was used. Three emergent themes formed the following unified description: The experience of waiting is intensifying ire while diversionary immersions reprieve amid unfolding becalming endurance.

Northrup, D. T. (2002). Time passing: A Parse research method study. *Nursing Science Quarterly, 15,* 318–326.

This study explored the meaning of time passing for nine HIV-positive men. Findings show that or study participants time passing is a lumbering-hastening tempo clarifying opportunities and constraints while focusing attention on gratifications amid expanding possibles.

Northrup, D. T., & Cody, W. K. (1998). Evaluation of the human becoming theory in an acute psychiatric setting. *Nursing Science Quarterly, 11,* 23–30.

This descriptive study evaluated Parse's theory of human becoming in practice in an acute psychiatric setting. A pre-mid-post implementation design served to generate qualitative data from nurses, patients, and hospital documentation that illuminated changes in the quality of nursing care on three diverse pilot units. Findings supported prior research except about job satisfaction reactions of nurses. Some nurses felt that to be in true presence with psychotic clients was nonproductive and was an inadequate guide to psychiatric nursing practice.

Ortiz, M.R. (2003). Lingering presence: A study using the human becoming hermeneutic method. *Nursing Science Quarterly, 16,* 146–154. The emergent meanings were (a) a lingering presence surfaces in the cherished remembered that changes moment to moment as new experiences arise in the now and shed different light on the was and will be; (b) a lingering presence is the lived in private ways, yet with others in a different alone-togetherness; and (c) a lingering presence is living with the familiar-unfamiliar in the now moment while moving beyond with different possibles.

Parse, R. R. (1997). Joy-sorrow: A study using the Parse research method. *Nursing Science Quarterly, 10,* 80–87.

This study found that the structure of the lived experience of joy-sorrow is the pleasure amid adversity emerging in the cherished contentment of benevolent engagements.

Parse, R. R. (1999). The lived experience of hope for family members of persons living in a Canadian chronic care facility. In R. R. Parse (Ed.), *Hope: An international perspective* (pp. 63–68). Boston: Jones & Bartlett.

The lived experience of hope for family members of persons in a Canadian chronic care home is an undaunting pursuit of the not-yet amid the wretched, as affable involvements arise with transfiguring.

Parse, R.R. (2001). The lived experience of contentment: A study using the Parse research method. *Nursing Science Quarterly, 14,* 330–338. The Parse research method, a phenomenological-hermeneutic method, was used to explore the meaning of the lived experience of contentment for 10 women. The major finding of this study is the following structure: *Contentment is satisfying calmness amid the arduous as resolute liberty arises within benevolent engagements.* The structure provides knowledge about contentment and its connection to health and quality of life.

Parse, R. R. (2003). The lived experience of felling very tired: A study using the Parse research method. *Nursing Science Quarterly, 16,* 319–325. The purpose of this study was to answer the research question, What is the structure of the lived experience of feeling very tired? The major finding of the study is the following structure: *The lived experience of feeling very tired is devitalizing languor arising with engaging endeavors amid pulsating moments of repose-revive.* The structure is discussed in light of the principles of human becoming.

Parse, R. R. (2006). Feeling respected: A Parse method study. *Nursing Science Quarterly, 19,* 51–56.

This study explored the feeling of being respected with 10 participants. The finding of this study is the following structure: *The lived experience of feeling respected is fortifying assuredness amid potential disregard emerging with the fulfilling delight of prized alliances.*

Parse, R. R. (2007). Hope in "Rita Hayworth and Shawshank Redemption": A human becoming hermeneutic study. *Nursing Science Quarterly, 20,* 148–154.

This human becoming hermeneutic method study on the above titled short story, screenplay, and film answered the research question, What is hope as humanly lived? Emergent meanings were discovered that enhanced knowledge and understanding of hope in general and expanded the human becoming school of thought.

Pilkington, F. B. (1999). A qualitative study of life after stroke. *Journal of Neuroscience Nursing, 31,* 336–347.

The purpose of this qualitative, descriptive exploratory study was to enhance understanding about quality of life after a stroke from the patient's own perspective. The guiding theoretical perspective was Parse's human becoming theory. Loosely structured interviews aimed at eliciting descriptions of quality of life were scheduled during the acute care stay and at one and three months after stroke onset. A total of 32 interviews were conducted with 13 participants, including nine men and four women, aged 40 to 91 years. Through a process of analysis/synthesis, four themes representing participants' descriptions were created: (1) suffering emerges amid unaccustomed restrictions and losses, (2) hopes for endurance mingle with dreams of new possibilities, (3) appreciation of the ordinary shifts perspectives, and (4) consoling relationships uplift the self.

Pilkington, F. B. (2000). Persisting while wanting to change: Women's lived experiences. *Health Care for Women International, 21,* 501–516.

This study explores the common lived experience of persisting while wanting to change. Parse's phenomenological-hermeneutic methodology was used to investigate the phenomenon as it is lived by women in an abusive relationship. Through dialogical engagement with the researcher, eight women described their experiences of persisting while wanting to change. The generated structure and central finding contained three core concepts: wavering in abiding with the burdensome-cherished, engaging-distancing with ameliorating intentions, and anticipating the possibilities of the new.

Pilkington, F. B. (2005). Grieving a loss: The lived experience for elders residing in an institution. *Nursing Science Quarterly, 18,* 233–242.

This phenomenological-hermeneutic study was an inquiry into the lived experience of grieving a loss. The nursing perspective was Parse's human becoming theory. The study finding specifies the structure of the lived experience of grieving a loss as *aching solitude amid enduring cherished affiliations, as serene acquiescence arises with sorrowful curtailments.*

Pilkington, F. B., & Millar, B. (1999). The lived experience of hope with persons from Wales, U.K. In R. R. Parse (Ed.), *Hope: An international perspective* (pp. 163–190). Boston: Jones & Bartlett.

The structure of the lived experience of hope for persons in Wales, United Kingdom, is anticipating cherished possibilities while persevering amid adversity with benevolent affiliations.

Pilkington, F. B., & Mitchell, G. J. (2004). Quality of life for women living with a gynecologic cancer. *Nursing Science Quarterly, 17,* 147–155.

The purpose of this study was to enhance understanding about the quality of life for women living with a gynecologic cancer. Four themes were identified, which provide the following unified description: *Quality of life is treasuring loving expressions while affirming personal worth, consoling immersions amid torment, emerge with expanding fortitude for enduring.*

Takahashi, T. (1999). Kibov: Hope for the person in Japan. In R. R. Parse (Ed.), *Hope: An international perspective* (pp. 115–128). Boston: Jones & Bartlett.

This study found that the structure of the lived experience of hope for persons in Japan is anticipation of expanding possibilities, while liberation amid arduous restriction arises with the contentment of desired accomplishments.

Toikkanen, T., & Muurinen, E. (1999). Toivo: Hope for persons in Finland. In R. R. Parse (Ed.), *Hope: An international perspective* (pp. 79–96). Boston: Jones & Bartlett.

This study found that the lived experience of hope for persons in Finland is persistent anticipation of contentment arising with the promise of nurturing affiliations, while inspiration emerges and easing the arduous.

Wang, C. H. (1999). Hope for persons living with leprosy in Taiwan. In R. R. Parse (Ed.), *Hope: An international perspective* (pp. 143–162). Sudbury, MA: Jones & Bartlett.

This study found that the structure of hope for persons living with leprosy is anticipating an unburdening serenity amid despair, as nurturing engagements emerge in creating anew with cherished priorities.

Welch, A. (2007). The phenomenon of taking life day-by-day using Parse's research methodology. *Advances in Nursing Science, 20,* 265–272.

The participants in this study were 10 men between 35 and 60 years who had experienced depressions and were willing to share their lived world of taking life day by day. Three core concepts were explicated from the participants' dialogues: enduring with the burdensome, envisioning the possibles, and sure-unsure.

Zanotti, R., & Bournes, D. A. (1999). *Speranza: A study of the lived experience of hope with persons from Italy.* In R. R. Parse (Ed.), *Hope: An international perspective* (pp. 97–114). Boston: Jones & Bartlett.

This study found that the structure of hope for persons from Italy is expectancy amid the arduous, as quiescent vitality arises with expanding horizons.

Dissertations Guided by the Human Becoming School of Thought (since 1997)

Bournes, D. A. (2000). *Having courage: A lived experience of human becoming.* Doctoral dissertation, Loyola University, Chicago, IL, Dissertation Abstracts.

Carroll, K. A. (2002). *Attentive presence: A lived experience of human becoming.* Doctoral dissertation, Loyola University, Chicago, IL, Dissertation Abstracts.

Dempsey, L. (2005). *A qualitative descriptive exploratory study of feeling confined using Parse's human becoming school of thought.* Unpublished doctoral dissertation, Loyola University, Chicago, IL.

Doucet, T. J. (2006). *The lived experience of having faith: A Parse method study.* Unpublished doctoral dissertation, Loyola University, Chicago, IL.

Hamalis, P. S. (2001). *Feeling peaceful: A lived experience of human becoming.* Unpublished doctoral dissertation, Loyola University, Chicago, IL.

Hanlon, A. (2004). *Feeling happy: A lived experience of human becoming.* Doctoral dissertation. Loyola University, Chicago, IL, Dissertation Abstracts.

Hayden, S. J. (2007). Laughing: A Parse research method study. *Dissertation Abstracts International, 68*(12B), 7928. Abstract retrieved December 1, 2009, from Dissertation Abstracts Online database.

Huffman, D. (2002). *Feeling unburdened: Research guided by Parse's human becoming theory.* Doctoral dissertation, Loyola University of Chicago, IL, Dissertation Abstracts.

Kagan, P. N. (2004). *Feeling listened to: A lived experience of human becoming.* Unpublished doctoral dissertation, Loyola University, Chicago, IL.

Karnick, P. M. (2003). *Feeling lonely: A lived experience of human becoming.* Unpublished doctoral dissertation, Loyola University, Chicago, IL.

Kostas-Polston, E. A. (2007). Persisting while wanting to change: A Parse method research study. *Dissertation Abstracts International, 69*(01B), 225. Abstract retrieved December 1, 2009, from Dissertation Abstracts Online database.

Milton, C. (1998). *Making a promise.* Unpublished doctoral dissertation, Loyola University, Chicago, IL.

Morrow, M. R. (2006). *Feeling unsure: A universal lived experience.* Unpublished doctoral dissertation, Loyola University, Chicago, IL.

Ortiz, M. R. (2001). *Lingering presence: A human becoming hermeneutic study.* Unpublished doctoral dissertation, Loyola University, Chicago, IL.

Perkins, J. B. (2004). *A cosmology of compassions for nursing explicated via dialogue with self, science and spirit.* Doctoral dissertation, University of Colorado Health Sciences Center, Boulder, CO.

Pilkington, F. B. (1997). *Persisting while wanting to change: Research guided by Parse's theory.* Unpublished doctoral dissertation, Loyola University, Chicago, IL.

Smith, S. M. (2006). The lived experience of doing the right thing: A Parse method study. *Dissertation Abstracts International, 67*(04B), 1921. Abstract retrieved December 1, 2009, from Dissertation Abstracts Online database.

Yancey, N. (2004). *Living with changing expectations: Research on human becoming.* Unpublished doctoral dissertation, Loyola University, Chicago, IL.

CHAPTER 20

The Modeling and Role-Modeling Theory

Helen Lorraine (Cook) Erickson, Evelyn M. Tomlin, Mary Ann P. Swain

Noreen Cavan Frisch
Susan Stanwyck Bowman

The Modeling and Role-Modeling Theory was developed by three individuals, Helen Lorraine (Cook) Erickson, Evelyn M. Tomlin, and Mary Ann P. Swain. The initial publication of the theory was presented in 1983 with the text Modeling and Role-Modeling: A Theory and Paradigm for Nursing. *A series of follow-up books edited by the principal author, Helen Erickson, has been planned to expand on the concepts within the theory. The first of these books was published in 2006 (H. L. Erickson, 2006a). The second and third books are in progress.*

Helen Lorraine (Cook) Erickson was born and raised in Michigan. She received her diploma in nursing from Saginaw General Hospital, Saginaw, Michigan (1957), and B.S. in nursing (1974), M.S. in psychiatric and medical-surgical nursing (1976), and Ph.D. in educational psychology (1984) from the University of Michigan, Ann Arbor. Her clinical practice has included emergency room and student health services in the United States and Puerto Rico; she has maintained an independent practice since 1976 and supervises health care providers interested in furthering their knowledge and skill in the use of Modeling and Role-Modeling as the theory base for practice. She held undergraduate and graduate nursing faculty and administrative positions at the University of Michigan and the University of South Carolina, Columbia, and is emeritus professor of nursing from the University of Texas, Austin. As a scholar, she initiated scientific testing of the theory, continues to work on articulating aspects of the theory, and has been involved in relating research findings and implications for practice through publications and numerous presentations. One of her current projects is to develop a Center for the Study and Practice of the Modeling and Role-Modeling theory and paradigm. She is a board member for the American Holistic Nurses Certification Corporation, which has guided the development and administration of the first national certification in holistic nursing. Her honors and awards include an Excellence in Nursing Award from Rho Chapter, Sigma Theta Tau in 1980; ADARA, Women's Leadership Society, University of Michigan and Amoco Foundation Good

Teaching Award (one of only two nursing faculty recipients in the 100-year history of the university) in 1982; Phi Kappa Phi membership in 1989; Faculty Teaching Award, University of Texas, in 1990; School of Nursing Graduate Teaching Award, University of Texas, in 1995; Honorary Lifetime Certification from the American Holistic Nurses Association in 1996; fellow, American Academy of Nursing in 1996; and establishment of the Helen L. Erickson Endowed Lectureship on Holistic Nursing, School of Nursing, University of Texas, in 1997. She was the first president of the Society for the Advancement of Modeling and Role-Modeling from 1986 to 1990.

Evelyn Tomlin received a baccalaureate degree in nursing from the University of Southern California, Los Angeles, and a master's degree in psychiatric nursing from the University of Michigan in 1976. She has extensive clinical practice experience both in the United States and in Afghanistan. She has been involved in staff nursing, critical care, home health, and independent practice as well as many areas of nursing education. In her retirement from "nursing for pay," Tomlin lives in Geneva, Illinois. She volunteers at a shelter for women and children, takes speaking engagements in Illinois and nearby states, and serves as a lay leader in several ministries (both in the United States and abroad), where she relates that remarkably expedited healings have been experienced through the power of sound teaching, truth-telling, and prayer within an interactive, interpersonal relationship with God. She published an article identifying an interface between Modeling and Role-Modeling and Judeo-Christian values in the first monograph published by the Society for the Advancement of Modeling and Role-Modeling (Tomlin, 1990).

Mary Ann Swain's educational background is in psychology with a B.A. degree from DePauw University in Greencastle, Indiana, and both an M.A. and a Ph.D. (1969) from the University of Michigan, Ann Arbor. Although not a nurse, much of Swain's career has been involved with nursing. She has taught research methods and statistics as well as psychology to nurses at DePauw University and the University of Michigan. Swain has held the positions of director of the doctoral program in nursing, chairperson of nursing research, professor of nursing research, and associate vice president for academic affairs at the University of Michigan. She is presently provost and vice president for academic affairs as well as director of the doctoral program, Decker School of Nursing, Binghamton University, part of the State University of New York. She has received many awards for academic excellence and is an honorary member of Sigma Theta Tau. She is active in the Society for the Advancement of Modeling and Role-Modeling and is a past president of the Society.

The book describing the theory of Modeling and Role-Modeling presents the theory in a very informal and readable style (H. C. Erickson, Tomlin, & Swain, 1983). It includes many case studies and clinical examples of the use of this theory in nursing. The basis of the theory is always to focus on the person receiving nursing care—not on the nurse, not on the care, and not on the disease. The concept of modeling a person's world is credited to Milton H. Erickson, M.D., who was the father-in-law of the principal author of this theory, Helen Erickson. Erickson credits her father-in-law with a great deal of influence on this theory. His initial beliefs in the mind–body connection in health, healing, and disease, as well as his belief that the most important thing a nurse can do to help a client is modeling that person's world, provided the underlying themes for this theory.

Erickson returned to graduate school after many years of clinical practice to "label and articulate" practice-based knowledge that she knew was important to and consistent in nursing. She believed this knowledge needed to be shared with other nurses. Both her master's thesis and her doctoral dissertation were instrumental in developing the theory of Modeling and Role-Modeling (H. Erickson, 1976; H. C. Erickson, 1984). Other early research that contributed to this theory was supported by two federal grants: "Influencing Compliance Among Hypertensives" from the National Heart, Lung, and Blood Institute (HL-17045) (H. Erickson, & Swain, 1977; Swain & Stickel, 1981) and "Health Promotion Among Diabetics: Comparing Nursing Systems" from the Division of Nursing (NU-00658). More recently, Dr. Erickson was the principal investigator for a major study at the University of Texas at Austin, "Modeling and Role-Modeling with Alzheimer's Patients," funded by the National Institutes of Health, the National Institute of Aging, and the National Center for Nursing Research (NIH Grant R01NR03032–01).

The combination of talents of the three authors who collaborated at the University of Michigan in the mid-1970s was advantageous for the development of a nursing theory that was useful and related to practice, education, and research. All three of the original authors have been involved in nursing education. Two are expert nursing clinicians and remain actively involved in clinical practice, and two remain active in research and scholarly pursuits.

THE THEORY OF MODELING AND ROLE-MODELING

Modeling and Role-Modeling is an interpersonal and interactive holistic theory of nursing that requires the nurse to assess (*model*), plan (*role-model*), and intervene (*five aims of intervention*) on the basis of the client's perspective of the world. The nurse always acknowledges the uniqueness and individuality of the client and appreciates that individuals, at some level, know what makes them ill and what makes them well (*self-care knowledge*). The nurse assesses the individual's ability to mobilize resources needed to contend with stressors (*adaptive potential*) and assists individuals to recognize and obtain resources (internal and external) that are important for their health and healing (*self-care resources*) and facilitates the use of these resources (*self-care action*). The nurse also acknowledges the individual's need to be dependent on support systems while simultaneously maintaining independence from these support systems (*affiliated individuation*). Concepts relating to the nurse who practices with a theory base of Modeling and Role-Modeling include *facilitation*, *nurturance*, and *unconditional acceptance*.

Modeling

Modeling is the process used by the nurse to develop an understanding of the client's world as the client perceives it. The model of a person's world is the representation of the unique aggregation of the way an individual perceives life and all of its aspects and components; the way an individual thinks, communicates, feels, believes, and behaves; and the underlying motivation and rationale for beliefs and behaviors. This concept is based on Milton Erickson's belief that an appreciation for a client's model of the world is a prerequisite for providing holistic care (H. C. Erickson et al., 1983). Modeling is both an art and a science. The art of modeling is the empathetic understanding of the present situation within the client's context of the world—that is, the development of a "model" of the situation from the client's perspective. The science of modeling is the analysis of the information collected about the client's world. To truly understand the client's model of the world, the nurse must have a strong theoretical base in the physical and social sciences. The client's perspective is analyzed on the basis of knowledge and theory in areas including human behavior, development, cultural diversity, interaction, pathophysiology, and human needs (H. C. Erickson et al., 1983).

Role-Modeling

Role-modeling is the facilitation of health. It is also both an art and a science. The art of role-modeling involves the individualization of care based on the client's model of the world; the science of role-modeling is the use of theoretical bases when planning and implementing nursing care. Role-modeling is the facilitation of the individual in attaining, maintaining, or promoting health through purposeful interventions based on the individual's perceptions as well as the theoretical base for the practice of nursing (H. C. Erickson et al., 1983).

Five Aims of Intervention

The aims of intervention are based on five principles pertaining to similarities among humans (see Table 20-1). Because each individual is unique and has his or her own model of the world, it is not possible to formulate standardized interventions. However, because all human beings have some similarities, the aims of intervention can be standardized. Individualized interventions are based on the client's model of the world and guided by the five aims of intervention, defined as follows.

BUILD TRUST   Nursing requires a trusting relationship. This relationship involves honesty, acceptance, respect, empathy, and a belief in the client's model of the world. Therapeutic communication skills are essential in building trust. Trust is basic to any interpersonal relationship and is easily threatened if clients perceive that nurses lack respect for their view of the world or feel that nurses consider the clients' concerns or beliefs to be invalid, unwarranted, erroneous, or inappropriate.

PROMOTE POSITIVE ORIENTATION   Nursing interventions need to promote each client's self-worth as well as the client's hope for the future. Reframing can be used to assist

TABLE 20-1   Relationship of Human Similarity Principles and Aims for Intervention

Principle	Aim
1. The nursing process requires that a trusting and functional relationship exist between nurse and client.	Build trust.
2. Affiliated-Individuation is dependent on the individual's perceiving that he or she is an acceptable, respectable, and worthwhile human being.	Promote client's positive orientation.
3. Human developement is dependent on the individual's perceiving that he or she has some control over his or her life, while concurrently sensing a state of affiliation.	Promote client's control.
4. There is an innate drive toward holistic health that is facilitated by consistent and systematic nurturance.	Affirm and promote client's strengths.
5. Human growth is dependent on satisfaction of basic needs and facilitated by growth-need satisfaction.	Set mutual goals that are health-directed.

From Erickson, H.C. Tomlin, E.M., A Swain, M. A. P. (1983) *Modeling and role-modeling: A theory and paradigm for nursing* (p. 170). Lexington, SC: Pine Press. Used with permission.

clients in changing their perception of a situation from one of threat to one of challenge, from one of hopelessness to one of hope, and from something negative to something positive. Promoting an individual's strengths promotes that individual's self-worth and perceived control. Promoting strengths also aids in building a trusting relationship between the client and the nurse.

PROMOTE PERCEIVED CONTROL   Human development depends on individuals' perceiving that they have some control over their lives. Nurses may understand that clients have control over what happens to them and may understand that clients are required to give informed consent for any procedure done to them. However, many clients do not perceive that they have any control. It is not enough for the nurse to promote client control; the nurse must promote the client's *perception* of control.

PROMOTE STRENGTHS   Identification and promotion of strengths is a means of assisting clients to mobilize resources. In the face of stressors, individuals may become overwhelmed with their perceived weaknesses and not be able to identify or use strengths.

SET MUTUAL GOALS THAT ARE HEALTH DIRECTED   Nurses must use the individual's innate drive to be as healthy as he or she can be. The nurse's and client's goals are the same—to meet the client's basic needs. When the nurse's and client's goals appear to differ, the nurse has most likely not fully modeled the client's world. Incomplete modeling can be the result of inadequate data gathering and empathy or a lack of knowledge for analysis and interpretation of the data collected. Incomplete modeling can also result from the nurse's focus on one subsystem (e.g., biophysical) rather than viewing the individual and health as truly holistic.

Self-Care

There are three aspects of self-care in the Modeling and Role-Modeling theory: *self-care knowledge, self-care resources*, and *self-care action*. Although the three aspects are interconnected (see Figure 20-1), they will be discussed individually.

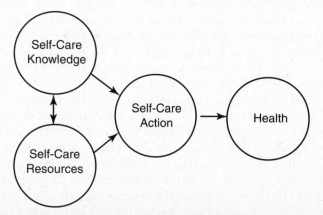

FIGURE 20-1   Self-care model for Modeling and Role-Modeling. (*Adapted from Hertz, J. E. (1991). The Perceived Enactment of Autonomy Scale: Measuring the potential for self care action in the elderly. Dissertation Abstracts International, 52(04B), 1953 (UMI No, 9128248).*)

SELF-CARE KNOWLEDGE   Self-care knowledge has been defined by Hertz and Baas (2006) as "the personal understanding of what is needed to help us grow, develop, or heal. It includes awareness of personal needs and goals, as well as strengths, capabilities, characteristics, values, and liabilities. It also includes recognition of what is not needed" (p. 98). In most situations, individuals can describe what they perceive to be their health problem; they can also identify what they think will make them feel better. According to H. C. Erickson et al. (1983), self-care knowledge is knowledge one has about "what has made him or her sick, lessened his or her effectiveness, or interfered with his or her growth. The person also knows what will make him or her well, optimize his or her effectiveness or fulfillment (given circumstances), or promote his or her growth" (p. 48). In an analysis of case studies reported by H. C. Erickson (1990a), the following four themes were found that relate to the nature of self-care knowledge:

1. An individual's perception of factors associated with his or her personal health problems are rarely obvious to the health care provider.
2. The individual's perceptions of what is needed to help him or her can best be defined by that person.
3. One nursing role is to facilitate clients to articulate what they perceive to be associated with their problem and what can be done to help them feel better.
4. Another nursing role is to assist the clients to resolve their problems in ways that meet personal needs and are health and growth directed. (p. 186)

SELF-CARE RESOURCES   All individuals have internal and external resources (strengths and support) that will help gain, maintain, and promote an optimum level of holistic health. The perception of adequate resources is itself a resource (Hertz & Baas, 2006). It is important for the nurse to assess these resources to assist the client in self-care action.

Primary internal self-care resources for each individual result from the person having successfully negotiated developmental challenges. Characteristics that result from appropriate need satisfaction (within the context of the human needs theory by Maslow [1970]) and positive resolution of the developmental tasks (within the context of the theory of psychosocial development by Erikson [1963]) leave the individual able to mobilize resources (H. C. Erickson, 1990a). Studies have been reported that describe and expand these characteristics in general and the use of specific internal resources such as autonomy, hope, control, purpose, wisdom, and spirituality as self-care resources (Baldwin, 1996; Baldwin & Herr, 2004; Beery, Baas, Fowler, & Allen, 2002; Curl, 1992; Hertz, 1996; Hertz & Anschutz, 2002; Hertz & Baas, 2006; Irvin &Acton, 1997; Jensen, 1995; Keck, 1989; MacLean, 1987, 1990, 1992; Miller, 1986).

Each individual identifies external self-care resources. Characteristics of external self-care resources are being explored. These characteristics include perceptions, social support, types of resources used when ill and well, and transitional objects, including technical devices. Kennedy (1991) discusses differences among individuals relating to perceptions of comfort and comforting care. Bowman (1998) reports that external resources used by persons when ill may be different than those used when well and identifies themes that characterize external resources used during healing from episodic illness at home, such as having things that are normal and familiar or associated with the past, viewing nature, and being pampered and treated. Transitional objects are external resources that may be utilized to facilitate the feelings of worthiness produced by secure attachments (H. C. Erickson, 1990b; M. E. Erickson, 2006). Beery and Baas (1996) describe the use of implanted technical devices such as pacemakers becoming "internal" transitional objects providing a secure attachment to facilitate health.

SELF-CARE ACTION   Self-care action is the development and use of self-care knowledge and self-care resources. The basis of nursing is assisting clients in self-care actions related to health. The concept of self-care is used differently in the Modeling and Role-Modeling theory than in Orem's (1995) Self-Care Deficit theory. Orem's theory focuses on delineating *when* nursing is needed. In Orem's theory, self-care is a universal need met through the ability to care for one's self; nurses assist clients in meeting self-care needs when there is a deficit in the clients' ability to meet their own needs. Self-care in Modeling and Role-Modeling focuses on the individual's personal knowledge about what makes him or her well or ill. All clients have self-care knowledge and self-care resources, and the nurse facilitates the client's identification and use of that knowledge and those resources. Self-care, then, in Modeling and Role-Modeling is used in planning implementations rather than for determining the *need* for nursing implementations, as is the situation in Orem's self-care theory.

Affiliated–Individuation

All individuals are seen as having simultaneous needs to be attached to other individuals and to be separate from them. This concept is described in Modeling and Role-Modeling as "affiliated–individuation" and considered to be a motivation for human behavior. "*Affiliated–individuation* occurs when a person perceives himself or herself as simultaneously close to and separate from a significant other" (H. C. Erickson et al., 1983, p. 68). According to M. E. Erickson, Erickson, and Jensen (2006), "When affiliation and individuation are in balance, we are able to find meaning in our life, work on our Life Purpose, and self-actualize" (p. 183). Affiliated–individuation is different from interdependence in that it is an intrapsychic phenomenon and can occur without being reciprocated. Affiliated–individuation is a resource for healing and an important component for well-being. Acton and Miller (1996) reported no decrease in affiliated–individuation for caregivers of persons with Alzheimer's disease, in spite of their continued caregiving, when the caregivers participated in a theory-based support group intervention.

Adaptive Potential

Adaptive potential refers to the individual's ability to mobilize resources to cope with stressors. Perception of stressors, availability of coping resources, and the ability to mobilize resources to deal with stress are very individual, and a basic understanding of the stressor-stress-coping process is necessary before being able to model another person's world (Benson, 2006). The Adaptive Potential Assessment Model (APAM) has three categories: *equilibrium, arousal*, and *impoverishment*. Equilibrium has two possibilities: *adaptive equilibrium* and *maladaptive equilibrium*. Arousal and impoverishment are both stress states. They differ in that those in impoverishment must deal with stress with diminished, if not depleted, resources (H. C. Erickson et al., 1983). Adaptive potential is dynamic, and individuals can move from any of the three states to any other of the states, as shown in Figure 20-2. Movement among the states is influenced by the individual's ability to cope. The APAM identifies states (not traits) of coping that can assist the nurse in planning interventions for

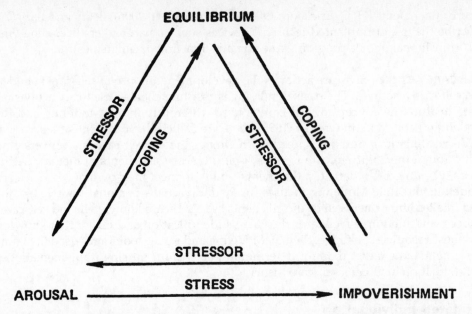

FIGURE 20-2   An illustration of the dynamic relationship among the states of the Adaptive Potential Assessment Model.   (*From Erickson, H., Tomlin, E., & Swain, M. A. (1983). Modeling and Role-Modeling: A theory and paradigm for nursing (p. 82). Lexington, SC: Pine Press. Used with permission.*)

the client. Assessment of adaptive potential has been well documented (Barnfather, Swain, & Erickson, 1989a, 1989b; Campbell, Finch, Allport, Erickson, & Swain, 1985; H. Erickson, & Swain, 1982). More recently, Hopkins (1994) has begun development of an Adaptive Potential Assessment Tool, and Benson (2003) designed a model for the assessment of adaptive potential in groups. Figure 20-3 identifies how interventions can be guided by the individual's ability to mobilize his or her own resources. A person who is impoverished is not in a situation to be an autonomous, independent person eager to learn and to perform self-care. An impoverished person requires that affiliation needs be met, internal strengths be promoted, and external resources be provided. A client in arousal is in a stress state and has difficulty mobilizing resources. This client has stronger individuation needs and responds to guidance, directions, assistance, and teaching that are all aimed at self-care. The client in equilibrium is in a nonstress state. Adaptive equilibrium is different from maladaptive equilibrium in that the adaptive client has all subsystems in harmony, whereas the maladaptive client places one or more subsystems in jeopardy to maintain equilibrium. The importance of equilibrium, whether adaptive or maladaptive, is that the client sees no reason to change because equilibrium already exists. Interventions for the client in maladaptive equilibrium need to focus on motivation strategies to develop a desire for change.

Modeling and Role-Modeling and Nursing's Metaparadigm

According to the theory, people are holistic beings with interacting subsystems (biophysical, psychological, social, and cognitive) and inherent genetic bases and spiritual drive (see Figure 20-4). "Holism" implies that the whole is greater than the sum of the parts and is differentiated from "wholism," which implies that a person is an aggregate of parts and the whole is equal to the sum of the parts (H. C. Erickson et al., 1983).

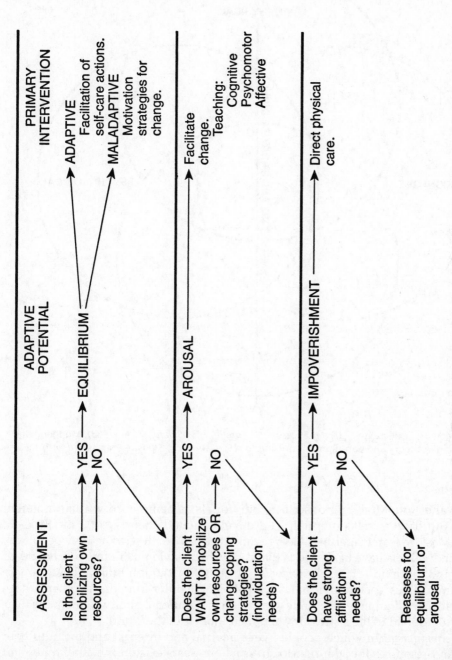

FIGURE 20-3 Adaptive potential as a guide to planning nursing interventions. *(From Bowman, S. S. (1992). Adaptive potential as a guide to planning nursing interventions. Presented at the Fourth National Modeling and Role-Modeling Conference. Boston, MA: Used with permission.)*

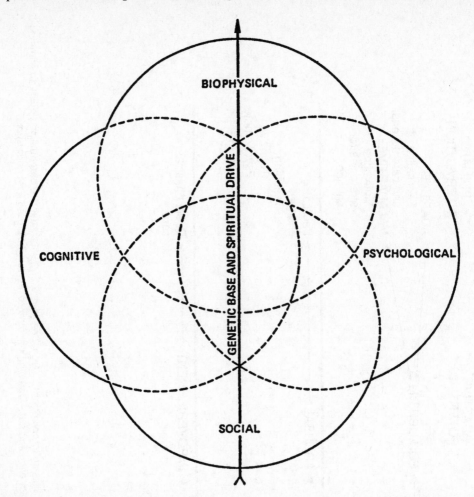

FIGURE 20-4   A holistic model.   (*From Erickson, H., Tomlin, E., & Swain, M. A. (1983).* Modeling and Role-Modeling: A theory and paradigm for nursing *(p. 45). Lexington, SC: Pine Press. Used with permission.)*

Modeling and Role-Modeling describes individuals as being born with an inherent desire to fulfill their self-potential. The developmental theories of Erik Erikson, Abraham Maslow, Jean Piaget, and George Engel are basic to describing how people are alike. All individuals have basic needs that motivate behavior, including a drive called affiliated–individuation (H. C. Erickson et al., 1983). Although human beings share these commonalities, each individual is unique. People differ from one another as a result of their individual inherited endowment, their situational ability to mobilize their resources to respond to life's stressors, and their models of the world.

The *environment* in which people live is internal and external and includes both stressors and resources for adapting to stressors. Stressors exist in life at all times and are necessary for overall growth and life enhancement. All individuals have both internal and external resources for dealing with stressors. Potential resources exist and individuals may need assistance in becoming aware of and constructively mobilizing them.

Consistent with the World Health Organization definition (World Health Organizaton, 1946), the theory views *health* as a state of physical, mental, and social well-being, not merely the absence of disease or infirmity. Modeling and Role-Modeling views health as a state of dynamic equilibrium among the various subsystems. This dynamic equilibrium implies an adaptive equilibrium whereby the individual learns to cope constructively with life's stressors by mobilizing internal and external coping resources and leaving no subsystem in jeopardy when adaptation occurs.

Nursing itself is a process between the nurse and the client and requires an interpersonal and interactive nurse–client relationship. Three characteristics of the nurse in this theory are facilitation, nurturance, and unconditional acceptance. Facilitation implies that the nurse aids the individual to identify, mobilize, and develop his or her own strengths. Rogers (1996, 1997) describes a new concept of "facilitative affiliation" that was developed within the framework of Modeling and Role-Modeling to express the essence of the nurse–client relationship. The attributes of facilitative affiliation include presence, needs assessment based on the client's self-care knowledge and perception of self-care resources, interventions based on the client's model of the world, selective normative disregard, mutual trust, nurturing, and advocacy by the nurse. Nurturance is the central nursing action that fuses and integrates the cognitive, psychological, and affective processes with the aim of assisting a client toward holistic health. Further, nursing actions must be carried out with unconditional acceptance, the acceptance of each individual as unique, worthwhile, and important with no strings attached. The Modeling and Role-Modeling definition of nursing as given by H. C. Erickson et al. (1983) is as follows:

> *Nursing* is the holistic helping of persons with their self-care activities in relation to their health. This is an interactive, interpersonal process that nurtures strengths to enable development, release, and channeling of resources for coping with one's circumstances and environment. The goal is to achieve a state of perceived optimum health and contentment. (p. 49)

Additional statements by H. C. Erickson et al. (1983) to define nursing are the following:

- Nursing is the nurturance of holistic self-care.
- Nursing is assisting persons holistically to use their adaptive strengths to attain and maintain optimum bio-psycho-socio-spiritual functioning.
- Nursing is helping with self-care to gain optimum health.
- Nursing is an integrated and integrative helping of persons to take better care of themselves. (p. 50)

In relation to the traditional view of nursing's metaparadigm, the concepts of person, environment, health, and nursing are fairly clear within this theory. Considering, however, that there are alternative and emerging developments in the metaparadigm, Modeling and Role-Modeling can be seen as a theory that utilizes additional concepts unique to the theory (*adaptive potential, affiliated individuation*) and, at the same time, uses concepts that may mirror contemporary ideas of nursing described by others. *Caring* as a concept has been used as a basis for several approaches, most notably Watson's (2005) theory and Leininger and McFarland's (2006) mandate of cultural care. Modeling and Role-Modeling defines the nursing role of providing comfort, support, and human-to-human contact as *nurturance*. *Nurturance* implies support for development and growth, something that provides sustenance, something that predicts change over time. Further, nurturance must be both given and received from within a context of unconditional acceptance (Sappington, 2003). Thus, this theory presents *nurturance* as a different but related concept to that of *caring*. *Self-care* is a concept foundational to other theories, most notably Orem's. In Modeling and Role-Modeling the meaning of *self-care* not merely reflects self-care action or agency but is tied directly to the concept of *self-care knowledge*—the view that the client knows at some level what is wrong and what he or she needs to achieve health. In Modeling and Role-Modeling, *self-care* incorporates five concepts: hope, control, satisfaction, physical health, and support (Baldwin, 2004). Thus, the theory is a *self-care theory* that was "created to listen to the client, model the client's circumstances, and role-model key behaviors" (Baldwin & Herr, 2004, p. 108).

In her most recent book reflecting on the use and development of the theory, Erickson devotes her first chapter to the notion of life purpose (H. L. Erickson, 2006b). The search for meaning and purpose is an overarching need for people as they move across the life span and reflect on their lived experiences. The theory invites reflection and requires the nurse to enter into relationships with clients that will inevitably change both the nurse and the client. In the array of contemporary, holistic theories, Modeling and Role-Modeling is a theory providing direction for nursing care and understanding of people in a developmental process.

CLINICAL APPLICATION OF MODELING AND ROLE-MODELING IN NURSING PRACTICE

Much discussion about nursing practice has been focused on the nursing process. Does that process have meaning in a holistic view of people? Does the process provide a limited reductionistic and mechanical view of nursing's work? Does the nursing process have a place in our discipline as nursing develops beyond the medical model? The authors of the Modeling and Role-Modeling theory acknowledged very early on that *nursing process* has two distinct meanings. The first is the formalized, step-by-step problem-solving process that includes gathering and analyzing data, planning and implementing interventions, and evaluating outcomes. The second is a more basic use of the term and refers to an interactive process—the exchange between nurse and patient in which the nurse has a purpose of nurturing and supporting the client's self-care. The step-by-step use of the nursing process is linear and, as such, a problem-solving method frequently used in teaching to help a novice learn to think logically about nursing care. The second meaning of the nursing process is a means of reflecting on the entire nurse–client encounter. This second view is more descriptive of nursing. It is represented by a circular rather than linear model. If one views nursing as an interaction, the nursing process is the means by which the nurse–client interaction takes place.

The Modeling and Role-Modeling theory reminds us that experienced nurses know that one never really applies the nursing process in a step-by-step fashion. One does not assess, then diagnose, and then devise outcomes and then plan, provide, and evaluate care in that order. One is diagnosing while assessing. As soon as a nurse walks into a client's room and begins interacting with a client, that nurse is intervening because the nurse's words, actions, and presence serve as nursing interventions and are part of nursing care. The Modeling and Role-Modeling theory liberates nurses from the endless debates over use of the nursing process—the linear view of the nursing process is useful in teaching and helping nurses to think logically about care; the circular view is the *process* of carrying out nursing care grounded in person-to-person interaction.

With the primary emphasis on the interactive, interpersonal nursing process, nursing involves an ongoing exchange of information, feelings, and behaviors. Thus, the nursing process begins with the first interaction between nurse and patient. The Modeling and Role-Modeling theory accepts the view, expressed by Lucille Kinlein (1977) in the 1970s, that nursing care begins with the first patient encounter because the nurse's immediate contributions to care include the nurse herself—the presence, the unconditional acceptance, and the support and comfort that are offered from one human being to another.

Because the theory directs the nurse to begin where the client is in modeling the client's world, a comprehensive assessment is rarely done to initiate nursing care. The client will always be asked to express his or her questions, concerns, and needs. Client concerns have utmost priority because a person whose immediate needs are unattended will not progress in other ways. Thus, the theory directs the nurse's priorities of care quite simply, beginning where the client requests care to begin, knowing that as one need is met, other unmet needs will emerge to direct care. At any point, assessment is dictated by client needs, and the nurse will gather whatever information is required to understand and care for the client's expressed concerns.

The interactive nursing process includes formal, logical thinking; H. C. Erickson et al. (1983) make it clear that they value scientific thinking. However, when using Modeling and Role-Modeling, there are no preset steps in applying the nursing process. The theorists write, "When we view the nursing process predominantly as an ongoing, interactive, interpersonal relationship that *includes* use of the formal scientific mode of thought, we can regard documentation of the nursing process primarily as a valuable way to communicate with others and keep records" (p. 105). In providing care, client data are gathered to model the client's world. An evaluation of the client's stress and adaptation, as well as information on self-care knowledge, resources, and actions, is essential. Diagnoses include adaptive potential, that is, the client's potential for mobilizing resources needed to contend with stressors.

H. C. Erickson, Tomlin, and Swain do not address the use of the nursing diagnoses taxonomy developed by the North American Nursing Diagnosis Association (NANDA) with Modeling and Role-Modeling. For many nurses in practice and in education, however, Modeling and Role-Modeling has been incorporated with the NANDA taxonomy and nursing care plans and case studies. In the early 1990s, the Brigham and Women's Hospital in Boston was the first institution in the country to adopt Modeling and Role-Modeling as the base for practice hospitalwide. Their lead was followed by Oregon Health Sciences Medical Center, where the theory is currently used as the basis for nursing practice. Staff articulate nursing concerns through the use of the theory and can use the concepts of the theory to communicate client needs. For example, the nurses may write a nursing diagnostic statement of "Fatigue r/t continued state of impoverishment secondary to stressors of hospitalization and isolation." In this way, the NANDA taxonomy can be used as an atheoretical labeling of a nursing concern; Modeling and Role-Modeling provides the theoretical base for understanding and intervening with that concern. A similar meshing of Modeling and Role-Modeling with NANDA has occurred at Humboldt State University, where Modeling and Role-Modeling is being used as the conceptual basis for nursing care in an undergraduate nursing curriculum. The case study of "Harold" presented in Table 20-2 provides an illustration of how nursing care

TABLE 20-2 "Harold" A Case Study Demonstrating the Difference Between the Atheoretical Use of Nursing Diagnoses and the Use of Nursing Diagnoses with Modeling and Role-Modeling as the Theoretical Base

CASE STUDY	Nursing Care Based on Admission Data:	Revised Nursing Care Based on Modeling and Role-Modeling:
Harold is a 72-year-old unemployed truck driver who was admitted to the hospital with severe COPD, unstable angina, and severe skin lesions on his legs. He is a homeless man who lives in a nonfunctioning car on the beach. He has been admitted 7 times in the past 6 months with exacerbations of COPD, R/O sepsis, and cellulitis. He presented at this admission with a TPR of 101, 138, and 44. Laboratory results demonstrated high WBCs, abnormal blood gases, and subtherapeutic digoxin and aminophylline serum levels. Harold was dirty, odorous, and had open, draining sores on his legs. The medical regimen was aminophylline, anti-inflammatory agents, antibiotics, and his routine medications, which consisted of digoxin, brethine, etc. He was receiving oxygen but was really uncomfortable. He was also very quiet.	INITIAL DIAGNOSES Ineffective breathing pattern Altered gas exchange Self-care deficit: Bathing and hygiene Altered health maintenance Fear	REVISED DIAGNOSES Impaired mobility Fatigue Powerless
Harold was seen as "difficult" by the nurses. The nurses were frustrated by his repeated admissions. Harold was frustrated because he thought people had "judged" him and that they wanted him to "change his whole life."	INITIAL INTERVENTIONS Positioning Maintaining oxygenation	REVISED INTERVENTIONS Increasing Harold's role in his care Increasing Harold's perceivbd control
Additional data were gathered to model Harold's world. Harold said that he came to the hospital because	Administering the appropriate medications Skin care: bathing and hygiene	Clustering nursing activities because of fatigue

TABLE 20-2   (Continued)

he was sick and didn't want to burden his friends. He said that he believed people at the hospital didn't like him because they wanted him to change things he didn't want to change—like where he lived. Harold said that he had always had skin problems with his legs, but the new problem was that his dog had sand fleas and that he couldn't seem to manage. He ran out of medication because his car didn't work and didn't take his theophylline because he thought it altered his sexual functioning. When asked what he saw as his major problem, he said: "I can't get to the shower because I'm so tired—then my legs get worse!"	Reassuring Harold	Discussing Harold's specific discharge planning (dog baths; medication delivery, etc.

How did Modeling and Role Modeling-based practice change Harold's nursing care?
- Harold got holistic, individualized care.
- Harold's attitude and self-esteem improved.
- Harold participated more in self-care activities.
- There was less frustration with the nurses.
- Harold increased his adherence to treatment.
- Ten months after discharge, he had still not been readmitted.

Adapted from a presentation at the Fourth National Modeling and Role-Modeling Conference. (1992) Developed by Wendy Woodward, Humboldt State University. Used with permission.

and diagnoses differ when using nursing diagnoses atheoretically and when using nursing diagnoses with Modeling and Role-Modeling as the theoretical base.

In carrying out nursing care, the nurse must use role-modeling, that is, help the client in attaining, maintaining, or promoting health through purposeful interventions that are consistent with the client's model of the world. Care is based on the five aims of interventions and is consistent with the client's adaptive potential (see Figure 20-3). The nurse's role is to facilitate, nurture, and provide unconditional acceptance while assisting the client to achieve health. Evaluation of nursing care is directed toward goals mutually determined between patient and client.

CRITIQUE OF THE THEORY OF MODELING AND ROLE-MODELING

1. *What is the historical context of the theory?*   Theories long studied by nursing students—Maslow, Erikson, Piaget, Selye, and Engel—emerge in a new perspective in Modeling and Role-Modeling as these psychosocial and developmental theories become useful and immediate in understanding the client's world. Modeling and Role-Modeling provides a sense of the true meaning of client-directed care, for the client is trusted as knowing what he or she needs from the nurse to achieve health. The theory provides a unique way of understanding nursing. The client is seen in a truly holistic manner, as a person with an understandable and individual worldview. Nursing's task becomes that of knowing the client, discovering the client's needs and concerns, affirming that the client is directing all health-related actions, and facilitating the client's striving toward health. Assumptions of the theory include that human beings are each unique, but with identifiable similarities; that each person is born with a genetic base and a spiritual drive; that the individual has bio-psycho-social components; and that the whole of any person is greater than the sum of his or her parts. Further, the assumption that each person has self-care knowledge and resources such that he or she knows on some level what made him or her ill and what is needed to make himself or herself better is a major divergence from traditional biomedical views of disease. This emphasis on self-care knowledge has its roots in the work of Milton Erickson.

2. *What are the basic concepts and relationships presented by the theory?*   Modeling and Role-Modeling provides a logical framework from which to understand nursing and from which to plan and provide care. Major concepts of the definition of the person, the meaning of health, and the client's responsibility for self-care are clear. The five aims of intervention emphasize the importance of the nurse–client relationship. Nurses who understand the interactive nature of what they are doing readily accept the view of the nursing process as an interpersonal process. H. C. Erickson (1990b) acknowledged the functional relationships among the concepts embedded within the theory, resulting in the following three major theoretical linkages:

1. Developmental task resolution and need satisfaction,
2. Basic need status, object attachment and loss, growth and development,
3. Adaptive potential and need satisfaction (p. 18).

Erickson also provided examples of theoretical propositions that can be derived from these linkages and used to direct care planning. These examples are the following:

1. Individuals' ability to contend with new stressors is directly related to the ability to mobilize resources needed.
2. Individuals' ability to mobilize resources is directly related to their need deficits and assets.
3. Distressors are related to unmet basic needs; stressors are related to unmet growth needs.
4. Objects that repeatedly facilitate the individual in need satisfaction take on significance for the individual. When this occurs, attachment to the object results.
5. Secure attachment produces feelings of worthiness.
6. Feelings of worthiness result in a sense of futurity.
7. Real, threatened, or perceived loss of the attachment object results in the grief process.

8. Basic need deficits coexist with the grief process.
9. An adequate alternative object must be perceived available in order for the individual to resolve the grief process.
10. Prolonged grief due to an unavailable or inadequate object results in morbid grief.
11. Unmet basic and growth needs interfere with growth processes.
12. Repeated satisfaction of basic needs is prerequisite to working through developmentaltasks and resolution of related developmental crises.
13. Morbid grief is always related to need deficits. (H. C. Erickson, 1990b, p. 18)

3. *What major phenomena of concern to nursing are presented?* **(***These phenomena may include* **but are not limited to** *human beings, environment, health, interpersonal relations, caring, goal attainment, adaptation, and energy fields***).**   The major phenomena of concern to Modeling and Role-Modeling are self-care knowledge, resources, and actions; affiliated–individuation; and adaptive-potential. These concepts direct the nurse's view of the client (i.e., one who has internal knowledge and perceptions of self that are essential to understand when working with the person to achieve health) and help in understanding behavior since actions (or nonactions) are based on an individual's state of adaptive potential. Further, the concept that a person has an innate spiritual drive is recognition of the spiritual essence of human beings. This aspect of the theory, while appealing intuitively to any holistic nurse, is less developed than the other concepts and has been identified by Erickson as one requiring further attention and development (H. C. Erickson, 1999). Walker and Erickson (2006) present an updated discussion of mind-body-spirit relations. Although energy concepts are implied in Modeling and Role-Modeling, the relationships between energy theories and modeling and role-modeling concepts are fully explored and discussed by Brekke and Schultz (2006).

4. *To whom does the theory apply? In what situations? In what ways?*   Theories should be relatively simple but generalizable. The simplicity of Modeling and Role-Modeling is its beauty. Trusting that clients know (at some level) what they need and planning nursing care based on each client's model of the world, as well as individual need deficits, need satisfaction, and ability to mobilize resources, is a simple yet profound idea. Beginning students in their first nursing course can readily understand the basic concepts, while the theory is still useful to advanced practitioners.

Modeling and Role-Modeling has been applied to clients who are individuals, families, and communities, and it has been applied to clients in all nursing specialty areas of practice. The theory can be used in assessing a family by determining both the adaptive potential of a family group and the adaptive potential of the individual family members (Frisch & Kelley, 1996). Many of the families referred to as "dysfunctional" are families living in maladaptive equilibrium. According to this theory, the family would need to be pushed into a state of arousal through some kind of crisis to be motivated for change. Further, individual members of the family may be in a state of impoverishment and require direct care and nurturance in order to mobilize resources to gain a healthy state of adaptation. The theory provides the nurse with a unique way of understanding a family and therefore suggests unique interventions. The concepts of the theory may also be used in work with groups or communities. For example, a work group (nurses on a hospital unit) may be understood in a manner similar to families. Likewise, a community can be assessed according to the APAM model and understood in an entirely different way. Benson (2003) developed the Group Adaptive Potential Assessment Model (G-APAM) for assessing adaptive potential of groups.

5. *By what method or methods can this theory be tested?* Methodological diversity has been demonstrated through scholarly inquiry of many areas within the theory. Acton, Irvin, Jensen, Hopkins, and Miller (1997) specify advantages of combining qualitative and quantitative techniques. Investigations have been reported that test or expand the concepts of adaptive potential (Barnfather, 1990; Barnfather et al., 1989a, 1989b; Benson, 2003; H. Erickson, & Swain, 1982; Finch, 1990), self-care (Baas, 2004; Beery & Baas, 1996; Bowman, 1998; H. C. Erickson, 1990a; Hertz & Anschutz, 2002; Kennedy, 1991; Rosenow, 1992), and affiliated–individuation (Acton, 1993; Acton & Miller, 1996). Studies are also reported that investigate the theoretical proposition derived from the major theoretical linkages embedded in the theory. These studies focus on developmental tasks, needs, and psychosocial developmental residual (Curl, 1992; Jensen, 1995; Keck, 1989; MacLean, 1987, 1990, 1992; S. H. Miller, 1986).

Acton et al. (1997) describe how five researchers involved in a large research project used different data subsets and different methods to explain or affirm middle range concepts and theories from Modeling and Role-Modeling. Acton (1993) found that affiliated–individuation was a significant predictor of well-being and further found, using Baron and Kenny's (1986) method to test for mediation, that affiliated–individuation is a resource used to mediate between the stress of caregiving and the well-being of the caregiver. Irvin (1993) investigated the relationships among perceived stress of caregivers and self-care resources using path analysis with regression procedures and found that responses to stressors were mediated somewhat by self-care resources such as hope, self-worth, and perceived social support. The study also supported that feelings of worthiness result in a sense of hope for the future. Irvin and Acton (1996) further employed Baron and Kenney's method to explore the mediating effect of self-care resources on stress and well-being and found that resources mediated the relationship between stress and well-being. Jensen (1995) used case study analysis to compare the actual responses to interventions with the response patterns predicted by the theory and found evidence of need satisfaction attainment, attachment, and resolution of loss and grief. Qualitative analysis of the case studies also showed a decrease in burden over time and an evidence of positive growth outcomes. Hopkins (1995) studied the concept of adaptive potential and utilized multivariate analysis of variance to demonstrate that caregivers in a state of equilibrium who were caring for adults with dementia showed perceived support and an increased sense of well-being. E. W. Miller's (1993) study used qualitative methods to expand knowledge of the inner spirit, and Acton and Miller (1996) pursued qualitative methods and demonstrated that support group interventions had some positive effect on affiliated individuation.

6. *Does this theory direct nursing actions that may lead to favorable outcomes?* The theory assists the nurse by giving direction and tools for action—beginning with the five aims of intervention. The nurse can then assess if trust has been achieved, if client strengths have been supported, and so on. Thus, the nurse has a framework to interpret and think about nursing actions. Critical thinking requires language to put into words and thoughts some of the areas of practice that can otherwise be relegated to intuition or spontaneity. Modeling and Role-Modeling directs the nurse to reflect on those intuitive moments and interpret and understand them on the basis of concepts such as adaptive potential, self-care knowledge, and modeling of another's world. Thus, practice through the use of the theory is both reflective and thoughtful.

The notion of five aims of intervention directs all nursing actions. While the five aims may seem simplistic, they provide a basis and a place to begin when a nurse is unsure of how to proceed. For example, in the setting of psychiatric nursing, nurses applying the theory became concerned with the notion of modeling the client's world, when the client's world was irrational and delusional. Returning to the five aims of intervention helped the nurses focus on what each knew is the basis of psychiatric nursing care—building trust and promoting positive orientation. Once the nurses adopted this focus, they began to understand that to model the client's world meant to understand the meaning of the delusions to the client. Thus, nursing interventions were based on building a positive and trusting relationship with the client and understanding the client's situations from within his own worldview.

The APAM is also useful for directing therapeutic nursing interventions. A client who is impoverished cannot be expected to initiate self-care actions. Interventions for a client who is in maladaptive equilibrium need to be aimed at motivation to change rather than teaching self-care. Teaching self-care would be appropriate for someone in arousal.

The three major federally funded research projects investigating this theory have all been intervention studies aimed at identifying the usefulness and cost-effectiveness of Modeling and Role-Modeling as the basis for practice. Helen Erickson has been the primary investigator for these projects, each of which has focused on a different population of clients with chronic health problems: hypertension, diabetes, and Alzheimer's disease. There have been many examples of the use of concepts from the theory directing therapeutic interventions (Frisch & Kelley, 1996; Holl, 1992; Kinney, 1990; Walsh, Vanden Bosch, & Boehm, 1989). The examples of theoretical propositions presented by Helen Erickson (1990b) are also useful in demonstrating how Modeling and Role-Modeling can be used to direct nursing interventions.

7. How contagious is the theory?   Since the initial publication of the theory in 1983, there has been increasing interest in and use of the theory. The theory has been used in multiple settings to guide nursing education, research, and practice throughout the United States. In education, the theory was adopted as the organizing framework for an undergraduate nursing curriculum in California in 1990. The theory is also used as an organizing framework in RN–BSN programs in Michigan and Minnesota. While many nurses use the theory to direct their own practice, Brigham and Women's Hospital in Boston adopted the theory as a housewide framework for nursing care in the early 1990s, and its lead was followed when the Oregon Health Sciences University adopted the theory for nursing practice in 2005. Research on the theory has been conducted in several medical centers and schools of nursing, including the University of Texas at Austin; Humboldt State University in Arcata, California; and the University of Cincinnati, Ohio. Another rather interesting application of the theory includes use of the theory to guide behavior modification programs for weight management (Folse, 2002; Lombardo & Roof, 2005; Timmerman & Acton, 2001), management of lifestyle issues associated with specific chronic diseases (Baas, 1992, 2004; Baas, Beery, Fontana, & Waggoner, 1999; Baldwin, 2004; Baldwin & Herr, 2004;

Beery et al., 2002; Bischof, 2006; Bowman, 1998; Daniels, 1994; H. Erickson & Swain, 1977; Holl, 1992; Hopkins, 1995; Keck, 1989; Kline Leidy, 1990; Landis, 1991; Leidy, 1989; Liddy & Traver, 1995; Perese, 1997; Robinson, 1992; Sofhauser, 1996), and caregiving (Acton, 1993, 1997; Acton & Miller, 1996; Baker, 1999; Irvin, 1993; Irvin & Acton, 1996, 1997; Jensen, 1995; E. W. Miller, 1993).

The Society for the Advancement of Modeling and Role-Modeling (SAMRM) held its charter meeting and the first theory conference in 1986 in Ann Arbor, Michigan. The Society continues to meet biennially at different locations throughout the United States for the purpose of disseminating knowledge relating to the theory acquired through research, practice, and teaching. The 11th national conference of the Society was held in Portland, Oregon, in conjunction with Oregon Health Sciences University Hospitals and Clinics in 2006. At that meeting, 26 presentations on the research and use of the theory were made in addition to a poster session. The 12th national conference was held in Chicago in 2008, and the 2010 conference is being planned for San Antonio, Texas. In providing a new way of understanding nursing, the Society stimulates evaluation and the study of nursing's effect on a client's health. The Society maintains a web page at http://www.mrmnursingtheory.org and a listserv at listserv@lists.ufl.edu, which is actively accessed by those using the theory in practice and conducting research on varying aspects of the theory. SAMRM will fund research, scholarship, or practice projects relating to the theory through a grant program begun in 2007. In the coming years, the focus of the society will be to develop a Center for the Study and Practice of Modeling and Role-Modeling theory and paradigm. The recent calls for a center for the advancement of the theory by those actively involved with the study and use of the theory further speak to the contagiousness of the theory.

The authors of this chapter note that the theory is not as well known as other nursing theories but that among those who have studied and used the theory, there is a growing and enthusiastic group of adherents who can no longer imagine practicing nursing without modeling their clients' worlds.

STRENGTHS AND LIMITATIONS

The theory has many strengths, including a strong holistic approach and emphasis on the nurse–client interaction and client-centeredness, as has been described. Its major limitation may be that it is relatively unknown and appears simplistic. Nurses coming to learn about the theory have felt that it merely describes what they have always done intuitively and that it is too simple merely to put the client in charge of his or her health care. A limitation in practice, particularly for inexperienced nurses, has been that the mandate to "model the client's world" leads, in some cases, to role confusion between being a caring professional and a caring friend.

Nurses at any level can quickly learn how to develop a model of the client's world and gain rewards from this practice. In practice, the development of empathetic assessment is so enticing that nurses may fail to develop the science of modeling. The science of modeling requires professional education. The scientific base for the analysis of data relating to the client's model of the world includes a broad understanding of both the physical and the social sciences. To be complete in modeling the client's world, the nurse must draw on many theories in other disciplines, such as psychology, sociology, cultural anthropology, physiology, and pathophysiology.

Summary

The Modeling and Role-Modeling theory suggests an interactive, interpersonal role for nursing. Modeling is the process used to develop an understanding of the client's world; role-modeling is the process of facilitating health-promoting behaviors. Nursing care is based on clients' adaptive potential and directed toward the five aims of intervention: building trust, promoting positive orientation, promoting perceived control, promoting strengths, and setting mutual, health-directed goals. From within this theory, the client is empowered to direct care, based on self-care knowledge, self-care resources, and self-care actions, as the client's perceived needs are addressed. The theory has been applied to work with clients who are individuals, families, and communities. Currently, the theory is being used in both practice and education, and research is being conducted to document and evaluate components of the theory.

Thought Questions

Discussion is based on the following case:

Two women are hospitalized for hysterectomies. They are both 48 years old with attentive husbands and grown children. They each have two sons and one daughter. After recovering from anesthesia, one of the women is ready to get up, get dressed, and go home. She is on the phone talking to her family to have them come and get her. She is directing the nursing staff that she will be leaving by 11 A.M. and is upset that they have not moved fast enough to meet her needs for discharge. Of course, she requires some assistance and is moving slowly and has requested some medication to help with pain control. The other woman is moaning quietly, does not want to move, and expresses that she has a great deal of pain and that she cannot possibly do her own hygiene care or get up and walk, even with assistance. She has no visitors and has asked her family not to come this morning but, rather, to let her rest.

Practicing from a Modeling and Role-Modeling perspective, consider the following:

- What questions would you ask of these women to model their worlds?
- Considering what you know and observe, how do you think they are alike and how do you think they are different in relation to developmental stage, internal and external resources, adaptive potential, and loss and grief?
- How will nursing interventions differ for these two women? How might the nurse intervene if not through role-modeling?
- Can you think of other situations where a nurse could model the client's world and then role-model nursing interventions?
- What happens when the nurse understands the model of the client's world but plans care on the basis of the nurse's model of the world, which is incongruent with that of the client's?

References

Acton, G. J. (1993). The relationships among stressors, stress, affiliated-individuation, burden, and well-being in caregivers of adults with dementia: A test of the theory and paradigm for nursing, Modeling and Role-Modeling. *Dissertation Abstracts International, 54*(05B), 2436. Abstract retrieved December 17, 2007, from Dissertation Abstracts Online database.

Acton, G. J. (1997). The mediating effect of affiliated-individuation in caregivers of adults with dementia. *Journal of Holistic Nursing, 15,* 336–357.

Acton, G. J., Irvin, B. L., Jensen, B. A., Hopkins, B. A., & Miller, E. W. (1997). Explicating middle-range theory through methodological diversity. *Advances in Nursing Science, 19*(3), 78–85.

Acton, G. J., & Miller, E. W. (1996). Affiliated-individuation in caregivers of adults with dementia. *Issues in Mental Health Nursing, 17,* 245–260.

Baas, L. S. (1992). The relationships among self-care knowledge, self-care resources, activity level and life satisfaction in persons three to six months after a myocardial infarction. *Dissertation Abstracts International, 53*(04B), 1780. Abstract retrieved December 27, 2007, from Dissertation Abstracts Online database.

Baas, L. S. (2004). Self-care resources and activity as predictors of quality of life in persons after myocardial infarction. *Dimensions of Critical Care Nursing, 23*(3), 131–138.

Baas, L. S., Beery, T. A., Fontana, J. A., & Wagoner, L. E. (1999). An exploratory study of developmental growth in adults with heart failure. *Journal of Holistic Nursing, 17*(2), 117–138.

Baker, C. (1999). Innovative new program. From chaos to order: A nursing-based psycho-education program for parents of children with attention-deficit hyperactivity disorder. *Canadian Journal of Nursing Research, 31*(2), 71–75.

Baldwin, C. M. (1996). Perceptions of hope: Lived experiences of elementary school children in an urban setting. *Journal of Multicultural Nursing and Health, 2*(3), 41–45.

Baldwin, C. M. (2004). Interstitial cystitis and self care: Bearing the burden. *Urologic Nursing, 24,* 111–112.

Baldwin, C. M., & Herr, S. W. (2004). The impact of self-care practices on treatment of interstitial cystitis. *Urological Nursing, 24*(2), 107–110, 113.

Barnfather, J. S. (1990). An overview of the ability to mobilize coping resources related to basic needs. In H. C. Erickson & C. K. Kinney (Eds.), *Modeling and Role-Modeling: Theory, practice and research,* monograph, 1(1), pp. 156–169. Austin, TX: Society for the Advancement of Modeling and Role-Modeling.

Barnfather, J. S., Swain, M. A. P., & Erickson, H. C. (1989a). Evaluation of two assessment techniques for adaptation to stress. *Nursing Science Quarterly, 2,* 172–182.

Barnfather, J. S., Swain, M. A. P., & Erickson, H. C. (1989b). Construct validity of an aspect of the coping process: Potential adaptation to stress. *Issues in Mental Health Nursing, 10,* 23–40.

Baron, R. M., & Kenny, D. A. (1986). The moderator-mediator variable distinction in social psychological research: Conceptual, strategic, and statistical considerations. *Journal of Personality and Social Psychology, 51,* 1173–1182.

Beery, T., & Baas, L. (1996). Medical devices and attachment: Holistic healing in the age of invasive technology. *Issues in Mental Health Nursing, 17,* 233–243.

Beery, T. A., Baas, L. S., Fowler, C., & Allen, G. (2002). Spirituality in persons with heart failure. *Journal of Holistic Nursing, 20,* 5–30.

Benson, D. S. (2003). Adaptive Potential Assessment Model applied to small groups. *Dissertation Abstracts International, 64*(12B), 6373. Abstract retrieved December 27, 2007, from Dissertation Abstracts Online database.

Benson, D. (2006). Adaptation: Coping with stress. In H. L. Erickson (Ed.), *Modeling and Role-Modeling: A view from the client's world* (pp. 240–271). Cedar Park, TX: Unicorns Unlimited.

Bischof, J. R. (2006). A comparison of quality of life in adult patients with heart failure in two medical settings: A heart failure clinic and a physician practice. *Dissertation Abstracts International, 67*(10B), 5660. Abstract retrieved December 1, 2009, from Dissertation Abstracts Online database.

Bowman, S. S. (1998). *The human-environment relationship in self-care when healing from episodic illness.* Unpublished doctoral dissertation, University of Texas at Austin. *Dissertation Abstracts International, 60*(07B), 3199. Abstract retrieved December 27, 2007, from Dissertation Abstracts Online database.

Brekke, M., & Schultz, E. (2006). Energy theories: Modeling and Role-Modeling. In H. L. Erickson (Ed.), *Modeling and Role-Modeling: A view from the client's world* (pp. 33–65). Cedar Park, TX: Unicorns Unlimited.

Campbell, J., Finch, D., Allport, C., Erickson, H. C., & Swain, M. A. P. (1985). A theoretical approach to nursing assessment. *Journal of Advanced Nursing, 10,* 111–115.

Curl, E. D. (1992). Hope in the elderly: Exploring the relationship between psychosocial developmental residual and hope. *Dissertation Abstracts International, 53*(04B), 1782. Abstract retrieved December 17, 2007, from Dissertation Abstracts Online database.

Daniels, R. D. (1994). Exploring the self-care variables that explain a wellness lifestyle in spinal cord injured wheelchair basketball athletes. *Dissertation Abstracts International, 55*(07B), 2654. Abstract retrieved December 17, 2007, from Dissertation Abstracts Online database.

Erickson, H. (1976). *Identification of states of coping utilizing physiological and psychological data.* Unpublished master's thesis, University of Michigan.

Erickson, H. C. (1984). Self-care knowledge: Relations among the concepts support, hope, control, satisfaction with daily life, and physical health status. *Dissertation Abstracts International, 45*(06B), 1731. Abstract retrieved December 27, 2007, from Dissertation Abstracts Online database.

Erickson, H. C. (1990a). Self-care knowledge: An exploratory study. In H. C. Erickson & C. K. Kinney (Eds.), *Modeling and Role-Modeling: Theory, research and practice,* monograph, 1(1), pp. 178–202. Austin, TX: Society for Advancement of Modeling and Role-Modeling.

Erickson, H. C. (1990b). Theory based practice. In H. C. Erickson & C. K. Kinney (Eds.), *Modeling and role-modeling: Theory, research and practice,* monograph, 1(1), pp. 1–27. Austin, TX: Society for Advancement of Modeling and Role-Modeling.

Erickson, H. C. (1999). Greetings. *Modeling and Role-Modeling Newsletter, 9,* 2, 1–2.

Erickson, H. L. (Ed.). (2006a). *Modeling and Role-Modeling: A view from the client's world.* Cedar Park, TX: Unicorns Unlimited.

Erickson, H. L. (2006b). Searching for life purpose: Discovering meaning. In H. L. Erickson (Ed.), *Modeling and Role-Modeling: A view from the client's world* (pp. 5–32). Cedar Park, TX: Unicorns Unlimited.

Erickson, H., & Swain, M. A. (1977). The utilization of a nursing care model for the treatment of essential hypertension. *Circulation* (abstract).

Erickson, H., & Swain, M. A. (1982). A model for assessing potential adaptation to stress. *Research in Nursing and Health, 5,* 93–101.

Erickson, H. C., Tomlin, E. M., & Swain, M. A. P. (1983). *Modeling and Role-Modeling. A theory and paradigm for nursing.* Lexington, SC: Pine Press.

Erickson, M. E. (2006). Attachment, loss, and reattachment. In H. L. Erickson (Ed.), *Modeling and Role-Modeling: A view from the client's world* (pp. 208–239). Cedar Park, TX: Unicorns Unlimited.

Erickson, M. E., Erickson, H. L., & Jensen, B. (2006). Affiliated–individuation and self-actualization: Need satisfaction as prerequisite. In H. L. Erickson (Ed.), *Modeling and Role-Modeling: A view from the client's world* (pp. 182–207). Cedar Park, TX: Unicorns Unlimited.

Erikson, E. (1963). *Childhood and society.* New York: Norton.

Finch, D. (1990). Testing a theoretically based nursing assessment. In H. C. Erickson & C. K. Kinney (Eds.), *Modeling and Role-Modeling: Theory, research and practice,* monograph, 1(1), pp. 203–213. Austin, TX: Society for Advancement of Modeling and Role-Modeling.

Folse, V. N. (2002). The Family Experience With Eating Disorders Scale: Psychometric analysis. *Dissertation Abstracts International, 63*(04B), 193. Abstract retrieved December 17, 2007, from Dissertation Abstracts Online database.

Frisch, N., & Kelley, J. (1996). *Healing life's crises: A guide for nurses.* Albany, NY: Delmar.

Hertz, J. E. (1996). Conceptualization of perceived enactment of autonomy in the elderly. *Issues in Mental Health Nursing, 17,* 261–273.

Hertz, J. E., & Anschutz, C. (2002). Relationships among perceived enactment of autonomy, self-care, and holistic health in community-dwelling older adults. *Journal of Holistic Nursing, 20,* 166–186.

Hertz, J. E., & Baas, L. (2006). Self-care: Knowledge, resources, and actions. In H. L. Erickson (Ed.), *Modeling and Role-Modeling: A view from the client's world* (pp. 97–120). Cedar Park, TX: Unicorns Unlimited.

Holl, R. M. (1992). The effect of role-modeled visiting in comparison to restricted visiting on the well-being of clients who had open heart surgery and their significant family members in the critical care unit. *Dissertation Abstracts International, 53*(08B), 4030. Abstract retrieved December 27, 2007, from Dissertation Abstracts Online database.

Hopkins, B. A. (1994). Development and validation of a content analysis tool to identify adaptive potential. *Dissertation Abstracts International, 55*(06B), 2156. Abstract retrieved December 29, 2007, from Dissertation Abstracts Online database.

Hopkins, B. A. (1995). *Adaptive potential of caregivers of adults with dementia.* Paper presented at the meeting of Sigma Theta Tau International, Detroit, MI.

Irvin, B. L. (1993). Social support, self-worth and hope as self-care resources for coping with caregiver status. *Dissertation Abstracts International, 54*(06B), 2995. Abstract retrieved December 17, 2007, from Dissertation Abstracts Online database.

Irvin, B. L., & Acton, G. (1996). Stress mediation in caregivers of cognitively impaired adults: Theoretical model testing. *Nursing Research, 45*(3), 160–166.

Irvin, B. L., & Acton, G. J. (1997). Stress, hope, and well-being of women caring for family members with Alzheimer's disease. *Holistic Nursing Practice, 11* (2), 69–79.

Jensen, B. J. A. (1995). Caregiver responses to a theoretically based intervention program: Case study analysis. *Dissertation Abstracts International, 56*(06B), 3127. Abstract retrieved December 17, 2007, from Dissertation Abstracts Online database.

Keck, V. E. (1989). Perceived social support, basic needs satisfaction, and coping strategies of the chronically ill. *Dissertation Abstracts International, 50*(09B), 3921. Abstract retrieved December 27, 2007, from Dissertation Abstracts Online database.

Kennedy, G. T. (1991). A nursing investigation of comfort and comforting care of the acutely ill patient. *Dissertation Abstracts International, 52*(12B), 6318. Abstract retrieved December 27, 2007, from Dissertation Abstracts Online database.

Kinlein, L. (1977). *Independent nursing practice with clients.* Philadelphia: Lippincott.

Kinney, C. K. (1990). Facilitating growth and development: A paradigm case for Modeling and Role-Modeling. *Issues in Mental Health Nursing, 11*, 375–395.

Kline Leidy, N. (1990). A structural model of stress, psychosocial resources, and symptomatic experience in chronic physical illness. *Nursing Research, 39*, 230–236.

Landis, B. J. P. (1991). *Uncertainty, spiritual well-being, and psychosocial adjustment to chronic illness.* Unpublished doctoral dissertation, University of Texas at Austin.

Leidy, N. (1989). A physiologic analysis of stress and chronic illness. *Journal of Advanced Nursing, 14*, 868–876.

Leidy, N. K., & Traver, G. A. (1995). Psychological factors contributing to functional performance in people with COPD: Are there gender differences? *Research in Nursing and Health, 18*, 535–546.

Leininger, M., & McFarland, M. R. (2006). *Culture care diversity and universality: A worldwide nursing theory.* Sudbury, MA: Jones & Bartlett.

Lombardo, S. L., & Roof, M. (2005). A case study applying the modeling and role-modeling theory to morbid obesity. *Home Healthcare Nurse, 23*(7), 425–428.

MacLean, T. (1987). Erikson's psychosocial development and stressors as factors in healthy lifestyle. *Dissertation Abstracts International, 48*, 1710A. (University Microfilms No. 87–20, 311)

MacLean, T. (1990). Health behaviors, developmental residual and stressors. In H. C. Erickson & C. K. Kinney (Eds.), *Modeling and Role-Modeling: Theory, research and practice,* monograph, 1(1), pp. 147–155. Austin, TX: Society for Advancement of Modeling and Role-Modeling.

MacLean, T. (1992). Influence of psychosocial development and life events on the health practices of adults. *Issues in Mental Health Nursing, 13*, 403–414.

Maslow, A.H. (1970). *Motivation and personality* (2nd ed.). New York: Harper & Row.

Miller, E. W. (1993). The meaning of encouragement and its connection with the inner spirit as perceived by caregivers of the cognitively impaired. *Dissertation Abstracts International, 55*(06B), 2157. Abstract retrieved December 27, 2007, from Dissertation Abstracts Online database.

Miller, S. H. (1986). The relationship between psychosocial development and coping ability among disabled teenagers. *Dissertation Abstracts International, 47*, 4113B. (University Microfilms No. 87–02, 793)

Orem, D. E. (1995). *Nursing: Concepts and practice* (5th ed.). St. Louis: Mosby.

Perese, E. F. (1997). Unmet needs of persons with chronic mental illnesses: Relationship to their adaptation to community living. *Issues in Mental Health Nursing, 18*, 19–34.

Robinson, K. R. (1992). Developing a scale to measure responses of clients with actual or potential myocardial infarctions. *Dissertation Abstracts International, 53*(12B), 6226. Abstract retrieved December 17, 2007, from Dissertation Abstracts Online database.

Rogers, S. (1996). Facilitative affiliation: Nurse–client interactions that enhance healing. *Issues in Mental Health Nursing, 17*, 171–184.

Rogers, S. (1997). Facilitative affiliation: A new NPR for the 21st century. *Proceedings of the First International Nursing Conference: Connecting Conversations of Nursing: Vol. 1, Nursing scholarship and practice* (pp. 217–221). Reykjavik: University Press, University of Iceland.

Rosenow, D. J. (1992). Multidimensional scaling analysis of self-care actions for reintegrating holistic health after a myocardial infarction: Implications for nursing. *Dissertation Abstracts International, 53*(04B), 1789. Abstract retrieved December 17, 2007, from Dissertation Abstracts Online database.

Sappington, J. Y. (2003). Nurturance: the spirit of holistic nursing. *Journal of Holistic Nursing, 21*, 8–19.

Sofhauser, C. D. (1996). The relations among hostility, self-esteem, self-concept, and psychosocial residual in persons with coronary heart disease. *Dissertation Abstracts International, 58*(01B), 138. Abstract retrieved December 17, 2007, from Dissertation Abstracts Online database.

Swain, M. A., & Stickel, S. B. (1981). Influencing adherence among hypertensives. *Research in Nursing and Health, 4*, 213–222.

Timmerman, G. A., & Acton, G. J. (2001). The relationship between basic need satisfaction and emotional eating. *Issues in Mental Health Nursing, 22*(7), 691–701.

Tomlin, E. M. (1990). Spiritual concerns in nursing: The interface of modeling and Role-modeling with professional nursing's Christian roots and values. In H. C. Erickson & C. K. Kinney (Eds.), *Modeling and Role-Modeling. Theory, practice and research*, monograph, 1(1), pp. 40–66. Austin, TX: Society for the Advancement of Modeling and Role-Modeling.

Walker, M. J., & Erickson, H. L. (2006). Mind-body-spirit relations. In H. L. Erickson (Ed.), *Modeling and Role-Modeling: A view from the client's world* (pp. 67–91). Cedar Park, TX: Unicorns Unlimited.

Walsh, K. K., Vanden Bosch, T. M., & Boehm, S. (1989). Modeling and Role-Modeling: Integrating nursing theory into practice. *Journal of Advanced Nursing, 14*, 775–761.

Watson, J. (2005). *Caring science as sacred science.* Philadelphia: F. A. Davis.

World Health Organization. (1946). *Preamble to the Constitution of the World Health Organization* as adopted by the International Health Conference, New York, 19 June–22 July 1946; signed on July 22, 1946, by the representatives of 61 states (Official Records of the World Health Organization, no. 2, p. 100) and entered into force on 7 April 1948. The definition has not been amended since 1948. Retrieved December 29, 2007, from http://www.who.int/suggestions/faq/en.

Bibliography

Acton, G., Mayhew, P., Hopkins, B., & Yauk, S. (1999). Communicating with person's with dementia: The impaired person's perspective. *Journal of Gerontological Nursing, 25*(2), 6–13.

Ashley, M. (1996). Differences between the attitudes and behaviors of oncology nurses: Inclusion of sexuality concerns as a component of care. *Masters Abstracts International, 35*(03), 786. Abstract retrieved December 27, 2007, from Dissertation Abstracts Online database.

Baldwin, C. M. M. (1998). An investigation of health outcomes for urban elementary children utilizing an innovative self-care health curriculum model as compared to the traditional health curriculum. *Dissertation Abstracts International, 59*(12A), 4372. Abstract retrieved December 17, 2007, from Dissertation Abstracts Online database.

Barnfather, J. S. (1987). Mobilizing coping resources related to basic need status in healthy, young adults. *Dissertation Abstracts International, 49*(02B), 360. Abstract retrieved December 17, 2007, from Dissertation Abstracts Online database.

Barnfather, J. S. (1993). Testing a theoretical proposition for Modeling and Role-Modeling: Basic need and adaptive potential status. *Issues in Mental Health Nursing, 14*, 1–18.

Barnfather, J. S., & Ronis, D. L. (2000). Test of a model of psychosocial resources, stress, and health among undereducated adults. *Research in Nursing and Health, 23*, 55–66.

Bischof, J. R. (2006). A comparison of quality of life in adult patients with heart failure in two medical settings: A heart failure clinic and a physician practice. *Dissertation Abstracts International, 67*(10B), 5660. Abstract retrieved December 17, 2007, from Dissertation Abstracts Online database.

Darling-Fisher, C. S. (1987). The relationship between mothers' and fathers' Eriksonian psychosocial attributes, perceptions of family support, and adaptation to parenthood. *Dissertation Abstracts International, 48*(06B), 1640. Abstract retrieved December 17, 2007, from Dissertation Abstracts Online database.

Emerson, E. A. (1992). Playing for health: The process of play and self-expression in children who have experienced a sexual trauma. *Dissertation Abstracts International, 53* (06B), 2784. Abstract retrieved December 17, 2007, from Dissertation Abstracts Online database.

Erickson, H. (1983). Coping with new systems. *Journal of Nursing Education, 22*, 132–135.

Erickson, H. (1988). Modeling and Role-Modeling: Ericksonian techniques applied to physiological problems. In J. Zeig & S. Lankton (Eds.), *Developing Ericksonian therapy: State of the art.* New York: Brunner/Mazel.

Erickson, H. (1990). Modeling and Role-Modeling with psychophysiological problems. In J. Zeig & S. Gilligan (Eds.), *Brief therapy: Myths, methods and metaphors* (pp. 473–491). New York: Brunner/Mazel.

Erickson, M. E. (1996). The relationships among need satisfaction, support, and maternal attachment in the adolescent mother. *Dissertation Abstracts International, 57*(06B), 3653. Abstract retrieved December 17, 2007, from Dissertation Abstracts International database.

Kinney, C., & Erickson, H. (1990). Modeling the client's world: A way to holistic care. *Issues in Mental Health Nursing, 11*, 93–108.

Parsons, C. M. (1992). Life satisfaction as perceived by the elderly home care client. *Masters Abstracts International, 21*(01), 280. Abstract retrieved December 17, 2007, from Dissertation Abstracts Online database.

Rogers, S. R. (2002). Nurse-patient interactions: what do patients have to say. *Dissertation Abstracts International, 64*(03B), 1183. Abstract retrieved December 17, 2007, from Dissertation Abstracts Online database.

Straub, H. G. (1993). The relationship among intellectual, psychosocial, and ego development of nursing students in associate, baccalaureate, and baccalaureate completion programs. *Dissertation Abstracts International, 55*(02B), 371. Abstract retrieved December 17, 2007, from Dissertation Abstracts Online database.

Weber, G. J. T. (1995). Employed mothers with preschool-aged children: An exploration of their lived experiences and the nature of their well-being. *Dissertation Abstracts International, 456*(06B), 3131. Abstract retrieved December 27, 2007, from Dissertation Abstracts Online database.

Annotated Bibliography

Baas, L. S. (2004). Self-care resources and activity as predictors of quality of life in persons after myocardial infarction. *Dimensions of Critical Care Nursing, 23*(3), 131–138.

This is a report of an ex post facto correlational study involving 86 subjects conducted to examine predictors of quality of life in persons three to six months after a myocardial infarction. Modeling and Role-Modeling provides a useful explanation of how self-care resources and self-care knowledge can be applied to persons recovering from myocardial infarction.

Erickson, H., & Swain, M. A. (1990). Mobilizing self-care resources: A nursing intervention for hypertension. *Issues in Mental Health Nursing, 11*, 217–235.

The purpose of this study was to investigate the potential for mobilizing self-care resources. Subjects were 10 persons with hypertension matched with 10 persons in a comparison group. Further research is needed with larger groups of subjects to validate the findings of this study that indicated treating the person rather than the symptom (hypertension) is likely to be helpful in dealing with stressors, reducing stress, and dealing with loss and grief.

Erickson, M. (2006). Developmental processes. In H. L. Erickson (Ed.), *Modeling and Role-Modeling: A view from the client's world* (pp. 121–181). Cedar Park, TX: Unicorns Unlimited. This chapter provides the most comprehensive review of human development in the nursing literature. M. Erickson begins by defining growth and development from within the Modeling and Role-Modeling theory and articulates the assumptions that developmental processes are continuous and predictable throughout the life span. She focuses her writing on psycho-social-spiritual development. After reviewing the major concepts of developmental theory (inherent development, chronological development, developmental residual), she moves on to explore a philosophical base for thinking about holistic development. She suggests that developmental stages can be expanded to include a stage before birth (integration) and after physical death (transformation). She discusses each stage in depth, presenting the developmental tasks and residuals, and explores factors that can facilitate or impede growth. Numerous case studies illustrate the ideas.

Frisch, N. C., & Kelley, J. (1996). *Healing life's crises: A guide for nurses*. Albany, NY: Delmar.

This book of approximately 150 pages is useful as a text or reference for nurses who are new to the use of Modeling and Role-Modeling as well as those who wish to further study the application of the theory to practice. After presenting an overview of the theory in the first chapter, each subsequent chapter includes a case study with an example of using Modeling and Role-Modeling to plan care. Although the majority of chapters address individuals as clients, the final three chapters demonstrate the use of Modeling and Role-Modeling in the unique situations of the family, nursing organizations, and conflict resolution.

Lombardo, S. L., & Roof, M. (2005). A case study applying the Modeling and Role-Modeling theory to morbid obesity. *Home Healthcare Nurse, 23*(7), 425–428.

An excellent demonstration, through case study, of the use of Modeling and Role-Modeling as the theoretical base to providing care. The case presented is of a 74-year-old woman who is wheelchair bound with a principal diagnosis of morbid obesity. The concepts of unconditional acceptance, developmental residual, self-care knowledge, and the five aims of intervention are all involved in the nurse–client interactions focused on improvement of the client's body image and self-esteem.

Schultz, E. D. (1998). Academic advising from a nursing theory perspective. *Nurse Educator, 23*(2), 22–25.

A unique application of the theory of Modeling and Role-Modeling in which the student is the client and the theory is the base for academic advising. Many of the major concepts of the theory are addressed, and specific activities related to the five aims of intervention are delineated.

Woodward, W. (2003). Preparing a new workforce. *Nursing Administration Quarterly, 27*(3), 215–222.

This is an excellent article for educators, clinicians, and administrators alike. The article addresses the importance and value of theory-based practice and specifically nursing practice based on the theory of Modeling and Role-Modeling. The author begins by debunking five myths about nursing theory, such as "nursing theory is for nursing educators to teach, not real nurses to use." The article succinctly defines all of the major components of Modeling and Role-Modeling and explains the specifics of teaching theory-based nursing practice in a baccalaureate nursing curriculum for over 10 years.

CHAPTER 21

Health Promotion Model

Nola J. Pender

Julia B. George

Nola J. Pender was born in 1941 in Lansing, Michigan. She received her diploma in nursing from the West Suburban Hospital School of Nursing, Oak Park, Illinois; B.S. in nursing and M.A. in human growth and Development from Michigan State University, East Lansing, Michigan; and Ph.D. in psychology and education from Northwestern University, Evanston, Illinois, all in the 1960s. She also did graduate-level work in community health nursing at Rush University, Chicago, Illinois.

Her experience in nursing practice was in medical-surgical nursing and pediatrics. She held faculty positions at Northern Illinois University, DeKalb, and the University of Michigan, Ann Arbor, and served as associate dean for research in the School of Nursing, University of Michigan, from 1990 to 2001 (Pender, 2006). She is Professor Emeritus in the University of Michigan School of Nursing and part-time Distinguished Professor, Loyola University, Chicago, Illinois (Graves, 2007). The focus of her research career has been health promotion.

Her awards and honors include the American Nurses Association Book of the Year for the fourth edition of Health Promotion in Nursing Practice; *recognition as distinguished alumni, Michigan State University; an honorary doctorate from Widener University, Chester, Pennsylvania; past president and recipient of the Distinguished Research Award from the Midwest Nursing Research Society; an American Psychological Association Award for outstanding contributions to nursing and health psychology; the Mae Edna Doyle Award for excellence in teaching, School of Nursing, University of Michigan, in 1998; fellow in and past president of the American Academy of Nursing; charter member of the National Advisory Council on Nursing Research; and member, Board of Directors of Research!America. She also served a four-year term on the U.S. Preventive Services Task Force and is on the Executive Committee of "Building Health Promotion into the National Agenda."*

Nola J. Pender (1969) began her research about how people make decisions with her doctoral dissertation. The initial version of her Health Promotion Model (HPM) was published in 1982. Pender, Murdaugh, and Parsons (2006) state that the HPM "proposed a framework for integrating nursing and behavioral science perspectives on factors influencing health behaviors. The framework offered a guide for exploration of the complex biopsychosocial processes that motivate individuals to engage in behaviors directed toward the enhancement of health" (p. 47). The initial model had seven cognitive-perceptual factors (importance of health, perceived control of health, definition of health, perceived health status, perceived self-efficacy, perceived benefits, and perceived barriers) and five modifying factors (demographic characteristics, biologic characteristics, interpersonal influences, situational influences, and behavioral factors). Pender, Murdaugh, and Parsons point out that this model is an approach- or competence-oriented model rather than one that includes fear or threat as a key concept.

As a result of analyzing research conducted on the HPM, Pender (1996) presented the HPM (revised). The research results empirically supported perceived self-efficacy, benefits, and barriers as predictors of health behaviors, and these factors were retained. Importance of health was not useful as a predictor, as all study participants had ranked health as high in value. Perceived control of health and definition of health did not contribute to explaining specific health behaviors. Perceived health status, while predictive of health behaviors, did not provide explanation of variance. Cues to action were identified as transient and had not been studied as variables in any of the research reviewed. Interpersonal, situational, and behavioral influences were recognized as of high theoretical importance and needing to be repositioned as having both direct and indirect effects on health-promoting behavior. Therefore, in the revised model, importance of health, perceived control of health, and cues to action were deleted from the HPM. Definition of health, perceived health status, and demographic and biologic characteristics were moved and included in a category labeled "personal factors." Three new variables, activity-related affect, commitment to a plan of action, and immediate competing demands and preferences, were added to the model. See Figure 21-1 for the HPM (revised).

THEORETICAL BASIS FOR THE HPM

Pender et al. (2006) identify the theoretical basis of the HPM as drawing upon social cognitive theory, expectancy value theory, and the nursing perspective of holistic human functioning. The social cognitive theory contribution might be considered the attitude of "I can do it . . ." and the expectancy value theory as ". . . and it will be worth it."

Social cognitive theory concepts were drawn from the works of Bandura (1977, 1985). This theory emphasizes self-direction, self-regulation, and perceptions of self-efficacy. Self-direction and self-regulation are the abilities to direct and control one's thinking and actions; perceptions of self-efficacy involve one's view of the personal ability to perform an identified set of actions. According to Pender et al. (2006), Bandura (1985) identifies the following basic human capabilities:

Symbolization—the ability to process and transform experiences to create internal models to guide action in the future

Forethought—the ability to anticipate possible consequences of potential actions and plan courses of action to achieve goals of value

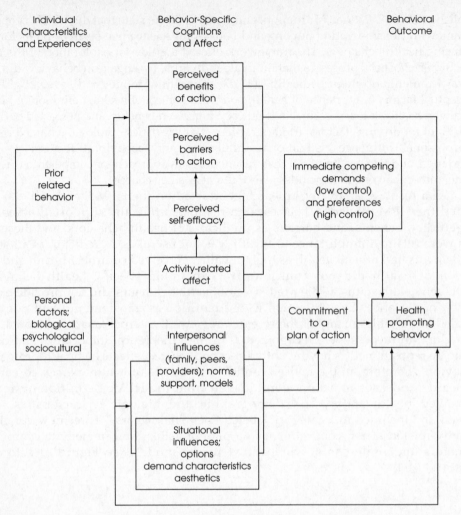

FIGURE 21-1   Health Promotion Model (revised). (*From Pender, N. J., Murdaugh, C. L., & Parsons, M. A. (2006). Health Promotion in Nursing Practice, (5th ed., p. 50). Upper Saddle River, NJ: Prentice Hall. Used with permission.*)

Vicarious learning—the ability to obtain rules for selecting actions through observation of others without having to use trial and error

Self-regulation—the ability to use internal standards and self-evaluation to inspire and adjust behavior and to arrange the external environment to construct encouragement for action

Self-reflection—the ability to consider one's own thought processes and change them

Other contributions to the HPM from Bandura include consideration of the interaction of inner forces and external stimuli and that self-beliefs (self-attribution, self-evaluation, self-efficacy) influence functioning.

TABLE 21-1   Assumptions of the Health Promotion Model (Revised)

- Persons seek to create conditions of living through which they can express their unique human health potential.
- Persons have the capacity for reflective self-awareness, including assessment of their own competencies.
- Persons value growth in directions viewed as positive and attempt to achieve a personally acceptable balance between change and stability.
- Individuals seek to actively regulate their own behavior.
- Individuals in all their biopsychosocial complexity interact with the environment, progressively transforming the environment and being transformed over time.
- Health professionals constitute a part of the interpersonal environment, which exerts influence on persons throughout their life span.
- Self-initiated reconfiguration of person–senvironment interactive patterns is essential to behavior change.

From Pender, N. J., Murdaugh, C. L., & Parsons, M. A. (2002). *Health Promotion in Nursing Practice* (4th ed., p. 63). Upper Saddle River, NJ: Prentice Hall.

TABLE 21-2   HPM Theoretical Propositions

- Prior behavior and inherited and acquired characteristics influence beliefs, affect, and enactment of health-promoting behavior.
- Persons commit to engaging in behaviors from which they anticipate deriving personally valued benefits.
- Perceived barriers can constrain commitment to action, a mediator of behavior, as well as actual behavior.
- Perceived competence or self-efficacy to execute a given behavior increases the likelihood of commitment to action and actual performance of the behavior.
- Greater perceived self-efficacy results in fewer perceived barriers to a specific health behavior.
- Positive affect toward a behavior results in greater perceived self-efficacy, which can, in turn, result in increased positive affect.
- When positive emotions or affect are associated with a behavior, the probability of commitment and action are increased.
- Persons are more likely to commit to and engage in health-promoting behaviors when significant others model the behavior, expect the behavior to occur, and provide assistance and support to enable the behavior.

Pender, N. J., Murdaugh, C. L., & Parsons, M. A. (2002). *Health Promotion in Nursing Practice* (4th ed., pp. 63–64). Upper Saddle River, NJ: Prentice Hall.

Expectancy value theory concepts were drawn from the work of Feather (1982). The contributions of expectancy value theory include that behavior is rational and economical. The undertaking and continuing of actions is based on those actions having positive personal value and includes the likelihood of achieving the desired outcome (based on available knowledge). There is a subjective value to change in that the greater the dissatisfactions with the current status, the greater the anticipated rewards and benefits of a favorable change.

For the assumptions on which the HPM (revised) is based, see Table 21-1. For theoretical propositions, derived from the HPM (revised), that provide a basis for research in relation to health behaviors, see Table 21-2.

HPM (REVISED) VARIABLES

The variables in the HPM (revised) include individual characteristics and experiences of prior related behavior and personal factors; behavior-specific cognitions and affect, including perceived benefits of action, perceived barriers to action, perceived self-efficacy, activity-related affect, interpersonal influences, and situational influences; commitment to a plan of action, immediate competing demands, and preferences; and finally, the behavioral outcome, hoped to be health-promoting behavior. Refer to Figure 21-1.

Individual Characteristics and Experiences

The combination of individual characteristics and experiences is unique to each person, and the importance of any characteristic, experience, or combination of them varies with the behavior(s) under consideration. The HPM (revised) seeks to provide flexibility in identifying the most important variable(s) in relation to a selected health behavior or in an identified target population. The individual characteristics and experiences are divided into prior related behaviors and personal factors.

Prior related behaviors are important because often the best predictor of future behavior is the frequency of the same or similar behaviors in the past. The person who has regularly exercised is more likely to continue to exercise than the person who has been a "couch potato." The direct effect of prior behavior is possibly that of habit formation since each time a behavior is performed, the habit is strengthened. The indirect effects of prior related behaviors are associated with perceptions of self-efficacy, perceived benefits and barriers, and positive or negative activity-related affect. Pender et al. (2006) indicate that the nurse can help the client move toward health-promoting behavior by focusing on the benefits of doing so and helping identify how to overcome recognized hurdles in the way of achieving the activity.

Personal factors are described as biological, psychological, and sociocultural. Biological factors include such aspects as "age, body mass index, pubertal status, menopausal status, aerobic capacity, strength, agility, or balance. Psychological factors include self-esteem, self-motivation, and perceived health status. Sociocultural factors include race, ethnicity, acculturation, education, and socioeconomic status" (Pender et al., 2006, p. 52). Only those factors that are theoretically relevant to the desired behavior should be considered for nursing intervention. It is important to remember that some of these factors cannot be changed. Those factors that cannot be changed are not a target for use in modifying behavior.

Behavior-Specific Cognitions and Affect

Behavior-specific cognitions and affect are viewed as of major motivational importance and are considered the core for intervention since they are the most amenable to change through nursing intervention. These cognitions and affect include perceived benefits of action, perceived barriers to action, perceived self-efficacy, activity-related affect, interpersonal influences, and situational influences, all of which lead to a commitment to a plan of action and consideration of immediately competing demands and preferences.

Perceived benefits of action have received moderate support in the research conducted on the HPM and HPM (revised) (Pender et al., 2006). Perceived benefits may moderate behavior both directly and indirectly. Prior personal experience with positive outcomes, or observations of others with such outcomes, increases the motivational importance of the target behavior and relates to the expectation of positive or negative outcomes. The benefits may be intrinsic (feeling better) or extrinsic (time to socialize while practicing the target behavior). "Beliefs in benefits or positive outcome expectations have generally been shown to be a necessary although not sufficient condition to engage in a specific health behavior" (p. 53).

Perceived barriers to action have been supported in HPM research as a determinant of participation in health-promoting behaviors (Pender et al., 2006). Perceived barriers may influence action directly by blocking that action or indirectly by decreasing any commitment to act. A key in this construct is that the barriers are perceived—they may be real as seen by others, or they may be imagined by the person. In either case, it is the perception of the barrier that influences the decision making about participating in the target behavior. Barriers may relate to degree of availability of access or resources, costs in money and time, and degree of perceived difficulty. Anticipation of loss of the satisfaction associated with such behaviors as smoking may also be seen as a barrier. Perceived barriers are more likely to lead to avoidance of a behavior. With low readiness and perceptions that barriers are high, change in behavior is not likely; with high readiness to act and perceptions of low levels of barriers, action in more likely.

Perceived self-efficacy, or one's judgment of one's ability to carry out an identified action, relates not to a person's skills but to that person's judgment about what can be accomplished with those skills. It is the perception of whether the person can achieve the desired behavior, not the perception of the potential consequences of the behavior. The perceived ability to achieve a behavior is perceived self-efficacy, or "can I do it?"; the potential consequences are outcome expectations, or "this is what will happen if I do it." The person who believes he or she can do it and do it satisfactorily will be encouraged to engage in the target behavior. Four types of information help form the perception of self-efficacy: having engaged in the behavior and met one's own standards or received positive feedback from others, having observed others successfully perform the behavior and be evaluated positively, being persuaded by others than one has the ability to successfully engage in the target behavior, and physiologic states such an calmness, anxiety, and fear that influence one's judgment of competency (Bandura, 1997, as cited in Pender et al., 2006). The HPM (revised) proposes that perceived self-efficacy is influenced by activity-related affect. However, Pender et al. (2006) indicate that there is a reciprocal relationship between perceived self-efficacy and activity-related affect. As affect becomes more positive, self-efficacy is viewed as greater; the more positive the view of self-efficacy, the more positive the affect. Also, as self-efficacy is perceived more positively, the perceptions of barriers decrease.

Activity-related affect may vary from mild to quite strong and will be cognitively labeled, remembered, and continue to be associated with thoughts about the particular behavior (Pender et al., 2006). There are three components to this affect: the act-related emotional arousal, the self-related self-acting, and the context-related environment in which the behavior occurs. Both repetition of the behavior and long-term continuance of the behavior are influenced by this affect. It is important to consider the affect before the action, during the action, and after the action. The target behavior may be approached with a negative affect of "I am only doing this because I have to." If the experience of the behavior is positive—"Gee, I really feel better"—the initially negative affect will become positive and be more likely to lead to continuing the behavior.

Interpersonal influences are the person's thoughts or beliefs about the behaviors, attitudes, and beliefs of others and may or may not accurately reflect those behaviors, attitudes, or beliefs (Pender et al., 2006). Sources of these influences include family, peers, and health care providers as primary sources and also include norms or expectation of significant others, social support (encouragement [or lack thereof] from others, both emotional and instrumental), and modeling or learning from watching others. All three of these influence a person's likelihood of engaging in health-promoting behaviors. Individuals will vary in the degree to which any of these influence their decision making and actions. Some people are more dependent upon the expectations and encouragement of others; other people may decide to participate because they observe others enjoying engaging in a health-promoting activity.

Situational influences include the options that are perceived as being available, demand characteristics, and environmental features (Pender et al., 2006). The options may include to participate or not participate or to participate in a variety of ways. When riding a motorcycle one can either wear a helmet or not wear a helmet, but when participating in a charity walk, one can walk all or some part of the distance and may speed up or slow down as desired. The degree of demand will also vary—if an employer expects everyone to participate in the charity walk, it is more likely that one will participate than if the employer simply mentions the charity walk will be happening. Environmental features can encourage or discourage an activity. "No smoking" signs are intended to discourage smoking or encourage not smoking. Readily available sinks for hand washing are intended to encourage cleanliness. When organizational policies specify regular hand washing (demand) and sinks are readily available (environment), it is more likely that any given employee will routinely engage in hand washing.

Commitment to a plan of action initiates the behavior (Pender et al., 2006). The underlying cognitive processes are a "commitment to carry out a specific action at a given time and place and with specified persons or alone, irrespective of competing preferences . . . and . . . identification of definitive strategies for eliciting, carrying out, and reinforcing the behavior" (p. 56). Both commitment and identified strategies are necessary. Commitment alone often can be characterized as those good intentions that create the paving stones to failure. Planning strategies for use at various points in the sequence of behaviors increases the likelihood of successful completion of the plan of action.

Immediate competing demands and preferences are "alternative behaviors that intrude into consciousness as possible courses of action immediately prior to the intended occurrence of a planned health-promoting behavior" (Pender et al., 2006, p. 56). Competing demands are behaviors over which the person has little control, such as work or family responsibilities, and are situations in which a failure to respond may have very negative consequences for the person or significant others. Competing preferences are behaviors over which the person likely has a high degree of control and that are powerfully reinforcing. The preference for a burger, fries, and a milkshake may overcome the intended behavior of eating a salad. Either or both competing demands and preferences can overturn a plan of action. Neither of these is identified as a barrier. The competing demand differs from a barrier because the alternative behavior occurs in response to an unanticipated external demand (called in to work in an emergency or a sick child). The competing preference differs from a barrier (such as it is too expensive) in that the alternative behavior is based on a last-minute urge. Strong commitment to the plan of action, with the exercise of self-regulation and control, will help deter the immediate competing demands and preferences from overturning the plan of action.

Behavioral Outcome

The desired behavioral outcome is *health-promoting behavior.* The purpose of the health-promoting behavior is for the client to realize positive health outcomes such as improved functional ability or improved quality of life. The intention is that by carrying out the plan of action, health-promoting behavior, as identified in the plan of action, will lead to better health for the client. Health-promoting behavior may involve increasing healthy behaviors already in place, replacing risky or unhealthy behaviors, or both of these.

HPM (REVISED) AND NURSING'S METAPARADIGM

Pender et al. (2006) recognize nursing's metaparadigm of humans, health, environment, and nursing. The focus of the HPM (revised) is on health promotion, and there is a detailed discussion about health and various definitions of health with a conclusion that a holistic definition that includes social aspects is important for an understanding of health. Otherwise, the four major concepts are not defined.

Health promotion is defined and differentiated from disease prevention, or health protection. Health promotion is defined as "behavior motivated by the desire to increase well-being and actualize human health potential" (Pender et al., 2006, p. 7). Whitehead (2005) takes issue with the use of this definition for teaching individuals to manage their own health and argues that health promotion involves community-driven health reform, collective health needs, and public health policies. He asserts the HPM should be called a health education model. It is interesting to note that the majority of the citations he uses to support his argument were published in England or Australia.

USING THE HPM (REVISED) IN NURSING CARE

The HPM (revised) can be a useful guide to nursing care in relation to assisting the recipients of nursing care in choosing and carrying out behaviors to increase well-being. It is not very helpful during the acute stages of an illness when the focus of care is on curing an illness or saving a life.

Assessment can be guided by the individual characteristics and experiences and the behavior-specific cognitions and affect. The *nursing diagnosis* would be derived from the data collected in relation to these areas but is not directly reflected in the model. *Planning* occurs in developing the plan of action to which the client commits; again, the planning process is not directly reflected in the model, although the outcome of that process is reflected in the plan of action. *Implementation* would draw upon the entire model, using the characteristics, experiences, cognitions, and affect information to identify how to support the commitment to a plan of action and how to encourage the client to seek to avoid competing demands and not become entangled by competing preferences. *Evaluation* would be based upon the performance of the target health-promoting behavior. An example is provided by the following case study.

You are working with Mrs. S., who recently had a minor myocardial infarction with no apparent permanent damage. She is interested in discussing lifestyle changes to help improve her health. She asks about an exercise plan and how to improve her nutrition.

PERSONAL FACTORS: Mrs. S. is a 62-year-old married female, with a body mass index of 28. She is postmenopausal and is moderately physically active. She enjoys water sports and swims and snorkels whenever she can. She has had no problems with agility or balance. She views her health status as satisfactory but worries about the implications of her parents' health histories in relation to high blood pressure and coronary problems. She is a highly motivated individual who has confidence in herself but expresses concern when others do not respond in the way she desires. She is Caucasian, was born and raised in Florida, and holds a graduate degree in social work. She and her husband own their own home as well as some rental properties. They are a double-income family; she is a social worker, and he is a computer consultant. Both of their children are grown, and the S.'s believe they have made adequate investments for retirement.

PRIOR RELATED BEHAVIOR: While she enjoys water sports, she has had no regular plan for exercise. She eats breakfast daily—usually juice, cereal with milk, and coffee. For lunch she often just "grabs something from the vending machine," and for dinner she indicates she is often too tired to cook so they order takeout of pizza or Chinese food.

PERCEIVED BENEFITS OF ACTION: Mrs. S. indicates she believes her heart attack is a wake-up call and that she needs to make some changes in her behavior to increase her well-being.

PERCEIVED BARRIERS TO ACTION: Mrs. S. states that her job has become more and more stressful, as the caseloads in her agency have increased without any increase in staff. She has found it harder and harder to meet the needs of her clients at a level that is satisfactory to her. Because of this she has been spending longer hours on the job and finding it a challenge to do things for herself.

PERCEIVED SELF-EFFICACY: Mrs. S. states she needs to regain control of her own health and that she can do that.

ACTIVITY-RELATED AFFECT: Mrs. S. reports she used to enjoy doing exercise on a regular basis, but she is a bit worried about how she can work it into her schedule. She also describes how the whole family ate healthy meals when her children were at home and that she needs to pull out some of those "old" recipes. If she could cook healthy meals while working and raising children, surely she can do it for just the two of them.

INTERPERSONAL INFLUENCES: Mr. S. is strongly in support of any changes Mrs. S. wishes to make so she will feel better; Mrs. S. remembers there are a few people at work who bring their own lunches and eat together, and she believes she would enjoy lunching with them.

SITUATIONAL INFLUENCES: Mrs. S. indicates the availability of a pleasant lunchroom at work will be helpful; she is concerned about the increasing demands of her work interfering with her ability to make the desired changes.

COMMITMENT TO A PLAN OF ACTION: With the information gathered above, you and Mrs. S. develop a plan of action to help her exercise regularly and to eat a low-fat, reduced-sodium diet. Mrs. S. states that she will begin to increase her exercise by parking at the end of the parking lot and taking the stairs instead of the elevator at work; she will pack a lunch daily of nutritious foods that are low in fat and sodium; she will prepare low-fat and low-sodium meals at hóme at least five nights a week.

You meet with Mrs. S. in three weeks to discuss how her plan of action is going. She has increased her exercise by parking at the end of the parking lot and taking the stairs instead of the elevator at work and is planning to begin swimming at least one day every weekend. She reports she has been less successful with changes in her eating patterns. She has packed her lunch as planned but the demands at work keep her at her desk "grabbing a bite now and again as I can"(IMMEDIATE COMPETING DEMAND). As a result, in the evening she is so exhausted that she rarely fixes a meal and they either snack or order takeout (IM-MEDIATE COMPETING PREFERENCES). She indicates that she is considering taking early retirement so she can "take better care of myself."

HEALTH-PROMOTING BEHAVIOR: Mrs. S. has been partially successful in achieving her desired health-promoting behavior, as she has increased her exercise. She has been less successful with her plans to change her nutrition and is considering other plans of action to increase her ability to make the desired changes.

CRITIQUE OF THE HPM (REVISED)

1. *What is the historical context of the theory?*   The assumptions of the HPM (revised) are presented in Table 21-1. Pender, Murdaugh, and Parsons (2002) assert that the assumptions reflect both nursing and behavioral science perspectives. They also indicate that the variables of the HPM (revised) were derived from social cognitive theory and expectancy-value theory and placed with a nursing perspective of holistic human functioning. Since both social cognitive theory and expectancy-value theory are from psychology, the HPM (revised) is based in psychology and nursing. The assumptions are clearly stated.

The HPM was introduced by Pender in 1982, with further discussion in 1987. The revised form of the HPM was introduced in1996; this revision was based upon research conducted on the original HPM.

While the HPM is based in nursing, with a holistic focus, it is more a theory to be used by nurses (theory for nursing to use) rather than a theory intended for exclusive use by nursing (theory about nursing).

2. *What are the basic concepts and relationships presented by the theory?*   The basic concepts are presented in the HPM (revised) (see Figure 21-1). The concepts are defined in the text of the various editions of *Health Promotion in Nursing Practice* in a consistent manner (Pender, 1982, 1987, 1996; Pender et al., 2002, 2006). The relationships are presented logically and are further illuminated in the stated theoretical propositions (see Table 21-2). The relationships of the original HPM were changed after a thorough review of research conducted on it (Pender, 1996).

3. *What major phenomena of concern to nursing are presented? (These phenomena may include* **but are not limited to** *human beings, environment, health, interpersonal relations, caring, goal attainment, adaptation, and energy fields.)*   The major phenomena of concern to nursing is apparent in the title of the model—health promotion. The HPM (revised) emphasizes the active role of the client in choosing and making lifestyle changes

to promote health and focuses on individual characteristics and experiences (prior related behavior and personal factors) and behavior-specific cognitions and affect (perceived benefits of action, perceived barriers to action, perceived self-efficacy, activity-related affect, interpersonal influences, situational influences) that lead to a commitment to action with a goal of health-promoting behavior. The concepts of immediate demands or preferences are also included.

4. *To whom does this theory apply? In what situations? In what ways?* The HPM (revised) is intended for use in any situation in which it is desirable for clients to seek changing their behavior and possibly changing the environment to support healthy behavior. It is not applicable in every nursing situation but in many of them. It is also of utility to other caring professionals interested in promoting health.

5. *By what method or methods can this theory be tested?* One of the ways in which the HPM (revised) is unique is that it is structured to be tested (see theoretical propositions in Table 21-2). The model was revised based upon an analysis of the research that had been conducted upon it. In 1996, Pender reported that 5 to 12 variables had been studied at any given time, with the effects of "cues to action" never having been tested. The range of variance explained in the studies reviewed was 19% to 59%. The strongest support was found for self-efficacy and barriers, with moderate support for benefits. In 2006, Pender et al. provided a more recent analysis of research results in relation to the HPM (revised). They reported the percentage of the studies that supported the importance of the variables in determining subsequent behavior as follows: self-efficacy 86%, perceived barriers 79%, prior related behavior 75%, perceived benefits 61%, interpersonal influences 57%, and situational influences 56%. They pointed out that since activity-related affect had been fairly recently added to the model, more research is needed on this variable.

Table 21-3 presents an overview of HPM-related research since 1996. Both quantitative and qualitative methods have been used, with descriptive studies being the most common.

6. *Does this theory direct nursing actions that lead to favorable outcomes?* Mendias and Paar (2007) report that results of research with the HPM have led to practice changes and health promotion activities. The intent of the model is provide guidance to nurses in identifying how to be most supportive to a client in planning and implementing a plan to make changes leading to health-promoting behavior. The Health Promoting Lifestyle Profile II (HPLPII) is useful for assessing a client's lifestyle as well as for use in research. The 52-item HPLPII consists of the six subscales of health responsibility, physical activity, nutrition, interpersonal relations, spiritual growth, and stress management (Pender et al., 2006). Use of this profile can assist in developing an individualized plan for health promotion that will enhance the attainment of favorable outcomes. Most of the published literature about the HPM (revised) reports research with stated implications for practice and for further research. More publications about use in practice would be helpful.

The model appears to assume that health-promoting behaviors will lead to healthy outcomes. Srof and Velsor-Friedrich (2006) believe this relationship has not been made explicit, particularly with adolescents.

TABLE 21-3   Health Promotion Model Research

Author/Year[*]	Topic	Subjects	Methodology
	DISSERTATIONS AND THESES		
Flores 1996	Multiple role stressors, health promotion activities	124 university female students	Comparative, descriptive
Kurtz 1996	Perceived health status, meaning of illness, health-promoting behaviors	215 women with rheumatoid arthritis	Survey correlational
Rothschild 1996	Health promoting behavior, perceived stress	50 new mothers; 38 in test–retest group	Descriptive correlational
Ryan 1996	Perceived health status, life satisfaction, self-esteem, happiness, stress, age, sex, education, cholesterol, smoking, alcohol intake, exercise	7,828 volunteers at a community health fair	Descriptive correlational
Tapler 1996	Health value, self-efficacy, health locus of control, health benefits, health barriers, health behavior practices	202 mothers, aged 25–45 years	Descriptive correlational and content analysis
White 1996	Individualized health promotion program, health-promoting behaviors	35 homebound older adults	Experimental, correlational
Wisnewski 1996	Health-promotion education, exercise	95 participants in diabetic education support group classes	Quasi experimental, pretest, posttest, correlational
Aalto 1997	Attitudes of women toward mammography screening (MS), attendance to MS, function of MS in health promotion, activity in breast self-examination	Women who did and did not participate in MS in Tampere, Finland in 1991 with follow-up in 1991, 1995; 13 radiographic technicians	Descriptive, phenomenography
Coviak 1998	Children's influence on parental physical activity	184 parents of children who participated in a study of exercise beliefs and habits	Survey, descriptive

(continued)

TABLE 21-3   Health Promotion Model Research (Continued)

Author/Year[*]	Topic	Subjects	Methodology
Egonu 1998	Race, perception of risk of pregnancy-induced hypertension	5 Afro-origin women diagnosed with pregnancy-induced hypertension	Descriptive, qualitative
C. R. Johnson 1998	Health-promoting lifestyles, breast cancer screening behaviors		Descriptive, correlational
Millard 1998	Health-promoting behavior in Seventh-day Adventists aged 65 and over	255 (163 women, 91 men) Seventh-Day Adventists 65 years and older	Descriptive, correlational
H-H. Wang 1998	Self-care, well-being	284 women, 60 years and older in rural Taiwan	Survey-interview, correlational
Yue 1998	Perceived benefits and barriers, health-promoting behaviors	46 post-cardiac event persons in rural southeastern New Mexico	Exploratory, cross-section survey
Al-Obeisat 1999	Perceived health status, definition of health, perceived benefits, perceived barriers, perceived self-efficacy, activity-related affect, age, education, socioeconomic status, parity, prenatal care utilization	124 newly delivered women in a hospital in northern Jordan	Correlational
McCullagh 1999	Hearing protector use among farmers	167 farmers	
Kalampakom 2000	Hearing protection use among construction workers	264 midwestern U.S. construction workers	Secondary analysis
Warner 2000	Parental role modeling of leisure-time activity, frequency of school-based physical education and level of leisure-time activity in twin children	84 same-sex twins, aged 8–17 years, and their parents (84 mothers, 65 fathers)	Secondary analysis
Willis 2001	Multiple roles, health promotion activities	College women with multiple roles	Descriptive

TABLE 21-3   Health Promotion Model Research (Continued)

Author/Year[*]	Topic	Subjects	Methodology
Hubbard 2002	Health-promoting curriculum, health promoting behaviors	74 nursing students, 98 non-nursing students in a community college	Pretest, posttest design
McMenamin 2002	Parental perceptions, use of peak flow meters in their children	20 parents, accessed through outpatient asthma allergy clinics	Descriptive correlational
Sakraida 2002	Divorce transition, coping responses, health-promoting behavior	154 recently divorced women; 24 later interviewed	Descriptive, qualitative
Sriyuktasuth 2002	Health-promoting behaviors	160 Thai women with systemic lupus erythematosus	Descriptive
Chandanasotthi 2003	Self esteem, stress, coping styles & health promoting behaviors	1,072 Thai adolescents	Descriptive
Deenan 2003	Exercise behavior	311 bilingual Thai adolescents	Survey, descriptive
Easom 2003b	Health promotion activities	80 rural, elderly caregivers, aged 65–84	Telephone interview;
Haus 2003	Medication management strategies	60 older adults living alone in Pittsburgh, PA	Correlational
Luther 2003	Health promotion behaviors	Women at risk for osteoporosis in Mississippi	Descriptive correlational
Sapp 2003	Personal characteristics and health-promoting lifestyle	99 adolescents with asthma	Descriptive correlational survey
Wilson 2003	Health practices	137 homeless women in Indiana	Cross-sectional, descriptive, non experimental

(continued)

TABLE 21-3 Health Promotion Model Research (Continued)

Author/Year[*]	Topic	Subjects	Methodology
Ammouri 2004	Exercise participation	300 subjects from the "Health Behaviors of Adolescents" Study; aged 10–19 years	Secondary data analysis—correlational
Cananub 2004	Personal factors, perceived benefits, perceived barriers, perceived self-efficacy, social support, prenatal care utilization	110 postpartum women in Thailand	Descriptive correlational ex post facto design
Edens 2004	Breast health education, clinical breast examination	101 women, 50 years or older, attending a rural Appalachian clinic	3 group posttest only, experimental
Gabry 2005	Health behavior during pregnancy and health locus of control	Abstract shortened by UMI—this information not included	Abstract shortened by UMI—this information not included
Ma 2005	Physical activity, personal factors, state anxiety, perceived life stress events, perceived benefits, perceived barriers, perceived self-efficacy, perceived family members' support, perceived friends' support	89 Taiwanese men and 150 Taiwanese women with anxiety	Model testing
Pichayapinyo 2005	Perceived benefits, perceived barriers, social support and sense of mastery	130 primiparous mothers in a Thailand hospital	Descriptive correlational
Yang 2005	Physical activity	121 Korean midlife immigrant in Texas	Relationship

TABLE 21-3   Health Promotion Model Research (Continued)

Author/Year[*]	Topic	Subjects	Methodology
Byam-Williams 2006	Age, gender, race, education, income, perceived self-efficacy, perceived barriers, interpersonal influences, health-promoting behaviors, health status	113 community-dwelling Whites and Blacks, 65 years and older in central Virginia	Descriptive correlational
Ordonez 2006	Lived experience of health	9 older Guatemalan women, living in South Florida	Phenomenology
	PUBLISHED RESEARCH ARTICLES		
Acton 2002	Health-promoting self care	Family caregivers and noncaregivers	Descriptive
Agazio, Ephraim, Flaherty, & Gurney 2002	Demographic characteristics, definition of health, perceived health status, perceived self-efficacy, resources, health promoting behaviors	141 active-duty women with children using military health services	Descriptive, exploratory, model testing
Bond, Jones, Cason, Campbell, & Hall 2002	Health-promoting lifestyle behaviors	230 Hispanic pregnant women	Descriptive correlational
Gasalberti 2002	Perceived barriers, health conception, Breast self examination	93 middle-aged women in New Jersey	Correlational
Grubbs & Carter 2002	Perceived benefits, perceived barriers, exercise	147 Undergraduate university students	Descriptive
Gu & Eun 2002	Health-promoting behaviors; young, middle aged and older adults	Young, middle aged and older adults in Korea	Descriptive
Hui 2002	Age, gender, income, employment status, levels of education, health-promoting lifestyles	169 undergraduate nursing students	Descriptive

(continued)

TABLE 21-3   Health Promotion Model Research (Continued)

Author/Year[*]	Topic	Subjects	Methodology
R. L. Johnson 2002	Racial identity, self-esteem, sociodemographics, health-promoting lifestyles	224 African Americans (108 males, 116 females) in southeastern United States	Descriptive correlational
Kerr, Lusk, & Ronis 2002	Hearing protection use, cognitive-perceptual factors	119 Mexican American workers in garment manufacturing plants	Descriptive correlational
Lambert, Fearing, Bell, & Newton 2002	Prostate screening health beliefs and practices	African American and Caucasian men	Comparative
McCullagh, Lusk, & Ronis 2002	Hearing protection use	139 farmers	Theory validation
McDonald, Wykle, Misra, Suwonnaroop, & Burant 2002	Social support, acceptance, health-promoting behaviors, glycemic control	63 African Americans with diabetes mellitus	Descriptive
Sohng, Sohng, & Yeom 2002	Self-efficacy, perceived health status, health-promoting behaviors	110 elderly Korean immigrants in the United States	Descriptive correlational
Suwonnaroop & Zauszniewski 2002	Social support, perceived health status, gender, race, education, income, health-promoting behaviors	121 adults, aged 55–105 years, in the United States	Survey
Tang & Chen 2002	Caregiver's personal factors, perceived self-efficacy, social support, reactions to caregiving, health promotion behaviors; care recipient's functional status	134 primary caregivers responsible for care of stroke patients in Taipei, Taiwan	Survey
Tashiro 2002	Health-promoting lifestyle behaviors, perceived health status and concerns	546 Japanese college women	Survey
Wu & Pender 2002	Physical activity, PHPM	969 eighth-grade students, aged 12–15 years, in Taipei, Taiwan	Cross sectional

TABLE 21-3   Health Promotion Model Research (Continued)

Author/Year*	Topic	Subjects	Methodology
Wu, Pender, & Yang 2002	Physical activity, cultures	969 middle school students in Taiwan; 286 late elementary and middle school students in the United States	Cross sectional, comparative
Wu, Ronis, Pender, & Jwo 2002	Perceived self-efficacy, perceived benefits, perceived barriers, adolescents' participation in physical activity	1079 Taiwanese adolescents	Instrument validation
Bujis, Ross-Kerr, Cousins, & Wilson 2003	Health promotion program for seniors	23 program participants (2 men, 21 women) aged 61–90 years	Qualitative evaluation
Frenn & Malin 2003	Diet and physical activity	221 middle school children	Descriptive
Frenn, Malin, & Bansal 2003	Diet and physical activity	117 urban middle school children	Quasi experimental pretest, posttest
Frenn, Malin, Bansal, Delgado, Greer, et al. 2003	Diet and physical activity	Middle school students	Pretest, posttest program evaluation
Lohnse 2003	Benefits and barriers to bicycle helmet use	Parents of first and second grade students who had a school-based bicycle safety education program	Descriptive comparative, program evaluation
Lusk, Ronis, Kazanis, Eakin, Hong, et al. 2003	Tailored intervention, hearing protection use	1325 factory workers	Randomized controlled design with pretest and posttest
McDonald & Wykle 2003	Health-promoting behavior	276 caregivers of impaired older adults	Secondary data analysis
Wu, Pender, & Noureddine 2003	Gender, physical activity	832 Taiwanese adolescents	Cross sectional

(continued)

TABLE 21-3 Health Promotion Model Research (Continued)

Author/Year*	Topic	Subjects	Methodology
Yates, Price-Fowlkes, & Agrawal 2003	Barriers and facilitators, physical activity	Cardiac patients	Cross sectional, correlational
S-Y. Chen 2004	Pelvic Floor Muscle Exercise Self-Efficacy Scale	106 women with urinary incontinence	Instrument development
Fowles & Feucht 2004	Barriers to Health Eating Scale	Pregnant women	Instrument validation
Jones, Kennedy-Malone, & Wideman 2004	Early detection of type 2 diabetes	20 African American adults 50 years and older	Descriptive correlational
Kanchana 2004	Knowledge and utilization of safety measures		Descriptive
Newton, Robinson, & Kozac 2004	Type of analgesia, pain scores, ambulation, hospital length of stay	98 females, post abdominal hysterectomy	Retrospective chart review
Stuifbergen, Harrison, Becker, & Carter 2004	Adapting wellness intervention for women with chronic diabling condition	Women with multiple sclerosis	Pretest, posttest
Tilokskulchai, Sitthimongkol, Prasopkiitikun, & Klainin 2004	Health promotion research	47 published studies using Pender's model in Thailand	Meta-analysis
Yoon & Horne 2004	Locus of control, perceived health competence, herbal product use	70 women (30 herbal users, 40 nonusers), age 65 years or older, in north-central Florida	Descriptive
Callaghan 2005a	Health behaviors, self-efficacy, self-care, basic conditioning factors	235 older adults	Secondary statistical analysis
Callaghan 2005b	Health-promoting self-care behaviors, self-care self-efficacy, self-care agency, spiritual growth	Adolescents	Descriptive

TABLE 21-3   Health Promotion Model Research (Continued)

Author/Year[*]	Topic	Subjects	Methodology
Campbell & Torrance 2005	Risk factors, patient's understanding	234 patients, 3–9 months post-coronary artery angioplasty, Melbourne, Australia	Descriptive survey
Chen, James, Hsu, Chang, Huang, et al. 2005	Health-related behaviors in adolescent mothers	37 adolescent mothers in rural Taiwan	Cross-sectional descriptive, survey
Hageman, Walker, & Pullen 2005	Promoting physical activity via the Internet	31 healthy women, aged 50–69 years	Pretest, posttest intervention evaluation
Han, Lee, Park, Park, & Cheol 2005	Quality of life, chronic cardiovascular disease, Korea	436 patients with chronic cardiovascular disease in a university hospital in Seoul, South Korea	Structural modeling
Hensley, Jones, Williams, Willsher, & Cain 2005	Outcomes for patients with diabetes and hypertension	115 patients in Louisiana	Retrospective chart review
Johnson, R. L. 2005	Gender, health-promoting lifestyles	223 African Americans in the southeastern United States	Descriptive comparative
R. L. Johnson & Nies 2005	Barriers, health-promoting behaviors	African Americans in two southeastern states in United States	Qualitative
Kahawong, Phancharoenworakul, Khampalikit, Taboonpong, & Chittchang 2005	Age, body mass index, duration of hyperlipidemia, perceived health risks, education, perceived self-efficacy, social support	263 Thai women with hyperlipidemia	Descriptive
McDonald, Brennan, & Wykle 2005	Perceived health status, health-promoting behaviors, age, gender, race and length of caregiving	393 African-American and White caregivers in northeastern Ohio	Secondary analysis

(continued)

TABLE 21-3 Health Promotion Model Research (Continued)

Author/Year[*]	Topic	Subjects	Methodology
Phuphaibul, Leucha, Putwattana, Nuntawan, Tapsart, et al. 2005	Adolescent health promotion behavior, family health promotion behavior, parent modeling	1,980 adolescents and their parents in Thailand	Descriptive, correlational
Sakraida 2005	See details in D &T, 2002		
Schlickau & Wilson 2005	Breastfeeding as health-promoting behavior	Hispanic women	Literature review
Wilson 2005	Health promoting behaviors	137 sheltered homeless women	Cross sectional
Wu & Pender 2005	Individual characteristics, cognitions, interpersonal influences and physical activity	Taiwanese adolescents	Test structural model
Arras, Ogletree, & Welshimer 2006	Perceived benefits, perceived barriers, self-efficacy, demographic factors, self-rated health, health-promoting behaviors	Middle-aged and older men	Survey
Callaghan 2006a	Basic conditioning factors, practice of healthy behaviors, self-efficacy beliefs, ability for self-care	256 adolescents	Secondary statistical analysis
Callaghan 2006b	Basic conditioning factors, practice of healthy behaviors, self-efficacy beliefs, self-care agency	379 adults	Secondary statistical analysis
Chanruengvanich, Kasemkitwattana, Charoenyooth, Towanabut, & Pongurgsorn 2006	Self-regulated exercise, program on physical fitness, risk factors for stroke	62 persons with history of transient ischemic attacks and minor strokes in Thailand	Randomized controlled trail

TABLE 21-3 Health Promotion Model Research (Continued)

Author/Year[*]	Topic	Subjects	Methodology
Costanzo, Walker, Yates, McCabe, & Berg 2006	Behavioral counseling, physical activity, muscle strengthening, stretching activity	46 women from an urban midwestern community	Pretest/posttest comparison group
Guarnero 2006	Health promotion behaviors	Gay and bisexual men, aged 18–29	Grounded theory
Hendricks, Murdaugh, & Pender 2006	Adolescent lifestyle behaviors	Adolescents	Instrument development
Kaewthummanukul, Brown, Weaver, & Thomas 2006	Exercise participation, personal factors, perceived benefits, perceived barriers, perceived self-efficacy, perceived social support, job demands, motivation	970 registered nurses, aged 18–60, working full-time in a Thai hospital	Correlational cross sectional
Lee & Lai 2006	Osteoporosis knowledge (exercise, calcium intake), osteoporosis health beliefs (susceptibility, seriousness, exercise benefits, calcium intake benefits, barriers to exercise and calcium intake, health motivation)	52 men in Hong Kong, aged 60 and over	Cross-sectional survey
McMurry 2006	Pharmacological and cognitive regimens, tobacco cessation relapse	40 military personnel participants in one of four tobacco cessation programs	Descriptive comparative
Milne & Moore 2006	Self-care and factors influencing it	Individuals with urinary incontinence	Qualitative, descriptive
Nies & Motyka 2006	Women's ability to maintain a walking program—benefits and barriers	97 women in a walking program	Qualitative analysis of field notes

(continued)

TABLE 21-3 Health Promotion Model Research (Continued)

Author/Year[*]	Topic	Subjects	Methodology
Olson & Berg 2006	Promoting perimenopausal bone health		Quasi-experimental
Robbins, Gretebeck, Kazanis, & Pender 2006	Use of computerized physical activity program	77 racially diverse sedentary girls in grade 6–8	Pretest/posttest control group
Ronis, Hong, & Lusk 2006	Fit and predictive usefulness of HPM and HPM (revised) in use of hearing protection devices	703 workers exposed to high noise	Model testing
Shin, Hur, Pender, Jang, & Kim 2006	Perceived exercise self-efficacy, exercise benefits, exercise barriers, commitment to a plan for exercise	154 Korean women diagnosed with either osteoporosis or osteoarthritis	Descriptive
A. B. Smith & Bashore 2006	Perceived health status, health-promoting behaviors	60 adolescent/ young adult cancer survivors, two years post-completion of cancer treatment	Descriptive
S. A. Smith & Michel 2006	Aquatic exercise program, perception of body image, participation in health-promoting behaviors, barriers to health-promoting participation, level of physical discomfort, mobility	40 nonexercising pregnant women	Two-group, pretest/posttest, quasi-experimental
Walker, Pullen, Hertzog, Boeckner, & Hageman 2006	Cognitive-perceptual determinants from HPM, physical activity, healthy eating	Rural women aged 50–69	Descriptive, correlational
Esperat, Feng, Zhang, & Owen 2007	Health behaviors	Low income pregnant Mexican American and African American women in southeastern Texas	Cross-sectional survey

TABLE 21-3   Health Promotion Model Research (Continued)

Author/Year[*]	Topic	Subjects	Methodology
Huang & Dai 2007	Weight retention predictors at six months postpartum	602 postpartum women in Taiwan	Descriptive, correlational
Kerr, Savik, Monsen, & Lusk 2007	Computer based interventions and use of hearing protection	343 construction workers	Evaluation research
Kwong & Kwan 2007	Influences on participation in physical activity, healthy dietary practices, stress management, barriers to these practices	896 community-dwelling Chinese adults, aged 60–98	Cross sectional, correlational
Mendias & Paar 2007	Perceived health and self-care learning needs, barriers, preferred leaning modalities	151 adult outpatients with HIV/AIDS	Survey
Murphy & Polivka 2007	Parental perceptions of childhood obesity, body mass index, school's role in prevention/treatment of obesity	Parents of school-aged children in a suburban latchkey program	Descriptive

[*]Full citations are in the reference list at the end of the chapter.

7. *How contagious is this theory?*   The HPM is reported as being used in practice in Swaziland (Makhubela, 2002) and the United States (Daggett & Rigdon, 2006; Easom, 2003a, 2003b) and in practice and education in the United States by Rothman, Lourie, Brian, and Foley (2005) and Torrens and Swan (2009). Research has been reported from around the world. The following list reflects examples of publications since 1995:

Australia: Campbell and Torrance, 2005
Brazil: Victor, de Oliveira Lopes, and Ximenes, 2005
Canada: Buijs, Ross-Kerr, Cousins, and Wilson, 2003; Keizer, 1995; Milne and Moore, 2006
Finland: Aalto, 1997
Hong Kong: Hui, 2002; Kwong and Kwan, 2007; Lee and Lai, 2006
India: Kanchana, 2004
Japan: Tashiro, 2002
Jordan: Al-Obeisat, 1999
Korea: Gu and Eun, 2002; Han, Lee, Park, Park, and Cheol, 2005; Shin, Hur, Pender, Jang, and Kim, 2006

Philippines: Cuevas, 2005; Evio, 2005
Taiwan: M. Chen, James, Hsu, Chang, Huang, and Wang, 2005; S-Y Chen, 2004; Huang and Dai, 2007; Ma, 2005; Tang and Chen, 2002; H-H Wang, 1998; R. Wang, and Chen, 2003, Wu and Pender, 2002, 2005; Wu, Pender, and Noureddine, 2003; Wu, Pender, and Yang, 2002; Wu, Ronis, Pender, and Jwo, 2002
Thailand: Cananub,   2004;   Chandanasotthi,   2003;   Deenan,   2003; Kaewthummanukul, Brown, Weaver, and Thomas, 2006; Kahawong, Phancharoenworakul, Khampalikit, Taboonpong, and Chittchang, 2005; Phuphaibul et al., 2005; Pichayapinyo, 2005; Sriyuktasuth, 2002; Tilokskulchai, Sitthimongkol, Prasopkiitikun, and Klainin, 2004

The HPM has also been used in other disciplines, such as health care management (Cunningham, 1989) and health education (Desmond, 1994; Marks, 1995). Research subjects have ranged in age from middle school students to the oldest old. Refer to Table 21-3 for an overview of the range of topics and variables studied.

STRENGTHS AND LIMITATIONS

A primary strength of the HPM is its strong base in research, as demonstrated in part by the revision in 1996. It is very flexible in that while it supports research, it also supports use in practice. The HPLPII is helpful for both activities.

The multitude of variables in the HPM (revised) is both a strength and a limitation. It is a strength for use in practice because looking at all of the variables provides a more complete picture of the client. This completeness in turn should enhance the possibilities of positive outcomes. It is a weakness for research as it is very difficult to measure, let alone test, all of the variables in one study. Without testing all of the variables at one time, it is impossible to ascertain fully how the variables influence each other as well how they influence the outcome.

While the HPM (revised) incorporates a holistic nursing focus, it is not limited to use by nurses. It depends upon one's worldview as to whether this is a strength or limitation.

A limitation within the model is that spiritual is not included under personal factors. Spiritual growth is a component, or subscale, of the HPLPII and described as an essential component of assessment. However, it is not specified in the model or in the discussion of the model itself.

Summary

The background of the HPM and HPM (revised) have been discussed, with a very brief summary of the social cognitive and expectancy-value theories that contribute to the model. The variables of the HPM (revised) have been presented—individual characteristics and experiences (prior related behavior, personal factors), behavior-specific cognitions and affect (perceived benefits of action; perceived barriers to action; perceived self-efficacy; activity-related affect; interpersonal influences, norms, support, models; situational influences), commitment to action, immediate competing demands and preferences, and the behavioral outcome of health-promoting behavior. Underlying assumptions and theoretical propositions have been included. The HPM (revised) was applied in a case study and critiqued with the standard questions for this text. An overview of research using the HPM (revised) was also included.

Thought Questions

1. Considering the subscales of the HPLPII, what additional information might be included in the case study in this chapter?
2. How might you help Mrs. S. deal with her immediate competing preferences in relation to her evening meal?
3. Identify two or three health-promoting behaviors you would like to (or think you should) enhance for yourself. Discuss how using the variables in the HPM (revised) could help you choose a behavior and develop a plan of action.
4. Describe a clinical situation you have experienced and identify how using the HPM (revised) might have led to a different outcome.
5. You are working with a client who says he really wants to develop a regular program of exercise. Using the HPM (revised), what do you want to know about him in order to help him develop a successful plan of action?

EXPLORE PEARSON mynursingkit™

MyNursingKit is your one stop for online chapter review materials and resources. Prepare for success with additional NCLEX®-style practice questions, interactive assignments and activities, web links, animations and videos, and more!

Register your access code from the front of your book at
www.mynursingkit.com.

References

Aalto, P. M. (1997). Rintasyopaseulonta: Odotukset ja kokemukset asiakas-ja hoitajankokulmasta [Finnish] Translated title: Mammography screening: Expectations and experiences. *Dissertation Abstracts International, 59*(03C), 0627. Translated abstract retrieved August 9, 2007, from Dissertation Abstracts Online database.

Acton, G. J. (2002). Health-promoting self-care in family caregivers. *Western Journal of Nursing Research, 24,* 73–86.

Agazio, J. G., Ephraim, P. M., Flaherty, N. B., & Gurney, C. A. (2002). Health promotion in active-duty military women with children. *Women and Health, 35*(1), 65–82.

Al-Obeisat, S. M. (1999). Prenatal care utilization among Jordanian women. *Dissertation Abstracts International, 60*(04B), 1525. Abstract retrieved August 9, 2007, from Dissertation Abstracts Online database.

Ammouri, A. A. (2004). Correlates of exercise participation in adolescents. *Dissertation Abstracts International, 66*(02B), 0806. Abstract retrieved August 9, 2007, from Dissertation Abstracts Online database.

Arras, R. E., Ogletree, R. J., & Welshimer, K. J. (2006). Health-promoting behaviors in mean age 45 and above. *International Journal of Men's Health, 5*(1), 65–79.

Bandura, A. (1977). Self efficacy: Toward a unifying theory of behavioral change. *Psychology Review, 84,* 191–215.

Bandura, A. (1985). *Social foundations of thought and action: A social cognitive theory.* Upper Saddle River, NJ: Prentice Hall.

Bandura, A. (1997). *Self-efficacy: The exercise of control.* New York: W. H. Freeman.

Bond, M. L. Jones, M. E., Cason, C., Campbell, P., & Hall, J. (2002). Acculturation effects on health promoting lifestyle behaviors among Hispanic origin pregnant women. *Journal of Multicultural Nursing and Health, 8*(2), 61–68.

Buijs, R., Ross-Kerr, J., Cousins, S. O., & Wilson, D. (2003). Promoting participation: Evaluation of a health promotion program for low income seniors. *Journal of Community Health Nursing, 20,* 93–107.

Byam-Williams, J. J. (2006). Factors influencing health status in community-dwelling older adults. *Dissertation Abstracts International, 67*(04B), 1914. Abstract retrieved August 9, 2007, from Dissertation Abstracts Online database.

Callaghan, D. (2005a). Health behaviors, self-efficacy, self-care, and basic conditioning factors in older adults. *Journal of Community Health Nursing, 22,* 169–178.

Callaghan, D. (2005b). The influence of spiritual growth on adolescents' initiative and responsibility for self-care. *Pediatric Nursing, 31*(2), 91–97, 115.

Callaghan, D. (2006a). Basic conditioning factors' influences on adolescents' healthy behaviors, self-efficacy, and self-care. *Issues in Comprehensive Pediatric Nursing, 29,* 191–204.

Callaghan, D. (2006b). The influence of basic conditioning factors on health behaviors, self-efficacy, and self-care in adults. *Journal of Holistic Nursing, 24,* 178–185.

Campbell, M., & Torrance, C. (2005). Coronary angioplasty: Impact on risk factors and patients' understanding of the severity of their condition. *Australian Journal of Advanced Nursing, 22*(4), 26–31.

Cananub, P. (2004). Factors that influence prenatal care utilization among Thai women. *Dissertation Abstracts International, 65*(09B), 4505. Abstract retrieved August 9, 2007, from Dissertation Abstracts Online database.

Chandanasotthi, P. (2003). The relationship of stress, self-esteem, and coping styles to health promoting behaviors of adolescents in Thailand. *Dissertation Abstracts International, 64*(03B), 1172. Abstract retrieved August 9, 2007, from Dissertation Abstracts Online database.

Chanruengvanich, W., Kasemkitwattana, S., Charoenyooth, C., Towanabut, S., & Pongurgsorn, C. (2006). RCT: Self-regulated exercise program in transient ischemic attack and minor stroke patients. *Thai Journal of Nursing Research, 10,* 165–179.

Chen, M., James, K., Hsu, L., Chang, S., Huang, L., & Wang, E. K. (2005). Health-related behavior and adolescent mothers. *Public Health Nursing, 22,* 280–288.

Chen, S-Y. (2004). The development and testing of the pelvic floor muscle exercise self-efficacy scale. *Journal of Nursing Research, 12,* 257–265.

Costanzo, C., Walker, S. N., Yates, B. C., McCabe, B., & Berg, K. (2006). Physical activity counseling for older women. *Western Journal of Nursing Research, 28,* 786–801.

Coviak, C. P. (1998). Child-parent reciprocal influences in exercise behavior. *Dissertation Abstracts International, 59*(02B), 0600. Abstract retrieved August 9, 2007, from Dissertation Abstracts Online database.

Cuevas, F. P. L. (2005). Correlates of physical activity determined by self-reports among DOH personnel. *Philippine Journal of Nursing, 75*(1), 14–19.

Cunningham, G. D. (1989). Health promoting self-care behaviors in the community older adult. *Dissertation Abstracts International, 50*(12B), 4968. Abstract retrieved August 9, 2007, from Dissertation Abstracts Online database.

Daggett, L. M., & Rigdon, K. L. (2006). A computer-assisted instructional program for teaching portion size versus serving size. *Journal of Community Health Nursing, 23*(1), 29–35.

Deenan, A. (2003). Testing the health promotion model with Thai adolescents. *Dissertation Abstracts International, 65*(04B), 1776. Abstract retrieved August 9, 2007, from Dissertation Abstracts Online database.

Desmond, L. M. H. (1994). Executive women: Perceived health status and health behaviors. *Dissertation Abstracts International, 55*(05A), 1195. Abstract retrieved August 9, 2007, from Dissertation Abstracts Online database.

Easom, L. R. (2003a). Concepts in health promotion: Perceived self-efficacy and barriers in older adults. *Journal of Gerontological Nursing, 29*(5), 11–19.

Easom, L. R. (2003b). Determinants of participation in health promotion activities in rural elderly caregivers. *Dissertation Abstracts International, 64*(02B), 0636. Abstract retrieved August 9, 2007, from Dissertation Abstracts Online database.

Edens, J. E. (2004). Outcome of an intervention clinical breast examination in rural Appalachian women. *Dissertation Abstracts International, 65*(12B), 6288. Abstract retrieved August 9, 2007, from Dissertation Abstracts Online database.

Egonu, D. M. (1998). Afro-origin women's perceived risks for pregnancy-induced hypertension. *Masters Abstracts International, 36*(06), 1599. Abstract retrieved August 9, 2007, from Dissertation Abstracts Online database.

Esperat, C., Feng, D., Zhang, Y., & Owen, D. (2007). Health behaviors of low-income pregnant minority women. *Western Journal of Nursing Research, 29,* 284–300.

Evio, B. D. (2005). The relationship between selected determinants of health behavior and lifestyle profile of older adults. *Philippine Journal of Nursing, 75*(1), 23–31.

Feather, N. T. (Ed.). (1982). *Expectations and actions: Expectancy-value models in psychology.* Hillsdale, NJ: Lawrence Erlbaum Associates.

Flores, K. A. (1996). Mother, spouse, employee, student: The effect of multiple roles on the health promotion activities of college women. *Masters Abstracts International, 35*(03), 0789. Abstract retrieved August 9, 2007, from Dissertation Abstracts Online database.

Fowles, E. R., & Feucht, J. (2004). Testing the Barriers to Health Eating Scale. *Western Journal of Nursing Research, 26,* 429–443.

Frenn, M., & Malin, S. (2003). Diet and exercise in low-income culturally diverse middle school students. *Public Health Nursing, 20,* 361–368.

Frenn, M., Malin, S., & Bansal, N. K. (2003). Stage-based interventions for low-fat diet with middle school students. *Journal of Pediatric Nursing, 18*(1), 36–45.

Frenn, M., Malin, S., Bansal, N., Delgado, M., Greer, Y., Havice, M., et al. (2003). Addressing health disparities in middle school students' nutrition and exercise. *Journal of Community Health Nursing, 20*(1), 1–14.

Gabry, H. (2005). Understanding the relationship between health behavior during pregnancy and health locus of control among Arab and non-Arab women to reduce high risk pregnancy. *Dissertation Abstracts International, 66*(03B), 1393. Abstract retrieved August 9, 2007, from Dissertation Abstracts Online database.

Gasalberti, D. (2002). Early detection of breast cancer by self-examination: The influence of perceived barriers and health conception. *Oncology Nursing Forum, 29,* 1341–1347.

Graves, D. (2007). *Pender packages powerful message.* Retrieved September 5, 2007, from South Dakota State University website at http://www3.sdstate .edu/Administration/UniversityRelations/ PublicationServices/Publications.

Grubbs, L., & Carter, J. (2002). The relationship of perceived benefits and barriers to reported exercise behaviors in college undergraduates. *Family and Community Health, 25*(2), 76–84.

Gu, M. O., & Eun, Y. (2002). Health-promoting behaviors of older adults compared to young and middle-aged adults in Korea. *Journal of Gerontological Nursing, 28*(5), 46–53.

Guarnero, P. A. (2006). Health promotion behaviors among a group of 18–29 year old gay and bisexual men. *Communicating Nursing Research, 39,* 298.

Hageman, P. A., Walker, S. N., & Pullen, C. H. (2005). Tailored versus standard Internet-delivered interventions to promote physical activity in older women. *Journal of Geriatric Physical Therapy, 28*(1), 28–33.

Han, K. S., Lee, S. J., Park, E. S., Park, Y., & Cheol, K. H.(2005). Structural model for quality of life of patients with chronic cardiovascular disease in Korea. *Nursing Research, 54,* 85–96.

Haus, C. S. (2003). Medication management strategies used by community-dwelling older adults living alone. *Dissertation Abstracts International, 64*(07B), 3188. Abstract retrieved August 9, 2007, from Dissertation Abstracts Online database.

Hendricks, C., Murdaugh, C., & Pender, N. (2006). The Adolescent Lifestyle Profile: Development and psychometric characteristics. *Journal of National Black Nurses' Association, 17*(2), 1–5.

Hensley, R. D., Jones, A. K., Williams, A. G., Willsher, L. B., & Cain, P. P. (2005). One-year clinical outcomes for Louisiana residents diagnosed with type 2 diabetes and hypertension. *Journal of the American Academy of Nurse Practitioners, 17,* 363–369.

Huang, T., & Dai, F. (2007). Weight retention predictors for Taiwanese women at six-month [sic] postpartum. *Journal of Nursing Research, 15*(1), 11–20.

Hubbard, A. B. (2002). The impact of curriculum design on health promoting behaviors at a community college in south Florida. *Dissertation Abstracts International, 63*(06A), 2112. Abstract retrieved August 9, 2007, from Dissertation Abstracts Online database.

Hui, W. C. (2002). The health-promoting lifestyles of undergraduate nurses in Hong Kong. *Journal of Professional Nursing, 18*(2), 101–111.

Johnson, C. R. (1998). The relationship between health promoting lifestyles and the practice of breast cancer screening behaviors in adult women. *Masters Abstracts International, 36*(05), 1328. Abstract retrieved August 9, 2007, from Dissertation Abstracts Online database.

Johnson, R. L. (2002). The relationships among racial identity, self-esteem, sociodemographics, and health-promoting lifestyles. *Research and Theory for Nursing Practice, 16,* 193–207.

Johnson, R. L. (2005). Gender differences in health-promoting lifestyles of African Americans. *Public Health Nursing, 22*(2), 130–137.

Johnson, R. L., & Nies, M. A. (2005). A qualitative perspective of barriers to health-promoting behaviors of African Americans. *ABNF Journal, 16*(2), 39–41.

Jones, E. D., Kennedy-Malone, L., & Wideman, L. (2004). Early detection of type 2 diabetes among older African Americans. *Geriatric Nursing, 25*(1), 24–28.

Kaewthummanukul, T., Brown, K. C., Weaver, M. T., & Thomas, R. R. (2006). Predictors of exercise participation in female hospital nurses. *Journal of Advanced Nursing, 54,* 663–675.

Kahawong, W., Phancharoenworakul, K., Khampalikit, S., Taboonpong, S., & Chittchang, U. (2005). Nutritional health-promoting behaviors among women with hyperlipidemia. *Thai Journal of Nursing Research, 9*(2), 92–102.

Kalampakom, S. (2000). Stages of construction workers' use of hearing protection. *Dissertation Abstracts International, 61*(07B), 3508. Abstract retrieved August 9, 2007, from Dissertation Abstracts Online database.

Kanchana, S. (2004). Assessment of knowledge and utilization of safety measures among workers on occupational health hazards. *Nursing Journal of India, 95*(2), 26.

Keizer, M. C. (1995). Relationships among provision of care, health and well-being, and engagement in health promoting activity of older adults who are the primary caregivers for spouses with cancer. *Dissertation Abstracts International, 34*(04), 1550. Abstract retrieved August 9, 2007, from Dissertation Abstracts Online database.

Kerr, M. J., Lusk, S. L., & Ronis, D. L. (2002). Explaining Mexican American workers' hearing protection use with the Health Promotion Model. *Nursing Research, 51,* 100–109.

Kerr, M. J., Savik, K., Monsen, K. A., & Lusk, S. L. (2007). Effectiveness of computer-based tailoring versus targeting to promote use of hearing protection. *Canadian Journal of Nursing Research, 39* (1), 80–97.

Kurtz, A. C. (1996). Correlates of health-promoting lifestyles among women with rheumatoid arthritis. *Dissertation Abstracts International, 57*(02B), 989. Abstract retrieved August 9, 2007, from Dissertation Abstracts Online database.

Kwong, E. W., & Kwan, A. Y. (2007). Participation in health-promoting behavior: Influences on community-dwelling older Chinese people. *Journal of Advanced Nursing, 57,* 522–534.

Lambert, S., Fearing, A., Bell, D., & Newton, M. (2002). A comparative study of prostate screening health beliefs and practices between African American and Caucasian men. *ABNF, 13*(3), 61–63.

Lee, L. Y-K., & Lai, E. K-F. (2006). Osteoporosis in older Chinese men: Knowledge and health beliefs. *Journal of Clinical Nursing, 15,* 353–355.

Lohnes, J. L. (2003). A bicycle safety program for parents of young children. *Journal of School Nursing, 19*(2), 100–110.

Luther, C. H. (2003). Living the coming of osteoporosis: Health promotion behaviors of women at risk for osteoporosis in Mississippi. *Dissertation Abstracts International, 64*(08B), 3746. Abstract retrieved August 9, 2007, from Dissertation Abstracts Online database.

Lusk, S. L., Ronis, D. L., Kazanis, A. S., Eakin, B. L., Hong, O., & Raymond, D. M. (2003). Effectiveness of a tailored intervention to increase factory workers' use of hearing protection. *Nursing Research, 52,* 289–295.

Ma, W-F. (2005). Predictors of regular physical activity among adults with anxiety in Taiwan. *Dissertation Abstracts International, 66*(05B), 2514. Abstract retrieved August 9, 2007, from Dissertation Abstracts Online database.

Makhubela, B. H. (2002). The self-care model of best practice: Home based care. *Africa Journal of Nursing and Midwifery, 4*(1), 35–37.

Marks, L. N. (1995). Health beliefs and health-promoting behaviors of older adults from the former Soviet Union. *Dissertation Abstracts International, 56*(11A), 4287. Abstract retrieved August 9, 2007, from Dissertation Abstracts Online database.

McCullagh, M. C. (1999). Factors affecting hearing protector use among farmers. *Dissertation*

Abstracts International, 61(02B), 780. Abstract retrieved August 9, 2007, from Dissertation Abstracts Online database.

McCullagh, M., Lusk, S. L., & Ronis, D. L. (2002). Factors influencing use of hearing protection among farmers: A test of the Pender Health Promotion Model. Nursing Research, 51, 33–39.

McDonald, P. E., Brennan, P. F., & Wykle, M. L. (2005). Perceived health status and health-promoting behaviors of African-American and white informal caregivers of impaired elders. Journal of National Black Nurses' Association, 16(1), 8–17.

McDonald, P. E., & Wykle, M. L. (2003). Predictors of health-promoting behavior of African-American and white caregivers of impaired elders. Journal of National Black Nurses' Association, 14(1), 1–12.

McDonald, P. E., Wykle, M. L., Misra, R., Suwonnaroop, N., & Burant, C. J. (2002). Predictors of social support, acceptance, health promoting behaviors, and glycemia control in African-Americans with type 2 diabetes. Journal of National Black Nurses' Association, 13(11), 23–30.

McMenamin, C. A. (2002). Parental perception concerning the use of peak flow meters to the child with asthma. Masters Abstracts International, 41(05), 1420. Abstract retrieved August 9, 2007, from Dissertation Abstracts Online database.

McMurry, T. B. (2006). A comparison of pharmacological tobacco cessation relapse rates. Journal of Community Health Nursing, 23(1), 15–28.

Mendias, E. P., & Paar, D. P. (2007). Perceptions of health and self-care learning needs of outpatients with HIV/AIDS. Journal of Community Health Nursing, 24(1), 49–64.

Millard, S. R. (1998). Factors related to health-promoting behaviors in Seventh-Day Adventist older adults. Dissertation Abstracts International, 59(06B), 2684. Abstract retrieved August 9, 2007, from Dissertation Abstracts Online database.

Milne, J. L., & Moore, K. N. (2006). Factors impacting self-care for urinary incontinence. Urologic Nursing, 26(1), 41–51.

Murphy, M., & Polivka, B. (2007). Parental perceptions of the schools' role in addressing childhood obesity. Journal of School Nursing, 23(1), 40–46.

Newton, S. E., Robinson, J., & Kozac, J. (2004). Balanced analgesia after hysterectomy: The effect on outcomes. MedSurg Nursing, 13, 176–199.

Nies, M. A., & Motyka, C. L. (2006). Factors contributing to women's ability to maintain a walking program. Journal of Holistic Nursing, 24(1), 7–14.

Olson, A. F., & Berg, J. A. (2006). Theoretical foundations of promoting perimenopausal bone health. Communicating Nursing Research, 39, 279.

Ordonez, M. de los A. (2006). The lived experience of health among older Guatemalan women. Masters Abstracts International, 44(05), 2278. Abstract retrieved August 9, 2007, from Dissertation Abstracts Online database.

Pender, N. J. (1969). A developmental study of conceptual, semantic differential, and acoustical dimensions as encoding categories in short-term memory. Dissertation Abstracts International, 30(10A), 4283. Abstract retrieved September 6, 2007, from Dissertation Abstracts Online database.

Pender, N. J. (1982). Health promotion in nursing practice. Norwalk, CT: Appleton-Century Crofts.

Pender, N.J. (1987). Health promotion in nursing practice (2nd ed.). New York: Appleton-Lange.

Pender, N. J. (1996). Health promotion in nursing practice (3rd ed.). Stamford, CT: Appleton-Century-Crofts.

Pender, N. J. (2006). Biographical sketch. Retrieved August 17, 2007, from University of Michigan, School of Nursing website: http://www.nursing.umich.edu/faculty/pender/pender_bio.html.

Pender, N. J., Murdaugh, C. L., & Parsons, M. A. (2002). Health promotion in nursing practice (4th ed.). Upper Saddle River, NJ: Prentice Hall.

Pender, N. J., Murdaugh, C. L., & Parsons, M. A. (2006). Health promotion in nursing practice (5th ed.). Upper Saddle River, NJ: Prentice Hall.

Phuphaibul, R., Leucha, Y., Putwattana, P., Nuntawan, C., Tapsart, C., Tachudhong, A., et al. (2005). Health promoting behaviors of Thai adolescents, family health related life styles and parent modeling. Thai Journal of Nursing Research, 9(1), 28–37.

Pichayapinyo, P. (2005). The relationship of perceived benefits, perceived barriers, social support, and sense of mastery on adequacy of prenatal care for first-time Thai mothers. Dissertation Abstracts International, 66(03B),

1400. Abstract retrieved August 9, 2007, from Dissertation Abstracts Online database.

Robbins, L. B., Gretebeck, K. A., Kazanis, A. S., & Pender, N. J. (2006). Girls on the Move program to increase physical activity participation. *Nursing Research, 55,* 206–216.

Ronis, D. L., Hong, O., & Lusk, S. L. (2006). Comparison of the original and revised structures of the Health Promotion Model in predicting construction workers' use of hearing protection. *Research in Nursing and Health, 29,* 3–17.

Rothman, N. L., Lourie, R. J., Brian, D., & Foley, M. (2005). Temple Health Connection: A successful collaborative model of community-based primary health care. *Journal of Cultural Diversity, 12*(4), 145–151.

Rothschild, S. L. (1996). Mental representations of attachment: Implications for health-promoting behavior and perceived stress. *Dissertation Abstracts International, 57*(02A), 879. Abstract retrieved August 9, 2007, from Dissertation Abstracts Online database.

Ryan, K. F. (1996). The relationships of perceived health status, cognitive-perceptual variables, and physiologic and demographic parameters to health behaviors. *Dissertation Abstracts International, 57*(08B), 5343. Abstract retrieved August 9, 2007, from Dissertation Abstracts Online database.

Sakraida, T. J. (2002). Divorce transition, coping responses, and health-promoting behavior of midlife women. *Dissertation Abstracts International, 62*(12B), 5646. Abstract retrieved August 9, 2007, from Dissertation Abstracts Online database.

Sakraida, T. J. (2005). Divorce transition differences of midlife women. *Issues in Mental Health Nursing, 26,* 225–249.

Sapp, C. J. (2003). Adolescents with asthma: Effects of personal characteristics and health-promoting lifestyle behaviors on health-related quality of life. *Dissertation Abstracts International, 64*(05B), 2131. Abstract retrieved August 9, 2007, from Dissertation Abstracts Online database.

Schlikcau, J. M., & Wilson, M. E. (2005). Breastfeeding as health-promoting behaviour for Hispanic women: Literature review. *Journal of Advanced Nursing, 52,* 200–210.

Shin, Y. H., Hur, H. K., Pender, N. J., Jang, H. J., & Kim, M. (2006). Exercise self-efficacy, exercise benefits and barriers, and commitment to a plan for exercise among Korean women with osteoporosis and osteoarthritis. *International Journal of Nursing Studies, 43*(1), 3–10.

Smith, A. B., & Bashore, L. (2006). The effect of clinic-based health promotion education on perceived health status and health promotion behaviors of adolescent and young adult cancer survivors. *Journal of Pediatric Oncology Nursing, 23,* 326–334.

Smith, S. A., & Michel, Y. (2006). A pilot study on the effects of aquatic exercises on discomforts of pregnancy. *JOGNN: Journal of Obstetric, Gynecologic, and Neonatal Nursing, 35,* 315–323.

Sohng, K., Sohng, S., & Yeom, H. (2002). Health promoting behaviors of elderly Korean immigrants in the United States. *Public Health Nursing, 19,* 294–300.

Sriyuktasuth, A. (2002). Utility of Pender's model in describing health-promoting behaviors in Thai women with systemic lupus erythematosus. *Dissertation Abstracts International, 63*(10B), 4599. Abstract retrieved August 9, 2007, from Dissertation Abstracts Online database.

Srof, B. J., & Velsor-Friedrich, B. (2006). Health promotion in adolescents: A review of Pender's Health Promotion Model. *Nursing Science Quarterly, 19,* 366–373.

Stuifbergen, A. K., Harrison, T. C., Becker, H., & Carter, P. (2004). Adaptation of a wellness intervention for women with chronic disabling conditions. *Journal of Holistic Nursing, 22*(1), 12–31.

Suwonnaroop, N., & Zauszniewski, J. (2002). The effects of social support, perceived health status, and personal factors on health-promoting behaviors among American older adults. *Thai Journal of Nursing Research, 6*(2), 41–55.

Tang, Y., & Chen, S. (2002). Health promotion behaviors in Chinese family caregivers of patients with stroke. *Health Promotion International, 17,* 329–339.

Tapler, D. A. (1996). The relationship between health value, self-efficacy, health locus of control, health benefits, health barriers, and health behavior practices in mothers. *Dissertation Abstracts International, 57*(05B), 3132. Abstract retrieved August 9, 2007, from Dissertation Abstracts Online database.

Tashiro, J. (2002). Exploring health promoting lifestyle behaviors of Japanese college women: Perceptions, practices, and issues. *Health Care for Women International, 23*(1), 59–70.

Tilokskulchai, F., Sitthimongkol, Y., Prasopkiitikun, T., & Klainin, P. (2004). Meta-analysis of health promotion research in Thailand [corrected] [published erratum appears in *Asian Journal of Nursing Studies*, 2004, 7(3)]. *Asian Journal of Nursing Studies, 7*(2), 18–32.

Victor, J. F., de Oliveira Lopes, M. V., & Ximenes, L. B. (2005). Analysis of diagram the Health Promotion Model of Nola J. Pender [Portuguese]. *Acta Paulista de Enfermagem, 18*, 235–240. Abstract retrieved August 8, 2007, from CINAHL Plus with Full Text.

Walker, S. N., Pullen, C. H., Hertzog, M., Boeckner, L., & Hageman, P. A. (2006). Determinants of older rural women's activity and eating. *Western Journal of Nursing Research, 28*, 449–468.

Wang, H-H. (1998). A model of self-care and well-being of rural elderly women in Taiwan. *Dissertation Abstracts International, 59*(06B), 2689. Abstract retrieved August 9, 2007, from Dissertation Abstracts Online database.

Wang, R., & Chen, C. (2003). Evaluating Pender's Health Promotion Model from literature review [Chinese], *Journal of Nursing, 50*(6), 62–68. Abstract retrieved August 9, 2007, from CINAHL Plus with Full Text.

Warner, K. D. (2000). Health-related lifestyle behaviors of twins: Interpersonal and situational influences. *Dissertation Abstracts International, 61*(03B), 1331. Abstract retrieved August 9, 2007, from Dissertation Abstracts Online database.

White, J. L. (1996). Outcomes of an individualized health promotion program for homebound older community residents. *Dissertation Abstracts International, 57*(12B), 7458. Abstract retrieved August 9, 2007, from Dissertation Abstracts Online database.

Whitehead, D. (2005). Letter to the Editor. *Research in Nursing and Health, 28*, 357–359.

Willis, J. L. (2001). The effect of multiple roles on the health promotion activities of college women. *Masters Abstracts International, 39*(05), 1382. Abstract retrieved August 9, 2007, from Dissertation Abstracts Online database.

Wilson, M. C. (2003). Health practices of homeless women. *Dissertation Abstracts International, 65*(02B), 660. Abstract retrieved August 9, 2007, from Dissertation Abstracts Online database.

Wilson, M. (2005). Health promoting behaviors of sheltered homeless women. *Family and Community Health, 28*(1), 51–63.

Wisnewski, C. A. (1996). A study of the health-promoting behavioral effects of an exercise educational intervention in adult diabetics. *Dissertation Abstracts International, 57*(05B), 3133. Abstract retrieved August 9, 2007, from Dissertation Abstracts Online database.

Wu, T., & Pender, N. (2002). Determinants of physical activity among Taiwanese adolescents: An application of the Health Promotion Model. *Research in Nursing and Health, 25*(1), 25–36.

Wu, T., & Pender, N. (2005). A panel study of physical activity in Taiwanese youth: Testing the revised health-promotion model. *Family and Community Health, 28*, 113–124.

Wu, T., Pender, N., & Noureddine, S. (2003). Gender differences in the psychosocial and cognitive correlates of physical activity among Taiwanese adolescents: A structural equation modeling approach. *International Journal of Behavioral Medicine, 10*, 93–105.

Wu, T., Pender, N., & Yang, K. (2002). Promoting physical activity among Taiwanese and American adolescents. *Journal of Nursing Research, 10*(1), 57–64.

Wu, T., Ronis, D. L., Pender, N., & Jwo, J. (2002). Development of questionnaires to measure physical activity cognitions among Taiwanese adolescents. *Preventive Medicine, 35*(1), 54–65.

Yang, K. (2005). Physical activities among Korean midlife immigrant women in the United States. *Dissertation Abstracts International, 66*(08B), 4159. Abstract retrieved August 9, 2007, from Dissertation Abstracts Online database.

Yates, B. C., Price-Fowlkes, T., & Agrawal, S. (2003). Barriers and facilitatiors of self-reported physical activity in cardiac patients. *Research in Nursing and Health, 26*, 459–469.

Yoon, S. L., & Horne, C. H. (2004). Holistic health care. Perceived health promotion practice by older women: Use of herbal products. *Journal of Gerontological Nursing, 30*(7), 9–15.

Yue, S. P. (1998). Assessing the needs of the post-cardiac event population in a rural southeastern New Mexico community. *Masters Abstracts International, 36*(06), 1594. Abstract retrieved August 9, 2007, from Dissertation Abstracts Online database.

Annotated Bibliography

Callaghan, D. M. (2003). Health-promoting self-care behaviors, self-care self-efficacy, and self-care agency. *Nursing Science Quarterly, 16,* 247–254.

This study explored the relationships among the four dimensions of self-care self-efficacy, the six dimensions of health-promoting self-care behaviors, and a set of variables including the four dimensions of self-care agency. Study participants were 387 adults, aged 18 to 65, from the greater Philadelphia area. The only concept identified as having an influence on self-care agency was spiritual growth.

Costanzo, C., Walker, S. N., Yates, B. C., McCabe, B., & Berg, K. (2006). Physical activity counseling for older women. *Western Journal of Nursing Research, 28,* 786–801.

In this study, 46 women were randomly assigned to a group to receive five behavioral counseling sessions or to a comparison group that received only one counseling session. The sessions incorporated the five As: ask, advise, assist, arrange, agree. The pretest and posttest measurements involved moderate-intensity physical activity, muscle strengthening, and stretching activity. The group that had five sessions showed a statistically significant increase in cardiorespiratory fitness. Time effects were demonstrated for both groups in increased left handgrip strength, increased leg strength, and increased flexibility.

Kaewthummanukul, T., Brown, K. C., Weaver, M. T., & Thomas, R. R. (2006). Predictors of exercise participation in female hospital nurses. *Journal of Advanced Nursing, 54,* 663–675.

This study investigated the relationship between participation in exercise, selected personal factors, perceived benefits, perceived barriers, perceived self-efficacy, perceived social support, job demands, and motivation. Subjects were 970 nurses employed in a Thai hospital. Findings were that an increased participation in exercise is related to perceptions of exercise, self-efficacy, social support as well as to motivation.

Kwong, E. W., & Kwan, A. Y. (2007). Participation in health-promoting behavior: Influences on community-dwelling older Chinese people. *Journal of Advanced Nursing, 57,* 522–534.

Face-to-face interviews with 896 community dwelling Chinese people, aged 60 to 98, in Hong Kong provided the data for this study about factors that influence participation in physical activity, healthy dietary practices, and stress management. The use of health-promoting behaviors was most strongly influenced by perceived self-efficacy, perceived benefits, and gender. The most frequently reported barriers were fatigue during and after physical activity, enjoyment of unhealthy foods, and lack of adequate social support from family and peers.

Newton, S. E., Robinson, J., & Kozac, J. (2004). Balanced analgesia after hysterectomy: The effect on outcomes. *MEDSUR Nursing, 13,* 176–180, 199.

This interesting application of the health promotion model investigated the type of postoperative analgesia used with 98 women who had had abdominal hysterectomies in relation to the health-promoting behaviors of low pain scores, greater mobility, and shorter hospital length of stay. Interestingly, there were no statistically significant differences found between the use of balanced analgesia and the use of morphine only. It is comforting to know that all women in the study apparently achieved adequate pain control. The balanced analgesia appeared to facilitate post-surgery mobility, but not at a statistically significant level.

Ronis, D. L., Hong, O., & Lusk, S. L. (2006). Comparison of the original and revised structures of the Health Promotion Model in predicting construction workers' use of hearing protection. *Research in Nursing and Health, 29,* 3–17.

This study compared the fit and usefulness of the original and revised versions of the HPM in relation to predicting construction workers' use of hearing protection. Subjects were 703 workers who identified themselves as being exposed to high noise levels. The results indicated that while both versions provided a good fit, the revised version was a better fit and explained more of the variance in the use of hearing protection.

CHAPTER 22

Philosophy of Caring and Expert Nursing Practice

Patricia Benner

Bobbe Ann Gray

Patricia Benner was born in Hampton, Virginia. Her childhood was spent in California, where she obtained both her early and her advanced education (Brykczynski, 2006). Benner received both her associate's degree in nursing and her bachelor's degree in nursing from Pasadena College in 1964. Her master's degree in medical-surgical nursing was received from the University of California, San Francisco, in 1970. Her Ph.D. was received from the University of California, Berkeley, in 1982, where she was an interdivisional student in education. Benner's doctoral work focused on stress, coping, and health in mid-career men (P. Benner, personal communication, October 24, 2006). During this time, she became heavily influenced by the work of Hubert Dreyfus and Richard Lazarus. She has nursing practice experience, as both a staff nurse and in management, in medical-surgical, emergency room, coronary care, intensive care, and home care nursing (Benner Associates, 2002).

Benner is currently director of the National Nursing Education Study for the Carnegie Foundation for the Advancement of Teaching. In addition, she is a professor in the Department of Social and Behavioral Sciences at the University of California, San Francisco, and holds the Thelma Shobe Endowed Chair in Ethics and Spirituality (P. Benner, personal communication, October 24, 2006).

Benner has authored numerous books, chapters, and articles. She has published in a number of international forums and has received several Book-of-the-Year awards from the American Journal of Nursing and other organizations. Her books have been translated into many languages and are influential worldwide on nursing practice and education. Benner's work has had a significant impact within the United States, Great Britain, Australia, and New Zealand. Among her many honors are induction as a fellow of the American Academy of Nursing in 1985 and as an honorary fellow of the Royal College of Nursing in the United Kingdom in 1994. Benner has received numerous awards in nursing for publications, research, leadership, education, and service (Benner Associates, 2002; P. Benner, personal communication, October 24, 2006; University of California, San Francisco Faculty Profiles, 2006).

Benner's recent projects include director of a National Nursing Education Research Project sponsored by the Carnegie Foundation for the Advancement of Teaching. This study is the first national study in 30 years to examine nursing education and is part of a larger project that is investigating the preparation for professionals. Other recent projects include a taxonomy of nursing errors for the National Council of State Boards of Nursing, development of a program to educate advanced practice nurses in genomics, a study of clinical knowledge development of nurses in combat operations environments, and a study of skill acquisition and clinical and ethical reasoning in critical care nurses (P. Benner, personal communication, October 24, 2006).

DEVELOPMENT OF BENNER'S PHILOSOPHY OF EXPERT NURSING PRACTICE

Benner identifies Virginia Henderson as a significant early influence on her nursing career (Benner & Wrubel, 1989). Benner's earlier work relating to expert nursing practice investigated the progression of skill acquisition for nurses based on the skill acquisition theory developed by philosopher Hubert Dreyfus and his brother, mathematician and systems analyst Stuart Dreyfus (Dreyfus & Dreyfus, 1980). It is important to clarify that Benner has consistently referred to this model as the "Dreyfus Model of Skill Acquisition." Benner, rather than developing a model of skill acquisition, merely validated and extended the existing Dreyfus model to exemplify the process of skill acquisition in nursing. In addition, much of Benner's writing is the result of collegial effort. For the sake of preventing redundancy, general references contained in this chapter to Benner's work must be assumed to refer to Benner and colleagues.

Benner served as project director for the *Achieving Methods of Intrapersonal Consensus, Assessment and Evaluation* project from 1979 through 1981. This project was designed to identify differences between beginning and expert nurses' clinical performance and situational appraisals (Benner, 1984/2001). A sample of 21 pairs of nurses in a preceptor relationship (newly graduated nurse and expert) was examined using an interpretive phenomenological method and structured using the Dreyfus Skill Acquisition Model (Dreyfus & Dreyfus, 1980). The pairs were interviewed separately and asked to describe a clinical incident that they had in common to determine if there were differences in the descriptions, indicating differing perceptions and approaches. In addition to the 21 pairs, 51 experienced nurses selected by administrators as being highly skilled, 11 new graduates, and five senior nursing students were interviewed (individual and small group) and/or observed to identify characteristics of performance in other skill levels of nurses. Six hospitals were represented. The results of this study are reported in *From Novice to Expert: Excellence and Power in Clinical Nursing Practice* (FNE). Findings indicated discernable differences in skill level between novices, advanced beginners, and competent, proficient, and expert nurses. Narrative descriptions were interpreted, and 31 nursing competencies were identified. These competencies were further examined and classified into seven domains of nursing practice. The information presented in *FNE* regarding skill acquisition domains of nursing practice provides a structure for later works in that frequent reference is made to the differences between inexperienced and expert nursing in terms of concepts such as critical thinking, intuition, and ethical agency.

While the levels of skill acquisition along with the related competencies and domains of nursing practice identified in *FNE* are frequently used as a framework for practice and education, Benner did not state an intent to develop an interpretive theory until the publication of *Primacy of Caring* (Benner & Wrubel, 1989). Here, Benner and Wrubel comment on the limitations of existing nursing theories in capturing the essential human issues that are central to nursing. They state, "A theory is needed that describes, interprets, and explains not an imagined ideal of nursing, but actual expert nursing as it is practiced day by day" (p. 5) with a goal to "make visible the hidden significant work of nursing as a caring practice" (p. xi). Benner and Wrubel note, "This book is devoted to an interpretive theory of nursing practice as it is concerned with helping people to cope with the stress of illness" (p. 7).

Primacy of Caring (Benner & Wrubel, 1989) contains further development of the distinguishing features of expert nurses begun in *FNE* as well as a description of the primary role of caring in nursing practice. Expert nursing practice, as presented in that work, is based on caring at multiple levels of practice. Caring is defined as a "basic way of being in the world" (p. xi) and nursing as a "caring practice whose science is guided by the moral art and ethics of care and responsibility" (p. xi). The descriptions contained in *Primacy of Caring* relate to the primacy of caring as a significant factor in stress and coping, nursing practice, and illness outcome. Expert nursing care is described related to specific situations such as chronic illness, cancer, and neurological illness. In addition, Benner discusses caregiving from a feminist perspective in her chapter on coping with caregiving.

Benner, Tanner, and Chesla (1996) present the findings of a study conducted between 1990 and 1996 in *Expertise in Nursing Practice: Caring, Clinical Judgment, and Ethics* (*ENP*). This work extended the original data of earlier studies. An additional 130 critical care nurses representing eight hospitals were interviewed in small groups, with 48 of those nurses individually interviewed and observed in practice. Benner states, "From this original study, we developed an ethnography of the practice of critical care nurses" (Benner, Hooper-Kyriakides, & Stannard, 1999, p. 6). *ENP* devotes several chapters to application of this information for improvement of nurse–physician relationships and implications for nursing education and administration.

Benner et al. (1999) published *Clinical Wisdom and Interventions in Critical Care: A Thinking-in-Action Approach* (*CWICC*) based on the findings of Phase 2 of the previously described study. Conducted between 1996 and 1997, Phase 2 extended the critical care focus to an additional 75 nurses working in a wide variety of critical care areas as well as advanced practice nurses. This book gives insight into the development of expert critical care nurses' ability to grasp a problem intuitively and plan ahead when in familiar clinical situations as well as excellent examples of Benner's nonlinear concept of nursing process. The work identified two habits of thought and actions of expert critical care nurses: (a) clinical grasp and clinical inquiry and (b) clinical forethought. In addition, nine domains of critical care nursing practice with nursing competencies specific to the critical care setting were delineated. Implications for the educational strategies to foster development of expertise are presented in *CWICC*.

PHILOSOPHY OF EXPERT NURSING PRACTICE

The exemplification of caring as primary in expert nursing practice differs according to the skill acquisition level of the nurse. It is therefore necessary to understand not only the nature of nursing care but also how that care differs according the individual nurse's professional development. In order to do this, Benner departs from the typical

Cartesian cognitive-rationality that splits the mind and body of the person. Benner cites Kuhn's (1970) and Polanyi's (1958) views that there is a difference between "knowing that" stemming from theoretical knowledge and "knowing how" stemming from practical knowledge. In order to discover how nurses "know how" to practice expertly, Benner adopted an interpretive or hermeneutic phenomenological approach. While nurses with a variety of experience levels and clinical focuses were included, the accumulated exemplars reported tend to be from narratives of expert nurses working in critical care units.

Use of the interpretive phenomenological approach enabled the researchers to identify numerous nursing competencies, which were then inductively grouped into a number of domains of nursing care. Benner explicitly states in a number of her writings that her work must be clearly understood to be useful. She cautions against "deifying" the domains of nursing described and the competencies attributed to those domains (Benner, 1984/2001, pp. xxii, xxv). She emphasizes the need to avoid trying to use her work as a template or set of rules, stating that it is a way of thinking or a method (Benner & Wrubel, 1989). Readers of Benner's work are cautioned to carefully consider the focus of the study from which the domains and competencies were derived. Thorough reading of Benner's body of work, as well as similar studies based on Benner's framework, reveals both expansions and contractions of the originally identified domains and varying competencies subsumed under those domains. Indeed, as an interpretive theory rather than an explanatory theory, those who wish to apply Benner's framework must first validate the domains and competencies for their unique clinical and staff situations.

Benner (1984/2001) divides nursing skill acquisition into five stages: novice, advanced beginner, competent, proficient, and expert. Novices are generally conceptualized as students. Advanced beginners are newly graduated nurses. Competent nurses have worked in a specialty for somewhere between one and a half and two years. Proficient nurses begin to rely less on theory and more on experientially learned knowledge. Expert nurses rely heavily on experientially learned knowledge and fall back on theory when the clinical picture is unclear.

Additional concepts were introduced in the books that followed. In *Primacy of Caring,* Benner and Wrubel (1989) discuss the importance of understanding the human in terms of the role of embodied intelligence, background meaning, human concern, situatedness, and temporality. Concepts such as stress, coping, life cycle, and health promotion are addressed. The stages of professional skill acquisition were further explicated in *ENP* (Benner et al., 1996), where the concepts and relationships among caring, clinical knowledge, clinical and ethical judgment, and social embeddedness are expanded. Benner et al. (1999) discussed clinical grasp, clinical inquiry, clinical forethought, expert nursing judgment, thinking, and clinical comportment in *CWICC.* In addition, the concepts of thinking and reasoning-in-action were discussed as well as skilled know-how, response-based practice, agency, perceptual acuity, ethical reasoning, and the role of emotions in nursing.

Key Concepts

Benner's work contains reference to a large number of significant concepts, as described next.

Agency refers to one's ability to influence the situation (Benner & Wrubel, 1989). Agency is affected by one's ability to see the possibilities within the situation based on one's experience level. New nurses feel little ability to impact the situation, whereas expert nurses have a realistic awareness of their ability to impact the situation (Benner & Wrubel; Benner et al., 1996).

Assumptions, expectations, and sets are beliefs generated from past experiences that orient and influence the nurse's perception of the patient situation. Sets are subtle and may not be completely explicit. These sets predispose the nurse to act in certain ways when involved in certain situations (Benner, 1984/2001).

Background meaning is part of context and is the culturally acquired set of meanings the person accumulates from birth. Background meaning is how the world is understood to "be" and influences one's perception of the factual world (Benner & Wrubel, 1989).

Caring is an essential skill of nurses and is "a basic way of being in the world" (Benner & Wrubel, 1989, p. xi). Caring means that "things," such as other people, events, and so on, matter. Some "things" matter more than others because we live in a differentiated world where priorities are evident. Caring is required to create personal concern.

Clinical forethought, or "future think," is anticipation of likely events and the actions required to prepare for those eventualities based on context. Clinical forethought allows the clinician to plan ahead based on the immediate situation, to anticipate and quickly prevent potential problems (Benner et al., 1999).

Clinical judgment implies recognizing salient, or important, aspects of the situation as they unfold and acting appropriately on that knowledge. The novice uses learned rules to make clinical judgments, whereas the expert nurse uses a more refined, engaged, practical reasoning based on subtle changes that are unseen by nurses functioning at a lower level. Clinical judgment in the expert nurse is based on experiential learning, moral agency, knowing the patient, emotional response to the situation, and intuition (Benner et al., 1996, 1999). Benner identifies six aspects of clinical judgment and skillful comportment: reasoning-in-transition, skilled know-how, response-based practice, agency, perceptual acuity and involvement, and links between clinical and ethical reasoning (Benner et al., 1999).

Clinical knowledge is practical knowledge. Benner (1984/2001) identifies six areas of practical knowledge: "(1) graded qualitative distinctions; (2) common meanings; (3) assumptions, expectations, and sets; (4) paradigm cases and personal knowledge; (5) maxims; and (6) unplanned practices" (p. 4).

Clinical reasoning is a process of understanding a particular patient's condition at a particular time based on the changes or transitions observed for that patient (Benner, 2003; Benner et al., 1996).

Clinical transitions are recognized when the clinician detects subtle or not-so-subtle changes in the patient's condition that require the clinician to reconsider the needs of the emerging situation (Benner et al., 1999).

Common meanings occur because nurses work within a health and illness situation. Nurses form common meanings with other nurses in their perspective on health- and illness-related issues commonly encountered. Nurses also learn what to expect from the situation by experience with patient and family responses. These meanings form a tradition that is used to compare specific patient situations and theory and further define the common meanings (Benner, 1984/2001).

Concern refers to a human way of being in the world, or being involved in one's world, which engages the person with the salient aspects of the world. This ability to be engaged in one's world is an essentially human aspect that allows one to determine what is "at stake" for the person. It explains why things matter to humans. Concern is situational, and the health care provider must be able to determine the concerns of persons within their culturally held meaning. Concern also has a temporal aspect as concerns change across time and situations (Benner & Wrubel, 1989).

Coping is defined consistently with Lazarus's beliefs that coping is reflected in the emotional and behavioral responses one has to stress (Benner & Wrubel, 1989; Lazarus & Folkman, 1984).

The **Dreyfus Model of Skill Acquisition** serves as the theoretical basis of Benner's work on identifying the professional development of nurses. This model identifies "five stages of qualitatively different perceptions of their [nurse's] task as skill improves" (Dreyfus & Dreyfus, 1996). These stages have been labeled novice, advanced beginner, competent, proficient, and expert. Dreyfus and Dreyfus caution, "There are, perhaps, no expert nurses, but certainly many nurses achieve expertise in the area of their specialization" (p. 35). This statement points to the situational and experiential aspects of expertise. Nurses may function as an expert in a situation where they have sufficient experience to intuitively grasp the nuances of the situation. However, if a nurse is confronted by a new situation, a new type of patient, or a new nursing unit, he or she will function at a lower level of expertise (Benner, 1984/2001). Dreyfus and Dreyfus also point out that closer examination of the stages may reveal substages; however, the five-stage model has been sufficient for their purposes. See Table 22-1 for a breakdown of the characteristics of each of the five stages of skill development for nurses.

Benner (1984/2001) states that the five levels reflect changes occurring in three aspects of skilled performance: (a) a movement from reliance on rules and abstract principles to the use of concrete past experiences as the basis of decision making, (b) increasing ability to see the situation as a whole or the "big picture," and (c) increasing involvement within the situation.

There are nurses who do not follow the trajectory outlined by the Dreyfus model. Aspects relevant to these nurses have been addressed by Rubin (1996). Rubin states that these nurses fail to follow the typical trajectory from the very beginning of their practice. She also makes clear that this failure to follow the typical trajectory is not an issue of personality differences. These nurses exhibit common patterns of behavior that cannot be attributed to common personality types or common psychological conditions. Classic narratives, or exemplars, derived from discussions with these nurses revealed: (a) a lack of ability to remember salient aspects of patient care situations; that is, seeing all patients as stereotypes; (b) perceiving that they do not use clinical knowledge and ethical judgment to make clinical decisions; (c) fuzzy boundaries between "patient" and "self," that is, assuming that the patient's thoughts and feelings are the same as one's own; (d) inability to see nuances in the situation; (e) confusion of the ethical and legal foundations of care; (f) shifting responsibility for decision making to others; and (g) feeling unimportant in the care of patients. Rubin states, "Whatever the psychological difficulties or moral shortcomings of these nurses, their fundamental problem is their lack of knowledge of the qualitative distinctions that are embodied in expert nursing practice" (p. 191).

Domains of practice are thematic groupings of clinical competencies identified in the narrative accounts of nurses. These domains of practice were not designed to be exhaustive or comprehensive (Benner, 1984/2001) but reflect the thoughts and actions of the nurses who participated in the study. Activity related to the domains of practice is not exclusive; that is, the nurse may be practicing in several domains simultaneously. The situation determines which domains take precedence, by necessity, over others (Benner et al., 1999).

TABLE 22-1   Benner's Descriptors of Nurses Based on the Dreyfus and Dreyfus Model of Skill Acquisition

Novice
- A complete beginner with no experience in that specialty area.[1]
- Practices using theoretical knowledge acquired through formal learning.[2]
- Relies on use of context-free rules for drawing conclusions based on recognizable, objective features of the situation.[1, 2]
- Behavior is extremely limited and inflexible, as learned rules cannot differentiate relevant versus nonrelevant aspects of the situation.[1]

Advanced Beginner
- The newly graduated nurse or the experienced nurse who has transferred to another specialty or dissimilar unit.[3]
- Performs at a marginally acceptable level after having gained experience coping with real situations.[2]
- Begins to notice situational elements in addition to the objective elements learned in formal situations.[2]
- Begins to see structure in the clinical setting.[3]
- Begins to realize the complexity of situations and feels overwhelmed, anxious, and exhausted in trying to identify all the relevant elements.[2, 3]
- Sees breakdowns in ability to provide care as lack of knowledge or poor organization.[3]
- Begins constructing more and more complex rules developed from actual practice to help guide actions.[2]
- Remains very task oriented with a physical/technological focus.[3]
- Goal orientation is the accomplishing of tasks in a timely fashion with elaborate organizational plans, often at the expense of not noticing what is occurring within the situation.[3]
- Sees clinical practice as a test of personal abilities, with a focus on personal goals rather than patient-centered goals.[3]
- Clinical agency has an external focus, with reliance on standards of care and orders for direction.[3]
- Decision making is referred up the clinical ladder, with extraordinary faith in the expertise of others.[3]
- Often makes decisions based on what has been done for the patient by other nurses on previous shifts.[3]
- Oriented to the present moment with little ability to see applicability of patient's past and future expectations on present care needs.[3]
- Begins to recognize changes in clinical state but lacks the experience to identify how to manage those changes.[3]

Competent
- The nurse who has about one and a half to two years of experience on a specific unit.[3]
- Differs from the advanced beginner primarily related to improved "clinical understanding, technical skills, organizational ability, and ability to anticipate the likely course of events" (p. 78).[3]
- Exemplifies "standard" nursing care.[3]
- A pivotal stage for progression to proficiency where pattern recognition begins to become established.[3]
- The overwhelming number of potentially relevant elements now recognized force the nurse to begin sorting the elements into a hierarchy of importance based on a conscious selection plan.[2]
- New rules are established to facilitate choice of plan.[2]
- The unlimited variety of potential plans of actions presents a frightening list of possibilities, which generates an exaggerated sense of responsibility in the nurse.[2]

(continued)

TABLE 22-1   Benner's Descriptors of Nurses Based on the Dreyfus and Dreyfus Model of Skill Acquisition (Continued)

- Goals remain predominantly focused on personal organization rather than immediate patient outcomes.[3]
- Emotional involvement increases and begins to be used as screening or alerting mechanism.[2,3]
- There is a gradual shift to a focus on clinical issues rather than self-performance.[3]
- The nurse begins to discriminate between skill levels of others involved in the clinical setting and recognizes the fallibility of others.[3]
- Extensive reading identifies the limits of theoretical knowledge, precipitating a crisis in the trust in that knowledge.[3]
- Clinical knowledge becomes integrated with theoretical knowledge to allow the nurse to begin to see the "big picture." [3]
- The temporal orientation increasingly shifts to the near future.[3]
- Ethical and clinical concerns may remain unaddressed due to lack of experiential wisdom.[3]
- Improved recognition of salient signs and symptoms and variations between patients develops.[3]
- Begins to deviate from standardized patient care practices to individualize to current demands.[3]
- Becomes more adept at presenting a clinical case for physician action.[3]

Proficient

- A transition stage that usually leads to expertise.[2,3]
- There is a qualitative, rather than incremental, leap in perceptual acuity and relational skills that shapes actions.[3]
- Experience results in development of synaptic pathways in the brain that alter the rule-and-principle-based responses to a more situationally associated response set of behaviors referred to as intuition.[2]
- This ability to intuitively discriminate between a variety of situations stems from a growing concern and involvement that helps differentiate important aspects of the situation.[2]
- There is improved reasoning-in-transition, sense of salience, and recognition of relevant changes. [3]
- Stress levels decrease as required actions becomes more clear and require less recourse to calculative reasoning.[2]
- Experience is still short of that required for expertise; thus, the proficient nurse still does not respond intuitively to situations without first giving conscious thought to the possible options.[2]
- The past becomes more critical to understanding the present and possibilities for the future.[3]
- The nurse exhibits a practical grasp and practical reasoning.[3]
- Practical grasp, emotional attunement, and involvement allow the nurse to develop an ethic of responsiveness to the current situation that allows the nurse to differentiate self from others.[3]
- The "big picture" now guides the nurse's care.[3]
- Actions demonstrate a smooth response-based approach and are situationally appropriate.[3]
- The nurse is able to read the situation and determine when changes have occurred but still lacks some skill in determining the correct course of action to take in response to changes.[3]
- The nurse begins to function as a change agent as sense of agency grows.[3]
- Responsibility is realistically examined, with a growing balanced awareness of the impact others have in the care given.[3]
- The focus shifts from self to patient outcomes.[3]
- Communication and negotiation skills increase in order to meet the situated needs of the patient and family.[3]
- Maxims, or rules based on subtle nuances within the situation, can now be developed and used. However, once the maxim is developed and the skill mastered, it is difficult for the nurse to remember the learning process that produced that maxim.[1,3]

TABLE 22-1	Benner's Descriptors of Nurses Based on the Dreyfus and Dreyfus Model of Skill Acquisition (Continued)

Expert

- There is an ability to notice both the unexpected and features that are absent in the situation, which alerts the expert nurses to give more detailed attention to the patient who fails to follow the expected trajectory.[4]
- The skill to discriminate when to act and when to wait becomes evident. This skill is based on "vigilant monitoring."[4]
- Expert nurses situate themselves within an observational distance of the patient in order to stay attuned to the changing needs and condition of the patient.[4]
- Attuning to changes and awareness of salient aspects of the situation are accomplished without conscious deliberation.[3]
- Discrimination between similar situations becomes more refined, allowing for ease of discrimination between courses of action.[3]
- An intuitive grasp of the situation based on extensive experience leads to a focus on actions rather than problems.[3]
- Expert nurses use "deliberative rationality" to reflect on goals and actions to achieve those goals rather than on formal rules and formulas.[3]
- Theory is understood at a deeper, applied level.[3]
- Moral agency is highly developed in expert nurses, as demonstrated by a highly developed concern for the personhood of the patient, protecting them in their vulnerability and helping them in ways that preserve the integrity of the person.[3]
- The "big picture" is future oriented for the patient and includes an awareness of people and activities occurring on the unit that add or detract from care. This future orientation is specific and contextually based.[1, 3]
- Expert nurses can take strong positions based on their experience and not only communicate effectively with other professionals, but use this communication to advocate for patients and to help redesign the system in caring ways.[3]
- Organizational expertise is evident as the expert nurse facilitates and directs care on multiple levels simultaneously within complex and sometimes rapidly changing environments.[1]
- Expert nurses are confident and able to keep their composure in the face of rapid shifts in patient change or system breakdown.[1]
- Experts develop sophisticated maxims for practice that are difficult to relate verbally to others.[1]

Note: [1] Benner (1984/2001); [2] Dreyfus and Dreyfus (1989); [3] Benner, Tanner, and Chesla (1996); [4] Benner, Hooper-Kyriakidis, and Stannard (1999).

The domains of practice identified in *FNE* have a somewhat broader applicability, as the nurses involved in that study represented a wider range of abilities and clinical specialties than in Benner's other studies. From that study, Benner (1984/2001) identified 31 competencies that lead to the inductive derivation of seven domains. These domains include "the helping role, the teaching-coaching function, the diagnostic and patient monitoring function, effective management of rapidly changing situations, administering and monitoring therapeutic interventions and regimens, monitoring and ensuring the quality of health care practices, and organizational and work role competencies" (Benner, 1984/2001, p. 46) (see Table 22-2).

TABLE 22-2   Domains of Nursing Practice and Related Competencies

The helping role
- "The healing relationship: Creating a climate for and establishing a commitment to healing
- Providing comfort measures and preserving personhood in the face of pain and extreme breakdown
- Presencing: Being with a patient
- Maximizing the patient's participation and control in his own recovery
- Interpreting kinds of pain and selecting appropriate strategies for pain management and control
- Providing comfort and communication through touch
- Providing emotional and informational support to patient's families
- Guiding a patient through emotional and developmental change: Providing new options, closing off old ones: Channeling, teaching, mediating
  - Acting as a psychological and cultural mediator
  - Using goals therapeutically
  - Working to build and maintain a therapeutic community" (Benner, 1984/2001, p. 50)

The teaching-coaching role
- "Timing: Capturing a patient's readiness to learn
- Assisting patients to integrate the implications of illness and recovery into their lifestyles
- Eliciting and understanding the patient's interpretation of his illness
- Providing an interpretation of the patient's condition and giving a rationale for procedures
- The coaching function: Making culturally avoided aspects of an illness approachable and understandable" (Benner, p. 79)

The diagnostic and patient-monitoring function
- "Detection and documentation of significant changes in a patient's condition
- Providing an early warning signal: Anticipating breakdown and deterioration prior to explicit confirming diagnostic signs
- Anticipating problems: Future think
- Understanding the particular demands and experiences of an illness: Anticipating patient care needs
- Assessing the patient's potential for wellness and for responding to various treatment strategies" (Benner, p. 97)

Effective management of rapidly changing situations
- "Skilled performance in extreme life-threatening emergencies: Rapid grasp of a problem
- Contingency management: Rapid matching of demands and resources in emergency situations
- Identifying and managing a patient crisis until physician assistance is available" (Benner, p. 111)

Administering and monitoring therapeutic interventions and regimes
- "Starting and maintaining intravenous therapy with minimal risks and complications
- Administering medications accurately and safely: Monitoring untoward effects, reactions, therapeutic responses, toxicity, and incompatibilities
- Combating the hazards of immobility: Preventing and intervening with skin breakdown, ambulating and exercising patients to maximize mobility and rehabilitation, preventing respiratory complications
- Creating a wound management strategy that fosters healing, comfort, and appropriate drainage" (Benner, p. 123)

Monitoring and ensuring the quality of health care practices
- "Providing a backup system to ensure safe medical and nursing care
- Assessing what can be safely omitted from or added to medical orders
- Getting appropriate and timely responses from physicians" (Benner, p. 137)

TABLE 22-2   Domains of Nursing Practice and Related Competencies (*Continued*)

Organizational and work-role competencies
- "Coordinating, ordering, and meeting multiple patient needs and requests: Setting priorities
- Building and maintaining a therapeutic team to provide optimum therapy
- Coping with staff shortages and high turnover:
  - Contingency planning
  - Anticipating and preventing periods of extreme work overload within a shift
  - Using and maintaining team spirit; gaining social support from other nurses
  - Maintaining caring attitude toward patients even in absence of close and frequent contact
  - Maintaining a flexible stance toward patients, technology, and bureaucracy" (Benner, p. 147)

Domains of practice are also identified in the narrative accounts of critical care nurses presented in *CWICC* (Benner et al., 1999). In that text, nine domains were identified from 46 competencies: "(1) diagnosing and managing life-sustaining physiologic functions in unstable patients; (2) the skilled know-how of managing a crisis; (3) providing comfort measures for the critically ill; (4) caring for patient's families; (5) preventing hazards in a technological environment; (6) facing death: end-of-life care and decision making; (7) communicating and negotiating multiple perspectives; (8) monitoring quality and managing breakdown; and (9) the skilled know-how of clinical leadership and the coaching and mentoring of others" (Benner et al., 1999, p. 3). As can be seen, the terminology differs to some extent and new domains were added. This points to the importance of identifying the domains present within the particular situation on a particular unit within a particular hospital before adopting these domains as anything other than suggested areas of competency.

Embodied knowledge is information that is learned and "known" by the body (Benner & Wrubel, 1989). Embodied knowledge affects the habits one develops related to attentiveness, thinking, and acting and is a method of learning and reasoning. Benner cites Merleau-Ponty's (1962) five dimensions of the ontological or "knowing" capacity of the body to be (a) the inborn skills of knowing (inborn complex); (b) the culturally and socially learned postures, gestures, and customs (habitual skilled body); (c) the way one normally acts in skilled comportment (projective body); (d) one's actual projection at the current time (actual projected body); and (e) the body's awareness of self (the existential body). Embodied knowledge allows us to grasp how humans make rapid, unconscious and seemingly reflex understandings of the significance of the world around them.

Emotions are recognized to play a key role in the nurse's ability to respond to situations in a engaged fashion and take morally sound action (Benner et al., 1999). Emotions give voice to the embodied knowledge and are useful to the nurse in terms of their qualitative content in understanding the meaning related to the particular situation (Benner & Wrubel, 1989).

Ethical judgment is the nurse's "fundamental disposition toward what is good and right" (Benner et al., 1996, p. 15). This disposition is shaped, or socially constructed, by both the discipline of nursing and the norms of the particular unit. Ethical judgment, as used by Benner, speaks to skillful and compassionate moral decisions and action on behalf of the patient and his or her family based on a specific situation (Benner et al., 1999).

Experience is an active rather than passive process. It does not depend on the passage of time but, rather, the transformation of expectations and perceptions (Benner et al., 1989). Preconceived notions and theory are refined in light of actual encounters, with many clinical situations adding a new richness to the theoretical basis. While theory can help guide the practitioner to the appropriate questions, experience adds to the necessarily limited and skeletal view provided by that theory (Benner, 1984/2001).

Graded qualitative distinctions are the subtle, context-dependent physiologic changes experienced by the patient that are recognizable to the expert nurse based on direct patient observation (Benner, 1984/2001). This recognition corresponds to Polanyi's (1958) concept of "connoisseurship," which is instrumental in uncovering clinical knowledge.

Intuition is a concept that has been much debated in the literature and is, perhaps, the most contentious of Benner's concepts (Bradshaw, 1995; Darbyshire, 1994; English, 1993; Paley, 1996; Thompson, 1999). Intuition, as used by Benner, is based on experiential learning and caring. Expert intuition involves pattern recognition of the salient aspects of a situation. This heightens the nurse's attentiveness to the situation (Benner & Tanner, 1987). This results in a sense of knowing without necessarily having a specific rationale (Benner et al., 1999). Benner et al. (1996) further clarify intuition in stating,

> To respond by intuition is not the same as thoughtless and automatic response–quite the contrary. We have found that while intuition is clearly possible when nurses don't know the patient, based on experiences with similar patients, knowing the patient and involvement with him supports the direct apprehension and understanding that we describe as intuition. (p. 10)

Knowing the patient implies knowledge of the patient's typical responses and enables the nurse to have a good clinical grasp and use expert clinical judgment even when the patient is in a transition phase. Benner et al. (1996) identify five aspects of knowing the patient: "(1) responses to therapeutic measures; (2) routines and habits; (3) coping resources; (4) physical capacities and endurance; and (5) body topology and characteristics" (p. 22). The importance of knowing the patient as a person assists to avoid stereotypes when making clinical decisions (Benner, 2003).

Maxims are described by Polanyi (1958) as instructions experts use to pass on explanations of their actions to others. However, these maxims are cryptic in nature, as one must have extensive experience in the situation to understand the subtle meanings and distinctions required to effectively interpret these instructions. The use of maxims makes it difficult for expert nurses to pass along their clinical wisdom to minimally experienced nurses (Benner, 1984/2001).

Paradigm cases and personal knowledge are past situations that stand out in the nurse's memory that allow for rapid perceptual grasp of the situation (Benner, 1984/2001, p. 7). This is an advanced type of clinical knowledge that provides a more comprehensive view of the situation than simple reliance on theory. Paradigm cases contain transferable knowledge that is useful in other situations (Benner, 1984/2001).

Reasoning-in-transition is habitually based thinking as situations change and unfold that takes into account past and present knowledge of the situation. Knowledge is gained or lost based on the unfolding situation, and the expert nurse develops the ability to recognize those gains and losses in knowledge in order to prevent errors (Benner et al., 1996, 1999).

Social embeddedness gives context to caring. Benner et al. (1996) state, "Caring for one another is social through and through. Both clinical and caring knowledge require the identification of salient situations and knowing how and when to act" (p. 194). This ability to identify salient aspects of a situation depends on the value systems within which professional development has occurred. The social mores and teaching style of the work unit help shape aspects the nurse will learn to see as valuable and salient to the situation.

Stress is viewed from a phenomenological standpoint as "the disruption of meanings, understanding, and smooth functioning so that harm, loss, or challenge is experienced, and sorrow, interpretation, or new skill acquisition is required" (Benner & Wrubel, 1989, p. 59).

Temporality refers to the relational events of past, present, and anticipated future. One never has the same experience twice because between those experiences lies other experiences that impact the "past" of any given situation (Benner & Wrubel, 1996).

Thinking-in-action is based on a pattern of thought learned initially through prototypical situations and expanded upon through experience and is directly tied to responding to patient and family needs (Benner et al., 1999).

Unplanned practices are practices that have been given to nurses by default. Many unplanned practices are the result of taking on more roles that were once the domain of other health care professionals. These practices are often unrecognized by others as skills performed by nurses. As these new skills are acquired, they influence nurse perceptions and add to clinical knowledge and thus impact clinical judgments (Benner, 1984/2001).

Relationships

In examining Benner's writing, many relationships are described in the exemplars derived from the discussions with nurses in various research studies. These relationships are complex and do not conform to the typical linear logic evident in cognitive-rationalist theories. The ability to draw a pictorial structure is neither feasible nor appropriate when describing this body of work as it is derived from phenomenological research. The themes and competencies identified must be appreciated within the context from which they are derived. Researchers using phenomenological methods do not seek to generalize their findings to the population at large. Narrative evidence within Benner's work lends support for many potential relationships among the variables. See Table 22-3 for a selection of relationships suggested to exist among concepts.

Assumptions

Benner bases her assumptions on the existential and phenomenological works of Merleau-Ponty, Kierkegaard, Heidegger, Charles Taylor, and Hubert Dreyfus. These assumptions are set forth in *Primacy of Caring* (Benner & Wrubel, 1989) and deal with the concept of person from an existential viewpoint. These assumptions are evident in Benner's discussions related to the metaparadigm. Selected assumptions are presented in Table 22-4.

TABLE 22-3   Selected Relationships Among Concepts Identified by Benner

---

- Experience within a supportive environment fosters progression of skill acquisition[1, 2]
- Experience allows for the development of caring, which is the basis of nursing practice[3]
- Experience fosters the intuitive grasp of the situation found in expert nurses[3, 4]
- Experience impacts agency[2, 3]
- Caring is socially embedded[2, 3]
- Caring allows for personal concern about the patient[2]
- Concern allows for the identification of stressors and potential coping options[2]
- Attending to the embodied knowledge and emotions elicited by the situation is required for ethical judgment to occur[2, 3]
- Expert-level nursing care is achieved through caring and concerned involvement; knowing the patient; awareness of temporal issues; ability to make clinical and ethical judgments; and use of intuitive clinical reasoning, reasoning-in-transition, and thinking-in-action[2, 3, 4]

Note: [1] Benner (1984/2001); [2] Benner and Wrubel (1989); [3] Benner, Tanner, and Chesla (1996); [4] Benner, Hooper-Kyriakidis, and Stannard (1999).

TABLE 22-4   Selected Assumptions of Benner's Work

- "Human wisdom is taken to be more than rational calculation" (p. 7).[1]
- "Theory is derived from practice" (p. 19).[1]
- Theory is a simplification of reality, and thus presents a limited picture of reality.[1]
- "Theory frames the issues and guides the practitioner in where to look and what to ask" (p. 21).[1]
- "Nursing practice is a systematic whole with a notion of excellence inherent in the practice itself (MacIntyre, 1981)" (p. 19).[1]
- Nurses can and do make a difference in the well-being of patients.[1]
- Caring is the core of nursing practice.[2]
- Caring is primary to nursing practice because: (a) caring creates possibility and is, therefore, essential for coping; (b) caring allows for concern, which is required for connectedness; (c) through caring, the possibility of giving and receiving care becomes possible.[1]
- Caring is always specific and is understood only in context.[1]
- "Caring is the basis of altruism" (p. 367).[1]
- "Caring is the essential requisite for all coping" (p. 1).[1]
- "Caring and interdependence are the ultimate goals of adult development" (p. 368).[1]
- "Concern is essential for the nurse to be situated." (p. 92).[1]
- Increased experience and mastery of the skill bring about a transforming improvement in performance.[3]
- Clinical performance cannot be understood in terms of "formal structural models, decision analysis, or process models" (p. 38).[3]
- "Regardless of the stage, no practitioner can practice beyond her experience, despite necessary attempts to make the practice as clear and explicit as possible."[2]

Note: [1] Benner and Wrubel (1989); [2] Benner (2000); [3] Benner (1984/2001).

EXPERT NURSING PRACTICE AND NURSING'S FOUR-CONCEPT METAPARADIGM

Person (or Being)

Benner draws from the phenomenological views of Heidegger (1962) in her interpretation of the person with additional references to Dreyfus and Dreyfus (1980) and Merleau-Ponty (1962). The human is to be viewed holistically. However, this view is not the typical "layered-on" holism described in nursing literature (Benner & Wrubel, 1989). The term "bio-psycho-social-spiritual being" frequently used in nursing breaks the human into four pieces that, when layered together, do not adequately represent the wholeness of the person. The question of "being" is extensively debated in the literature, with questions regarding whether Benner is, in fact, using a Heideggarian definition (Benner, 1996; Benner & Wrubel, 2001; Bradshaw, 1995; Cash, 1995; Darbyshire, 1994; Edwards, 2001; Horrocks, 2000, 2002, 2004). However, regardless of the validity or lack of validity of those arguments, Benner makes important observations about the humanness of persons. The person is a whole who cannot be reduced to mind–body dualism (Benner & Wrubel, 1989). The person's way of being in the world affects his or her thoughts and understandings of the world because "a person is a self-interpreting being, that is, a person does not come into the world predefined but becomes defined in the course of living a life" (Benner & Wrubel, 1989, p. 41). This person is situated in a world that has a personal meaning. The situatedness of the person allows him or her to grasp the world through embodied knowledge, background meanings, concern about things that matter, and the ability to participate in the environment and world. The person cannot be understood out of context (Benner & Wrubel, 1989).

Well-Being

The term "well-being" is preferred by Benner over the term "health" because "health" has typically been associated with physiological and psychological measures. She takes a phenomenological view, selecting the term "well-being" as it "reflects the lived experience of health, just as the term illness reflects the lived experience of disease" (Benner & Wrubel, 1989, p. 160). Benner goes on to define well-being as "congruence between one's possibilities and one's actual practices and lived meanings as is based on caring and feeling cared for" (p. 160). Well-being is both contextual and relational. She goes on to say, "Health, as well-being, comes when one engages in sound self-care, cares, and feels cared for—when one trusts the self, the body, and others" (p. 161). In addition, health or well-being can be promoted by effective use of the patient's formal beliefs, deliberate choices and planning, understanding and being guided by emotional responses, awareness and use of embodied intelligence, investigating meanings and concerns, and identifying and understanding the situational aspects impacting well-being.

Benner and Wrubel (1989) differentiate health, illness, and disease by stating, "Health is not the absence of illness, and illness is not identical with disease. Illness is the human experience of loss or dysfunction, whereas disease is the manifestation of aberration at the cellular, tissue, or organ level" (p. 8). Disease and illness have a bidirectional flow, with each impacting the other. The human experience of illness impacts disease since humans assign meaning to the disease and respond emotionally to that meaning. Disease, in turn, affects illness from a biophysical standpoint, giving rise to signs and symptoms that are then perceived by the person as an interruption, an inconvenience, or a worry.

Situation

People are situated in a world that gives meaning to their being. Benner and Wrubel (1989) state, "The term situation is used as a subset of the more common nursing term environment because the former term connotes a peopled environment. Environment is a broader more neutral term, whereas situation implies a social definition and meaningfulness" (p. 80). The ways in which people experience "being" in a situated world impacts how they understand that world, which impacts their experience of the world. This experience is shaped by context and influenced by the background meanings given to that context. Context implies the many ways in which people are connected to the world. Temporality is part of context. People understand themselves and the world in relation to past and present with possibilities for the future.

Benner and Wrubel (1989) note that people can feel "situationless" when placed in a new and unfamiliar situation. There is a lack or loss of meaning to draw upon. Nurses often work with people who are experiencing new, unfamiliar situations and are instrumental in helping the person to regain a feeling of situatedness. The nurse, situated in a familiar world, informs and coaches the patient through active involvement with that person.

Nursing

Benner and Wrubel (1989) define nursing as "a caring practice whose science is guided by the moral art and ethics of care and responsibility" (p. xi). Further, they state that "nursing is concerned with health promotion and treatment of illness and disease" (p. 303). In addition, nursing is a

> science that studies the relationships between mind, body, and human worlds. . . . Nursing is concerned with the social sentient body that dwells in finite human worlds: that gets sick and recovers; that is altered during illness, pain, and suffering; and that engages with the world differently upon recovery. (Benner, 1999, p. 315)

Nurses are knowledgeable practitioners who are central to the promotion of health and well-being of patients. Expert nurses understand the theoretical basis of health, illness, and disease as well as have experientially based, practical understanding of the typical patterned responses of humans to situations of well-being and illness. Cognitive, relational, and technical skills and understanding are acquired through experience with real patients in real situations over extended periods of time (see earlier description of novice to expert levels). These skill competencies comprise the domains of nursing (Benner, 1984/2001; Benner & Wrubel, 1989).

EXPERT NURSING PRACTICE AND THE NURSING PROCESS

The linear nursing process is viewed by Benner as insufficient to meet the needs of expert nursing practice. Benner (1984/2001) states that this view oversimplifies nursing transactions because it leaves out context and content. As an oversimplification, the formal steps do not capture all of the expert nurse's thought processes as he or she interacts in a therapeutic manner with the patient and family. As stated by Benner et al. (1999), "Classification systems may work for information management and record retrieval, but they do not present an accurate account of the habits of thought, thinking-in-action, or reasoning-in-transition involved in actual clinical practice" (p. 66). The linear process does not allow for the intuitive grasp and flexibility required of the nurse in rapidly changing situations, nor does it not account for the interrelatedness of the steps. When expert nurses recognize a problem, it is already diagnosed with treatment options already selected and implementation begun.

However, given the criticisms noted, the nursing process is viewed as a sound method for the development of patterns of thought for novices and advanced beginners. In addition, when faced with a new or unique situation, it is a tool that can be effectively used by the more advanced nurse (Benner et al., 1999).

Assessment. Benner (1984/2001) maintains that assessment "is so central and contains so much content and skill in its own right that much of the skill and content are overlooked if this domain is seen solely as the first step of a linear process" (p. 107). Symptoms are to be viewed in terms of the patient's past and present context and are never experienced in isolation. Thus, the nurse must learn to utilize the patient's embodied knowledge to assist with assessment. Benner and Wrubel (1989) caution that patients become experts in the assessment of their own state of well-being. A great fear of these "expert patients" is that their expertise will be discounted, and practitioners will intervene in less-than-expert ways. Thus, the nurse must learn to know the patient in terms of his typical response patterns and be able to make qualitative distinctions between the patient's typical state and the current state.

Learning these assessment skills is not an easy task. Inexperienced practitioners have not yet developed the skill of differentiating the most salient symptoms within a situation. They therefore try to interpret every symptom demonstrated in terms of their understanding of disease (Benner & Wrubel, 1989). Observational, or monitoring, skills are primary to assessment. In learning to be a skilled observer, the nurse must gain experience and expertise in distinguishing changes from the patient's typical pattern and the expected pattern given the situation as well as understanding the meanings inherent in that change.

Diagnosis. The concept of nursing diagnosis is meant to serve a wide variety of purposes within the framework of nursing process. Benner et al. (1996) state that the purposes espoused by nursing for nursing diagnoses are many and varied and that "no single dimension of a professional practice can achieve all that nursing diagnosis as a concept and as a taxonomic effort was intended to do" (pp. 27–28).

The use of an established taxonomy for diagnosis can have the negative effect of putting the nurse into a mind-set where diagnosis leads to focus on certain symptoms at the expense of others that may be present within the situation (Benner & Wrubel, 1989). Symptoms, by nature, are ambiguous and present an unclear picture. However, attending to these vague symptoms can occur because of embodied knowledge. For example, a nurse may encounter a patient, sense an odor, and understand that the patient has an infection. The question of where and what organism is then left to be determined through skilled observation and technology. The simplistic label "potential for infection" lacks specificity because of an unknown etiology and gives little direction to determine which signs and symptoms may be salient in that situation. Thus, the partial diagnosis does not convey enough information for the experienced nurse to respond to the patient and family's needs. The experienced nurse relies on other means.

Prioritization of diagnoses is an additional problem exemplified by the traditional view of nursing process. Salience of symptoms and diagnoses is situated in time and place. Consequently, priorities may change rapidly, or two diagnoses may have comparable weight at any given time. Lack of observational skills or problem solving on the part of the nurse can compromise prioritization. Benner et al. (1999) state that "being a good problem solver is not sufficient if the most critical problem is overlooked or the problem is framed or defined in misguided ways" (pp. 14–15).

Expert nurses, rather than relying on labels, base clinical judgments on experience, knowing the typical trajectory of disease states within their specialty, knowing the patient as a temporally situated being, and making observations guided by theoretical, practical, and embodied knowledge (Benner et al., 1996, 1999).

Planning, implementation, and evaluation. Benner and colleagues have established through their qualitative study of nurses that while the less experienced nurse attempts to follow the structured nursing process, the more expert nurse engages in an intuitively based process of interpreting care needs that is not well captured by the steps labeled planning, implementation, and evaluation. Expert nurses engage in essentially response-based action based on experience and individualization to the specific patient at that specific time and place (Benner et al., 1996). These actions are intuitively based and imply a simultaneous, multidirectional, and multidimensional grasp of what needs to be done at any given time (Benner, 1999; Benner et al., 1996).

Nursing action is goal directed. For the expert nurse, goals are patient focused, whereas less experienced nurses focus extensively on personal goals to be accomplished during their shift, and these personal goals inhibit them from focusing on the goals of the patient (Benner et al., 1996). Experienced nurses understand the importance of realistic, individualized goals in establishing and maintaining the patient's commitment for, perhaps, long periods of time (Benner, 1984/2001). Goals are established through knowing the patient. This allows goals to be congruent with the person's view of what is possible and desirable (Benner et al., 1999).

Expert nurses intuitively design interventions to avoid known hazards. They are vigilant to safety needs of the patient and are assertive in changing the plan as needed should circumstances change. Plans are seen as flexible and evolving and are subject to ongoing review and questioning. Priorities shift as the patient situation changes. Thus, needs may be conflicting at times. Benner speaks of the "fuzzy recognition" of changes in clinical status. Intervention may well be delayed until additional information is acquired to have sufficient understanding to guide intervention. One feature of the expert nurse is that he or she is willing to wait before taking action (Benner et al., 1996).

In evaluation of the effectiveness of care, the nurse is sometimes required to determine which of conflicting interventions is the most salient to the current situation. Evaluation based on situated knowledge enables the nurse to determine when to reprioritize, when to change interventions, and when to discontinue orders that are no longer relevant (Benner, 1984/2001).

An example of care given by an advanced beginner and an expert can be found in the story of Sara.

Sara's Story

Sara is 24-year-old gravida 1 para 1 who delivered late yesterday evening. She has an unremarkable medical history and had an uneventful pregnancy, although she did just recently move to this area, resulting in a need to change her primary care provider in the 8th month of her pregnancy.

Sara is an elementary school teacher. Her husband is a sculptor and painter who just accepted a position at the local college as an art instructor.

Maria R.N. is caring for Sara from 7 A.M. to 11 A.M. Maria has been working on postpartum since graduation from nursing school seven months ago. The night nurse reports that Sara is in stable condition with no outstanding problems other than having a hard time getting the baby to latch on for breastfeeding. Following report, Maria organizes her day according to the nursing needs she identified from night shift's report. Around 8:15, Maria stops by Sara's room and notes that Sara is nursing the baby. Maria introduces herself and asks how Sara is feeling this morning. Other than a few aches and some pain from the third-degree episiotomy, Sara says she is feeling fine. Maria then proceeds to inquire about breastfeeding problems. Sara indicates that she has finally been able to get the baby to latch on and that the baby seems to be sucking effectively. Maria checks the latch, mentally going over her growing list of "tips and tricks for proper breastfeeding," and assures Sara that the baby is well latched. She instructs the new mother on how to assess for a proper latch-on. Maria then asks if Sara would mind delaying the rest of the baby's feeding until she finishes her morning assessments. Sara agrees, unlatches the baby, and Maria efficiently finishes her postpartum and neonatal assessments. During this time, Maria notes that Sara seems to have been crying recently, as her eyes are puffy. Maria gives positive reinforcement for Sara's good breastfeeding technique and assures her that the initial frustrations of breastfeeding are well worth the final results. She then makes a mental note to have the lactation consultant stop by to in order to identify any breastfeeding issues that she may have missed in her inexperience. Maria asks Sara if she would like some pain medication for her episiotomy pain. After providing the medication and making sure that the baby is again well latched, Maria leaves Sara's room confident that she has performed good nursing care.

At 11 A.M., Maria gives report to Jessie R.N. Jessie, an energetic nurse who has worked on postpartum for 15 years, is well known for her insight into clinical situations and her ability to manage even the most unexpected events. Shortly after report, Jessie stops by Sara's room. Again, Sara is breastfeeding her baby. Jessie smiles warmly and looks Sara in the eyes as she introduces herself and asks how things are going. Sara looks tired and somewhat withdrawn as she remarks that the baby is feeding well and her stitches are still sore. Jessie notes that there are a number of used tissues accumulated on the bedside table. She sits down on the chair next to Sara's bed, leans forward, and gently asks her about the tissues.

Sara looks grateful that someone seems interested in her "real" pain. She tearfully begins her story by saying that she wasn't happy about moving to this town a few weeks ago. However, the fall semester was starting and her husband had to start work. She didn't want to stay in her old home because it was a six-hour trip and she was afraid her husband wouldn't be able to be present for the birth. In her home town, she had been planning a natural birth in the home-like birthing suite. Unfortunately, only one obstetrician in the new town was accepting patients. She had gone into labor, been sentenced to continuous fetal monitoring, and was restrained in the labor bed with monitor belts. She couldn't walk or use a whirlpool, so her labor pattern became sluggish and oxytocin was started to augment the contractions. The oxytocin worked well, and labor became very painful since Sara couldn't change positions easily in bed without causing problems with the labor tracing. She finally asked for an epidural. When it came time to deliver, Sara couldn't push effectively. After a failed vacuum extraction, forceps were used to deliver the baby. Her episiotomy had ripped into a third-degree tear. Sara hadn't slept well following the delivery, as there were seven times during the night when staff members came into her room. Sara stated that she wanted to go home right now, but she was told that the pediatrician wouldn't release the baby in less than 48 hours post-birth and she wasn't going home alone. She stated that she felt very lonely, as the baby had spent so much time in the nursery and her husband would be at work until 4 P.M.

Jessie recognized the acute grieving Sara was experiencing for her lost dreams and plans of a fulfilling labor. She recognized that Sara was feeling overwhelmed with the imposed power structure in the hospital and was feeling out of control. After listening to the story, Jessie expressed her sorrow that things had worked out so differently than Sara had planned. Jessie suggested that Sara had a number of options that they could implement to give Sara a better sense of control over the hospitalization. Sara was encouraged to get dressed into her normal daywear. Jessie suggested that Sara call her husband and ask him to bring in her favorite takeout food for dinner and Sara's favorite bedtime snack. Jessie gave Sara several nonpharmacological options for pain control as well as informing her about the variety of pain medications Sara could request. Noting the small cross on Sara's necklace, Jessie inquired whether Sara would like to speak with her clergy or whether she would like to speak to one of the hospital clergy representatives. A sign was put onto Sara's door instructing staff to not bother Sara except at 4, 8, and 12 so that Sara could get uninterrupted time for proper sleep. The nursery was informed that the baby would be rooming-in, per Sara's request, for the remainder of the stay and that all infant assessments and procedures should be done in the mother's room only at 4, 8, or 12 if possible. Noting that Sara was smiling and her eyes were now brighter, Jessie asked if Sara could think of anything else that would make the rest of her stay more pleasant. Jessie left the room stating that she would check with the pediatrician about an earlier discharge for the baby. As Jessie walked to the nurses' station, she reflected on Sara's experience and what the unit could learn from Sara's story. Identifying several points of concern, Jessie planned to speak with the policies committee to be sure that evidence-based care and national standards for family-centered maternity care were truly reflected in the unit's policies and orientation plan.

EXPERT NURSING PRACTICE AND THE CHARACTERISTICS OF A THEORY

1. *What is the historical context of the theory?* According to Benner, understanding the historical context of her work requires a return to the mind-set of the late

1970s and early 1980s. During this time, the grand theories of nursing were extensively taught and debated in nursing schools. Nursing theory was espoused in nursing education programs as a way of structuring and understanding the science and practice of nursing. Most nursing theorists focused on the science of nursing and building a scientific basis to legitimize nurse's existence as a distinct profession. These grand theories were hoped to be templates that could be used to guide nursing science development as well as nursing practice. However, restrained by traditional views of theory development, these theorists encountered difficulties in capturing aspects of the lived experience of nursing. Attempts to use the theories as templates resulted in devaluing of the clinical knowledge possessed by the individual nurse (Benner & Wrubel, 1989).

Predominantly female occupations such as nursing and teaching were striving to be recognized as professions despite their historical deviation from the generally accepted professional development pathways. Feminist theory was being applied to understand aspects of these typically female professions. Traditional views of science, as laid down by Socrates, Descartes, and other early philosophers, were viewed with dissatisfaction by professions where cognitive-rational deductive theory did not take into account the human element. The mechanistic view of people as orderly, predictable, measurable entities did not reflect the day-to-day reality experienced by professions such as nursing. Academic discussions on science offered by Kuhn (1970) and Polanyi (1962) appeared in nursing literature as well as nursing classrooms. The question of "knowing-how" without being clearly aware of the reasoning behind that "know-how" left unsettling questions for nurse theorists. Alternative perspectives were sought in the philosophy of other disciplines.

Benner's work reflects the search for a more congruent philosophical stance on the profession of nursing. Influenced by the feminist movement and the phenomenological philosophy of Heidegger (1962), Merleau-Ponty (1962), Taylor (1985), and others, as well as by Hubert and Stuart Dreyfus and Richard Lazarus's views on stress and coping, Benner sought to discover the knowledge and wisdom embedded in the practice of nursing in order to address the many contextual issues challenging nurses of the time. Accounts of nursing shortages, the rising impact of technology and resulting dehumanizing of the health care environment, poor caregiving practices, and devaluation of nurses within the health care system plagued the formative professional years of Benner (Benner & Wrubel, 1989). These issues continue today. New challenges have occurred during the years since the first publication of Benner's work. The increasing existence of large conglomerates controlling numerous health institutions, insurance company control of health care availability, mushrooming new categories of health care workers seeking licensure, and rising standards in education level for advanced practice nurses make articulating the basis of quality nursing care imperative for the continued development of the profession. The work of Benner, then, continues to be relevant today.

Benner's work takes the stand that theory arises from practice and practice subsequently uses theory to change practice. Theory, according to Heidegger (1962), either confirms or disconfirms practice. As such, theory is then subject to modification based on the new possibilities within the situation that extend practice knowledge. An understanding of the writing of Heidegger and phenomenology is useful for understanding many of the concepts discussed by Benner. In addition, an appreciation of feminist theory can assist the reader to grasp the fundamental importance of this body of work. The ability to give voice to nurses in order to articulate their knowledge and wisdom is, perhaps, the most significant achievement of Benner.

2. *What are the basic concepts and relationships presented by the theory?* Benner's efforts were aimed at developing a scientific basis for nursing based on the lived experience of the nurse that encompassed the lived experience of the person experiencing illness (Benner & Wrubel, 1989). Caring became the pivotal concept. Although caring had been addressed by other nurse theorists such as Lydia Hall, Madeleine Leininger, and Jean Watson, Benner sought a phenomenological understanding of how caring develops and is exemplified by expert nurses. Thus, differentiating between the thoughts and actions of nurses as different skill levels becomes a necessary foundation.

Benner discusses a large number of concepts in her works. The concepts are defined in terms that are continually expanded. Relationships between concepts are well explicated through the use of exemplars and demonstrate a complex fabric to nursing expertise. Few assumptions are explicitly stated. The reader can hypothesize a number of assumptions, however, based on the recurrence of thoughts throughout the works.

3. *What major phenomena of concern to nursing are presented? (These phenomena may include* but are not limited to *human beings, environment, health, interpersonal relations, caring, goal attainment, adaptation, and energy fields.)* Benner clearly discusses the four concepts of the metaparadigm although she does make changes to the terminology to person, well-being, situation, and nursing. These concepts are covered extensively and consistently. As stated previously, caring is a primary focus and differs in approach from the works of other nursing theorists.

Benner's work does provide insight into critical thinking as an evolutionary process that becomes more intuitive as experience is gained. Elements of this critical thinking are identified as clinical reasoning, clinical judgment, clinical forethought, reasoning-in-transition, and thinking-in-action. Development of critical thinking skills can be fostered or hindered by the unit culture where this experience is gained. Thus, administrators have responsibility to demonstrate positive leadership and assist the system to develop into professionally nurturing environments.

This is not to imply that Benner finds no place for traditional models of critical thinking. Benner et al. (1996) note, "Calculative reasoning, requiring analysis of particular situations, consulting research and theoretical literature for possible interpretations and solutions, and explicitly weighing of possible outcomes and consequences of each potential action, does and should figure prominently in the practice of experienced clinicians" (p. 12).

4. *To whom does this theory apply? In what situations? In what ways?* Over 175 research based articles citing Benner's work as the framework were identified in a recent CINAHL search. Benner's work is applicable in nursing education, nursing practice, nursing administration, and nursing research. There is extensive information contained in her books suggesting appropriate education methods for nurses at different levels of skill acquisition. Benner's descriptions of professional development and domains of practice have been used to guide nursing curricula and to give direction to staff development programs (Carlson, Crawford, & Contrades, 1989; Gatley, 1992). Nurse administrators are given direction in how to create an environment that fosters expertise. In addition, an understanding of how to individualize the domains of nursing practice to a particular institution fostered the development of Clinical Practice Development Model (Haag-Heitman, 1999) and similar models used within a number of hospital systems across the country. Researchers have further investigated Benner's domains of nursing skill acquisition and competencies in other settings (Brykczynski, 1998; Noyes, 1995; Urs, Van Rhyn, Gwele, McInerney, & Tanga, 2004).

Benner's work focuses on the question of how nurses intervene as they do rather than the questions of what nurses need to do in any given situation. Nurses intervene as they do because they are beings who care. The novice nurse's focus of care is on how he or she, the nurse, performs. This self-focus gradually shifts as experience is gained to a mature ability to care about the patient. Expert caring leads to concern, and concern allows the nurse to identify salient aspects of the situation. Concern is influenced by the nurse's background meanings, embodied intelligence, reasoning processes, and future focus. These factors lead to an intuitive grasp that allows the nurse to first start with interventions that have worked most of the time for patients in similar circumstances. Vigilant monitoring then dictates whether changes are made to the intervention plan based on expert observational skills.

5. *By what method or methods can this theory be tested?* Benner's conclusions have been tested, for the most part, using qualitative methods to determine whether the domains of nursing practice, as identified by Benner, are evident in other settings. Qualitative methods are most appropriate as the concepts are most amenable to analysis of narrative information and observation. Quantitative attempts have been made to design and validate competency assessment forms (Meretoja, Erickson, & Leino-Kilpi, 2002; Meretoja, Isoaho, & Leino-Kilpi, 2004).

6. *Does this theory direct nursing actions that lead to favorable outcomes?* Benner did not investigate client outcomes except that many of the exemplars from the nurses focused on a significant occasion when the nurse believed she made a difference. The domains of nursing practice can, however, give direction to nursing actions. The competencies identified with a particular domain of practice gives guidance to the nurse in terms of what is expected of her within that practice setting. In addition, important aspects emphasized in Benner's work that direct attention to a means for favorable outcomes include the concepts of ethical judgment and moral agency.

7. *How contagious is this theory?* A CINHAL search in mid-2006 using the keywords "Benner," and "Novice to Expert" yielded just over 1,500 publications either citing Benner or having a major focus on Benner's work. These citations include a number in international journals. Benner's work has been translated into many languages and has been the source of many nursing conferences. Nursing curricula receive guidance from Benner's work. In addition, many hospital systems have instituted clinical ladders based on the Dreyfus model as applied to nursing. Internationally, Benner's work has been influential at national levels in countries such as the United Kingdom, New Zealand, and Australia in structuring nursing education and practice guidelines.

STRENGTHS AND LIMITATIONS OF THE THEORY

The narrative detail evident in Benner's work makes it easy for nurses to validate whether Benner's conclusions seem reasonable. While there are a large number of concepts, they complement each other to tell the story of expert nursing practice. Benner's work can be understood in a simple form, such as skill levels of novice to expert, or can be applied in a more expanded form in terms of understanding critical thinking and caring practices.

Benner's work has been tremendously influential in nursing in several areas. Her work has drawn renewed attention to the pivotal role played by caring in nursing practice. Nursing practice is, in essence, caring. In a society that values a rational, logical, positivistic view of science, Benner reawakened the desire to examine the profession from a more humanist view in order to see nursing's wisdom in a fresh new light.

Benner repeatedly cautions the reader to question the representativeness of her works and to carefully examine the applicability of her ideas to the specific situation (Benner, 1984/2001). A limitation noted repeatedly in the literature is the inappropriate use of Benner's work as a template in situations where the framework has not been validated (Benner & Benner, 1999). Institutions that are truly interested in effectively using Benner's ideas must assess their own situation to see if modifications to her domains are in order.

Other concerns have been noted in the literature. An excellent review is provided by Padgett (2000), who notes questions regarding the appropriate interpretation of her philosophical foundations, the limitation of the majority of her work to the examination of expert nurses without equal focus on the other levels of practice, the practice of selection of expert research participants by administrators, and the methodological limitations of using a predetermined framework to structure her qualitative, phenomenological studies.

Summary

The work of Benner and colleagues has had a significant impact on nursing within the United States and abroad. The questions of what is a nurse and what is nursing have been debated and described for decades. The question of what is an expert practitioner requires an examination of the day-to-day activity of nurses in real situations. Here, one needs to begin to step back to fundamentals that can be supplied only by the nurses themselves. Thus, practice generates knowledge and knowledge contributes to practice.

Thought Questions

1. In Sara's story, identify examples of how the practice of the advanced beginner and the expert nurse varied.
2. Given Benner's conceptualization of the competent nurse, what is the impact of mandatory annual "competency" testing on the motivation of nurses to attain proficient or expert levels of practice?
3. Benner cautions against using her qualitatively identified domains of practice and competencies as a template. How can staff development nurses examine the appropriateness of Benner's work for the development of a clinical advancement model for a particular hospital? Would factors within particular units of the hospital require variations of the proposed model?

4. Benner focuses extensively on the concept of caring as a basic concept in the development of nursing expertise. What are the implications of role conflict between a desire to care and the economic considerations of time and resource management on the professional development of nurses?

5. Benner states that expert nurses use maxims to explain the rationale for their nursing actions. These maxims are cryptic instructions based on subtle experiential learning that are difficult to verbalize; thus, it is difficult to pass along clinical wisdom to newer nurses. What implications does this have for the orientation of advanced beginners as they enter the work environment?

6. Given that Benner states that the clinical reasoning and decision making of expert nurses does not follow the traditional nursing process taught to novices, what modifications may be in order for the teaching of critical thinking skills in nursing education programs?

EXPLORE PEARSON **mynursingkit**™

MyNursingKit is your one stop for online chapter review materials and resources. Prepare for success with additional NCLEX®-style practice questions, interactive assignments and activities, web links, animations and videos, and more!

Register your access code from the front of your book at
www.mynursingkit.com.

References

Benner, P. (1996). A response by P. Benner to K. Cash (1995), Benner and expertise in nursing: A critique. *International Journal of Nursing Studies, 33*(6), 669–674.

Benner, P. (1999). New leadership for the new millennium: Claiming the wisdom and worth of clinical practice. *Nursing and Health Care Perspectives, 20*(6), 312–319.

Benner, P. (2000). The wisdom of our practice. *American Journal of Nursing, 100*(10), 99–105.

Benner, P. (2001). *From novice to expert: Excellence and power in clinical nursing practice* (com. ed.). Upper Saddle River, NJ: Prentice Hall. [Original work published 1984, Menlo Park, CA: Addison-Wesley]

Benner, P. (2003). Beware of technological imperatives and commercial interests that prevent best practices. *American Journal of Critical Care, 12*(5), 469–471.

Benner, P., & Benner, R. V. (1999). The clinical practice development model: Making the clinical judgment, caring, and collaborative work of nurses visible. In B. Haag-Heitman (Ed.), *Clinical practice development: Using novice to expert theory* (pp. 17–42). Gaithersburg, MD: Aspen.

Benner, P., Hooper-Kyriakides, P., & Stannard, D. (1999). *Clinical wisdom and interventions in critical care: A thinking-in-action approach.* Philadelphia: Saunders.

Benner, P., & Tanner, C. A. (1987). Clinical judgment: How expert nurses use intuition. *American Journal of Nursing, 87*(1), 23–31.

Benner, P., Tanner, C., & Chesla, C. A. (1996). *Expertise in nursing practice: Caring, clinical judgment and ethics.* New York: Springer.

Benner, P., & Wrubel, J. (1989). *The primacy of caring: Stress and coping in health and illness.* Menlo Park, CA: Addison-Wesley.

Benner, P., & Wrubel, J. (2001). Response to: Edwards S. D. (2001) Benner and Wrubel on caring in nursing. *Journal of Advanced Nursing, 33*(2), 172–174.

Benner Associates. (2002). Short resume of Patricia Benner. Available online at http://home.earthlink.net/~bennerassoc/patricia.html.

Bradshaw, A. (1995). What are nurses doing to patients? A review of theories of nursing past and present. *Journal of Clinical Nursing, 4*, 81–92.

Brykczynski, K. A. (1998). Clinical exemplars describing expert staff nursing practices. *Journal of Nursing Management, 6*, 351–359.

Brykczynski, K. A. (2006). Patricia Benner. From novice to expert: Excellence and power in clinical nursing practice. In A. M. Tomey & M. R. Alligood (Eds.), *Nursing theorists and their work* (6th ed., pp. 140–166). Philadelphia: Mosby.

Carlson, L., Crawford, N., & Contrades, S. (1989). Nursing student novice to expert–Benner's research applied to education. *Journal of Nursing Education, 28*(4), 188–190.

Cash, K. (1995). Benner and expertise in nursing: A critique. *International Journal of Nursing Studies, 32*(6), 527–534.

Darbyshire, P. (1994). Skilled expert practice: Is it "all in the mind"? A response to English's critique of Benner's novice to expert model. *Journal of Advanced Nursing, 19*, 755–561.

Dreyfus, S. E., & Dreyfus, H. L. (1980). *A five-stage model of the mental activities involved in directed skill acquisition.* Unpublished report supported by the Air Force Office of Scientific Research (AFSC), USAF (Contract F49620-79-c-0063), University of California at Berkley.

Dreyfus, H. L., & Dreyfus, S. E. (1996). The relationship of theory and practice in the acquisition of skill. In P. Benner, C. Tanner, & C. Chesla (Eds.), *Expertise in nursing practice: Caring, clinical judgment, and ethics* (pp. 29–47). New York: Springer.

Edwards, S. D. (2001). Benner and Wrubel on caring in nursing. *Journal of Advanced Nursing, 33*(2), 167–171.

English, I. (1993). Intuition as a function of the expert nurse: A critique of Benner's novice to expert model. *Journal of Advanced Nursing, 18*, 387–393.

Gatley, E. P. (1992). From novice to expert: The uses of intuitive knowledge as a basis for district nurse education. *Nurse Education Today, 12*, 81–87.

Haag-Heitman, B. (Ed.). (1999). *Clinical practice development, using novice to expert theory.* Gaithersburg, MD: Aspen.

Heidegger, M. (1962). *Being in time* (J. MacQuarrie & E. Robinson, Trans.). New York: Harper & Row.

Horrocks, S. (2000). Hunting for Heidegger: Questioning the sources in the Benner/Cash debate. *International Journal of Nursing Studies, 37*, 237–243.

Horrocks, S. (2002). Edwards, Benner and Wrubel on caring. *Journal of Advanced Nursing, 40*(1), 36–41.

Horrocks, S. (2004), Saving Heidegger from Benner and Wrubel. *Nursing Philosophy, 5*, 175–181.

Kuhn, T. S. (1970). *The structure of scientific revolutions* (2nd ed.). Chicago: University of Chicago Press.

Lazarus, R. S., & Folkman, S. (1984). *Stress, appraisal, and coping.* New York: Springer.

MacIntyre, A. (1981). *After virtue.* Notre Dame, IN: University of Notre Dame Press.

Meretoja, R., Erickson, E., & Leino-Kilpi, H. (2002). Indicators for competent nursing practice. *Journal of Nursing Management, 10*, 95–102.

Meretoja, R., Isoaho, H., & Leino-Kilpi, H. (2004). Nurse Competence Scale: Development and psychometric testing. *Journal of Advanced Nursing, 47*(2), 124–133.

Merleau-Ponty, M. (1962). *Phenomenology of perception* (C. Smith, Trans.). London: Routledge and Kegan Paul.

Noyes, J. (1995). An explanation of the differences between expert and novice performance in the administration of an intramuscular injection of an analgesic agent to a patient in pain. *Journal of Advanced Nursing, 22*, 800–807.

Padgett, S. M. (2000). Benner and the critics: Promoting scholarly dialogue. *Scholarly Inquiry for Nursing Practice: An International Journal, 14*(3), 249–266.

Paley, J. (1996). Intuition and expertise: Comments on the Benner debate. *Journal of Advanced Nursing, 23*(4), 665–671.

Polanyi, M. (1958). *Personal knowledge.* Chicago: University of Chicago Press.

Rubin, J. (1996). Impediments to the development of clinical knowledge and ethical judgment in critical care nursing. In P. Benner, C. Tanner, & C. Chesla (Eds.), *Expertise in nursing practice: Caring, clinical judgment, and ethics* (pp. 170–192). New York: Springer.

Taylor, C. (1985). Theories of meaning. In C. Taylor, *Human agency and language: Philosophical papers* (Vol. 1, pp. 248–292). Cambridge: Cambridge University Press.

Thompson, C. (1999). A conceptual treadmill: The need for "middle ground" in clinical decision making theory in nursing. *Journal of Advanced Nursing, 30*(5), 1222–1229.

University of California, San Francisco (2008). Faculty Profiles: Patricia Benner. Available online at http://www.nurseweb.ucsf.eud/www/ffbennp.htm.

Urs, L. R., Van Rhyn, L. L., Gwele, N. S., McInerney, P. & Tanga, T. (2004). Problem-solving competency of nursing graduates. *Journal of Advanced Nursing, 48*(5), 500–509.

Selected Bibliography (2002–2007)

Ali, N. S., Hodson-Carlton, K., Ryan, M., Flowers, J., Rose, M. A., & Wayda, V. (2005). Online education: Needs assessment for faculty development. *Journal of Continuing Education in Nursing, 36*(1), 32–38.

Benner, P. (2003). Attending death as a human passage: Core nursing principles for end-of-life care. *American Journal of Critical Care, 12,* 558–561.

Benner, P. (2003). Avoiding ethical emergencies. *American Journal of Critical Care, 12*(1), 71–72

Benner, P. (2003). Beware of technological and commercial interests that prevent best practices. *American Journal of Critical Care, 12,* 469–471.

Benner, P. (2003). Enhancing patient advocacy and social ethics. *American Journal of Critical Care, 12,* 374–375.

Benner, P. (2003). Reflecting on what we care about. *American Journal of Critical Care, 12,* 165–166.

Benner, P. (2004). Designing formal classification systems to better articulate knowledge, skills, and meaning in nursing practice. *American Journal of Critical Care, 13,* 426–430.

Benner, P. (2004). Seeing the person beyond the disease. *American Journal of Critical Care, 13,* 75–78.

Benner, P. (2005). Extending the dialogue about classification systems and the work of professional nurses. *American Journal of Critical Care, 14,* 242–244.

Benner, P. (2005). Honoring the good behind rights and justice in healthcare when more than justice is needed. American *Journal of Critical Care, 14,* 152–156.

Benner, P., Sheets, V., Uris, P., Malloch, K., Schwed, K., & Jamison, D. (2002). Individual, practice, and system causes of errors in nursing. A taxonomy. *JONA, 32,* 509–523.

Benner, P., & Sutphen, M. (2007). Learning across the professions: The clergy, a case in point. *Journal of Nursing Education, 46*(3), 103–108.

Cathcart, E. B. (2008). The role of the chief nursing officer in leading the practice: Lessons from the Benner tradition. *Nursing Administration Quarterly, 32*(2), 87–91.

Chang, S. U., & Corgan, N. L. (2006). A partnership model for the teaching nursing home project in Taiwan. *Nursing Education in Practice, 6,* 78–86.

Christensen, M., & Hewitt-Taylor, J. (2006). From expert to tasks, expert nursing practice redefined? *Journal of Clinical Nursing, 15,* 1531–1539.

Dunn, K. S., Otten, C., & Stephens, E. (2005). Nursing experience and the care of dying patients. *Oncology Nursing Forum, 32*(1), 97–104.

Floyd, B. O., Kretschmann, S., & Young, H. (2005). Facilitating role transition for new graduate RNs in a semi-rural healthcare setting. *Journal for Nurses in Staff Development, 21*(6), 284–290.

Larew, C., Lessans, C., Spunt, D., Foster, D., & Coving, B. G. (2005). Application of Benner's theory in an interactive patient care simulation. *Nursing Education Perspectives, 27*(1), 16–21.

Lathan, C. L., & Fahey, L. J. (2006). Novice to expert advanced practice nurse role transition: Guided student self-reflection. *Journal of Nursing Education, 45*(1), 46–48.

Meretoja, R., Eriksson, El, & Leino-Kilpi, H. (2002). Indicators for competent nursing practice. *Journal of Nursing Management, 10,* 95–102.

Richards, J., & Hubbert, A. O. (2007). Experiences of expert nurses in caring for patients with postoperatiave pain. *Pain Management Nursing, 8*(1), 17–24.

Robinson, J. A., Flynn, V., Canavan, K., Cerreta, S., & Krivak, L. (2006). Evaluating your evaluation plan. Are you meeting the needs of nurses? *Journal for Nurses in Staff Development, 22*(2), 65–69.

Weiss, S. M., Malone, R. E., Merighi, J. R., & Benner, P. (2002). Economism, efficiency, and the moral ecology of good nursing practice. *Canadian Journal of Nursing Research, 34*(2), 59–119.

Annotated Bibliography

Barrett, C., Borthwick, A., Bugeja, S., Parker, A., Vis, R., & Hurworth, R. (2005). Emotional labour: Listening to the patient's story. *Practice Development in Health Care, 4*(4), 213–223.

This article discusses the dissociation between "patient" and "person" found in expert nurses when doing program evaluation using an empowerment evaluation strategy. The authors report that expert nurses developed a level of cynicism that sometimes prevented them from hearing the patient's story and seeing them as unique human beings. The authors state that while expert nurses desired to function as described by Benner, the realities of health care encouraged cynicism as a protective mechanism against burnout.

Bonner, A., & Greenwood, J. (2006). The acquisition and exercise of nephrology nursing expertise: A grounded theory study. *Journal of Clinical Nursing, 15,* 480–489.

This grounded theory study of 11 expert nurses and six non-expert nurses examined skill acquisition by nephrology nurses on an Australian renal unit. Three levels of skill were identified: non-expert, experienced non-expert, and expert. Comparisons with Benner's five stages of skill acquisition are provided.

Evans, R. J., & Donnelly, G. W. (2006). A model to describe the relationship between knowledge, skill, and judgment in nursing practice. *Nursing Forum, 41*(4), 150–157.

This article introduces a model showing the relationships between knowledge, skill and judgment built upon the work by Benner. Allowance is made for varying levels of skill acquisition.

Fennig, T., Bender, J., Colby, H., & Werner, R. R. (2005). Genesis of a professional development tool for ambulatory pediatric nursing practice. *Health Care Manager, 24,* 369–373.

Benner's work is used as the basis for development of a performance review tool used in a children's hospital in Wisconsin. Job descriptions and rating tools were developed for use in the orientation program and evaluation of staff.

Gobet, F., & Chassy, P. (2007). Towards an alternative to Benner's theory of expert intuition in nursing: A discussion paper. *International Journal of Nursing Studies.* Retrieved June 14, 2007, from http://www.sciencedirect.com.

Benner's concept of expert intuition is reviewed in light of numerous published discussions of the concept. An alternative model is suggested along with a discussion of areas of agreement and disagreement with Benner's work.

Johns, C. (2005). Dwelling with Alison: A reflection on expertise. *Complementary Therapies in Clinical Practice, 11,* 37–44.

This article discusses the concepts of reflection and clinical judgment in expert practice. Using the work of both Benner and Carper's fundamental patterns of knowing in nursing, the author presents a case study and discusses the role of reflection for making conscious efforts to improve expertise as a complementary therapist.

King, L., & Clark, J. M. (2002). Intuition and the development of expertise in surgical ward and intensive care nurses. *Journal of Advanced Nursing, 37,* 322–329.

The authors use a qualitative study design to identify levels of expertise for 61 postoperative nurses, with particular attention to the concept of intuition. Findings are divided into advanced beginner, competent, proficient, and expert nursing levels of practice. Both intuition and analytical thinking were evident at all levels of practice. Ability to use intuition skillfully was more characteristic of expert nurses.

Meretoja, R., Isoaho, H., & Leino-Kilpi, H. (2004). Nurse Competence Scale: Development and psychometric testing. *Journal of Advanced Nursing, 47*(2), 124–133.

The authors present a discussion of the development of the Nurse Competence Scale that was derived from Benner's work on skill acquisition in nursing. The resulting 73-item scale consisted of seven subcategories and showed good internal consistency. The tool is suggested to be useful in a variety of hospital work environments.

Robinson, K., Eck, C., Kech, B., & Wells, N. (2003). The Vanderbilt professional nursing practice program. Part 1: Growing and supporting professional nursing practice. *JONA, 33*(9), 441–450.

A career advancement model is presented based on Benner's work on professional development in nursing. Four levels of practice are identified (advanced beginner to expert) along with related behaviors.

Schoessler, M., & Waldo, M. (2006). The first 18 months of practice. A developmental transition model for the newly graduated nurse. *Journal for Nurses in Staff Development, 22*(2), 47–52.

Benner's work is used as the basis for a transition model for newly graduated nurses. Other aspects are included in the model drawn from transition management and learning theory. The model was developed using an interpretive phenomenological study of graduate nurses. Themes identified include relationships with patients, their families, and coworkers; organizational ability; and marker events. Three time phases are presented.

Spichiger, E., Wallhagen, M., & Benner, P. (2005). Nursing as a caring practice from a phenomenological perspective. *Scandinavian Journal of Caring Sciences, 19,* 303–309.

This article expands on Benner's pivotal concept of caring in nursing practice. The concepts of caring, practice, and caring practices are examined from a phenomenological viewpoint.

Simpson, E., Butler, M., Al-Somail, S., & Courtney, M. (2006). Guiding the transition of nursing practice from an inpatient to a community-care setting: A Saudi Arabian experience. *Nursing and Health Sciences, 8,* 120–124.

Benner's work on novice to expert nursing practice was used by the authors as the basis of the Transitional Practice Model in order to provide a smooth transition for nurses into the community setting. The model includes dimensions, domains of practice, and evaluation methods for each of the five stages of skill acquisition identified by Benner.

Twycross, A., & Powls, L. (2006). How do children's nurses make clinical decisions? Two preliminary studies. *Journal of Clinical Nursing, 15,* 1324–1335.

Nurses' decision making regarding postoperative pain management for children is examined across experience levels. All 27 nurses involved, regardless or experience level or setting (medical or surgical), tended to use the same type of decision-making skills in contrast to Benner's assertion that decision-making skills change as nurses progress in professional skill development. In comparing the decision-making outcomes, more experienced nurses did not always make better decisions than less experienced nurses.

Uys, L. R., Gwele, N. S., McInerney, P., van Rhyn, L., & Tanga, T. (2004). The competence of nursing graduates from problem-based programs in South Africa. *Journal of Nursing Education, 43,* 352–361.

This qualitative study described the examination of the competency of 49 graduates from four nursing programs designed as problem-based learning programs compared to three conventional nursing programs in South Africa between six and nine months after graduation. Examples of behaviors indicative of each of the Benner's novice, advanced beginner, competent, and proficient levels of skill acquisition were evident in the behaviors. No differences were found between the two groups related to level of practice.

CHAPTER **23**

Other Theories of the 1980s

Julia B. George
Janet S. Hickman

Other nursing theories developed during the 1980s include Fitzpatrick's Life Perspective Rhythm Model, Mercer's theory of Maternal Role Attainment (now "Becoming a Mother"), Meleis's theory of transitions, and Mishel's theory of uncertainty in illness. Of these, development continues in relation to Becoming a Mother, transitions, and uncertainty in illness. These three theories will be the focus of this chapter.

MATERNAL ROLE ATTAINMENT/ BECOMING A MOTHER

Ramona T. Mercer

Ramona T. Mercer received her diploma in nursing in 1950 from Saint Margaret's School of Nursing, Montgomery, Alabama; bachelor of science in nursing from the University of New Mexico (UNM), Albuquerque, in 1962; master of science in maternal child nursing from Emory University, Atlanta, Georgia; and Ph.D. in maternal nursing from the University of Pittsburgh, Pennsylvania. She is Professor Emeritus, Department of Family Health Care Nursing, at the University of California, San Francisco (UCSF). Her career has focused on maternal–child nursing. Her research on high-risk situations and transition to the maternal role has spanned over 30 years. She currently lectures, consults, and writes. Dr. Mercer was the 1984 recipient of the UCSF School of Nursing Helen Nahm Lecture Award, the 1988 recipient of the Western Society for Research in Nursing Distinguished Research Lectureship Award, and the 1990 recipient of the American Nursing Foundation's Distinguished Contribution to Nursing Science Award and, in 2004, was the first recipient of the UNM College of Nursing Distinguished Alumni Award. She is a fellow in the American Academy of Nursing (AAN) and was named an AAN Living Legend in 2003. She is the author of *Nursing Care for Parents at Risk* (1977), *Perspectives on Adolescent Health Care* (1979), *First-Time Motherhood: Experiences from Teens to Forties* (1986a), *Parents at Risk* (1990), and *Becoming a Mother: Research on Maternal*

Identity from Rubin to the Present (1995) (http//:www.nurses.info/nursing_theory_ midrange_theories_ramona_mercer.htm).

MATERNAL ROLE ATTAINMENT/ BECOMING A MOTHER   Mercer's theory of Maternal Role Attainment (MRA)/Becoming a Mother (BAM) is based on her extensive education, experience, and research in maternity nursing. While a doctoral student at the University of Pittsburgh, Mercer was mentored by Reva Rubin, who is well known for her work in defining and describing maternal binding-in with the infant and achieving comfort in the maternal role (Rubin, 1977, 1984). In addition to Rubin, Mercer based her research on role, developmental, and systems theories. Initially, Mercer (1980, 1981, 1985, 1986a, 1986b) conducted a series of studies that focused on maternal role attainment (MRA) in situations during the first 8 to 12 months of motherhood. Thornton and Nardi's (1975) four stages of role acquisition—anticipatory, formal, informal, and personal identity—were used to describe the process of MRA. The *anticipatory stage*, pregnancy, is a time of psychosocial preparation for the new role. At birth, the mother moves to the *formal stage* of identifying her infant's uniqueness and begins the caretaking tasks by copying expert mothering behaviors and asking advice. During the *informal stage*, the new mother progresses from rigidly following the advice of others to using her own judgment about how to best care for her baby. The *stage of personal or maternal identity* is characterized by the mother's sense of harmony, confidence, satisfaction in the maternal role, and attachment to her infant. The new mother feels a congruence of self and motherhood (Mercer, 1981, 1985, 2004).

Mercer's theory and model of MRA was introduced in 1991 at a research symposium. The theory was refined and presented in her 1995 book *Becoming a Mother: Research on Maternal Identity from Rubin to Present.* This book describes her theory of MRA and her framework for studying the variables that affect the maternal role.

The Mercer's MRA is depicted inside nested circles labeled microsystem, mesosytem, and macrosystem. The *microsystem* is the immediate environment in which maternal attainment occurs. It includes factors such as the father's role, family function and relationships, family support systems, economic status, values, and stressors. All of the microsystem elements affect the transition to motherhood and are the most influential on MRA (Mercer, 1990, 1995).

The *mesosystem* is comprised of the social systems that surround the microsystem. Interactions between the microsystem and the larger mesosystem influence the developing maternal role and the child. The mesosystem includes school, church, day care, and other social systems within the immediate community (Mercer, 1995).

The *macrosystem* refers to the larger culture surrounding the family. It includes the social, political, and cultural influences on the other two systems. It also includes the health care system and health policies that may affect MRA (Mercer, 1995).

Mercer (1981, 1986b) identified variables that influence MRA. These include maternal age, socioeconomic status, perception of their birth experience, early mother–infant separation, social stress, social support, personality traits, self-concept, child-rearing attitudes, perception of the infant, role strain, and health status. Infant variables affecting MRA included temperament, appearance, responsiveness, and health status.

Self-reported maternal behavior, observed maternal behavior, attachment to the infant, and gratification in the maternal role were constructs of MRA used to compare three age-groups of women during their first year of motherhood. The majority (64%) had achieved a maternal identity by four months; at one year, 4% had not achieved it. The patterns of self-reported maternal behaviors, feelings of attachments for the baby, and observed maternal competence did not differ by age-group, although their levels of achievement differed (Mercer, 1985, 1986b). Mercer's research also includes the role of the father and parental attachment and competence (Ferketich & Mercer, 1995a, 1995b, 1995c; Mercer, 1995; Mercer & Ferketich 1990a, 1990b).

Mercer (2004) states, "Women's descriptions of the life-transforming experience in becoming a mother with the concomitant growth, development, and new self-definition are not adequately encompassed in MRA terminology. The maternal persona continues to evolve as the child's developmental challenges and life's realities lead to disruptions in the mother's feelings of competence and self-confidence. The argument is made to replace 'maternal role attainment' with 'becoming a mother' to connote the initial transformation and continuing growth of the mother identity" (p. 231). Thus, Mercer revised her theory and retired the term *maternal role attainment* (MRA). The revised theory focuses on the woman's transitions in *becoming a mother* (BAM), which involve an extensive change in life space and require ongoing development. Mercer asserts that becoming a mother is more than assuming a role; it is an unending and evolving event (Mercer, 2004).

Mercer uses her own research and that of others to refine her theory. Her 2004 article provides a review of the nursing research related to maternal role attainment. After the literature review, she presents new names for the stages in the process of establishing a maternal identity in BAM: (a) *commitment, attachment, and preparation* (pregnancy); (b) *acquaintance, learning, and physical restoration* (first two to six weeks following birth); (c) *moving toward a new normal* (two weeks to four months); and (d) *achievement of the maternal identity* (around four months). She states that active involvement in the first stage has been consistently linked to a positive adaptation to motherhood. She also states that the timelines for achieving the last three stages are highly variable and may overlap and that they are influenced by maternal and infant variables as well as the social environmental context.

While BAM continues to use idea of nested environments, the environments have been renamed as *family and friends, community,* and *society at large* to emphasize that they are living environments. In the revised model the center of the nested environments consists of the interactions of the mother–father–infant triad (Mercer as cited in Meighan, 2006, p. 614). The center is first surrounded by the family and friends environment and includes the variables of social support, family values, cultural guidelines for parenting, family functioning, and family stressors. Moving outward, the next living environment is the community in which the variables are child care settings, places of worship, schools, health care settings, and recreational, work, and cultural settings. The outermost living environment is society at large and includes the variables of maternal-child legislation, reproductive science and genetics, and national health programs (Meighan, 2006).

METAPARADIGM, RESEARCH, AND PRACTICE USING MRA/BAM   While Mercer does not specifically define the four concepts in nursing's metaparadigm, she does incorporate each of them in her discussions. Table 23-1 demonstrates an example for each of the concepts.

Several researchers have investigated aspects of MRA/BAM or have conducted studies which support Mercer's work. Some examples are discussed in the following paragraphs.

TABLE 23-1	Maternal Role Attainment/Becoming a Mother and Nursing's Metaparadigm
Nursing	"Nurses are the health professional having the most sustained and intense interaction with women in the maternity cycle" (1995, p. xii).
Person	"The self or self core is separate from the roles that are played" (1985).
Health	The parents' perception of their prior health, current health, health outlook, resistance-susceptibility to illness, health worry or concern, sickness orientation, and rejection of the sick role" (1986)
Environment	"Systems perspective of person–environment interrelationship" (1995).

Walker, Crain, and Thompson (1986a) identified three aspects of MRA: maternal identity and perceived and demonstrated role attainment. Both primiparas' and multiparas' attitudes about themselves as mothers were correlated with attitudes toward their infants within and among the test periods at one to three days and at four to six weeks after birth. First-time mothers' formation of the mother–infant relationship and their gaining of self-confidence in the parenting role appeared to be interdependent. Walker, Crain, and Thompson (1986b) found that primiparas' self-confidence was moderately correlated with observed maternal behavior, maternal age, education, and socioeconomic status at four to six weeks postpartum. Multiparas' self-confidence during the first three days was related to observed maternal behavior at four to six weeks; however, their self-confidence was related only to maternal age and infant size.

Koniak-Griffin (1993) questioned the existence of discrete cognitive-affective and behavioral dimensions of MRA in her historical and empirical review of the theory. Zabielski (1994) reported that she did not find support for separation of maternal identity from perceived role performance among mothers of preterm and term infants. Britton, Gronwaldt, and Britton (2001) report findings that indicate that early-observed maternal behavior reflected the mother's emotional involvement with her baby and that this early behavior was predictive of later mothering and infant behavior. They conclude, though, that only the mother can provide the data about her own perceptions of self as a mother and of her infant for conclusions about her assimilation of a maternal identity.

Mercer (2004) reports that several researchers have focused on the importance of mothers' work during pregnancy in preparation for becoming a mother and the variables influencing this transition. Swedish mothers' prenatal attachment to their unborn babies predicted observed mother–infant relationships at 12 weeks postpartum (Siddiqui & Hägglöf, 2000). Expectant mothers' ideas about their own mothers mediated their prenatal attachment to their babies (Priel & Besser, 2001), while mothers' current relationships with their own mothers tended to be re-created in their relationships with their infants (Kretchmar & Jacobvitz, 2002).

Mothers' memories of maternal and paternal acceptance or rejection as children were also found to be predictors of depressive symptoms and maternal sensitivity when their infants were five to six months old (Crockenberg & Leerkes, 2003). Fowles (1998) found that women with postpartum depression had more negative perceptions of their infants and of themselves as mothers at two to three months postpartum. Women who reported higher levels of depression, anxiety, and marital ambivalence and conflict during pregnancy reported less efficacy in the parenting role (Porter & Hsu, 2003).

Clark, Kochanska, and Ready (2000) validated the bidirectionality of the early parent–child relationship. Maternal personality alone and in interaction with the infant's emotionality predicted future parenting behaviors. A study of Finnish mothers' adjustment of their personal goals during pregnancy and at one and three months postpartum showed that an increase in family-related goals predicted a decline in depressive symptoms (Salmela-Aro, Nurmi, Saisto, & Halmesmäki, 2001). Pancer, Pratt, Hunsberger, and Gallant (2000) found that mothers who demonstrated higher levels of complexity of thinking during pregnancy about their future experiences as parents and at six months postpartum about their experiences as mothers were better adjusted than were mothers with simpler expectations.

Nelson (2003), in her synthesis of nine qualitative studies of mothers, identified two overlapping processes in the transition to motherhood. The primary process is engagement, defined as making a commitment, striving, and being engrossed in mothering through active involvement in the child's care. At the same time this engagement leads to a woman's growth and transformation as a mother. Hartrick (1997) reports that mothers of children aged 3 to 16 years old identified self-definition as a continual process.

Mercer's theory of MRA/BAM has been used extensively in nursing research and to guide nursing practice. It has been used as the basis for numerous doctoral dissertations and masters theses (e.g., Best, 1988; Fowles, 1994; Reiha, 2005; Russell, 2006; Sank, 1991; Washington, 1996), as well as serving as a starting point for other exploratory studies, some of which have been described in this chapter. Mercer's theory of BAM translates easily to the clinical setting and provides a structure for assessment, planning/implementation, and evaluation of nursing care. It is helpful for both students and practitioners. Meighan (2006) provides a case study example using Mercer's theory.

TRANSITIONS

Afaf I. Meleis

Afaf I. Meleis was born in Egypt, graduated magna cum laude from the University of Alexandria in 1961, and earned an M.S. in nursing (1964), an M.A. in sociology (1966), and a Ph.D. in medical and social psychology (1968) from the University of California, Los Angeles (UCLA) (http://www.nursing.upenn.edu/faculty). She has held faculty positions at UCLA and the University of California, San Francisco (UCSF). She is the Margaret Bond Simon Dean of Nursing at the University of Pennsylvania School of Nursing, professor of nursing and sociology, and director of the school's WHO Collaborating Center for Nursing and Midwifery Leadership, Philadelphia. Her teaching, research, and publications focus on theoretical nursing, the organization and structure of nursing knowledge, coping and living with transitions, and international health and nursing. She has mentored hundreds of students, clinicians, and researchers from Thailand, Brazil, Egypt, Jordan, Israel, Colombia, Korea, and Japan. Her many honors include fellow, American Academy of Nursing; fellow, Royal College of Nursing, United Kingdom (2006); and fellow, College of Physicians of Philadelphia. In 1990, she received the Medal of Excellence for professional and scholarly achievements from President Hosni Mubarak of Egypt; in 2000 she was awarded the Chancellor's Medal, University of Massachusetts, Amherst; and in 2001, she received the Chancellor's Award for the Advancement of Women, UCSF, in recognition of her worldwide activism on behalf of women's issues. In 2004 the Pennsylvania Commission for Women granted its award to her in celebration of Women's History Month; that same year she received the Special Recognition Award in Human Services from the Arab American Family Support Center, New York, and in 2006 the Penn Professional Women's Network recognized her advocacy of women with the Robert E. Davies Award. She is a member of the Institute of Medicine, the Forum of Executive Women, and the Pennsylvania Women's Forum; a trustee of the National Health Museum; and a board member of the Global Health Council; CARE (a global intervention group); the Nurses Education Fund, Inc.; and Life Science Career Alliance. She is counsel general of the International Council on Women's Health Issues (http://www.icowhi.org), an international nonprofit association dedicated to the goal of promoting health, health care, and well-being of women throughout the world through participation, empowerment, advocacy, education, and research. She has received many honorary doctorates and distinguished and honorary professorships worldwide (http://www.nursing.upenn.edu/faculty).

TRANSITIONS—A MIDDLE-RANGE THEORY   Meleis (1975, 1985, 1986, 1991; Schumacher & Meleis, 1994) describes transition as a central concept for nursing. She identifies that nurses and patients often meet during a time of change or transition for the patient. These changes, which may be developmental, situational, or related to health, affect the individual as well as that person's significant others and have implications for well-being. Meleis and Trangenstein (1994) state that "nursing . . . is concerned with the process and the experience of human beings undergoing transitions where health and perceived well-being is the outcome" (p. 257).

Chick and Meleis (1986) began developing a theory of transitions by doing a concept analysis. In this analysis they first defined transitions as "a passage or movement from one state, condition, or place to another" (Schumacher & Meleis, 1994, p. 119). They proposed properties for transition and looked at relationships between transition and the metaparadigm concepts of person, nursing, health, and environment. Schumacher and Meleis (1994) further extended this work through a review of the nursing literature published since 1986. This review was conducted to identify the types of transitions addressed in the nursing literature and the conditions influencing these transitions as well as to define the characteristics of a healthy transition.

Chick and Meleis (1986) identified three types of transitions: developmental, situational, and health–illness. The *developmental transition* receiving the most attention in the literature was becoming a parent. Adolescence and midlife were also identified as transitions. While the majority of the work on transitions related to development had focused on individuals, dyads (mother–daughter) and families had been addressed.

Situational transitions that have received attention in the nursing literature include transitions in educational and professional roles. Changes such as completion of educational programs and changes in clinical practice roles or settings have been addressed (Schumacher & Meleis, 1994). Other identified situational transitions include changes in family situations such as divorce and widowhood, nursing home entry, caregiving, immigration, homelessness, moving out of abusive relationships, and near-death experiences (Schumacher & Meleis, 1994).

The third type of transition, *health–illness*, has been explored in the nursing literature in relation to individuals and families in many illness contexts. Articles describe transitions through levels of care, from critical care to step-down units, to rehabilitation, and back to the community (Schumacher& Meleis, 1994).

Schumacher and Meleis (1994) add a fourth type of transition, *organizational transition*. Organizational transitions occur with environmental changes that may be related to social, political, or economic alterations in the environment external to the organization or alterations in the structure or dynamics of the organization itself. These transitions encompass changes in leadership, role changes, the adoption of new policies and procedures, and the introduction of new technology. Transitions affecting the nursing profession such as changes in educational preparation, curricular content, and research methods have also been of interest to authors. Community transitions are also organizational transitions. Schumacher and Meleis caution that transitions are not mutually exclusive but rather complex processes where many transitions may be occurring simultaneously during a given period of time. A more recent concept analysis (Meleis, Sawyer, Im, Messias, & Schumacher, 2000) also supports the idea of transitions as patterns of multiplicity and complexity. *Patterns of transitions* include single, multiple, sequential, simultaneous, related, and unrelated. See Figure 23-1.

Despite the diversity of transitions, Meleis et al. (2000) identify commonalities that may be considered *properties* of the transition experience. These include the following:

- *Awareness*, which is associated with how the person perceives, knows about, and recognizes the experiences associated with the transition. The level of awareness is associated with how well what is known about the transitions agrees with what is expected of those undergoing such a transition. It remains a question as to whose awareness, the nurse's or the client's, triggers the start of the transition process.

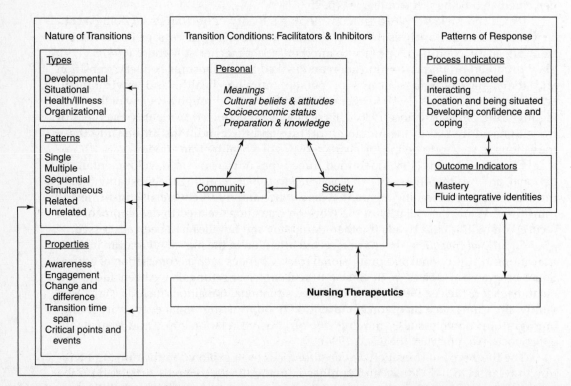

FIGURE 23-1 Transitions: A middle-range theory. *(From Meleis, A. F., et al (2000). Experiencing transitions: An emerging middle-range theory. Advances in Nursing Science. 23(1), p. 17. Used with permission.)*

- *Engagement* is the extent to which the person is involved in the processes that naturally occur as part of the transition. Level of awareness and engagement are closely associated, as engagement, or active participation in the processes, cannot occur unless the person is aware of the transition. Examples of engagement include seeking out information and actively planning ahead.
- *Change and difference* are also necessary to transitions. While all transitions include change, not all changes are transitions. Understanding the effects and meanings of the changes is necessary to understanding the transition process. Aspects to be considered include the kind of change as well as the perceptions of the timing, importance or severity of the change, and expected responses associated with the change. Another element of transitions is dealing with difference, whether that difference occurs through expectations that are not met or are not the same, through feeling different, or through being perceived as different.
- *Time span* is a property that is characterized by movement and flow over time (Meleis & Trangenstein, 1994). Research results suggest that the time span for transitions is more fluid than concrete.
- *Critical points and events* are properties of transitions. Some transitions are associated with marker events, such as birth or onset of menopause, while in others a specific marker event is less evident. Research findings indicate that the majority of transitions are associated with critical turning points or events. These events frequently involve a heightened perception of change or difference or result in increased activity in the behaviors associated with engagement. In addition, final critical points were noted to differentiate transitions. These critical points represent a time of newly developed stability that involves new skills, habits, and activities. For example, Schumacher (1994), in her study of family caregiving during chemotherapy, identified the four critical periods of during diagnosis, times when side effects were intensive, times of change between treatment modalities, and completion of the treatment.

TRANSITION CONDITIONS: FACILITATORS AND INHIBITORS   The achievement of health transitions may be facilitated or inhibited by a number of conditions, both personal and environmental. The theory of transitions discusses personal, community, and societal conditions.

PERSONAL CONDITIONS   *Meanings* are subjective and are associated with one's view of either a transition that is thought likely to occur or one that has occurred. Meanings also involve the evaluation of the anticipated effect(s) of the transition. Meanings may be positive, negative, or neutral and can be either facilitators or inhibitors of health transition. The transition may or may not be either desired or a result of personal choice. For persons to understand their experience and its consequences, they must be aware of the meanings associated with the transition. The importance of the perspective of the person living the transition is emphasized by the inclusion of meanings in the theory of transitions. Meaning may also have an existential connotation of searching for meaning during a transition (Meleis et al., 2000; Schumacher & Meleis, 1994).

   Cultural beliefs and attitudes will hinder a healthy transition when they attach a stigma to the transition experience. In particular, the expression of emotional states associated with the transition is likely to be inhibited. A lack of stigma facilitates a healthy transition (Meleis et al., 2000).

Socioeconomic status can be an inhibitor. Research indicates that persons of low socioeconomic status are more likely to report negative psychological symptoms. Thus, low socioeconomic status is likely to be an inhibitor of healthy transitions (Meleis et al., 2000).

Preparation and knowledge can facilitate or inhibit. The transition experience can be facilitated through anticipatory preparation; in contrast, lack of such preparation will inhibit the transition. Preparation and knowledge relevant to a transition are another personal condition that influences health outcomes and may or may not be sufficient to meet the demands of a new situation. Necessary to adequate preparation for a healthy transition are information about both what to expect and what to do to manage the changes (Meleis et al., 2000).

COMMUNITY CONDITIONS   Transitions may also be facilitated or inhibited by resources in the community. Examples can be found in Sawyer's (1996) study of transitions to motherhood in a group of African American women. Participants in this study identified the following community conditions to be *facilitators* of healthy transition:

- Family and partner support, especially from the women's mothers and other significant females.
- Pertinent information provided by health care personnel in whom the women had confidence and from classes and written materials.
- Recommendations from sources they respected
- Role models
- Informative and appropriate responses to questions

Community *inhibitors* included not having adequate resources or support to deal with pregnancy and motherhood, negative responses from others, classes offered at inconvenient times, negative advice, stereotyping, and receiving contradictory information.

SOCIETAL CONDITIONS   The larger society beyond the community also can be a facilitator or an inhibitor of healthy transitions. Viewing a transitional event as a stigma with stereotyped meanings interferes with healthy transitions. In a study by Im (1994), immigrant Korean women were marginalized both by the host society and their own culture. Both cultural attitudes about the body and gender inequities were other societal inhibiting factors to a healthy transition.

PATTERNS OF RESPONSE   Meleis et al. (2000) state that a healthy transition is characterized by both process and outcomes indicators. As a transition unfolds over time, the identification of process indicators that move the patient toward health (or vulnerability and risk) allows for early nursing assessment and intervention.

PROCESS INDICATORS
Feeling Connected.   During times of transition, feeling and staying connected are prominent features of the experience. Research findings indicated that persons who utilized support networks, either social contacts or health care providers, had healthy transitions (Meleis et al., 2000).

Interacting.   Interaction and reflection were found to be positive indicators of healthy transitions. Interaction allowed those in transition to discover the meaning of the transition experience. Interaction also provided for exploration of behaviors developed as a result of the transition and for the clarification and acknowledgment of both the transition and the new behaviors (Meleis, et al., 2000).

Location and Being Situated.   In most cases, where the transition occurs is important. The importance of location is obvious in cases where the transition involves moving to a new place, such as for immigrants. Comparisons are one way people "situate" themselves in terms of time, space, and relationships. Comparing to situate is a way to explain and perhaps justify a new life (Meleis et al., 2000).

Developing Confidence and Coping.   Another indicator of healthy transitions is the development of an increasing level of confidence. In the healthy transitions process the person will exhibit a progressive development of confidence (Meleis et al., 2000).

OUTCOME INDICATORS   Schumacher and Meleis (1994) found more emphasis in the nursing literature on the process of transition than on the outcome(s) of transition. They state, however, that the identification of outcomes is critical in order to facilitate research about transitions and to evaluate clinical interventions. They identify indicators of healthy transitions but caution that the outcome(s) can occur at any point in the transition process. An example they provide is that mastery will occur at various times during the transition process, depending upon the individual and the transition. Meleis et al. (2000) state that if outcomes are assessed too early in the transition process, they may be in fact process indicators. In the studies reported in their 2000 article, mastery of new skills and having a new sense of a fluid integrative identity reflected healthy outcomes of the transition process.

Mastery.   A healthy transition outcome is determined by the degree to which the person can use the skills and behaviors needed to deal with the new situation or environment. These skills will likely be a blend of previously established skills and those more newly developed and can include taking action, making decisions, adjusting behaviors, and utilizing resources (Meleis et al., 2000).

Fluid Integrative Processes.   Transition experiences have been described as resulting in reforming an identity. Messias's (1997) research findings about immigrants support the idea that reformulated identities are more likely to be *fluid* than stable, which implies a degree of ambiguity (Meleis et al., 2000).

Transitions Practice and Research

Meleis (2007) identifies the concepts central to the domain of nursing as the nursing client, transitions, interaction, nursing process, environment, nursing therapeutics, and health. The *nursing client* is the recipient, or potential recipient, of nursing care and is defined as "a human being with needs who is in constant interaction with the environment and has an ability to adapt to that environment but, due to illness, risk, or vulnerability to potential illness, is experiencing disequilibrium or is at risk of experiencing disequilibrium . . . manifested in unmet needs, inability to take care of oneself, and nonadaptive responses" (p. 469). *Transitions* have been defined and discussed in this chapter. *Interaction* involves both exchanges between the person and the environment and between the nurse and the patient. *Nursing process* involves the acts of assessing, diagnosing, planning, and evaluating and includes defining and attaining goals, with a focus on the patient's perceptions. *Environment* "includes but is not limited to immediate client settings, family, significant others, health care professionals, and the socioeconomic and political contexts of the client's families and communities" (p. 476, citing Hedin, 1986). *Nursing therapeutics* are "all nursing activities and actions deliberately designed to care for nursing clients" and take into account both the content and goals of nursing interventions (p. 477, citing Barnard, 1980, 1983). *Health* is viewed from the perspective of many authors as Smith's (1983) view as absence of disease, Johnson's (1980) discussion of health as homeostatis, Roy's (1984) definition of health as adaptation, Orem's (1988) view of health as the ability to perform tasks and functions, Paterson and Zderad's (1976) view of health as an existential phenomenoma, Rogers's (1970) and Newman's (1986) inclusion of space/time/energy, and multiple authors' inclusion of cultural, social, and political aspects.

Meleis states that most of the care that nurses provide happens during a transition the patient or client is experiencing and that the goal of nursing care is to enhance healthy outcomes (2007). Meleis and Trangenstein (1994) define nursing as the art and science of facilitating the transition of populations' health and well-being. They also define nursing as "being concerned with the processes and the experiences of human beings undergoing transitions where health and perceived well-being is the outcome" (p. 257). Meleis (2007) states that nurses do not deal with transitions, whether those of an individual, a family, or a community, in isolation from an environment, but rather nurses assess how persons respond to transitions and how the environment affects those responses.

Schumacher and Meleis (1994) identified three nursing therapeutics for use during transitions. The first therapeutic is *assessment of readiness*, which should include assessment of all of the conditions of transition. The second therapeutic is *preparation* for transition. The primary method of preparation is education to help create the conditions to optimize the transition. Adequate preparation requires enough time to support the assumption of new responsibilities gradually. Another modality for preparing patients or staff for transition is the creation of special transitional units where individuals can practice and learn new skills in a supportive environment The third nursing therapeutic is *role supplementation*, which uses education and practice to facilitate the transitional process. Role supplementation is any intentional process in which role insufficiency, real or potential, is recognized by the role incumbent and significant others. Nurses help people to understand the new roles and identities that they may need to develop, provide opportunities for knowledge to clarify the new role(s), and facilitate the application of new knowledge and abilities to assume the new role(s) (Meleis, 2007; Meleis et al., 2000).

Meleis's work on transitions has been both based in research and generated research. Some examples include the following:

Childless to first-time mother: Fowles, 1994

College: Coburn, 2003

Developmental transitions: Im, 1994; Lenz, 2002; Pearson, 2002

Education to practice: McMillen, 2002; Sadler, 1997

Family caregiving: Schumacher, 1994

Geographic relocation: Puskar and Martsolf, 1994

Grandmotherhood: Bee, 2007; Dallas, 2004

Health to disease transition: Martins and Zagonel, 2003

Hospice caregiving: Hehn, 1985

Illness–wellness transition: Bramwell, 1984; Dallaire, 2005; Hedstrom, 1998; Skärsäter and William, 2006; Weiss et al., 2007

Motherhood: Missal, 2003; O'Brien-Barry, 2003

Multiple role stress: Gigliotti, 2004, 2007; Hattar-Pollara, Meleis, and Nagib, 2003

Pregnancy: Batty, 1999

Pregnancy loss: Van and Meleis, 2003

Residential relocation: Almendarez, 2007; Rossen, 1998; Rossen and Knafl, 2003; Messias, 1997

Role integration: Kim, 1993

Examples of cultures involved in transition studies include the following:

African American: Bee, 2007; Dallas, 2004; Van and Meleis, 2003

Arab: Missal, 2003

Brazil: Martins and Zagonel, 2003; Messias, 1997

Canada: Batty, 1999; Dallaire, 2005; Hedstrom, 1998

Egyptian: Hattar-Pollara, Meleis, and Nagib, 2003

Korean-American: Im, 1994; Kim, 1993

Mexican-American: Almendarez, 2007

Sweden: Skärsäter and William, 2006

Watson and Pulliam (2000) have discussed the use of the concepts of transition in transgenerational health promotion, and Young, Sikma, Trippett, Shannon, and Blachly (2006) have linked transitions theory to gerontological nursing practice. More literature is needed on the use of this theory in practice.

UNCERTAINTY IN ILLNESS

Merle H. Mishel

Merle H. Mishel earned a bachelor's degree from Boston University and an M.A. in 1961; a master's degree in psychiatric nursing from the University of California, Los Angeles (UCLA), in 1966; and a master's degree (1976) and Ph.D. (1980) in social psychology from the Claremont Graduate University, Claremont, California. She has had faculty appointments at UCLA; California State University, Los Angeles, and University of Arizona, Tucson, and has been at the University of North Carolina, Chapel Hill, since 1991, where she is the Kenan Professor of Nursing and director of the Doctoral and Post-Doctoral Programs (http://nursing.unc.edu/muic/Mishelbio.html). Dr. Mishel's honors and awards include the Friends of the National Institute of Nursing Research's Research Merit Award (1997); Kenan Professorship (1994); fellow, American Academy of Nursing (1990); the Mary Wolanin Research Award (1986); and first alternate, Fulbright Award, Sigma Theta Tau Nurse Research Predoctoral Fellowship, 1977–1979.

Theories of Uncertainty in Illness

UNCERTAINITY IN ILLNESS THEORY   Mishel's original Uncertainty in Illness Theory (UIT) was published in 1988 (see Figure 23-2). "It was developed to address uncertainty during the diagnostic and treatment phases of an illness or an illness with a determined

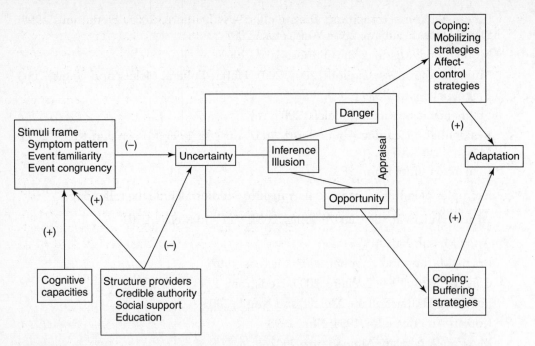

FIGURE 23-2 Model of perceived uncertainty in illness. *(From Mishel, M. H. (1988). Uncertainty in illness. Image, The Journal of Nursing Scholarship. 20, 226. Used with permission.)*

downward trajectory. . . . [It] proposes that uncertainty exists in illness situations that are ambiguous, complex, unpredictable, and when information is inconsistent or not available" (Mishel & Clayton, 2003, p. 25). The major concepts of the UIT are uncertainty and cognitive schema (Mishel, 1988; Mishel & Clayton, 2003). Mishel and Clayton define *uncertainty* "as the inability to determine the meaning of illness-related events occurring when the decision maker is unable to assign definite value to objects or events and/or is unable to accurately predict outcomes" (p. 29). It is a cognitive state that occurs "when an individual cannot adequately structure or categorize an illness event because of insufficient cues" (Mishel & Clayton, 2003, p. 25). *Cognitive schema* is defined as "the person's subjective interpretation of illness-related events" (p. 29). The UIT is applicable in both acute and chronic illnesses, prior to diagnosis as well as during diagnosis and treatment. The focus of the UIT is on the ill individual and the family of that individual. The three major themes of the theory are the *antecedents of uncertainty*, the *appraisal of uncertainty*, and *coping with uncertainty*.

Mishel has identified the *antecedents of uncertainty* as the stimuli frame, cognitive capacity, and structure providers (Mishel & Clayton, 2003). The elements of *stimuli frame* are symptom pattern, event familiarity, and event congruence. *Symptom pattern* occurs when symptoms are consistently present to the extent that a pattern can be identified. When symptoms form a pattern, the person will experience less uncertainty and especially will have less ambiguity about the illness (Mishel & Braden, 1988). Inconsistent symptoms cannot be used to gauge reliably the state of illness, and therefore they generate uncertainty. *Event familiarity* relates to the extent of recognition of the cues in the health care environment, including if the situation is a repeat of a previous experience or even has the characteristics of being a habit. Note that symptom pattern relates to the arrangement of physical sensations and that event familiarity relates to experiences within the health care environment. Event familiarity requires experience in the health care setting over time, and its development will be slowed by experiences in new or novel settings and by events that are more complex (Mishel, 1988). *Event congruence* relates to how well the expected illness-related events match the experienced events. When the experience does not match the expectation, the person will question how well future events may be predicted as well as how consistent the experiences will be (Mishel, 1988).

Each of the three parts of the stimuli frame are influenced by cognitive capacity and structure providers. *Cognitive capacity* refers to the ability of the person to process information. Physiological malfunctions have a detrimental effect on cognitive abilities, especially those that require attention. When demands for attention occur, the processing of the stimuli frame is disrupted, and uncertainty results. Other negative impacts on the ability to be attentive include drugs, pain, poor nutrition, and lack of sleep (Mishel, 1988).

Structure providers are the resources available to help the individual interpret the stimuli frame and include education, social support, and credible authority. *Education* is a structure provider with both a direct and an indirect relationship to uncertainty. Education is directly related to uncertainty when it helps build the knowledge base needed to identify meaning and context to the experienced events (Mishel, 1988; Mishel & Clayton, 2003). Education's indirect relationship to uncertainty occurs when it influences the stimuli frame rather than the experience of uncertainty itself. *Social support* provides structure in that it acts to prevent uncertainty in various life crises by supplying feedback on the meaning of events. Social support can also function as a means of avoiding uncertainty by establishing a network of information resource persons (Mishel, 1988). *Credible authority,* the degree of trust and confidence that patients and their families have in health care providers, also provides structure. Credible authority strengthens the stimuli frame by providing relevant information about the events of the illness. When the authority of the health care provider is deemed to be highly credible, uncertainty is lessened. Cues residing in the health care environment are best addressed by a credible authority such as the physician or the nurse, while cues residing in the patient are best addressed by interactions with significant others (Mishel, 1988).

The second theme, the *appraisal of uncertainty*, is defined as "the process of placing a value on the uncertain event or situation" (Mishel & Clayton, 2003, p. 30). This process is made up of inference and illusion. *Inference* occurs when past experiences and related knowledge are used to evaluate events; *illusion* occurs when the beliefs that are formed from the uncertain situation relate to a positive outlook. The outcome of appraisal is deciding if the uncertainty is a danger or an opportunity (Mishel, 1988; Mishel & Clayton, 2003).

The third theme, *coping with uncertainty*, includes the concepts of danger, opportunity, coping, and adaptation. *Danger* and *opportunity* refer to the view of the possible outcome, with danger being associated with a negative outcome and opportunity associated with a positive outcome. *Coping* occurs with either appraisal. With an appraisal of danger, coping will try to reduce the uncertainty and manage the emotions associated with the danger. With an appraisal of opportunity, coping is likely to try to maintain uncertainty. *Adaptation* involves all the behaviors of the person, biologically, psychologically, and socially, as they occur within that person's usual range of behavior (Mishel, 1988; Mishel & Clayton, 2003).

RECONCEPTUALIZED UNCERTAINTY IN ILLNESS THEORY   As research was conducted on the UIT, particularly the collection of data from chronically ill individuals, Mishel and her colleagues began to identify limitations of the UIT (Mishel & Clayton, 2003). Among these limitations was the lack of recognition of life changes as a result of living with chronic illness and of changes over time. As a result, the Reconceptualized Uncertainty in Illness Theory (RUIT) was developed. While the RUIT includes the UIT definition of uncertainty and the major themes of the UIT, it adds two concepts to better address living with the uncertainty of a chronic illness and its ongoing management or with an illness that could recur. The two added concepts are self-organization and probabilistic thinking. *Self-organization* begins with integrating continuous uncertainty into one's self-structure that leads to the formation of a new sense of order for oneself with the result that uncertainty becomes a natural rhythm of life. *Probabilistic thinking* is "a belief in a conditional world in which the expectation of uncertainty and predictability is abandoned" (p. 31). In the RUIT, four factors, prior life experiences, physiological status, social resources, and providers of health care, affect the person's development of a new perspective of life. The desired outcome from RUIT is growth to a new value system, while the desired outcome for the UIT is return to the previous level of functioning (Mishel, 1990: Mishel & Clayton, 2003).

METAPARADIGM, RESEARCH, AND PRACTICE WITH THE THEORIES OF UNCERTAINTY IN ILLNESS   Mishel's theories of uncertainty in illness provide a foundation for nursing practice and research on the responses of individual and their families to illness. Use of either of these theories with groups or communities is not appropriate (Mishel & Clayton 2003).

In relation to the four major concepts in nursing's metaparadigm, Mishel's theories are clearly tied to *nursing*, as they describe and explain human responses to illness and nursing care is included in the concept of structure providers. Although they focus on the illness experience and *health* is not specifically defined, the theories are pertinent to all health experiences throughout the life span. Mishel and Clayton (2003) identify that the *environment* is included as part of the stimuli frame. The structure providers are also part of the environment. The *person* is the focus of the theories, as it is the person who has cognitive capacity and experiences uncertainty.

The UIT was developed after Mishel's personal experience with her father's coping with cancer led her to consider the importance and effects of uncertainty. She identified that individuals who were experiencing some aspect of illness frequently reported feelings of uncertainty. During her doctoral study she developed and tested a measure of uncertainty. She used the works of Norton (1975), who identified eight dimensions of uncertainty, and of Moos and Tsu (1977) as the framework for interviews that provided the basis for the Mishel Uncertainty in Illness Scale (Mishel & Clayton, 2003). Her early ideas were also influenced by Bower's (1978) and Shalit's (1977) descriptions of "uncertainty as a complex cognitive stressor" (Mishel & Clayton, 2003, p. 27). She also mentions Budner's (1962) view that stimuli that are ambiguous, either through novelty or complexity, lead to uncertainty. She points out that the ideas of these cognitive psychologists led her to view uncertainty as a cognitive state rather than as an emotional response and that this distinction was important in her theory development. Additionally, Shalit (1977) and Lazarus (1974) contributed the view of uncertainty as a stressor or a threat, and Lazarus also influenced the view of the response of coping as both a primary and a secondary appraisal. Mishel's (1981) measurement model of uncertainty included these ideas to develop a concept of uncertainty and to create the Uncertainty in Illness Scale (Michel & Clayton, 2003).

The publication of the Mishel Uncertainty in Illness Scale (MUIS) led to nursing research that resulted in further development of the antecedents of uncertainty described in the measurement model (Mishel, 1983, 1984; Mishel & Braden, 1987, 1988; Mishel, Hostetter, King, & Graham, 1984; Mishel & Murdaugh, 1987). The variable of stimuli frame, consisting of both familiarity with and congruence of events, was developed through research findings on uncertainty in illness and cognitive psychology. The third component of the stimuli frame, named symptom pattern and developed from qualitative studies (Mishel & Murdaugh, 1987), describes the importance of symptoms being both consistent and predictable for the person to be able to identify a pattern (Mishel & Clayton, 2003).

The appraisal of uncertainty was initially developed in the 1981 model. Later expansion was based on clinical data indicating that some people could prefer uncertainty as well as on discussions with colleagues who encouraged consideration of personality variables in evaluating uncertainty. These influences led to the inclusion of the two phases of appraisal, inference and illusion, as well as to support and definition of the phases and of coping strategies through research in nursing and psychology (Mishel & Braden, 1987; Mishel & Murdaugh, 1987). Mishel states that uncertainty is a neutral state until it is appraised and value assigned (Mishel & Clayton, 2003).

The RUIT was developed after identification of limitations of the UIT, especially in relation to changes over time. The RUIT maintains both the UIT's definition of uncertainty and its major themes and uses chaos theory as the basis of reconceptualization. The RUIT includes *disorganization* (jagged lines in Figure 23-3) and *reformulation* (patterned circular lines in Figure 23-3) of a new stability that explain how an individual with continuing uncertainty develops a new life view that embraces multiple contingencies as preferred and possible. The line at the bottom of the diagram signifies that change occurs over time (Mishel, 1990; Mishel & Clayton, 2003).

Since the publication of MUIS (Mishel, 1981), there has been a great deal of research into individuals' experiences with uncertainty arising from either acute or chronic illnesses. Mast (1995), Mishel (1997, 1999), and Stewart and Mishel (2000) have all published comprehensive reviews of research that summarized and critiqued the current state of knowledge on uncertainty in illness.

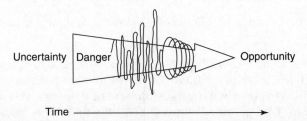

FIGURE 23-3 Reconceptualized model of uncertainty in chronic illness. *(From Bailey, D. E. & Stewart, J. L. (2006). Merle H. Mishel: Uncertainty in Illness Theory. In Tomey, A. M. & Alligood, M. R. (Eds). Nursing theorists and their work (6th ed., p. 629) St. Louis: Mosby. Used with permission.)*

Mishel and Clayton (2003) report that a number of studies have investigated the antecedents of stimuli frame and structure providers. They indicate that severity of illness, erratic symptoms, and ambiguous symptoms all cause uncertainty. Both illness severity and ambiguity correspond to the stimuli frame and erratic symptoms corresponds to event congruence within the stimuli frame. Mishel (1997) indicates that while studies have supported severity of illness as a predictor of uncertainty, the indicators of illness severity have varied across studies. Among patients with acute illnesses such as cardiovascular disease (Christman et al., 1988) and cancer (Galloway & Graydon, 1996; Hilton, 1994) and in parenting of severely ill children (Tomlinson, Kirschbaum, Harbaugh, & Anderson, 1996), severity of illness was positively associated with uncertainty.

Other examples of use of the UIT or RUIT in research include with cardiac patients (Haugh & Salyer, 2006; Kang, 2006), with cancer patients in the United States and Ireland (Bailey, Wallace, & Mishel, 2007; DiBiase & Rice, 2007; Mishel & Sorenson, 1991; Wallace & Hegerty, 2007), with people diagnosed with fibromyalgia (Anema, 2006; Bowers, 2006; Johnson, Zautra, & Davis, 2006; Reich, Johnson, Zautra, & Davis, 2006), and in genetic counseling (Guadalupe, 2007).

The MUIS has been used in many countries and with many populations. Examples include the following:

China
    Cancer: Lai, Lin, and Yeh, 2007

Sweden
    Cardiac: Flemme, Bolse, and Fridlund, 2006

Taiwan
    Childhood cancer survivors: Lee, 2006

United States
    Cancer: Bertram, 2004; Coxon, 1989; Decker, Haase, and Bell, 2007; Hockett, 2005; Owens, 2007; Weber, Roberts, Chumbler, Mills, and Algood, 2007

    Cardiac: Jurgens, 2006; Sossong, 2007

    Childhood cancer survivors: Lee, Santacroce, and Sadler, 2007; Santacroce and Lee, 2006

    Family of critically ill patients: Kloos, 2004

    Multiple sclerosis: Sorenson, 2002; Sorenson, Janusek, and Mathews, 2006

    Pregnancy: Giurgescu, Penckofer, Maurer, and Bryant, 2006; Handley and Crow, 2006

It is of interest to note that of the large volume of published literature about the UIT, RUIT, and MUIS, there is a paucity of literature about the use of the theories to guide practice. This is ironic when the development of these theories was stimulated by clinical observations. Mishel and Clayton (2003) state that: "it is in the area of practice that more work on using the theory is needed. Planning care to address uncertainty, or attempting to use different approaches in the clinical setting to prevent uncertainty, would encourage the application of the theories to practice. Since uncertainty is a clinical phenomenon, it is in the clinical setting where it should be addressed" (p. 43).

References for Mercer

Best, M. A. (1988). Interrole conflict in working mothers: Relationship to maternal identity, competence in the maternal role, and global self-esteem during the first year of motherhood. *Dissertation Abstracts International, 49*(07B), 2553. Abstract retrieved December 3, 2007, from Dissertation Abstracts Online database.

Britton, H. L., Gronwaldt, V., & Britton, J. R. (2001). Maternal postpartum behaviors and mother-infant relationship during the first year of life. *Journal of Pediatrics, 138*, 905–909.

Clark, L. A., Kochanska, G., & Ready, R. (2000). Mothers' personality and its interaction with child temperament as predictors of parenting behavior. *Journal of Personality and Social Psychology, 79*, 274–285.

Crockenberg, S. C., & Leerkes, E. M. (2003). Parental acceptance, postpartum depression, and maternal sensitivity: Mediating and moderating processes. *Journal of Family Psychology, 17*, 80–93.

Ferkitich, S. L., & Mercer, R. T. (1995a). Paternal-infant attachment of experienced and inexperienced fathers during infancy. *Nursing Research, 44*, 31–37.

Ferkitich, S. L., & Mercer, R. T. (1995b). Predictors of paternal role competence by risk status. *Nursing Research, 43*, 80–85.

Ferkitich, S. L., & Mercer, R. T. (1995c). Predictors of role competency for experienced and inexperienced fathers. *Nursing Research, 44*, 89–95.

Fowles, E. R. (1994). The relationship between prenatal maternal attachment, postpartum depressive symptoms and maternal role attainment. *Dissertation Abstracts International, 55*(01B), 6578. Abstract retrieved December 3, 2007, from Dissertation Abstracts Online database.

Fowles, E. R. (1998). The relationship between maternal role attainment and postpartum depression. *Health Care for Women International, 19*, 83–94.

Hartrick, G. A. (1997). Women who are mothers: The experience of defining self. *Health Care for Women International, 18*, 263–277.

Koniak-Griffin, D. (1993). Maternal role attainment. *Image: Journal of Nursing Scholarship, 25*, 257–262.

Kretchmar, M. D., & Jacobvitz, D. B. (2002). Observing mother–child relationship across generations: Boundary patterns, attachment, and the transmission of caregiving. *Family Process, 41*, 351–374.

Meighan, M. (2006). Maternal role attainment—Becoming a mother. In A. M. Tomey & M. R. Alligood (Eds.), *Nursing theorists and their work* (6th ed., pp. 605–622). St. Louis: Mosby Elsevier.

Mercer, R. T. (1977). *Nursing care for parents at risk.* Thorofare, NJ: Charles B. Slack.

Mercer, R. T. (1979). *Perspectives on adolescent health care.* Philadelphia: Lippincott.

Mercer, R. T. (1980). Teenage motherhood: The first year. *Journal of Obstetric, Gynecologic, and Neonatal Nursing, 9*, 16–27.

Mercer, R. T. (1981). A theoretical framework for studying factors that impact on the maternal role. *Nursing Research, 30*, 73–77.

Mercer, R. T. (1985). The process of maternal role attainment over the first year. *Nursing Research, 34*, 198–204.

Mercer, R. T. (1986a). *First time motherhood: Experiences from teens to forties.* New York: Springer.

Mercer, R. T. (1986b). The relationship of developmental variables to maternal behavior. *Research in Nursing and Health, 9*, 25–33.

Mercer, R. T. (1990). *Parents at risk.* New York: Springer.

Mercer, R. T. (1991). *Maternal role: Models and consequences.* Paper presented at the International

Research Conference, Council of Nurse Researchers and American Nurses Association, Los Angeles, CA.

Mercer, R. T. (1995). *Becoming a mother: Research on maternal identity from Rubin to the present.* New York: Springer.

Mercer. R. T. (2004). Becoming a mother versus maternal role attainment. *Journal of Nursing Scholarship, 36,* 226–238.

Mercer, R. T., & Ferketich, S. L. (1990a). Predictors of family functioning eight months following birth. *Nursing Research, 39,* 76–82.

Mercer, R. T., & Ferketich, S. L. (1990b). Predictors of parental attachment during early parenthood. *Journal of Advanced Nursing, 15,* 268–280.

Nelson, A. M. (2003). Transition to motherhood. *Journal of Obstetric, Gynecologic, and Neonatal Nursing, 32,* 465–477.

Pancer, S. M., Pratt, M., Hunsberger, B., & Gallant, M. (2000). Thinking ahead: Complexity of expectations and the transition to parenthood. *Journal of Personality, 68,* 253–280.

Porter, C. L., & Hsu, H. (2003). First-time mothers' perceptions of efficacy during the transition to motherhood: Links to infant temperament. *Journal of Family Psychology, 1,* 54–64.

Priel, B., & Besser, A. (2001). Bridging the gap between attachment and object relations theories: A study of the transition to motherhood. *British Journal of Medical Psychology, 74,* 85–100.

Reiha, J. (2005). An examination of the relationship between perceived spousal social support and mood state of primiparous postpartum women, and the subsequent effect on maternal role identity. *Masters Abstracts International, 44,* 317. Abstract retrieved December 3, 2007, from Dissertation Abstracts Online database.

Rubin, R. (1977). Binding-in in the postpartum period. *Maternal Child Nursing Journal, 6,* 67–75.

Rubin, R. (1984). *Maternal identity and the maternal experience.* New York: Springer.

Russell, K. (2006). Maternal confidence of first-time mothers during their child's infancy. *Dissertation Abstracts International, 67*(03B), 1377. Abstract retrieved December 3, 2007, from Dissertation Abstracts Online database.

Salmela-Aro, K., Nurmi, J. E., Saisto, T., & Halmesmäki, E. (2001). Goal reconstruction and depressive symptoms during the transition to motherhood: Evidence from two cross-lagged longitudinal studies. *Journal of Personality and Social Psychology, 81,* 1144–1159.

Sank, J. C. (1991). Factors in the prenatal period that affect parental role attainment during the postpartum period in Black American mothers and fathers. *Dissertation Abstracts International, 52*(07B), 3533. Abstract retrieved December 3, 2007, from Dissertation Abstracts Online database.

Siddiqui, A., & Hägglöf, B., (2000). Does maternal prenatal attachment predict postnatal mother-infant interaction? *Early Human Development, 59,* 13–25.

Thornton, R., & Nardi, P. M. (1975). The dynamics of role acquisition. *American Journal of Sociology, 80,* 870–885.

Walker, L. O., Crain, H., & Thompson, E. (1986a). Maternal role attainment and identity in the postpartum period: Stability and change. *Nursing Research, 35,* 68–71.

Walker, L. O., Crain, H., & Thompson, E. (1986b). Mothering behavior and maternal role attainment during the postpartum period. *Nursing Research, 35,* 352–355.

Washington, L. J. (1996). Learning needs of adolescent mothers when identifying fever and illnesses in infants less than twelve months of age. *Dissertation Abstracts International, 57*(12B), 7458. Abstract retrieved December 3, 2007, from Dissertation Abstracts Online database.

Zabielski, M. T. (1994). Recognition of maternal identity in preterm and fullterm mothers. *Maternal-Child Nursing Journal, 22,* 2–36.

References for Meleis

Almendarez, B. L. (2007). Mexican American elders and nursing home transition. *Dissertation Abstracts International, 68*(07B), 4384. Abstract retrieved March 31, 2008, from Dissertation Abstracts Online database.

Barnard, K. (1980). Knowledge for practice: Directions for the future. *Nursing Research, 29,* 208–212.

Barnard, K. (1983). Social policy statement can move nursing ahead. *American Nurse, 15*(1), 4–14.

Batty, M. L. E. (1999). Pattern identification and expanding consciousness during the transition of "low-risk" pregnancy: A study embodying Newman's health as expanding consciousness. *Masters Abstracts International, 39*(03), 826.

Abstract retrieved December 6, 2007, from Dissertation Abstracts Online database.

Bee, A. M. (2007). The transition to grandmother-hood of co-residing African American grandmothers with first-time parenting adolescent daughters. *Dissertation Abstracts International, 68*(04A), 1343. Abstract retrieved December 6, 2007, from Dissertation Abstracts Online database.

Bramwell, L. (1984). The relationship of role clarity and empathy to support role performance and anxiety during an illness-wellness transition. *Dissertation Abstracts International, 45*(12B), 3769. Abstract retrieved March 31, 2008, from Dissertation Abstracts Online database.

Chick, N., & Meleis, A.I. (1986). Transitions: A nursing concern. In P. L. Chinn (Ed.), *Nursing research methodology: Issues and implementation* (pp. 237–257). Gaithersberg, MD: Aspen.

Coburn, K. B. (2003). The effects of ego identity status and level of role integration on college adjustment among traditional and nontraditional college students. *Dissertation Abstracts International, 65*(04B), 2089. Abstract retrieved December 6, 2007, from Dissertation Abstracts Online database.

Dallaire, M. (2005). Description de la transition en postchirurgie cardiaque de l'hopital vers le domicile: Les perceptions des patients et des infirmieres. *Masters Abstracts International, 44*(03), 13333. Abstract retrieved December 6, 2007, from Dissertation Abstracts Online database.

Dallas, C. (2004). Family matters: How mothers of adolescent parents experience adolescent pregnancy and parenting. *Public Health Nursing, 21,* 347–353.

Fowles, E. R. (1994). The relationship between prenatal maternal attachment, postpartum depressive symptoms and maternal role attainment. *Dissertation Abstracts International, 55*(01B), 6578. Abstract retrieved March 31, 2008, from Dissertation Abstracts Online database.

Gigliotti, E. (2004). Etiology of maternal-student role stress. *Nursing Science Quarterly, 17*(2), 156–164.

Gigliotti, E. (2007). Improving external and internal validity of a model of midlife women's maternal-student role stress. *Nursing Science Quarterly, 20,* 161–170.

Hattar-Pollara, M., Meleis, A. I., & Nagib, H. (2003). Multiple role stress and patterns of coping of Egyptian women in clerical jobs. *Journal of Transcultural Nursing, 14*(2), 125–133.

Hedin, B. A. (1986). Nursing, education, and emancipation: Applying the critical theoretical approach to nursing research. In P. L. Chinn (Ed.), *Nursing research methodology: Issues and implementation.* Rockville, MD: Aspen.

Hedstrom, V. A. (1998). Activities of daily living outcomes of hospital discharge planning for people 55 years of age and older living in Yukon. *Masters Abstracts International, 37*(02), 0589. Abstract retrieved December 6, 2007, from Dissertation Abstracts Online database.

Hehn, D. M. (1985). Hospice care: Critical role behaviors related to self-care and role supplementation. *Dissertation Abstracts International, 46*(08B), 2623. Abstract retrieved March 31, 2008, from Dissertation Abstracts Online database.

Im, E. O. (1994). An analytical study of the relationship between menopausal symptoms and the stress of life events. *Journal of Korean Community Health Nursing Academic Society, 8*(2), 1–34.

Johnson, D. E. (1980). The Behavioral System Model for Nursing. In J. P. Riehl & C. Roy (Eds.), *Conceptual models for nursing practice* (2nd ed., pp. 207–216). New York: Appleton-Century-Crofts.

Kim, S. (1993). Ethnic identity, role integration, quality of life, and mental health in Korean American women. *Dissertation Abstracts International, 54*(12B), 6134. Abstract retrieved December 6, 2007, from Dissertation Abstracts Online database.

Lenz, B. K. (2002). Correlates of tobacco use and non-use among college students at a large university: Application of a transition framework. *Dissertation Abstracts International, 63*(06B), 2789. Abstract retrieved December 6, 2007, from Dissertation Abstracts Online database.

Martins, M., & Zagonel, I. P. S. (2003). The health-to-disease transition experienced by hypertensive pregnant women mediated by educative care in nursing [Portuguese]. *Texto & Contexto Enfermagem, 12,* 298–306. Abstract in English retrieved March 31, 2008, from CINAHL Plus with Full Text database.

McMillen, E. S. (2002). Education to Practice Questionnaire: A content analysis. *Masters Abstracts International, 41*(01), 192. Abstract retrieved December 6, 2007, from Dissertation Abstracts Online database.

Meleis, A. I. (1975). Role insufficiency and role supplementation: A conceptual framework. *Nursing Research, 24,* 264–271.

Meleis, A. I. (1985). *Theoretical nursing: Development and progress.* Philadelphia: Lippincott.

Meleis, A. I. (1986). Theory development and domain concepts. In P. Moccia (Ed.), *New approaches to theory development* (pp. 3–21). New York: National League for Nursing.

Meleis, A. I. (1991). *Theoretical nursing: Development and progress* (2nd ed.). Philadelphia: Lippincott.

Meleis, A. I., & Trangenstein, P. A. (1994). Facilitating transitions: Redefinition of the nursing mission. *Nursing Outlook, 42*(6), 255–259.

Meleis, A. I., Sawyer, L. M., Im, E., Messias, D. K. H., & Schumacher, K. (2000). Experiencing transitions: An emerging middle-range theory. *Advances in Nursing Science, 23*(1), 12–28.

Messias, D. K. H. (1997). Narratives of transnational migration, work, and health: The lived experience of Brazilian women in the United States. *Dissertation Abstracts International, 58*(08B), 4142. Abstract retrieved November 20, 2007, from Dissertation Abstracts Online database.

Missal, B. E. (2003). The Gulf Arab woman's transition to motherhood. *Dissertation Abstracts International, 64*(06B), 2594. Abstract retrieved November 20, 2007, from Dissertation Abstracts Online database.

Newman, M. (1986). *Health as expanding consciousness.* St. Louis: Mosby.

O'Brien-Barry, P. (2003). The contribution of sex-role orientation and role commitment to inter-role conflict in working first-time mothers at 6 to 9 months postpartum. *Dissertation Abstracts International, 64*(04B), 1687. Abstract retrieved December 6, 2007, from Dissertation Abstracts Online database.

Orem, D. E. (1988). *Nursing: Concepts of practice* (3rd ed.). New York: McGraw-Hill.

Paterson, J. G., & Zderad, L. T. (1976). *Humanistic nursing.* New York: Wiley.

Pearson, G. S. (2002). "Growing up in pieces": Adolescents with pervasive developmental disorder transitioning into adulthood. *Dissertation Abstracts International, 63*(02B), 742. Abstract retrieved December 6, 2007, from Dissertation Abstracts Online database.

Puskar, K. R., & Martsolf, D. S. (1994). Adolescent geographic relocation: Theoretical perspective. *Issues in Mental Health Nursing, 15*, 471–481.

Rogers, M. E. (1970). *An introduction to the theoretical basis of nursing.* Philadelphia: F. A. Davis.

Rossen, E. K. (1998). Older women in relocation transition. *Dissertation Abstracts International, 59*(12B), 6265. Abstract retrieved December 6, 2007, from Dissertation Abstracts Online database.

Rossen, E. K., & Knafl, K. A. (2003). Older women's response to residential location: Description of transition styles. *Qualitative Health Research, 13*(1), 20–36.

Roy, C. (1984). *Introduction to nursing: An adaptation model* (2nd ed.). Englewood Cliffs, NJ: Prentice Hall.

Sadler, M. E. (1997). Professional role expectations for entry-level graduate nurses: Characteristics, differences, and change over time. *Dissertation Abstracts International, 58*(10B), 5331. Abstract retrieved December 6, 2007, from Dissertation Abstracts Online database.

Sawyer, L. M. (1996). Engaged mothering within a racist environment: The transitions to motherhood for a group of African American women. *Dissertation Abstracts International, 58*(03B), 1217. Abstract retrieved November 20, 2007, from Dissertation Abstracts Online database.

Schumacher, K. L. (1994). Shifting patterns of self-care and caregiving during chemotherapy. *Dissertation Abstracts International, 56*(01B), 0175. Abstract retrieved March 31, 2008, from Dissertation Abstracts Online database.

Schumacher, K. L., & Meleis, A. I. (1994). Transitions: A central concept in nursing. *Image, Journal of Nursing Scholarship, 26*, 119–127.

Skärsäter, I., & William, A. (2006). The recovery process in major depression: An analysis employing transitions framework for deeper understanding as a foundation for nursing interventions. *Advances in Nursing Science 29*, 245–259.

Smith, J. A. (1983). *The idea of health: Implications for the nursing professional.* New York: Teachers College, Columbia University.

Van, P., & Meleis, A. I. (2003). Coping with grief after involuntary pregnancy loss: Perspectives of African-American women. *Journal of Obstetric, Gynecologic, and Neonatal Nursing, 32*(1), 28–39.

Watson, N., & Pulliam, L. (2000). Transgenerational health promotion. *Holistic Nursing Practice, 14*(4), 1–11.

Weiss, M. E., Piacentine, L. B., Lokken, L., Ancona, J., Archer, J., Gresser, S., et al. (2007). Perceived readiness for hospital discharge in adult medical-surgical patients. *Clinical Nurse Specialist, 21*(1), 31–42.

Young, H. M., Sikma, S. K., Trippett, L. S. J., Shannon, J., & Blachly, B. (2006). Linking theory and gerontological nursing practice in senior housing. *Geriatric Nursing, 27*, 346–354

Bibliography for Meleis

Brooten, D. K. H., & Naylor, M. D. (1999). Transitional environments. In A. S. Hinshaw, S. L. Feetham, & J. Shaver (Eds.), *Handbook of clinical nursing research* (pp. 641–653). Thousand Oaks, CA: Sage.

Davidson, P. M., Meleis, A. I., Daly, J., & Douglas, M. (2003). Globalization as we enter the 21st century: Reflections and directions for nursing education, science, research and clinical practice. *Advances in Contemporary Transcultural Nursing, 15,* 162–174.

De Leon Siantz, M. L., & Meleis, A. I. (2007). Integrating cultural competence into nursing education and practice: 21st century action steps. *Journal of Transcultural Nursing, 18*(1, Suppl.), 86S–90S.

Dracup, K., Cronenwett, L., Meleis, A. I., & Benner, P. E. (2005). Reply to letter to the editor on reflections on the doctorate of nursing practice. *Nursing Outlook, 53,* 269.

Dracup, K., Cronenwett, L., Meleis, A. I., & Benner, P. E. (2005). Reflections on the doctorate of nursing practice. *Nursing Outlook, 53,* 177–182.

Hall, J. M. (1999). Marginalization revisited: Critical, postmodern, and liberation perspectives. *Advances in Nursing Science, 22*(2), 88–102.

Hall, J. M., Stevens, P. E., & Meleis, A. I. (1994). Marginalization: A guiding concept for valuing diversity in nursing knowledge development. *Advances in Nursing Science, 16*(4), 23–41.

Im, E. (1997). Neglecting and ignoring menopause within a gender and multiple transition context: Low income Korean immigrant women. *Dissertation Abstracts International, 58*(07B), 3557. Abstract retrieved November 20, 2007, from Dissertation Abstract Online database.

Im, E., & Meleis, A. I. (1999). A situation-specific theory of Korean immigrant women's menopausal transition. *Image: Journal of Nursing Scholarship, 31,* 333–338.

Im, E., & Meleis, A. I. (1999). Situation-specific theories: Philosophical roots, properties, approach. *Advances in Nursing Science, 22*(2), 11–24.

Im, E., & Meleis, A. I. (2001). An international imperative for gender-sensitive theories in women's health. *Image: Journal of Nursing Scholarship, 33,* 309–314.

Im, E., & Meleis, A. I. (2001). Women's work and symptoms during midlife: Korean immigrant women. *Women and Health, 33*(1/2), 83–103.

Jones, P. S., Jaceldo, K. B., Lee, J. R., Zhang, X. E., & Meleis, A. I. (2001). Role integration and perceived health in Asian-American women caregivers. *Research in Nursing and Health, 24,* 133–144.

Jones, P. S., Zhang, X. E., Jaceldo-Siegl, K., & Meleis, A. I. (2002). Caregiving between two cultures: An integrative experience. *Journal of Transcultural Nursing, 13,* 202–209.

Jones, P. S., Zhang, X. E., & Meleis, A. I. (2003). Transforming vulnerability. *Western Journal of Nursing Research, 25,* 835–853.

Meleis, A. I. (1992). Directions for nursing theory development in the 21st century. *Nursing Science Quarterly, 5,* 112–117.

Meleis, A. I. (1998). Revisions in knowledge development: A passion for substance. *Scholarly Inquiry for Nursing Practice: An International Journal, 12*(1), 65.

Meleis, A. I. (2007). *Theoretical nursing: Development and progress* (4th ed.). Philadelphia: Lippincott Williams & Wilkins.

Meleis, A. I. (Ed.). (2001). *Women's work, health and quality of life.* Binghamton, NY: Haworth Press.

Meleis, A. I. (2001). Scholarship and the R01 (Editorial). *Journal of Nursing Scholarship, 33,* 104–105.

Meleis, A. I. (2001). Small steps and giant hopes: Violence on women is more than wife battering (Editorial). *Health Care for Women International, 23,* 313–315.

Meleis, A. I. (2001). Women's work, health and quality of life: It is time we redefine women's work. *Women and Health, 33*(1/2), xv–xviii.

Meleis, A. I. (2002). Whither international research? (Editorial). *Journal of Nursing Scholarship, 34,* 4–5.

Meleis, A. I. (2003). Brain drain or empowerment. *Journal of Nursing Scholarship, 35,* 105.

Meleis, A. I. (2005). Arab Americans. In J. Lipson & S. Dibble (Eds.), *Culture and clinical care: A practical guide* (pp. 42–57). San Francisco: UCSF Nursing Press.

Meleis, A. I. (2005). Safe womanhood is not safe motherhood: Policy implications. *Health Care for Women International, 26,* 464–471.

Meleis, A. I. (2005). Shortage of nurses means a shortage of nurse scientists. (Editorial). *Journal of Advanced Nursing, 49,* 111.

Meleis, A. I. (2006). Human capital in health care: A resource crisis or a caring crisis? *Global HealthLink, 139,* 6–7, 21–22.

Meleis, A. I. (2005). Foreword. In B. A. Powers & T. R. Knapp (Eds.), *Dictionary of nursing theory and research* (3rd ed.). New York: Springer.

Meleis, A. I., & Dracup, K. (2005). The case against the DNP: History, timing, substance, and marginalization. *The Online Journal of Issues in Nursing, 10(3),* Manuscript 2.

Meleis, A. I., & Fishman, J. (2001). Rethinking the work in health: Gendered and cultural expectations (Editorial). *Health Care for Women, International, 22,* 195–197.

Meleis, A. I., & Im, E. (2002). Grandmothers and women's health: From fragmentation to coherence. *Health Care for Women, International, 23,* 207–224.

Meleis, A. I., & Lipson, J. (2003). Cross-cultural health and strategies to lead development of nursing practice. In J. Daly, S. Speedy, & D. Jackson (Eds.), *Nursing leadership* (pp. 69–88). Philadelphia: Churchill Livingstone.

Meleis, A. I., & Lindgren, T. G. (2001). World Health: Show me a woman who does not work! *Journal of Nursing Scholarship, 33,* 209–210.

Meleis, A. I., & Lindgren, T. (2002). Man works from sun to sun, but woman's work is never done: Insights on research and policy. *Health Care for Women, International, 23,* 742–753.

Meleis, A. I., Lipson, J. G., Muecke, M., & Smith, G. (1998). *Immigrant women and their health: An olive paper.* Indianapolis: Center for Nursing Press, Sigma Theta Tau.

Meleis, A. I., & Rogers, S. (1987). Women in transition: Being versus becoming or being and becoming. *Health Care for Women International, 8(4),* 199–217.

Meleis, A. I., & Schumacher, K. L. (1998). Transitions and health. In J. J. Fitzpatrick (Ed.), *Encyclopedia of nursing research* (pp. 570–571). New York: Springer.

Messias, D. K. H., Hall, J. M., & Meleis, A. I. (1996). Voices of impoverished Brazilian women: Health implications of roles and resources. *Women and Health, 24(1),* 1–20.

Messias, D. K. H., Im, E., Page, A., Regev, H., Spier, J., Yoder, L., et al. (1997). Defining and redefining work: Implications for women's health. *Gender and Society, 11,* 296–323.

Robinson, P. R., Ekman, S. L., Meleis, A. I., Winblad, B., & Wahlund, L. (1997). Suffering in silence: The experience of early memory loss. *Health Care in Later Life, 2,* 107–120.

Schaeffer, D., Moers, M., Steppe, H., & Meleis, A. I. (1997). *Plegethorien.* Bern: Verlag Hans Huber.

Schumacher, K. L., Jones, P. S., & Meleis, A. I. (1999). Helping elderly persons in transition: A framework for research and practice. In E. Swanson & T. Tripp-Reimer (Eds.), *Life transitions in older adults: Issues for nurses and other health professionals* (pp. 1–26). New York: Springer.

Shih, F., Meleis, A. I., Yu, P., Hu, W., Lou, M., & Huang, G. (1998). Taiwanese patients' concerns and coping strategies: Transition to cardiac surgery. *Heart and Lung, 27(2),* 82–98.

St. Hill, P., Lipson, J., & Meleis, A. I. (Eds.). (2002). *Caring for women cross-culturally: A portable guide.* Philadelphia: F. A. Davis.

References for Mishel

Anema, C. L. (2006). Spiritual well-being in individuals with fibromyalgia syndrome: Relationships with symptom pattern variability, uncertainty and psychosocial adaptation. *Dissertation Abstracts International, 67(03B),* 1372. Abstract retrieved December 6, 2007, from Dissertation Abstracts Online database.

Bailey, D. E., Wallace, M., & Mishel, M. H. (2007). Watching, waiting and uncertainty in prostate cancer. *Journal of Clinical Nursing, 16,* 734–741.

Bertram, C. C. (2004). Uncertain knowledge of a certain virus. Human papillomavirus and abnormal pap smears: An Internet survey of knowledge and beliefs among a university population in Hawai'i. *Dissertation Abstracts International, 65(10B),* 5084. Abstract retrieved December 6, 2007, from Dissertation Abstracts Online database.

Bower, G. H. (1978). *The psychology of learning and motivation: Advances in research and theory.* New York: Academic Press.

Bowers, R. J. (2006). Uncertainty and social support as predictors of coping in women experiencing fibromyalgia: A structural model. *Dissertation Abstracts International, 67*(10B), 6046. Abstract retrieved December 6, 2007, from Dissertation Abstracts Online database.

Budner, S. (1963). Intolerance of ambiguity as a personality variable. *Journal of Personality, 30,* 29–50.

Christman, N. J., McConnell, E. A., Pfeiffer, C., Webster, K. K., Schmitt, M., & Ries, J. (1988). Uncertainty, coping, and distress following myocardial infarction: Transition from hospital to home. *Research in Nursing and Health, 11,* 71–82.

Coxon, V. J. (1989). Subjective perceptions of the demands of hospitalization and anxiety in bone marrow transplant patients. *Dissertation Abstracts International, 51*(05B), 2285. Abstract retrieved December 6, 2007, from Dissertation Abstracts Online database.

Decker, C. L., Haase, J. E., & Bell, C. J. (2007). Uncertainty in adolescents and young adults with cancer. *Oncology Nursing Forum, 34,* 681–688.

DiBiase, R. J., & Rice, V. (2007). Chemotherapy education: Effects on knowledge and uncertainty in cancer patients. *Oncology Nursing Forum, 34*(1), 238.

Flemme, I., Bolse, K., & Fridlund, B. (2006). Quality of life related to shocks in ICD-recepientsa [*sic*] 5-year follow-up. *European Journal of Cardiovascular Nursing, 5*(Suppl. 1), S20.

Galloway, S. C., & Graydon, J. E. (1996). Uncertainty, symptom distress, and information needs after surgery for cancer of the colon. *Cancer Nursing, 19,* 112–117.

Giurgescu, C., Penckofer, S., Maurer, M. C., & Bryant, F. B. (2007). Impact of uncertainty, social support, and prenatal coping on the psychological well-being of high-risk pregnant women. *Nursing Research, 55,* 356–365.

Guadalupe, K. A. (2007). The role of uncertainty in decision making about genetic counseling. *Dissertation Abstracts International, 68*(03B), 1556. Abstract retrieved December 6, 2007, from Dissertation Abstracts Online database.

Handley, M. C., & Crow, C. S. (2006). Emotional responses to pregnancy based on geographical classification of residence. *Online Journal of Rural Nursing and Health Care, 6*(2), 16 pages. Abstract retrieved May 18, 2007, from CINAHL Plus with Full Text database.

Haugh, K. H., & Salyer, J. (2006). Mastering uncertainty in end-stage cardio-pulmonary disease: A comparison between patients awaiting transplant and those medically managed. *Progress in Cardiovascular Nursing, 21*(2), 108.

Hilton, B.A. (1994). The Uncertainty Stress Scale: Its development and psychometric properties. *Canadian Journal of Nursing Research, 26*(3), 15–30.

Hockett, K. A. (2005). The effects of a comprehensive post-treatment recovery program for breast cancer survivors. *Dissertation Abstracts International, 66*(09B), 4725. Abstract retrieved December 6, 2007, from Dissertation Abstracts Online database.

Johnson, L. M., Zautra, A. J., & Davis, M. C. (2007). The role of illness uncertainty on coping with fibromyalgia symptoms. *Health Psychology, 25,* 696–703.

Jurgens, C. Y. (2006). Somatic awareness, uncertainty, and delay in care-seeking in acute heart failure. *Research in Nursing and Health, 29*(2), 74–86.

Kang, Y. (2006). Effect of uncertainty on depression in patients with newly diagnosed atrial fibrillation. *Progress in Cardiovascular Nursing, 21*(2), 83–88.

Kloos, J. A. (2004). Effect of family-maintained progress journal on families of critically ill patients. *Dissertation Abstracts International, 65*(05B), 2343. Abstract retrieved December 6, 2007, from Dissertation Abstracts Online database.

Lai, H., Lin, S., & Yeh, S. (2007). Exploring uncertainty, quality of life and related factors in patients with liver cancer [Chinese]. *Journal of Nursing [China], 54*(6), 41–52. Abstract in English retrieved March 12, 2008 from CINAHL Plus with Full Text database.

Lazarus, R. S. (1974). Psychological stress and coping in adaptation and illness. *International Journal of Psychiatry in Medicine, 5,* 321–333.

Lee, Y. (2006). The relationships between uncertainty and posttraumatic stress in survivors of childhood cancer. *Journal of Nursing Research, 14*(2), 133–142.

Lee, Y. L., Santacroce, S. J., & Sadler, L. (2007). Predictors of health behaviour in long-term survivors of childhood cancer. *Journal of Clinical Nursing, 16*(11c), 285–295.

Mast, M. E. (1995). Adult uncertainty in illness: A critical review of research. *Scholarly Inquiry for Nursing Practice, 9*(1), 3–29.

Mishel, M. H. (1981). The measurement of uncertainty in illness. *Nursing Research, 30,* 258–263.

Mishel, M. H. (1983) Parent's perception of uncertainty concerning their hospitalized child. *Nursing Research 32,* 324–330.

Mishel, M. H. (1984). Perceived uncertainty and stress in illness. *Research in Nursing and Health, 7,* 163–171.

Mishel, M. H. (1988). Uncertainty in illness. *Image: The Journal of Nursing Scholarship, 20,* 225–232.

Mishel. M. H. (1990). Reconceptualization of the Uncertainty in Illness Theory. *Image: The Journal of Nursing Scholarship, 22,* 256–262.

Mishel, M. H. (1997). Uncertainty in acute illness. In J. J. Fitzpatrick (Ed.), *Annual review of nursing research, 15* (pp. 57–80). New York: Springer.

Mishel, M. H. (1999) Uncertainty in acute illness. In J. J. Fitzpatrick (Ed.), *Annual review of nursing research, 17* (pp. 269–294). New York: Springer.

Mishel, M. H., & Braden, C. J. (1987). Uncertainty: A mediator between support and adjustment. *Western Journal of Nursing Research, 9,* 43–57.

Mishel, M. H., & Braden, C. J. (1988). Finding meaning: Antecedents of uncertainty in illness. *Nursing Research, 37,* 98–103, 127.

Mishel, M. H., & Clayton, M. F. (2003). Theories of uncertainty in illness. In M. J. Smith & P. R. Liehr (Eds.), *Middle range theory for nursing* (pp. 25–48). New York: Springer.

Mishel, M. H., Hostetter, T., King, B., & Graham, V. (1984). Predictors of psychosocial adjustment in patients newly diagnosed with gynecological cancer. *Cancer Nursing, 7,* 291–299.

Mishel, M. H., & Murdaugh, C. L. (1987). Family adjustment to heart transplantation: Redesigning the dream. *Nursing Research, 36,* 332–338.

Mishel, M. H., & Sorenson, D. S. (1991). Uncertainty in gynecological cancer: A test of the mediating functions of mastery and coping. *Nursing Research, 40,* 167–171.

Moos, R., & Tsu, V. (1977). The crisis of physical illness: An overview. In R. Moos (Ed.), *Coping with physical illness* (pp. 3–25). New York: Plenum.

Norton, R. (1975). Measurement of ambiguity tolerance. *Journal of Personal Assessment, 39,* 607–619.

Owens, B. (2007). A test of the Self-Help Model and use of complementary and alternative medicine among Hispanic women during treatment for breast cancer. *Oncology Nursing Forum, 34*(4), Online Exclusive: E42-50. Abstract retrieved March 12, 2008, from CINAHL Plus with Full Text database.

Reich, J. W., Johnson, L. M., Zautra, A. J., & Davis, M. C. (2006). Uncertainty of illness relationships with mental health and coping processes in fibromyalgia patients. *Journal of Behavioral Medicine, 29,* 307–316.

Santacroce, S. J., & Lee, Y. (2006). Uncertainty, posttraumatic stress, and health behavior in young adult childhood cancer survivors. *Nursing Research, 55,* 259–266.

Shalit, B. (1977). Structural ambiguity and limits to coping. *Journal of Human Stress, 3,* 32–45.

Sorenson, M. R. (2002). Psychological stress, coping, and illness uncertainty in individuals with multiple sclerosis: Relationship with cytokine production. *Dissertation Abstracts International, 63*(01B), 182. Abstract retrieved December 6, 2007, from Dissertation Abstracts Online database.

Sorenson, M. R., Janusek, L., & Mathews, H. L. (2006). Perceived stress, illness uncertainty, and disease symptomatology in multiple sclerosis. *SCI Nursing Journal, 23*(1). Retrieved March 13, 2008, from http://www.unitedspinal.org/publications/nursing/2006/05/01/perceived-stress-illness-uncertainty-and-disease-symptomatology-in-multiple-sclerosis.

Sossong, A. (2007). Living with an implantable cardioverter defibrillator: Patient outcomes and the nurse's role. *Journal of Cardiovascular Nursing, 22*(2), 99–104.

Stewart, J. L., & Mishel, M. H. (2000). Uncertainty in childhood illness: A synthesis of the parent and child literature. *Scholarly Inquiry for Nursing Practice, 14,* 299–319, 321–326.

Tomlinson, P. S., Kirschbaum, M., Harbaugh, B., & Anderson, K. H. (1996). The influence of illness severity and family resources on maternal uncertainty during critical pediatric hospitalization. *American Journal of Critical Care, 5,* 140–146.

Wallace, M., & Hegerty, J. (2007). Quality of life and uncertainty in men with prostate cancer undergoing watchful waiting: An Irish-American comparative study. *Oncology in Nursing Forum, 34*(1), 250.

Weber, B. A., Roberts, B. L., Chumbler, N. R., Mills, T. L., & Algood, C. B. (2007). Urinary, sexual, and bowel dysfunction and bother after radical prostatectomy. *Urologic Nursing, 27,* 527–533.

Selected Additional References for Mishel (After 1997)

Badger, T. A., Braden, C. J., & Mishel, M. H. (2001). Depression burden, self-help interventions, and side effect experience in women receiving treatment for breast cancer. *Oncology Nursing Forum, 28,* 567–574.

Badger, T. A., Braden, C. J, Longman, A. J., & Mishel, M. H. (1999). Depression burden, self-help interventions, and social support in women receiving treatment for breast cancer. *Journal of Psychosocial Oncology, 17*(2), 17–35.

Bailey, D. E., Mishel, M. H., Belyea, M., Stewart, J. L., & Mohler, J. (2004). Uncertainty intervention for watchful waiting in prostate cancer. *Cancer Nursing, 27,* 339–346.

Braden, C. J., Mishel, M. H., Longman, A. J., & Burns, L. R. (1998). Self Help Intervention Project: Women receiving breast cancer treatment. *Cancer Practice, 6*(2), 87–98.

Brashers, D. E., Heidig, J. L., Russell, J. A., Cardillo, L. W., Haas, S. M., Dobbs, L. K., et al. (2003). The medical, personal, and social causes of uncertainty in HIV illness. *Issues in Mental Health Nursing, 24,* 497–522.

Calvin, R. L., & Lane, P. L. (1999). Perioperative uncertainty and state anxiety of orthopaedic surgical patients. *Orthopaedic Nursing, 18* (6), 61–66.

Carroll, D. L., Hamilton, G. A., & McGovern, B. A. (1999). Changes in health status and quality of life and the impact of uncertainty in patients who survive life-threatening arrhythmias. *Heart and Lung, 28,* 251–260.

Clayton, M. F. (2006). Testing a model of symptoms, communication, uncertainty, and well-being in older breast cancer survivors. *Research in Nursing and Health, 29*(1), 18–39.

Flemme, I., Edvardsson, N., Hinic, H., Jinhage, B., Dalman, M., & Fridlund, B. (2006). Long-term quality of life and uncertainty in patients living with an implantable cardioverter defibrillator. *Heart and Lung, 34,* 386–392.

Frain, M. P., Bishop, M., Tschopp, M. K., Ferrin, M. J., & Frain, J. (2009). Adherence to medical regimens: Understanding the effects of cognitive appraisal, quality of life, and perceived family resiliency. *Rehabilitation Counseling Bulletin, 52,* 237–250.

Germino, B. B., Mishel, M. H., Belyea, M., Harris, L., Ware, A., & Mohler, J. (1998). Uncertainty in prostate cancer: Ethnic and family patterns. *Cancer Practice, 6*(2), 107–113.

Gil, K. M., Mishel, M. H., Germino, B., Porter, L. S., Carlton-LaNey, I. E., & Belyea, M. (2005). Uncertainty management intervention for older African American and Caucasian long-term breast cancer survivors. *Journal of Psychosocial Oncology, 23,* 3–21.

Hommel, K. A., Chaney, J. M., Wagner, J. L., White, M. M., Hoff, A. L., & Mullins, L. L. (2003). Anxiety and depressions in older adolescents with long-standing asthma: The role of illness uncertainty. *Children's Health Care, 32*(1), 51–63.

Horner, S. D. (1997). Uncertainty in mothers' care for their ill children. *Journal of Advanced Nursing, 26,* 658–663.

Kang, Y., Daly, J., & Kim, J. (2004). Uncertainty and its antecedents in patients with atrial fibrillation. *Western Journal of Nursing Research, 26,* 770–783.

Kang, Y. (2005). Effects of uncertainty on perceived health status inpatients with atrial fibrillation. *Nursing in Critical Care, 10*(4), 184–191.

Lien, C., Lin, H., Kuo, I., & Chen, M. (2009). Perceived uncertainty, social support and psychological adjustment in older patients with cancer being treated with surgery. *Journal of Clinical Nursing, 18,* 2311–2319.

Lemaire, G. S. (2004). More than just menstrual cramps: Symptoms and uncertainty among women with endometriosis. *Journal of Obstetric, Gynecologic, and Neonatal Nurses, 33*(1), 71–79.

Liu, L., Li, C., Tang, S. T., Huang, C., & Chiou, A. (2006). Role of continuing supportive cares in increasing social support and reducing perceived uncertainty among women with newly diagnosed breast cancer in Taiwan. *Cancer Nursing, 29,* 273–282.

Longman, A. J., Braden, C. J., & Mishel, M. H. (1997). Pattern of association over time of side-effects burden, self-help and self-care in women with breast cancer. *Oncology Nursing Forum, 24,* 1555–1560.

Longman, A., Braden, C. J., & Mishel, M. H. (1999). Side effects burden, psychological adjustment and life quality in women with breast cancer: Pattern of association over time. *Oncology Nursing Forum, 26,* 909–915.

Madar, H., & Bar-Tal, Y. (2009). The experience of uncertainty among patients having peritoneal dialysis. *Journal of Advanced Nursing, 65,* 1664–1669.

Mast, M. E. (1998). Survivors of breast cancer: Illness uncertainty, positive reappraisal, and emotional distress. *Oncology Nursing Forum, 25,* 555–562.

McCormick, K. M., Naimark, B. J., & Tate, R. B. (2006). Uncertainty, symptom distress, anxiety, and functional status in patients awaiting coronary bypass surgery. *Heart and Lung, 35*(1), 34–45.

Mishel, M. H. (1998). Methodological studies: Instrument development. In P. Brink & M. Woods (Eds.), *Advanced design in nursing research* (2nd ed., pp. 235–282). Beverly Hills, CA: Sage.

Mishel, M. H., Germino, B., Belyea, M., Stewart, J. L., Bailey, D. E., Mohler, J., et al. (2003). Moderators of an uncertainty management intervention for men with localized prostate cancer. *Nursing Research, 52*(2), 89–97.

Mishel, M. H., Belyea, M., Germino, B., Stewart, J. L. Bailey, D., Robertson, C., et al. (2002). Helping patients with localized prostate cancer manage uncertainty and treatment side effects: Nurse delivered psycho-educational intervention via telephone. *Cancer, 94,* 1854–1866.

Mullins, L. L., Cote, M. P., Fuemmeler, B. F. Jean, V. M., Beatty, W. W., & Paul, R. H. (2001). Illness intrusiveness, uncertainty, and distress in individuals with multiple sclerosis. *Rehabilitation Psychology, 46,* 139–153.

Neville, K. (1998). The relationships among uncertainty, social support, and psychological distress in adolescents recently diagnosed with cancer. *Journal of Pediatric Oncology Nursing 15*(1), 37–46.

Neville, K. L. (2003) Uncertainty in illness: An integrative review. *Orthpaedic Nursing, 22,* 206–214.

Northouse, L. L., Mood, D., Tempin, T., Mellon, S., & George, T. (2000). Couples' patterns of adjustment to colon cancer. *Social Science and Medicine, 50,* 271–284.

Ritz, L. O., Nissen, M. J., Swenson, K. K., Farrell, J. B., Sperduto, P. W., Sladek, M. L., et al. (2000). Effects of advanced nursing care on quality of life and cost outcomes of women diagnosed with breast cancer. *Oncology Nursing Forum, 27,* 923–932.

Rosen, N. O., & Knäuper, B. (2009). A little uncertainty goes a long way: State and trait differences in uncertainty interact to increase information seeking but also increase worry. *Health Communication, 24,* 228–238.

Sammarco, A. (2009). Quality of life of breast cancer survivors: A comparative study of age cohorts. *Cancer Nursing, 32,* 347–358.

Sanders-Dewey, N. E. J., Mullins, L. L., & Chaney, J. M. (2001). Coping style, perceived uncertainty in illness, and distress in individuals with Parkinson's disease and their caregivers. *Rehabilitation Psychology, 46,* 363–381.

Santacroce, S. J. (2000). Support from health care providers and parental uncertainty during the diagnosis phase of perinatally acquired HIV infection. *Journal of the Association of Nurses in AIDS Care, 11*(2), 63–75.

Santacroce, S. J. (2003). Paternal uncertainty and posttraumatic stress in serious childhood illnesses. *Journal of Nursing Scholarship, 35*(1), 45–51.

Sexton, D. L., Calcasola, S. L., Bottomley, S. R., & Funk, M. (1999). Adults' experience with asthma and their reported uncertainty and coping strategies. *Clinical Nurse Specialist, 13*(1), 8–17.

Sorenson, M. R. (2002). Psychological stress, coping, and illness uncertainty in individuals with multiple sclerosis: Relationship with cytokine production. *Dissertation Abstracts International, 63*(01B), 182. Abstract retrieved December 6, 2007, from Dissertation Abstracts Online database.

Taylor-Piliae, R., & Molassiotis, A. (2001). An exploration of the relationships between uncertainty, psychological distress and type of coping strategy among Chinese men after cardiac catheterization. *Journal of Advanced Nursing, 33*(1), 79–88.

Wallace, M. (2003). Uncertainty and quality of life of older men who undergo watchful waiting for prostate cancer. *Oncology Nursing Forum, 30,* 303–309.

Weiss, M. E., Saks, N. P., & Harris, S. (2002). Resolving the uncertainty of preterm symptoms: Women's experiences with the onset of preterm labor. *Journal of Obstetric, Gynecologic, and Neonatal Nursing, 33*(1), 66–76.

Wineman, N. M., Schwetz, K. M., Zeller, R., & Cyphert, J. (2003) Longitudinal analysis of illness uncertainty, coping, hopefulness, and mood during participation in a clinical drug trial. *Journal of Neuroscience Nursing, 35*(2), 100–106.

Wonghongkul, T., Dechaprom, N., Phamiviehuvate, L., & Losawatkul, S. (2006). Uncertainty appraisal coping and quality of life in breast cancer survivors. *Cancer Nursing, 29,* 250–257.

Wonghongkul, T., Moore, S. M., Musil, C., Schneider, S., & Deimling, G. (2000). The influence of uncertainty in illness, stress appraisal, and hope on coping in survivors of breast cancer. *Cancer Nursing, 23,* 422–429.

Wunderlich, R. J., Perry, A., Lavin, M., & Katz, B. (1999). Patients' perceptions of uncertainty and stress during weaning from mechanical ventilation. *Dimensions of Critical Care Nursing, 18*(1), 2–10.

Examples of Dissertations Using Mishel's Theory of Uncertainty in Illness

Amertil, N. P. (1997). Self-management in adult clients with sickle cell disease. *Dissertation Abstracts International, 58*(06B), 2954. Abstract retrieved December 6, 2007, from Dissertation Abstracts Online database.

Bailey, D. E. (2002). Uncertainty and watchful waiting in men with prostate cancer. *Dissertation Abstracts International, 63*(03B), 1263. Abstract retrieved December 6, 2007, from Dissertation Abstracts Online database.

Cuvar, K. M. (2004). The relationship of health-related hardiness, uncertainty, social support on coping in post-cardiac transplant recipients. *Dissertation Abstracts International, 65*(05B), 2340. Abstract retrieved December 6, 2007, from Dissertation Abstracts Online database.

Davis, L. A. (1997). Hardiness, social support, uncertainty, and adjustment in women clinically free of breast cancer. *Dissertation Abstracts International, 58*(09B), 4719. Abstract retrieved December 6, 2007, from Dissertation Abstracts Online database.

Forester, Z. D. (1998). Knowledge and attitudes of Virginia clinical nurse specialists about menopause. *Dissertation Abstracts International, 59*(11B), 5785. Abstract retrieved December 6, 2007, from Dissertation Abstracts Online database.

Handley, M. C. (2002). Uncertainty in pregnancy. *Dissertation Abstracts International, 63*(05B), 1268. Abstract retrieved December 6, 2007, from Dissertation Abstracts Online database.

Haugh, K. H. (2005). Mastering uncertainty in end-stage cardiopulmonary disease: A comparison between patients awaiting transplant and those medically managed. *Dissertation Abstracts International, 66*(02B), 812. Abstract retrieved December 6, 2007, from Dissertation Abstracts Online database.

Hockett, K. A. (2005). The effects of a comprehensive post-treatment recovery program for breast cancer survivors. *Dissertation Abstracts International, 66*(09B), 4725. Abstract retrieved December 6, 2007, from Dissertation Abstracts Online database.

Jurgens, C. Y. (2003). Somatic awareness, uncertainty, and delay in care-seeking in acute heart failure. *Dissertation Abstracts International, 64*(06B), 2591. Abstract retrieved December 6, 2007, from Dissertation Abstracts Online database.

Kang, Y. (2002). The relationship among uncertainty, seriousness of illness, social support, appraisal of uncertainty, health locus of control, and perceived health status in patients newly diagnosed with atrial fibrillation. *Dissertation Abstracts International, 63*(07B), 3231. Abstract retrieved December 6, 2007, from Dissertation Abstracts Online database.

Maliski, S. L. (1997). The experience of recurrent breast cancer: A case study. *Dissertation Abstracts International, 58*(12B), 6489. Abstract retrieved December 6, 2007, from Dissertation Abstracts Online database.

Mauro, A. M. P. (1998). The relation between uncertainty and psychosocial adjustment among recipients of an implantable cardioverter defibrillator. *Dissertation Abstracts International, 59*(09B), 4729. Abstract retrieved December 6, 2007, from Dissertation Abstracts Online database.

Sall, J. L. (2000). The effect of prostate cancer support groups on uncertainty in prostate cancer. *Masters Abstracts International, 38*(06), 1589. Abstract retrieved December 6, 2007, from Dissertation Abstracts Online database.

Sammarco, A. T. (1998). The relationship between perceived social support, uncertainty, and quality of life among younger women who have had breast cancer. *Dissertation Abstracts International,* 60(06B), 2621. Abstract retrieved December 6, 2007, from Dissertation Abstracts Online database.

Santacroce, S. J. (1997). Uncertainty and mothering the HIV seropositive infant. *Dissertation Abstracts International,* 58(04B), 1806. Abstract retrieved December 6, 2007, from Dissertation Abstracts Online database.

Sossong, A. E. (2004). The relationship between implantable cardioverter defibrillator, uncertainty, and quality of life in individuals living with an ICD. *Dissertation Abstracts International,* 65(03B), 1252. Abstract retrieved December 6, 2007, from Dissertation Abstracts Online database.

Wagner, L. C. (1998). A preliminary investigation of uncertainty in illness, coping, and social support in women with acquired immune deficiency syndrome. *Dissertation Abstracts International,* 59(07B), 3353. Abstract retrieved December 6, 2007, from Dissertation Abstracts Online database.

Wallace, M. (2001). The quality of life of older men who are receiving the watchful waiting treatment for prostate cancer. *Dissertation Abstracts International,* 62(02B), 787. Abstract retrieved December 6, 2007, from Dissertation Abstracts Online database.

Winters, C.A. (1998). Heart failure: Living with uncertainty. *Dissertation Abstracts International,* 59(08B), 4023. Abstract retrieved December 6, 2007, from Dissertation Abstracts Online database.

Wonghongkul, T. (1999). Uncertainty, appraisal, hope, and coping in breast cancer survivors. *Dissertation Abstracts International,* 6(11B), 5439. Abstract retrieved December 6, 2007, from Dissertation Abstracts Online database.

CHAPTER **24**

Other Nursing Theories from the 1990s

Janet Hickman
Julia B. George

During the 1990s other theories, those focusing both on a specific area and on a general scheme, were developed. This chapter will provide overviews for Juliet Corbin and Anselm Strauss's Chronic Illness Trajectory Framework Nursing Model, Anne Boykin and Savina O. Schoenhofer's grand theory of nursing as caring, and Kathy Kolcaba's comfort theory.

CHRONIC ILLNESS TRAJECTORY FRAMEWORK

Juliet M. Corbin and Anselm Leonard Strauss

Juliet M. Corbin reports that she played doctor and nurse as a child and, since she could not afford medical school, planned to attend a three-year diploma nursing program. Fortunately, a wise high school counselor guided her to a four-year degree program. After completing her baccalaureate degree in nursing, she first worked on a medical-surgical unit and then in maternal–child public health care in Arizona. In the 1970s she earned a master's degree in public health nursing with a maternal–child focus from San Jose State University, California (SJSU), and in 1981 a doctorate in nursing science from the University of California, San Francisco (UCSF). Because of her interest in qualitative research, she also did post-doctoral work with Anselm Strauss at UCSF. After completing her master's degree, she accepted a position at SJSU teaching maternal–child health nursing. After completing her doctorate, in addition to her work with Strauss, she taught and practiced at SJSU in a nursing managed center. The clinical work led her to complete a family nurse practitioner program (Meetoo, 2007). Her research and publications have focused on qualitative research, chronic illness, chronic pain, maternal care, and aging. She is a frequent speaker on qualitative research. Corbin is emeriti faculty at SJSU and an adjunct professor in the International Institute for Qualitative Methodology, University of Alberta, Canada (http://www.uofaweb .ualberta.ca/iiqm).

Anselm Leonard Strauss was born December 18, 1916, and grew up in Mount Vernon, New York. He died September 5, 1996, in San Francisco, California, after a long and illustrious career in medical sociology. He received a B.S. in biology from the University of Virginia, Charlottesville, in 1939, and an M.A. in sociology (1942) and Ph.D. in sociology (1945) from the University of Chicago, Illinois. After completing his Ph.D. he was a lecturer at Lawrence University, Appleton, Wisconsin (1946–1952); an assistant professor at the University of Chicago, Illinois (1952–1958); and director of research, Institute for Psychosomatic and Psychiatric Research and Training, Michael Reese Hospital, Chicago, Illinois (1958–1960). In 1960, he was convinced by Dean Helen Nahm to found the Department of Social and Behavioral Sciences in the School of Nursing at UCSF. He served as chair of that department from 1960 to 1980 and professor from 1980 to 1987, when he "retired" and became Professor Emeritus. He continued to teach a qualitative research seminar until his death. He also served as invited visiting professor at universities in England, France, Germany, and Australia. He published (both solely and in collaboration) many articles and 32 books, which have been translated into eight languages. In addition to cofounding the grounded theory methodology of qualitative research, his areas of interest included searching for identity, the experience of dying, professional work, how hospitals function, chronic illness, and chronic pain. His awards include election as a fellow of the American Association for the Advancement of Science (1980); the Charles H. Cooley Award, Society for the Study of Symbolic Interaction (1980); Leo G. Reeder Award for distinguished scholarship in medical sociology, Medical Sociology Section, American Sociological Association (1981); Helen Nahm Research Lecturer, School of Nursing, UCSF (1985); George H. Mead Award (a career award), Society for the Study of Symbolic Interaction (1985); Campus Faculty Research Lecturer, UCSF (1986–1987); and the Cooley-Mead Award, Social Psychology Section, American Sociological Association (1994) (Curriculum vitae, 2003; Bainton, 1995).

CHRONIC ILLNESS TRAJECTORY FRAMEWORK   When Juliet Corbin graduated with her doctorate, her focus on chronic illness during pregnancy in her dissertation had convinced her that her research focus would continue to be on chronic illness (Corbin, 1981; Meetoo, 2007). Her 15-year collaboration with Anselm Strauss began during her postdoctoral studies of chronic illness with him. Strauss (1985) indicated he began development of the concept of "trajectory" during his work with Barney Glaser in the 1960s. His curriculum vitae (2003) indicates he first published about chronic illness in 1973. In 1975, Strauss and Glaser published a framework for chronic illness. Thus, a foundation was laid for the development of the nursing model Chronic Illness Trajectory Framework. During the 1980s and into the 1990s, Corbin and Strauss (1984, 1985a, 1985b, 1987, 1988, 1990, 1991; Strauss & Corbin, 1988) published about various facets of chronic illness. In 1992, Corbin and Strauss presented the nursing model for chronic illness management, built upon their work and that of others (Fagerhaugh & Strauss, 1977; Strauss, Fagerhaugh, Suzeck, & Weiner, 1981, 1985). In 1992, when the first book with the nursing model was published, there were eight phases in the trajectory (Corbin & Strauss, 1992; Woog, 1992). In 1998, Corbin published an update of the model in which she placed greater emphasis on health promotion and illness prevention and sought to increase the focus on global influences on health care. In 2001, Corbin presented the model with nine phases in a book that includes chapters specific to individual phases (Corbin, 2001; Hyman & Corbin, 2001).

Concepts. The major and unifying concept of the Chronic Illness Trajectory Framework Nursing Model is trajectory. Other important concepts include trajectory phasing and subphasing, trajectory projection, trajectory scheme, conditions influencing management, trajectory management, biographical and everyday living impact, and reciprocal impact. It is also important to define chronic illness. Corbin (2001) defines *chronic illness* as "any physical or mental condition that require long-term (over 6 months) monitoring and/or management to control symptoms and to shape the course of the disease" (p. 1). *Trajectory* is defined as "a course of illness over time, *plus the actions* taken by patients, families, and health professionals to manage or shape that course"(p. 3).

Trajectory phasing and subphasing make up what is perhaps the most useful aspect of the model. They represent the many fluctuations in status that can occur over time in a chronic illness. Within each phase, there may be subphases that represent the potential for daily fluctuations, even to the extent of seeming to reverse the trend of the overall phase, that is, to move downward in an upward phase or upward in a downward phase (Corbin & Strauss, 1992). The phases are displayed in Table 24-1.

Other concepts are defined by Corbin and Strauss (1992). A *trajectory projection* is the personal vision of the course of the illness—what the illness means, what the symptoms will be like, how it will affect one's life (biography), and what the time frame is. Individuals with the same medical diagnosis may have totally different trajectory projections. For example, some may see the illness as meaning inevitable death and decide to make amends with those with whom they have strained relationships in what they see is the short time left. Others may see the meaning of inevitable death and decide to seek to squeeze the most pleasure possible out of the available time, while others may see this meaning and choose to withdraw from the world. *Trajectory scheme* is the plan to deal with three things—shaping the course of the illness, controlling immediate symptoms, and handing any disability. *Conditions influencing management* range from the very personal to the broadly social and include technology (type, amount and duration of use, number and type of side effects), resources, past experiences, motivation, setting, lifestyle, interaction and relationship style, type of illness and physical involvement, the nature of the symptoms, and the political and economic climate in relation to health care legislation. *Trajectory management* is how the course of the illness is shaped by the trajectory scheme; it is important that the plans in the scheme be specific to each trajectory phase. *Biography* in this model means the course of one's life; *biographical impact* relates to changes in that life course due to the illness or its management. This impact includes what Corbin and Strauss call "coming to terms" or making the changes or adaptations needed to live with the chronic condition. An example could be retraining for employment that requires less physical activity when faced with physical limitations. *Everyday life activities* include those usual activities of daily living that are necessary to keep us going. These may require "limitations management" or changes to be able to carry out the activities. Limitations management may be something as simple as sitting on the side of the bed for a few moments when arising for those with postural hypotension. The final concept is *reciprocal impact*, the purpose of which is to help us be aware that the illness, the biography, and everyday life activities will interact and create complex challenges for management of the chronic illness, to the point of compounding problems that arise.

Corbin (2001) discusses that nurses are the only professionals who provide care during all phases of the chronic illness trajectory, as well as in all the settings of the

TABLE 24-1 Chronic Illness Trajectory Framework Nursing Model Phases

Phase	When	Characteristics	Biography	Everyday Activity	Where	Goal
Pretra-jectory	Before symptoms	Genetic or lifestyle factors create risk of chronic condition				Prevent occurrence of chronic illness
Trajectory onset	Noticeable symptoms appear	Include diagnostic workup and announcement	In limbo—seeking to discover and cope with implications of the diagnosis	Degree of disruption will depend on the symptoms	May be inpatient or out-patient, depending on the symptoms	Develop trajectory projection and scheme that is appropriate
Stable	Course of illness and its symptoms are under control		Managed within limitations created by the illness		Illness manage-ment likely to be at home	Maintain stability in all areas
Unstable	Either the symptoms cannot be kept under control or the illness reactivates		Disrupted	Hard to carry out normal activities	Regimen adjustments made; usually at home	Return to stable
Acute	Symptoms are severe, unrelieved, or illness complications lead to hospitalization or bed rest		Either drastically cut back or totally placed on hold		Hospital or bed rest at home	Regain control over illness; resume normal life and activities
Crisis	Critical or life-threat-ening symptoms or events	Emergency treatment or care required	Suspended until crisis passes		Likely to be hospi-talized	Remove the threat to life

TABLE 24-1   Chronic Illness Trajectory Framework Nursing Model Phases (*Continued*)

Phase	When	Characteristics	Biography	Everyday Activity	Where	Goal
Comeback	Return to acceptable way of life	Gradual; within limits imposed by illness or disability; physical healing involved with stretching limitations through rehabilitation; psychosocially, coming to terms is needed	Reengaging in life	Making necessary adjustments	Returning home	Get trajectory projections and scheme going again
Downward	Ill again	Physical decline—may be rapid or gradual; symptoms increasingly difficult to control; disability increasing	Each major step downward leads to biographical adjustment and to alterations in everyday life activities		Probably home	Adapt to increasing disability
Dying	Final days or weeks before death	Body processes shutting down—may be rapid or gradual	Disengage-ment and closure	Relinquishment	Home or hospital	Achieve closure, let go, peaceful death

Adapted from Corbin, J. M. (2001). *Introduction and overview: Chronic illness and nursing.* In R. B. Hyman, & J. M. Corbin (Eds.), *Chronic illness: Research and theory for nursing practice* (pp. 4–5). New York: Springer.

model. Nurses are uniquely situated and prepared to identify nuances of change and to provide the holistic care needed.

PRACTICE AND RESEARCH WITH THE CHRONIC ILLNESS TRAJECTORY   Corbin and Strauss (1992) discussed the four major concepts in nursing's metaparadigm. *Persons* of any ages may develop a chronic illness and, except during hospitalizations, the care needed is provided by the person or significant others. Thus, people are active participants in both prevention and management, including making choices about how to live the personal biography and carry out everyday life activities. *Health* obviously is not the absence of disease in this framework; neither is the focus on curing the illness but rather on managing and living with the illness to achieve the desired quality of life. *Environment* is identified as the home as the center of care, with health care facilities seen as backup resources. The goal of *nursing* is to help the persons "shape the illness course while . . . maintaining quality of life" (p. 20). The focus of nursing care will be to prevent illness and, when illness does occur, to manage chronic conditions properly with appropriate attention to biographical and everyday living activity needs. Clients are individuals, families, communities, and society. Nursing activities include direct care, "teaching, counseling, making referrals, making arrangements, and monitoring" (p. 21). It is important to assist both individuals and families with the transitions between environments, such as home to hospital to home again.

Since the Chronic Illness Trajectory Nursing Model was developed through qualitative research using the grounded theory methodology, it is based in research. Since much of that research occurred in practice settings, it is also based in practice. The framework has been used in research studies, both by nurses and other professionals, in many countries and with many chronic illnesses. Examples include the following:

Australia:
     Traumatic injury: Halcomb, 2005

Brazil:
     Elderly: Vargas and Gonçalves, 2000

Canada:
     Children: La Salle, 1997; Steele, 2000
     Chronic fatigue syndrome: Edgar Brotherston,[*] 1996
     HIV: Gurevich,[**] 1996
     Knowledge building: Burke, 1999
     Parent's perceptions of trajectories: Burke, Kauffmann, LaSalle, Harrison, and Wong, 2000

United Kingdom:
     Stroke rehabilitation: Burton, 2000
     Use in practice: Nolan and Nolan, 1995

Germany:
     Chronic pain: Kessler-Berther, 2003

United States:
     Adherence: Granger, Moser, Harrell, Sandelowski, and Ekman, 2007
     Adult learning: Massoni,[***] 2000
     Chronically ill elderly: Robinson et al., 1993
     Congestive heart failure: Barber, 1999
     Elderly post-surgical cancer patients: Hughes, Hodgson, Muller, Robinson and McCorkle, 2000; Robinson, Nuamah, Cooley, and McCorkle, 1997
     HIV/AIDS: Nokes, 1998; Ross, 1995
     Home parenteral nutrition: Fitzgerald, 2004
     Intensive care: Limerick, 2007
     Mental illness: Holub,[**] 1996
     Multiple sclerosis: Miller, 1993
     Outcomes measurement tool: Cherry, 1997
     Post stroke: Vanhook, 2007
     Theory analysis: Cooley, 1999

[*]social work
[**]clinical psychology
[***]education

NURSING AS CARING

Anne Boykin and Savina O. Schoenhofer

Anne Boykin (b. 1944) received her bachelor of science in nursing from Alverno College, Milwaukee, Wisconsin, in 1966; M.S. in adult nursing from Emory University, Atlanta, Georgia, in 1972; and Ph.D. in higher education administration with a nursing emphasis from Vanderbilt University, Nashville, Tennessee, in 1981. She has practiced nursing in acute care as well as community settings. She has held faculty positions at Clemson University, Clemson, South Carolina; Valdosta State College, Valdosta, Georgia; Marquette University, Milwaukee, Wisconsin; and Florida Atlantic University, Boca Raton. She is professor and dean of the Christine E. Lynn College of Nursing, Florida Atlantic University, and has served as president of the International Association for Human Caring. She is active in numerous professional associations, including the National League for Nursing, the American Association of Colleges of Nursing, and the Southern Council on Collegiate Education. Her publications are in the areas of caring in nursing education and practice and nursing as a discipline. Her awards include Woman of Distinction Lifetime Achievement Award from Soroptimist International of Boca Raton/Deerfield Beach, Florida, in 2003; election as a Distinguished Practitioner by the National Academies of Practice in 2004; and a Lifetime Achievement Award in Nursing from *Nursing Spectrum/Nurseweek* in 2005.

Savina O. Schoenhofer (b. 1940) holds a B.A. in psychology, a B.S. in nursing, an M.Ed. in guidance and counseling, and a master's degree in nursing from Wichita State University, Wichita, Kansas, and a Ph.D. in higher education administration from Kansas State University, Manhattan. She has practiced nursing in community mental health and migrant health care. She has held faculty and administrative positions at Wichita State University, Florida Atlantic University, and the University of Mississippi, Jackson. She is professor of graduate nursing at the Cora S. Balmat School of Nursing, Alcorn State University, Natchez, Mississippi. She has published in the areas of nursing home management, advanced practice, nursing values, caring, and touch in nursing in critical care settings.

NURSING AS CARING THEORY   Boykin and Schoenhofer (1993) propose a grand theory of nursing as caring. They argue that an overarching grand nursing theory offers an organizing perspective for the selection of middle-range theories to "create a coherent conceptual pattern for nursing practice" (Boykin, Schoenhofer, Baldwin, & McCarthy, 2005, p. 16). Major influences in the development of the theory are Mayeroff's (1971) generic discussion of caring and Roach's (1984, 1987, 1992) discussions of caring person and caring in nursing. Roach's view of caring as process, rather than Mayeroff's view of caring as end, is incorporated in the theory of nursing as caring. Caring is a process of daily becoming, not a goal to be attained (Beckerman, Boykin, Folden, & Winland-Brown, 1994). Parker (1993) describes this theory as one that is personal rather than abstract and advises that one must know oneself as caring person to live the theory. She also points out that the theory of nursing as caring focuses on living caring rather than on achieving an end product and may be used alone or with other theories.

Gaut (1993) identifies the process of theory development used by Boykin and Schoenhofer as that of intension as described by Kaplan (1964). She characterizes such knowledge growth as being comparable to the gradual illumination of a room that occurs as people with lights enter a dark room. The first to enter perceive in general what is in the room. As additional people bring more light, details become clearer and clearer. Knowledge developed by intension begins with general awareness of the whole and progresses to more and more in-depth identification and awareness of the specifics. Boykin and Schoenhofer (1993) write that work on their theory of nursing as caring began in 1983 as they worked together in curriculum development (a general view) and progressed over time to an identification of a level of detail that led them to the label of a general theory of nursing.

Supporting Structures and Assumptions. Mayeroff's (1971) caring ingredients are drawn on in the theory of nursing as caring. Boykin and Schoenhofer (1993) state that "when we have gone outside the discipline [of nursing] to extend possibilities for understanding, we have made an effort to go beyond application, to think through the nursing relevance of ideas that seemed, on the surface to be useful" (p. xiv). Boykin and Schoenhofer summarize Mayeroff's caring ingredients as follows (page numbers within the quotation refer to Mayeroff's work):

Knowing—Explicitly and implicitly, knowing that and knowing how, knowing directly and knowing indirectly (p. 14).

Alternating rhythm—Moving back and forth between a narrower and a wider framework, between action and reflection (p. 15).

Patience—Not a passive waiting but participating with the other, giving fully of ourselves (p. 17).

Honesty—Positive concept that implies openness, genuineness, and seeing truly (p. 18).

Trust—Trusting the other to grow in his or her own time and own way (p. 20).

Humility—Ready and willing to learn more about other and self and what caring involves (p. 23).

Hope—"An expression of the plenitude of the present, alive with a sense of a possible" (p. 26).

Courage—Taking risks, going into the unknown, trusting (p. 27). (pp. xiv–xv, italics added)

Boykin and Schoenhofer present two major perspectives for the theory of nursing as caring. Their perspectives are a perception of persons as caring and a conception of nursing as discipline and profession.

Perception of Persons as Caring. The basic premise of nursing as caring is that *all persons are caring* (Boykin & Schoenhofer, 1993, p. 3). Seven major assumptions underlie the theory, as follows:

- Persons are caring by virtue of their humanness
- Persons are caring, moment to moment
- Persons are whole or complete in the moment
- Personhood is a process of living grounded in caring
- Personhood is enhanced through participating in nurturing relationships with caring others
- Nursing is both a discipline and a profession (Boykin & Schoenhofer, 1993, p. 3)
- Persons are viewed as already complete and continuously growing in completeness, fully caring and unfolding caring possibilities moment-to-moment (p. 21)

Fundamental assumptions are person-as-person, person-as-whole in the moment, and person-as-caring (Boykin & Schoenhofer, 2000). The capacity for caring grows throughout one's life. Although the human is innately caring, not every human act is caring. Knowing oneself as caring person leads to a continuing commitment to know self and other as caring. This in turn leads to a moral obligation, the quality of which is a "measure of being 'in place' in the world" (Boykin & Schoenhofer, 1993, p. 7). The ways in which one expresses caring are continually developing. The more opportunities one exercises fully to know oneself as caring, the easier it becomes to allow oneself (and others) the space and time to further develop caring. This enhances the awareness of self and consciousness that caring is lived moment to moment and directs one's "oughts." The emerging question becomes "How ought I act as caring person?" (p. 7). The degree of authentic awareness of self as caring person influences how one is with others. It requires the courage to let go of the present to discover new meaning about self and other.

Personhood, a process of living grounded in caring, recognizes the possibilities for caring in every moment and is enhanced through caring relationships with others. Caring is living in the context of relational responsibilities—responsibilities for self and other. The heart of the caring relationship is the importance of person-as-person (Boykin & Schoenhofer, 1993).

Drawing on Pribram's (1971) discussion of the uniqueness of a hologram as being that any part of a broken hologram is capable of reconstructing the total image, Boykin and Schoenhofer (1993) speak of the necessity to view the person as a whole. The person as a whole is a significant value that communicates respect for all that person is at the moment. Using the holographic perspective, it is recognized that any aspect or dimension of the person reflects the whole. Viewing the person as a whole, as caring and complete, is intentional and does not provide for dividing the other into parts or segments, such as mind, body, or spirit, at any time. The person, both self and other, is at all times whole. Unless the person is encountered as a whole, there is only a failed encounter. The person can be fully known only as a whole.

To understand the person as caring, one needs to focus on valuing, to celebrate the wholeness of humans, to view humans as both living and growing in caring, and to actively seek engagement on a personal level with others. The caring perspective of humans is basic to a view of nursing as an undertaking that focuses on humans, provides service from person to person, exists because of a social need, and is a human science (Boykin & Schoenhofer, 1993).

Conception of Nursing as a Discipline and Profession.   The theory of nursing as caring is derived from a belief that nursing is both a discipline and a profession. The discipline of nursing originates in the unique social call to which nursing is a response and involves being, knowing, living, and valuing all at once. As a discipline, nursing is a unity of science, art, and ethic. Discipline relates to all aspects of the development of nursing knowledge.

The profession of nursing is based on understanding the social need from which the call for nursing originates and the body of knowledge that is used in creating the response known as nursing. Professions are based in everyday human experiences and responses to one another. Boykin and Schoenhofer (1993) discuss the relationship between the nurse and the nursed as a social contract that involves recognition that a basic need is present in conjunction with the availability of the knowledge and skill required to meet that need. The social call is for a group in society to make a commitment to acquire and use this knowledge and skill for the good of everyone. They also believe that nursing is in transition from social contract relationships to covenantal relationships. In contrast to the impersonal, legalistic emphasis in a social contract, the covenantal relationship emphasizes personal commitment and an always present freedom to choose commitments. The covenantal relationship leads to knowledge that each of us is related to all others as well as to the universe and that caring relationships lead to harmony. While discipline develops knowledge, as a profession nursing uses that knowledge to respond to specific human needs.

General Theory of Nursing as Caring.   The focus of nursing is *"nurturing persons living caring and growing in caring"* (Boykin & Schoenhofer, 1993, p. 21). Nursing is the response to the unique human need to be recognized as, and supported in being, a caring person. The nurse must know the person as a caring person and take those nursing actions that seek to nurture the person in living and growing in caring.

The focus of nurturing persons living, caring, and growing in caring is broad in statement but specific to the individual situation in practice. As the nurse seeks to know the nursed who is living and growing in caring, the individual's unique ways of living caring become known. Although it is easy to identify instances of noncaring, it is the nurse's commitment to discover the unique caring individual. For example, the nurse connects with the hope that underlies despair, hopelessness, fear, and anger and recognizes these emotions as personal expressions of the caring value. The nurse enters the world of the nursed with the intention and commitment to know the other as a caring person. It is in knowing the other in this way that calls for nursing are heard (Boykin & Schoenhofer, 1993). Knowing *how* the other is living caring and expressing aspirations for growing in caring is as important as knowing the other as a caring person. "The call for nursing is a call for acknowledgment and affirmation of the person living caring in specific ways in this immediate situation" (p. 24). The nursing response to this call is a caring nurturance evidenced by specific caring responses to sustain and enhance the nursed in living caring and growing in caring in the immediate situation. Boykin and Schoenhofer liken this being in relationship to a dance of caring persons (see Figure 24-1). The circle represents relating with respect for and valuing of the other in the basic dance to know self and other as caring persons. Each dancer in the circle makes a contribution and moves within the dance as the nursing situation evolves. There is always room for more in the circle, and dancers may move in or out as the nursed calls for services. While dancers may or may not connect by holding hands, eye-to-eye contact facilitates knowing other as caring.

The *nursing situation* is defined by Boykin and Schoenhofer (1993) as "a *shared lived experience in which the caring between nurse and nursed enhances personhood*" (p. 24). The nursing situation is the context in which nursing exists. It is through the study of the nursing situation that the content and structure of nursing knowledge is known. The nursing situation is composed whenever a nurse engages in a situation from a nursing focus. It is the intention with which the situation is approached and caring is expressed that creates the nursing situation and demonstrates nursing as caring. "As an expression of nursing, *caring is the intentional and authentic presence of the nurse with another who is recognized as person living caring and growing in caring. Here, the nurse endeavors to come to know the other as caring person and seeks to understand how that person might be supported, sustained, and strengthened in their* [sic] *unique process of living caring and growing in caring*" (p. 25).

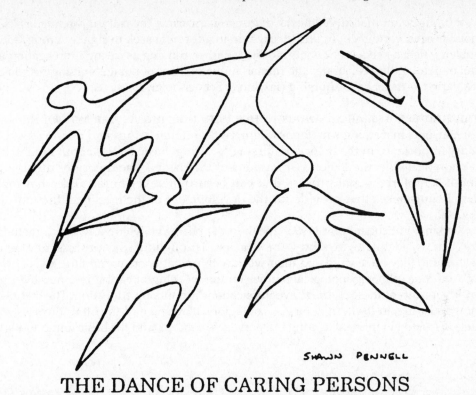

SHAWN PENNELL

THE DANCE OF CARING PERSONS

FIGURE 24-1   The dance of caring persons. (*From Boykin, A., & Schoenhofer, S. (1993). Nursing as caring: A model for transforming practice. New York: National League for Nursing Press.) (Used with permission from Anne Boykin, Florida Atlantic University.)*

The call for nursing comes from persons who are living caring and aspiring to grow in caring. The call is for nurturance through personal expressions of caring. The nurse responds to the call of caring person, not to a lack of caring or to noncaring. The nurse brings to this response a deliberately developed, or expert, knowledge of what it means to be human and to be caring; the nurse has made a commitment to recognize and nurture caring in all situations. The nurse risks entering the other's world, comes to know how the other is living caring in the moment, discovers unfolding possibilities for growing in caring, and thus transforms the general knowledge brought to the situation through an understanding of the uniqueness of the specific situation.

Every nursing situation is original and differs from all others because each is a lived experience that involves two individuals who do not have duplicates. The nature of this lived experience is one of reciprocity, with personal investment from both the nurse and the nursed. Knowing self and other as caring, which is the crux of the nursing situation, involves a constant and mutual unfolding to discover the living of caring in the moment and the possibilities. For the nurse to enter the world of another, the other must allow such entrance. It is only through openness and willingness from both the nurse and the nursed that true presence in the situation occurs. Boykin and Schoenhofer (1993) identify the phenomenon that develops through the encountering of the nurse and the nursed as *caring between*. When caring between occurs, personhood is nurtured.

It is important that in the theory of nursing as caring, the call for nursing is based on neither need nor deficit. In this theory nursing does not seek to right a wrong, solve a problem, meet a need, or alleviate a deficit. Rather, nursing as caring is an egalitarian model of helping that celebrates the human in the fullness of being. Nursing responses are as varied as the calls for nursing (Boykin & Schoenhofer, 1993).

METAPARADIGM, RESEARCH, AND PRACTICE WITH NURSING AS CARING   Of the four major concepts in nursing's metaparadigm, two—human beings and nursing—are of primary importance in the theory of nursing as caring. Basic beliefs about human beings are reflected in the major assumptions of the theory. The theory of nursing as caring is an interpersonal process that can occur wherever nurse and other meet under circumstances that provide for the development of the nursing situation. See Table 24-2.

Boykin and Schoenhofer (1993) speak to the need to develop a research methodology that is adequate to study this theory. Throughout the process of theory development, they have validated their work with practitioners of nursing. Beck (1994) reports on three phenomenological studies on the meaning of caring in a nursing program. The results of these studies have implications for nursing education. The theory of nursing as caring, in itself, may be less contagious than some of the other theories and models discussed in this text. Caring is a pervasive concept, and the basic foundations of

TABLE 24-2   Nursing as Caring and Nursing's Metaparadigm

Metaparadigm Concept	Nursing as Caring definition
Nursing	*Nursing* involves the nurse knowing self as a caring person and coming to know the other as caring. Each expresses unique ways of living and growing in caring. The other expresses a call for caring to which the nurse attends. Nursing includes creating caring responses that nurture personhood and exists when the nurse actualizes personal and professional commitment to the belief that all persons are caring. Not all that a nurse does may express nursing. Any interpersonal experience has potential to become a nursing situation. The nursing situation occurs when the nurse presents self as offering the professional service of nursing and the other presents self as seeking, wanting, and/or accepting such professional service.
Person	*Human beings* are persons who are caring from moment to moment and are whole and complete in the moment and enhanced through their participation in nurturing relationships with caring others. All persons are caring, although not all actions are caring.
Health	Not defined as part of the theory—assumed to be defined by each individual.
Environment	Not defined as part of the theory—environmental aspects are important to the extent they influence the expression of caring.

nursing as caring are often included in discussions that do not reference Boykin and Schoenhofer but may reference those works upon which they drew. Some examples of use of the work of Boykin and Schoenhofer follow.

Boykin and Schoenhofer (1991, 1993) believe that the telling of stories of nursing situations makes evident the service of nursing. Anderson (1998) supports storytelling for the practice of genetics nurses as practitioners of holistic nursing. The three reasons given include that holistic practice assumes the patient is known as a whole person, that the goal in genetics of informed decision making is based on the assumption that people make the best decisions for themselves when they can integrate their values and beliefs with new knowledge, and that considering the context of being human and living a life provides a different orientation for genetics nurses in relation to the predictive value of the genetics information to be obtained. In a similar vein, Herrington (2002) investigated the meaning of caring from the perspective of homeless women who described caring as a way of being, of being authentic, of helping others to grow, and of allowing interconnectedness and enhancement to the meaning of life.

Bulfin (2005) discusses the transformations in patient care and in staff relationships when nursing as caring was the basis for the implementation of a nursing model in a community hospital. Other such transformations are described in Boykin et al. (2005); Boykin, Bulfin, Baldwin, and Southern (2004); and Boykin, Schoenhofer, Smith, St. Jean, and Aleman (2003). Boykin and Schoenhofer (2001) and Boykin et al. (2005) also speak to the vital role played by nurse administrators in creating caring environments. Dunphy and Winland-Brown (1998) applied the transformative model to advanced practice nursing. Thomas, Finch, Schoenhofer, and Green (2004) investigated caring in the practice of nurse practitioners and found that spirituality was a significant component and that caring enhanced the personhood of the nurse practitioners and of the nursed.

Use of nursing as caring in education is discussed in Fletcher and Coffman's (1999) description of a baccalaureate nursing course on case management. The framework for this course was nursing as caring with a focus on case managers coming to know their clients and creating a climate for growth and change. Woodward (2000) speaks to the need for the incorporation of caring in the education of nurse midwives in the United Kingdom as a result of her comparative study of palliative care nurses and nurse midwives. The palliative care nurses were described as responsive to the person of the other; the nurse midwives delivered care that was routine, oriented to tasks, and at times not responsive to the needs of the clients. Drumm (2006) describes the student's experience of learning caring as having the two major themes of innate knowing of self as caring and caring in the curriculum.

In Sweden, Hansebo and Kihlgren's (2000) study of nursing home caregivers telling of patient life stories supported nursing as caring. Included in their findings was that the life stories can act as a mediator between the patient and the caregiver in the nursing situation, and thus create a lived experience. In the United States, Touhy, Strews, and Brown (2005) found, in their project in a unit in a skilled nursing care facility to create a model of nursing care grounded in caring, that caring led to attention to the "little things" and resulted in patients and families sharing stories that reflected feeling more respected and cared about.

A strength of nursing as caring is the focus on caring, rather than problem solving, in the practice of nursing. The emphasis on the importance and strength of the client as caring provides a focus that has often been ignored or forgotten and that has been described as not being valued by the environment in which health care is delivered, in spite of the apparent value to the client.

Locsin (1998) presents a case for technologic competence as caring in nursing. She argues that it is not the knowledge of technology held by the nurse that should be important; it is the use of this knowledge in authentic presence that should take precedence. Also, competence may be described as performance or viewed as a state of being and thus a characteristic of the practitioner. This latter meaning allows for a description of competence that is distinctive to nursing as caring. Schoenhofer and Boykin (1998) support that competent participation in the use of life-sustaining technologies is an expression of caring. In the same vein, Purnell (1998) argues that nursing is being challenged to care meaningfully for the whole person in an environment that does not support this value. She points out that the expression of a personal commitment to caring by a nurse includes a commitment to caring for self. It is the mutuality of need that provides for authentic nursing technology in which harmony is promoted.

Another strength rests in the description of nursing as caring as a general theory and the encouragement to use the theory in conjunction with other theories. The novice nurse particularly may find more direction and support for the knowledge that is needed in the nursing situation when combining nursing as caring with another nursing theory, particularly with a more specific middle range theory.

A limitation may be found in the qualitative nature of the theory and its approach to nursing practice. While the discussion of nursing as a discipline and a profession identifies the importance of the knowledge the nurse brings to the nursing situation, the theory itself does not provide any structure as to what that knowledge might be. Those who need structure and guidance for their nursing actions may be uncomfortable with the lack of specific structure within this theory. It does not provide an answer to the question, What am I supposed to do next?

COMFORT THEORY AND PRACTICE

Katharine Kolcaba

Katharine Kolcaba (b. 1944) earned a diploma in nursing from St. Luke's Hospital School of Nursing, Cleveland, Ohio, in 1965; a master's degree in nursing from Case Western Reserve University, Cleveland, in 1987; and a Ph.D. in nursing from Case Western Reserve University in 1997. She holds American Nurses Association certification in gerontology and has received numerous awards and honors. These include the Marie Haug Student Award for Excellence in Aging Studies from Case Western Reserve University in 1997, Links2Go Resource Award in 1999 for the Comfort Line website, the Mary Hanna Memorial Journalism Award from the American Academy of Perianesthesia Nurses in 2003, the Advancement of Science Award from the Midwest Nursing Research Society in 2003, and the Harford Institute and American Association of Colleges of Nursing 3rd Annual Award for Excellence in Baccalaureate Gerontology Curriculum.

Dr. Kolcaba is an associate professor at the University of Akron, Ohio, where she teaches an undergraduate course titled Nursing Care of Older Adults and graduate courses in research, theory, professional roles, and domains of nursing knowledge. Her areas of expertise include gerontology, end-of-life and long-term care interventions, comfort studies, instrument development, nursing theory, nursing research, and magnet status (http://www.thecomfortline.com).

The Comfort Line is Dr. Kolcaba's website, which provides information and resources about her theory of comfort. It also documents current research and provides personal information and photographs.

COMFORT THEORY   Kolcaba (2004) reminds us that Nightingale recognized that comfort was essential for patients. Nightingale stated, "It must never be lost sight of what observation is for. It is not for the sake of piling up miscellaneous information or curious facts, but for the sake of saving life and increasing health and comfort" (1859, p. 70). Kolcaba points out that Nightingale implies that the relationship between health and comfort is dependent.

Kolcaba (2004) goes on to discuss the concept of comfort in the 20th-century context of nursing practice. She cites Aiken (1908) and Harmer (1928), both of whom speak to the provision of patient comfort as a nursing role. Goodnow (1935) devoted a chapter of her nursing text to patient comfort. Prior to the advent of effective analgesic medications, comfort measures were treatment oriented (massage, heat, compresses, and so on). While the provision of physical comfort is prominent in the literature, the psychosocial-spiritual realm is recognized in the expectation that the nurse "comforts" or provides "comforting" to patients. An overview of the major concepts and definitions in Kolcaba's comfort theory can be found in Table 24-3.

Concept Analysis—Types of Comfort.   A concept analysis of comfort resulted in the development of three types of comfort: relief, ease, and transcendence (originally termed *renewal*; Kolcaba & Kolcaba, 1991). "*Relief* . . . [is] defined . . . as the experience of a patient who has had a specific comfort need met. *Ease* . . . [is] defined as a state of calm or contentment. . . . *Transcendence* . . . [is] defined as a state in which one rises above problems or pain" (Kolcaba, 2003, p. 9).

Contexts of the Human Experience of Comfort.   The first context of the human experience of comfort identified by Kolcaba is *physical comfort*. She states that this is the most obvious and most agreed upon context of comfort. Kolcaba synthesized Hamilton's (1989) findings about comfort and those of later authors into a definition of physical comfort as "pertaining to bodily sensations and homeostatic mechanisms that may or may not be related to specific diagnoses" (2003, p. 12).

The second context that Kolcaba identifies is *psychospiritualcomfort*. This context is defined as "whatever gives life meaning for an individual and entails self esteem, self-concept, sexuality, and one's relationship to a higher order or being" (2003, p. 12). The definition is synthesized from the works of Hamilton (1989), Howarth (1982), Labun (1988), and Reed (1987).

The third context of human experience is *environmental comfort*. This context is defined as "pertaining to external surroundings, conditions, and influences" (Kolcaba, 2003, p. 13). This definition is synthesized from the works of Levine (1967), Fuller (1978), and Wolanin and Phillips (1981). Included in this definition are color, noise, light, ambience, temperature, views from windows, access to nature, and natural versus synthetic elements (Kolcaba, 1991).

The fourth context is *sociocultural comfort*. Kolcaba defines this as "pertaining to interpersonal, family, and societal relationships including finances, education and support" (2003, p. 14). The idea of culture includes family histories, traditions, language, clothes, and customs.

TABLE 24-3   Overview of Comfort Theory Definitions

Concepts	Definitions
Comfort	The immediate experience of being strengthened by having needs for relief, ease, and transcendence addressed in the four contexts (physical, psychospiritual, sociocultural, and environmental). Comfort is much more than the absence of pain and discomfort.
Comfort care	A philosophy of health care that addresses physical, psychospiritual, sociocultural, and environmental comfort needs of patients. Comfort care has three components: 1. an appropriate and timely intervention; 2. a mode of delivery that projects caring and empathy; 3. the intent to comfort.
Comfort measures	Interventions designed to enhance patient/family comfort.
Comfort needs	Patients' or families' desire for or deficit in relief/ease/transcendence in physical, psychospiritual, sociocultural, and environmental contexts of human experience.
Health-seeking behaviors (HSB)	Behaviors in which patients or families engage consciously or subconsciously, moving them toward well-being. HSBs can be internal, external, or dying peacefully.
Institutional integrity	The quality or state of health care organizations as complete, whole, sound, upright, professional, and ethical providers of health care.
Intervening variables	Positive or negative factors over which nurses or institutions have little control, but that affect the direction and success of comfort care plans or comfort studies.

From Kolcaba, K. (2004). Comfort. In S. J. Peterson & T. S. Bredow (Eds.), *Middle range theories: Application to nursing research* (p. 255). Philadelphia: Lippincott, Williams, & Wilkins. Used with permission

The Taxonomy.   Kolcaba juxtaposes the three types of comfort with the four contexts of human experience, which results in the 12-cell grid in Figure 24-2 (1991). From this structure as well as literature reviews, Kolcaba formulated a definition of holistic comfort: *Comfort is the immediate experience of being strengthened by having needs for relief, ease, and transcendence met in four contexts* (Kolcaba, 1992). She reminds the reader that comfort is an essential outcome for health care, that it is both holistic and complex, and that the aspects of comfort are interrelated. Kolcaba goes on to say that the goal of health care is to enhance comfort when compared to some previous baseline. Comfort care can be quantified by pre- and post-intervention comfort scores.

The Theory of Comfort.   The assumptions that a theorist makes are the beginning point or base of a theory. Kolcaba's (1994) theoretical assumptions are the following:

1. Human beings have holistic responses to complex stimuli.
2. Comfort is a desirable holistic outcome that is germane to the discipline of nursing.

	Relief	Ease	Transcendence
Physical			
Psychospiritual			
Environmental			
Sociocultural			

FIGURE 24-2 Taxonomic structure of comfort. *(From Kolcaba, K. (2004). The theory of comfort. In S. J. Peterson, & T. S. Brednow (Eds.),* Middle range theories: Application to nursing research *(pp. 259). Philadelphia: Lippincott, Williams and Wilkins. Used with permission.)*

3. Human beings strive to meet, or to have met, their basic comfort needs. It is an active endeavor.
4. Comfort is more than the absence of pain, anxiety, and other discomfort.

Kolcaba (2003) describes her theory as being a mid-range theory, a theory meant to be easily grasped and applied. She states that the theory is normative, describing what nurses and other health team members *should* do, and descriptive, what nurses and other health care team members *actually* do if they subscribe to the theory. The theory of comfort also states that patients who are comfortable are more likely to engage in health-seeking behaviors (HSBs), which determine their level of wellness or peacefulness of death. Comfort theory can be applied to individuals, families, or communities in any setting. Propositions for the first part of theory include the following:

1. Nurses identify patients' comfort needs that have not been met by existing support systems.
2. Nurses design interventions to address those needs.
3. Intervening variables are taken into consideration in designing the interventions and in determining whether they will be successful.
4. If the intervention is appropriate and delivered in a caring manner, the patient experiences the immediate outcome of enhanced comfort. Comfort care entails an appropriate intervention delivered in a caring manner, with the goal of enhanced comfort. (p. 82)

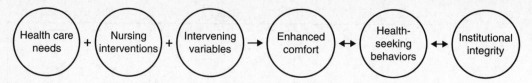

FIGURE 24-3   Conceptual framework- theory of comfort. *(Modified from Kolcaba, K. (2007) Conceptual framework for comfort theory. Retrieved December 7, 2007 from www.thecomfortline.com. Used with permission.)*

Propositions for the second part of theory include the following:

5. Patients and nurses agree upon desirable and realistic HSBs.
6. If enhanced comfort is achieved, patients are strengthened to engage in HSBs that further enhance comfort. (p. 82)

Kolcaba's theory of comfort is depicted in Figure 24-3.

Comfort Care and Comfort Measures.   Kolcaba (2003) details three types of comfort measures that she hopes all nurses will employ whether or not they subscribe to her theory. *Technical comfort measures* are those nursing interventions that maintain homeostasis and manage pain. These measures include the administration of medications and monitoring of physiological functioning. *Coaching* includes interventions that relieve anxiety, provide reassurance and information, instill hope, listen, and help the patient plan realistically for the expected future. *Comfort food for the soul* refers to nursing interventions that are unexpected but appreciated by patients. Suggestions for these types of interventions include massage, environmental adaptations, guided imagery, music therapy, therapeutic touch, and presence.

General Comfort Questionnaire.   Flowing from the taxonomic structure of the comfort care theory, Kolcaba developed the General Comfort Questionnaire (GCQ), which she refined throughout her doctoral study. This questionnaire is a 48-item instrument with a 5-point Likert scale response ranging from strongly disagree to strongly agree. The instrument, as well as directions for adapting it to specific populations, is available in her 2003 publication and on the Comfort Line website. Kolcaba herself modified the GCQ for use with breast cancer patients for her dissertation research, a result of which was the Radiation Therapy Comfort Questionnaire (RTCQ) (1998, 2003).

Adaptations of the General Comfort Scale include the Visual Analog Scales (VAS), Urinary Incontinence and Frequency Comfort Questionnaire (UIFCQ), and the Hospice Comfort Questionnaire (HCQ): Family and Patient (Kolcaba, 2004). In order to assess the comfort of patients who cannot use questionnaires, the Comfort Behavior Checklist (CBC) was developed. The nurse rates the patient's comfort based on 30 observable behaviors. The questionnaires may be downloaded in a choice of formats from http://www .thecomfortline.com

METAPARADIGM, RESEARCH, AND PRACTICE WITH THE COMFORT THEORY   Both Kolcaba's website and her text (2003, p. 68) provide her definitions of the metaparadigm concepts. These are shown in Table 24-4.

While this theory is fairly new, it can be applied to individuals, families, and communities in any setting. The concepts are clear and easy to define. Nurses are "comfortable" with the idea of comfort being an integral part of nursing care. These aspects all promote the use of this mid-range theory by nurses in clinical practice.

TABLE 24-4   Theory of Comfort and Nursing's Metaparadigm

Metaparadigm Concept	Theory of Comfort Definition
Nursing	*Nursing:* the intentional assessment of comfort needs of patients, families, or communities; design of comfort measures to address comfort needs, including reassessment of comfort level after implementation of comfort measures, compared to a previous baseline.
Person	*Patient:* an individual, family, or community in need of health care, including primary, tertiary, or preventive care.
Health	*Health:* optimum function of a patient/family/community facilitated by the enhanced comfort.
Environment	*Environment:* aspects of patient/family/community surroundings that affect comfort and can be manipulated to enhance comfort.

The nursing literature documents several studies that have used comfort theory as a guiding framework:

- Nurse midwifery (Schuiling & Sampselle, 1999)
- Labor and delivery (Koehn, 2000)
- Cardiac catheterization (Hogan-Miller, Rustad, Sendelbach, & Goldenberg, 1995)
- Critical care (Jenny & Logan, 1996; Kolcaba & Fisher, 1996)
- Hospice (Schoerner & Krysa, 1996)
- Radiation therapy (Cox, 1998; Kolcaba & Fox, 1999)
- Oncology patients (Bortolusso, Boscolo, & Zampieron, 2007)
- Orthopedic nursing (Panno, Kolcaba, & Holder, 2000; Santy, 2001)
- Perioperative nursing (Wilson & Kolcaba, 2004)
- Hospitalized elderly (Robinson & Benton, 2002)
- Urinary incontinence (Dowd, Kolcaba, & Steiner, 2000, 2002, 2003)
- Emergency nursing (Hawley, 2000)
- Post-surgical areas (McCaffrey & Good, 2000)
- Postpartum (Collins, McCoy, Sale, & Weber, 1994)
- Pain control (Taylor, 1992)

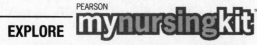

EXPLORE   PEARSON   **mynursingkit**™

MyNursingKit is your one stop for online chapter review materials and resources. Prepare for success with additional NCLEX®-style practice questions, interactive assignments and activities, web links, animations and videos, and more!

Register your access code from the front of your book at
www.mynursingkit.com.

References for Corbin and Strauss

Bainton, D. F. (1995). Nomination for Distinguished UCSF Professor Emeritus Award. Retrieved April 2, 2008, from http://www.ucsf.edu/anselmstrauss/pdf/award-emeritus.pdf.

Barber, M. L. (1999). Community-focused nurse case management by telephone for patients with congestive heart failure. *Masters Abstracts International, 37*(06), 1814. Abstract retrieved December 6, 2007, from Dissertation Abstracts Online database.

Burke, S. O. (1999). Trajectories and transferability: Building nursing knowledge about chronicity. *Canadian Journal of Nursing Research, 30*, 243–247.

Burke, S. O., Kauffmann, E., LaSalle, J., Harrison, M. B., & Wong, C. (2000). Parent's [sic] perceptions of chronic illness trajectories. *Canadian Journal of Nursing Research, 32*(3), 19–36.

Burton, C. R. (2000). Re-thinking stroke rehabilitation: The Corbin and Strauss chronic illness trajectory framework. *Journal of Advanced Nursing, 32*, 595–602.

Cherry, J. C. (1997). Testing of the Corbin and Cherry Evaluation Tool for Chronic Illness Management. *Masters Abstracts International, 36*(03), 0780. Abstract retrieved December 6, 2007, from Dissertation Abstracts Online database.

Cooley, M. E. (1999). Analysis and evaluation of the trajectory theory of chronic illness management. *Scholarly Inquiry for Nursing Practice, 13*(2), 75–95, 97–103, 105–109.

Corbin, J. M. (1981). Protective governing: Strategies for managing a pregnancy-illness. *Dissertation Abstracts International, 43*(02B), 0382. Abstract retrieved April 2, 2008, from Dissertation Abstracts Online database.

Corbin, J. M. (1998). The Corbin and Strauss Chronic Illness Trajectory Model: An update. *Scholarly Inquiry for Nursing Practice, 12*, 33–41.

Corbin, J. M. (2001). Introduction and overview: Chronic illness and nursing. In R. B. Hyman & J. M. Corbin (Eds.), *Chronic illness: Research and theory for nursing practice*. New York: Springer.

Corbin, J., & Strauss, A. L. (1984). Collaboration: Couples working together to manage chronic illness. *Image, 16*, 109–115.

Corbin, J. M., & Strauss, A. L. (1985a). Issues concerning regimen management in the home. *Aging and Society, 5*, 249–265.

Corbin, J., & Strauss, A. L. (1985b). Managing chronic illness at home: Three lines of work. *Qualitative Sociology, 8*, 224–247.

Corbin, J., & Strauss, A. L. (1987). Accompaniment of chronic illness: Changes in body, self, biography, and biographic time. *Research in the Sociology of Health Care, 6*, 249–281.

Corbin, J., & Strauss, A. L. (1988). *Unending work and care: Managing chronic illness at home.* San Francisco: Jossey-Bass. [Translated into German in 1991 by Weiter-Leben Lernen. *Chronisch Kranke in der Familie.* München: Piper Verlag]

Corbin, J., & Strauss, A. L. (1990). Making arrangements: The key to home care. In J. Gubrium & A. Sanker (Eds.), *The home care experience: Ethnography and policy* (pp. 59–73). Newbury Park, CA: Sage.

Corbin, J., & Strauss, A. L. (1991). Comeback: The process of overcoming disability. *Advances in Medical Sociology, 2*, 137–159.

Corbin, J. M., & Strauss, A. (1992). A nursing model for chronic illness management based upon the trajectory framework. In P. Woog (Ed.), *The Chronic Illness Trajectory Framework: The Corbin and Strauss nursing model* (pp. 9–28). New York: Springer.

Curriculum Vitae, Anselm L. Strauss (2003). Retrieved April 2, 2008, from www.ucsf.edu/anselmstrauss/cv.html.

Edgar Brotherston, N. F. (1996). Adolescence and myalgic encephalomyelitis/chronic fatigue syndrome: Journeys with the dragon. *Masters Abstracts International, 35*(06), 1666. Abstract retrieved December 6, 2007, from Dissertation Abstracts Online database.

Fagerhaugh, S., & Strauss, A. (1977). *The politics of pain management.* Menlo Park, CA: Addison-Wesley.

Fitzgerald, K. A. (2004). The psychological and social impact of home parenteral nutrition. *Dissertation Abstracts International, 65*(03B), 1246. Abstract retrieved December 6, 2007, from Dissertation Abstracts Online database.

Granger, B. B., Moser, D., Harrell, J., Sandelowski, M., & Ekman, I. (2007). A practical use of theory to study adherence. *Progress in Cardiovascular Nursing, 22*(3), 152–158.

Gurevich, M. (1996). Identity renegotiation in HIV-positive women. *Dissertation Abstracts International, 58*(07B), 3967. Abstract retrieved December 6, 2007, from Dissertation Abstracts Online database.

Halcomb, E. (2005). Using the Illness Trajectory Framework to describe recovery from traumatic injury. *Contemporary Nurse: A Journal for the Australian Nursing Profession, 19*(1–2), 232–241.

Holub, E. A. (1996). Family experience in the caring for a seriously mentally ill family member: A qualitative study. *Dissertation Abstracts International, 57*(02B), 1443. Abstract retrieved December 6, 2007, from Dissertation Abstracts Online database.

Hughes, L. C., Hodgson, N. A., Muller, P., Robinson, L. A., & McCorkle, R. (2000). Information needs of elderly postsurgical cancer patients during the transition from hospital to home. *Journal of Nursing Scholarship, 32*(1), 25–30.

Hyman, R. B., & Corbin, J. M. (Eds.). (2001). *Chronic illness: Research and theory for nursing practice.* New York: Springer.

Kessler-Berther, G. (2003). Up and down—The experience of women suffering from the rheumatic disease fibromyalgia [German]. *Pflege, 16*(4), 184–191. Abstract in English retrieved June 6, 2007, from CINAHL Plus with Full Text database.

La Salle, J. M. (1997). Developmental reactions to repeated hospitalizations within life-threatening and chronic illness trajectory frameworks. *Masters Abstracts International, 36*(02), 0511. Abstract retrieved December 6, 2007, from Dissertation Abstracts Online database.

Limerick, M. H. (2007). The process used by surrogate decision makers to withhold and withdraw life-sustaining measures in an intensive care environment. *Oncology Nursing Forum, 34*, 331–339.

Massoni, M. (2000). A case study of a health-related Internet discussion group as a venue for adult learning. *Dissertation Abstracts International, 61*(04A), 1255. Abstract retrieved December 6, 2007, from Dissertation Abstracts Online database.

Meetoo, D. D. (2007). *Interview with Juliet M. Corbin.* Retrieved April 2, 2008, from http://www.journalofadvancednursing.com/docs/JulietCorbinInterview.pdf.

Miller, C. M. (1993). Trajectory and empowerment theory applied to care of patients with multiple sclerosis. *Journal of Neuroscience Nursing, 25*(6), 343–348.

Nokes, K. M. (1998). Revisiting how the Chronic Illness Trajectory Framework can be applied for persons living with HIV/AIDS. *Scholarly Inquiry for Nursing Practice, 12*(1), 27–31.

Nolan, M., & Nolan, J. (1995). Responding to the challenge of chronic illness. *British Journal of Nursing, 4*(3), 145–147.

Robinson, L. A., Bevil, C., Arcangelo, V., Reifsnyder, J., Rothman, N., & Smeltzer, S. (1993). Operationalizing the Corbin & Strauss Trajectory Model for elderly clients with chronic illness. *Scholarly Inquiry for Nursing Practice, 7*(4), 253–268.

Robinson, L., Nuamah, I. F., Cooley, M. E., & McCorkle, R. (1997). A test of the fit between the Corbin and Strauss Trajectory Model and care provided to older patients after cancer surgery. *Holistic Nursing Practice, 12*(1), 36–47.

Ross, T. L. (1995). The lived experience of hope in young mothers with human immunodeficiency virus infection: A phenomenological inquiry. *Dissertation Abstracts International, 56*(07B), 3696. Abstract retrieved December 6, 2007, from Dissertation Abstracts Online database.

Steele, R. G. (2000). Trajectory of certain death at an unknown time: Children with neurodegenerative life-threatening illnesses. *Canadian Journal of Nursing Research, 32*(3), 49–67.

Strauss, A. L. (1973). Chronic illness. *Trans-action, 10*(6), 33–39.

Strauss, A. L. (1985). *Research on chronic illness and its management* (The Fifth Helen Nahm Research Lecture, University of California, San Francisco, June 7, 1985). Retrieved April 3, 2008, from http://www.ucsf.edu/anselmstrauss/pdf/award-nahm1985.pdf.

Strauss, A. L., & Corbin, J. M. (1988). *Unending work and care: Managing chronic illness at home.* New York: Wiley.

Strauss, A., Fagerhaugh, S., Suzeck, B., & Weiner, C. (1981). Patients' work in the technologized hospital . . . illness is more than passive suffering. *Nursing Outlook, 29*, 404–412.

Strauss, A., Fagerhaugh, S., Suzeck, B., & Weiner, C. (1985). *The social organization of medical work.* Chicago: University of Chicago Press.

Strauss, A. L., & Glaser, B. (1975). *Chronic illness and the quality of life.* St. Louis: Mosby.

Vanhook, P. M. (2007). Comeback of Appalachian female stroke survivors: The interrelationships of cognition, function, self-concept, and interpersonal and social relationship. *Dissertation Abstracts International, 68*(06B), 3697. Abstract retrieved April 2, 2008, from Dissertation Abstracts Online database.

Vargas, D. R. M., & Gonçalves, L. H. T. (2000). Corbin and Strauss's trajectory reference framework of chronic conditions in a situation of caring for aged people [Portuguese]. *Texto & Contexto Enfermagem, 9,* 251–263. Abstract in English retrieved June 6, 2007, from CINAHL Plus with Full Text database.

Woog, P. (Ed.). (1992). *The Chronic Illness Trajectory Framework: The Corbin and Strauss Nursing Model.* New York: Springer.

Bibliography for Corbin and Strauss

Corbin, J. (2008). Is caring a lost art in nursing? *International Journal of Nursing Studies, 45*(2), 163–165.

Corbin, J., & Strauss, A. (1988). Carers: Working together. *Nursing Times, 84*(15), 48–49.

Corbin, J., & Strauss, A. (1988). Ted and Alice . . . families are the major care-givers of the chronically ill. *Nursing Times, 84*(14), 32–33.

Corbin, J., & Strauss, A. (1990). Grounded theory research: Procedures, canons, and evaluative criteria. *Qualitative Sociology, 13*(1), 3–21.

Corbin, J., & Strauss, A. (1990). Grounded theory research: Procedures, canons, and evaluative criteria. *Zeitschrift fur Soziologie, 19,* 418–427.

Corbin, J., & Strauss, A. L. (1993). The articulation of work through interaction. *The Sociological Quarterly, 34,* 71–83.

Corbin, J. M., & Strauss, A. L. (1996). Analytic ordering for theoretical purposes. *Qualitative Inquiry, 2*(2), 139–150.

Corbin, J. M., & Strauss, A. L. (2008). *Basics of qualitative research: Techniques and procedures for developing grounded theory* (3rd ed.). Thousand Oaks, CA: Sage.

Strauss, A. L., & Corbin, J. M. (1988). *Shaping a new health care system: The explosion of chronic illness as a catalyst for change.* New York: Wiley.

Strauss, A. L., & Corbin, J. (1990). *Basics of qualitative research: Grounded theory procedures and techniques.* Newbury Park, CA: Sage. [Translated into Korean, 1995; German, 1996; Chinese, 1997]

Strauss, A. L., & Corbin, J. (1994). Grounded theory methodology: An overview. In N. K. Denzin & Y. S. Lincoln (Eds.), *Handbook of qualitative research* (pp. 273–285). Newbury Park, CA: Sage.

Strauss, A. L., & Corbin, J. (Eds.). (1997). *Grounded theory in practice.* Thousand Oaks, CA: Sage

Strauss, A. L., & Corbin, J. M. (2005). *Basics of qualitative research: Techniques and procedures for developing grounded theory* (2nd ed.). Thousand Oaks, CA: Sage.

Swanson, J. M., & Corbin, J. (1983). The contraceptive context: A model for increasing nursing's involvement in family health. *Maternal-Child Nursing Journal, 12*(3), 169–183.

References for Boykin and Schoenhofer

Anderson, G. (1998). Storytelling: A holistic foundation for genetic nursing. *Holistic Nursing Practice, 12*(3), 64–76

Beck, C. T. (1994). Researching experiences of living caring. In A. Boykin (Ed.), *Living a caring-based program* (pp. 93–126) (Pub. No. 14–2536). New York: National League for Nursing Press.

Beckerman, A., Boykin, A., Folden, S., & Winland-Brown, J. (1994). The experience of being a student in a caring-based program. In A. Boykin

(Ed.), *Living a caring-based program* (pp. 79–92) (Pub. No. 14-2536). New York: National League for Nursing Press.

Boykin, A., Bulfin, S., Baldwin, J., & Southern, S. (2004). Transforming care in the emergency department. *Topics in Emergency Medicine, 26,* 331–336.

Boykin, A., & Schoenhofer, S. (1991). Story as link between nursing practice, ontology, epistemology. *Image: Journal of Nursing Scholarship, 23,* 245–248.

Boykin, A., & Schoenhofer, S. (1993). *Nursing as caring: A model for transforming practice* (Pub. No. 15-2549). New York: National League for Nursing Press. [re-released 2001, Sudbury, MA: Jones & Bartlett]

Boykin, A., & Schoenhofer, S. (2000). Invest in yourself. *Nursing Forum, 35*(4), 36–38.

Boykin, A., & Schoenhofer, S. (2001). The role of nursing leadership in creating caring environments in health care delivery systems. *Nursing Administration Quarterly, 25,* 1–7.

Boykin, A., Schoenhofer, S. O., Baldwin, J., & McCarthy, D. (2005). Living caring in practice: The transformative power of the theory of nursing as caring. *International Journal for Human Caring, 9*(3), 15–19.

Boykin, A., Schoenhofer, S. O., Smith, N., St. Jean, J., & Aleman, D. (2003). Transforming practice using a caring-based nursing model. *Nursing Administration Quarterly, 27,* 223–230.

Bulfin, S. (2005). Nursing as caring theory: Living caring in practice. *Nursing Science Quarterly, 18,* 313–319.

Drumm, J. T. (2006). The student's experience of learning caring in a college of nursing grounded in a caring philosophy. *Dissertation Abstracts International, 67*(06B), 3059. Abstract retrieved December 6, 2007, from Dissertation Abstracts Online database.

Dunphy, L. M., & Winland-Brown, J. E. (1998). The Circle of Caring: A transformative model of advanced practice nursing. *Clinical Excellence for Nursing Practitioners, 2,* 241–247.

Fletcher, I. L., & Coffman, S. (1999). Case management in the nursing curriculum. *Journal of Nursing Education, 38,* 371–377.

Gaut, D. A. (1993). Introduction. In A. Boykin & S. Schoenhofer (Eds.), *Nursing as caring: A model for transforming practice* (pp. xvii–xxix) (Pub. No. 15-2549). New York: National League for Nursing Press.

Hanesbro, G., & Kihlgren, M. (2000). Patient life stories and current situation as told by carers in nursing home wards. *Clinical Nursing Research, 9,* 260–279.

Herrington, C. L. (2002). The meaning of caring: From the perspective of homeless women. *Masters Abstracts International, 41*(01), 191. Abstract retrieved December 6, 2007, from Dissertation Abstracts Online database.

Kaplan, A. (1964). *The conduct of inquiry.* San Francisco: Chandler Publishing.

Locsin, R. C. (1998). Technologic competence as caring in critical care nursing. *Holistic Nursing Practice, 12*(4), 50–56.

Mayeroff, M. (1971). *On caring.* New York: Harper & Row.

Parker, M. (1993). Foreword. In A. Boykin & S. Schoenhofer (Eds.), *Nursing as caring: A model for transforming practice* (pp. ix–xii) (Pub. No. 14-2549). New York: National League for Nursing Press.

Pribham, K. H. (1971). *Languages of the brain: Experimental paradoxes and principles in neuropsychology.* Upper Saddle River, NJ: Prentice Hall.

Purnell, M. J. (1998). Who really makes the bed? Uncovering technologic dissonance in nursing. *Holistic Nursing Practice, 12*(4), 12–22.

Roach, S. (1984). *Caring: The human mode of being, implications for nursing.* Toronto: Faculty of Nursing, University of Toronto.

Roach, S. (1987). *The human act of caring.* Ottawa: Canadian Hospital Association.

Roach, S. (1992). *The human act of caring (Rev. ed.).* Ottawa: Canadian Hospital Association.

Schoenhofer, S. O., & Boykin, A. (1998). Discovering the value of nursing in high-technology environments: Outcomes revisited. *Holistic Nursing Practice, 12*(4), 31–39.

Thomas, J. D., Finch, L. P., Schoenhofer, S. O., & Green, A. (2004). The caring relationships created by nurse practitioners and the ones nursed: Implications for practice. *Topics in Advanced Practice Nursing e-Journal, 4*(4).

Touhy, T. A., Strews, W., & Brown, C. (2005). Expressions of caring as lived by nursing home staff, residents, and families. *International Journal for Human Caring, 9*(3), 31–37.

Woodward, V. (2000). Caring for women: The potential contribution of formal theory to midwifery practice. *Midwifery, 16*(1), 68–75.

References for Kolcaba

Aiken, C. (1908). Making the patient comfortable. *Canadian Nurse and Hospital Review, 4*, 422–424.

Bortolusso, V., Boscolo, A., & Zampieron, A. (2007). Survey about the comfort livel [*sic*] according to Kolcaba on a sample of oncologic patients [Italian]. *Professioni Infermieristiche, 60*(3), 166–169. Abstract retrieved November 30, 2009, from CINAHL Plus with Full Text database.

Collins, B. A., McCoy, S. A., Sale, S., & Weber, S. E. (1994). Descriptions of comfort by substance-abusing and nonusing postpartum women. *Journal of Obstetric, Gynecologic and Neonatal Nursing, 23*, 293–300.

Cox, J. (1998). Assessing patient comfort in radiation therapy. *Radiation Therapist, 5*(2), 119–125.

Dowd, T., Kolcaba, K., & Steiner, R. (2000). Using cognitive strategies to enhance bladder control and comfort. *Holistic Nursing Practice, 14*(2), 91–102.

Dowd, T., Kolcaba, K., & Steiner, R. (2002). Correlations among six measures of bladder function. *Journal of Nursing Measurement, 10*(1), 27–38.

Dowd, T., Kolcaba, K., & Steiner, R. (2003). The addition of coaching to cognitive strategies. *Journal of Ostomy and Wound Management, 30*(2), 90–99.

Fuller, S. (1978). Holistic man and the science of nursing. *Nursing Outlook, 26*, 700–704.

Goodnow, M. (1935). *The technic of nursing.* Philadelphia: Saunders.

Hamilton, J. (1989). Comfort and the hospitalized chronically ill. *Journal of Gerontological Nursing, 15*(4), 28–33.

Harmer, B. (1928). *Text-book of the principles and practice of nursing.* New York: Macmillan.

Hawley, M. P. (2000). Nurse comforting strategies: Perceptions of emergency department patients. *Clinical Nursing Research, 9*, 441–459.

Hogan-Miller, E., Rustad, D., Sendelbach, S., & Goldenberg, I. (1995). Effects of three methods of femoral site immobilization on bleeding and comfort after coronary angiogram. *American Journal of Critical Care, 4*(2), 143–148.

Howarth, F. 1982). A holistic view of middle management. *Nursing Outlook, 30*, 522–552.

Jenny, J., & Logan, J. (1996). Caring and comfort metaphors used by patients in critical care.

Image: The Journal of Nursing Scholarship, 28, 349–352.

Koehn, M. (2000). Alternative and complementary therapies for labor and birth: An application of Kolcaba's theory of holistic comfort. *Holistic Nursing Practice, 15*(1), 66–77.

Kolcaba, K. (1991). A taxonomic structure for the concept comfort: Synthesis and application. *Image: Journal of Nursing Scholarship, 23*, 237–240.

Kolcaba, K. (1992). Holistic comfort: Operationalizing the construct as a nurse-sensitive outcome. *Advances in Nursing Science, 15*(1), 1–10.

Kolcaba, K. (1994). A theory of comfort for nursing. *Journal of Advanced Nursing, 19*, 1178–1184.

Kolcaba, K. (1998). The effects of guided imagery on comfort in women with breast cancer choosing conservative therapy. *Dissertation Abstracts International, 58*(07), 3558. Abstract retrieved December 5, 2007, from Dissertation Abstracts Online database.

Kolcaba, K. (2003). *Comfort theory and practice: A vision for holistic health and research.* New York: Springer.

Kolcaba, K. (2004). The theory of comfort. In S. J. Peterson & T. S. Brednow (Eds.), *Middle range theories: Application to nursing research* (pp. 255–273). Philadelphia: Lippincott Williams & Wilkins.

Kolcaba, K., & Fisher, E. (1996). A holistic perspective on comfort care as an advance directive. *Critical Care Quarterly, 18*(4), 66–76.

Kolcaba, K., & Fox, C. (1999). The effects of guided imagery on comfort of women with early-stage breast cancer going through radiation therapy. *Oncology Nursing Forum, 26*(1), 67–71.

Kolcaba, K., & Kolcaba, R. (1991). An analysis of the concept of comfort. *Journal of Advanced Nursing, 16*, 1301–1310.

Labun, E. (1988). Spiritual care: An element in nursing care planning. *Journal of Advanced Nursing, 13*, 314–320.

Levine, M. (1967). The four conservation principles of nursing. *Nursing Forum, 6*, 45–49.

McCaffrey, R. G., & Good, M. (2000). The lived experience of listening to music while recovering from surgery. *Journal of Holistic Nursing, 18*, 378–390.

Nightingale, F. (1859). *Notes on nursing.* London: Harrison.

Panno, J., Kolcaba, K., & Holder, C. (2000). Acute Care for Elders (ACE): A holistic model for geriatric nursing. *Orthopaedic Nursing, 19*(6), 53–60.

Reed, P. (1987). Spirituality and well-being in terminally ill hospitalized adults. *Research in Nursing and Health, 10,* 335–344.

Robinson, S., & Benton, G. (2002). Warmed blankets: An intervention to promote comfort for elderly hospitalized patients. *Geriatric Nursing, 23,* 320–323.

Santy, J. (2001). An investigation of the reality of nursing work with orthopaedic patients. *Journal of Orthopaedic Nursing, 5*(1), 22–29.

Schoerner, C., & Krysa, L. (1996). The comfort and discomfort of infertility. *Journal of Obstetrical, Gynecological, and Neonatal Nurses, 25*(2), 167–172.

Schuilling, K., & Sampselle, C. (1999). Comfort in labor and midwifery art. *Image: The Journal of Nursing Scholarship, 31*(1), 77–81.

Taylor, B. (1992) Relieving pain through ordinariness in nursing: A phenomenological account of a comforting nurse-patient relationship. *Advances in Nursing Science, 15*(1), 33–43.

Wilson, L., & Kolcaba, L. (2004) Practical application of comfort theory in the perianesthesia setting, *Journal of Perianesthesia Nursing, 19*(3), 164–173.

Wolanin, M., & Phillips, L. (1981). *Confusion: Prevention and care.* St. Louis: Mosby.

Bibliography for Kolcaba

Dowd, T. (2006). Katharine Kolcaba: Theory of comfort. In A. Tomey & M. Alligood (Eds.), *Nursing theorists and their work* (6th ed., pp. 726–742). St. Louis: Mosby Elsevier

Dowd, T., Kolcaba, K., Steiner, R., & Fashinpaur, D. (2007). Comparison of a healing touch, coaching, and a combined intervention on comfort and stress in younger college students. *Holistic Nursing Practice, 21*(4), 194–202.

Fox, C., & Kolcaba, K. (1996). Decision making in unsafe practice situations. *Revolution: The Journal of Nurse Empowerment,* Spring, 68–69.

Kinion, E., & Kolcaba, K. (1992). Plato's model of psyche. *Journal of Holistic Nursing, 10,* 218–230.

Kolcaba, K. (1987). Reaching optimum function us realistic goal for elderly (Letter to the Editor). *Journal of Gerontological Nursing, 13*(12), 36.

Kolcaba, K. (1988). A framework for the nursing care of demented patients. *Mainlines, 9*(6), 12–13.

Kolcaba, K. (1992). The concept of comfort in an environmental framework. *Journal of Gerontological Nursing, 18*(6), 33–38.

Kolcaba, K. (1995). The process and product of comfort care, merged in holistic nursing art. *Journal of Holistic Nursing, 13*(2) 117–131.

Kolcaba, K. (1995). The art of comfort care. *Image: The Journal of Nursing Scholarship, 27,* 293–295.

Kolcaba, K. (1998). Comfort. In J. Fitzpatrick (Ed.), *The encyclopedia of nursing research* (pp. 102–104). New York: Springer.

Kolcaba, K. (2001). Evolution of the mid range theory of comfort for outcomes research. *Nursing Outlook, 49*(2), 86–92.

Kolcaba, K. (2006). Comfort theory: A unifying framework to enhance the practice environment. *Journal of Nursing Administration, 36,* 538–544.

Kolcaba, K., & DiMarco, M. A. (2005). Comfort theory and its application to pediatric nursing. *Pediatric Nursing, 31*(3), 187–194.

Kolcaba, K., & Dowd, T. (2000) Kegel exercises: Strengthening the weak pelvic floor muscles that cause urinary incontinence. *American Journal of Nursing, 100*(11), 59.

Kolcaba, K., Dowd, T., & Steiner, R. (2006) Development of an instrument to measure holistic client comfort as an outcomes of healing touch. *Holistic Nursing Practice, 20*(3), 122–129.

Kolcaba, K., Dowd, T., Steiver, R., & Mitzel, A. (2004). Efficacy of hand massage for enhancing comfort of hospice patients. *Journal of Hospice and Palliative Care, 6*(2), 91–101.

Kolcaba, K., & Kolcaba, R. (1994) Health maintenance as a responsibility for self. *Philosophy in the Contemporary World, 1*(2), 266–269.

Kolcaba, K., & Kolcaba R. (2003). Fiduciary decision-making using comfort care. *Philosophy in the Contemporary World, 101*(1), 81–86.

Kolcaba, K., & Miller, C. (1989). Geropharmacology: A nursing intervention. *Journal of Gerontological Nursing, 15*(5), 29–35.

Kolcaba, K., Schirm, V., & Steiner, R. (2006). Effects of hand massage on comfort of nursing home residents. *Geriatric Nursing, 27*(2), 85–91.

Kolcaba, K., & Steiner, R. (2000). Empirical evidence for the nature of holistic comfort. *Journal of Holistic Nursing, 18*(1), 46–62.

Kolcaba, K., & Wilson, L. (2002). Comfort care: A framework for perianesthesia nursing. *Journal of PeriAnesthesia Nursing, 17*(2), 102–114.

Kolcaba, K., & Wykle, M. (1994). Health promotion in long-term care facilities. *Geriatric Nursing, 15,* 266–269.

Kolcaba, K., & Wykle, M. (1997). Comfort research: Spreading comfort around the world. *Reflections, 23*(2), 12–13.

Kolcaba, R. (1997). The primary holisms in nursing. *Journal of Advanced Nursing, 25,* 290–296.

McIlveen, K. H., & Morse, J. M. (1995). The role of comfort in nursing care: 1900–1980. *Clinical Nursing Research, 4,* 127–148.

Morse, J. M. (1992). Comfort: The refocusing of nursing care. *Clinical Nursing Research, 1*(1), 91–106.

Novak, B., Kolcaba, K., Steiner, R., & Dowd, T. (2001). Measuring comfort in caregivers and patients during end of life care. *American Journal of Hospice and Palliative Care, 13*(3), 170–180.

Palmer, R., Landefeld, S., Kresevic, D., & Kowal, J. (1994). A medical unit for the acute care of the elderly. *Journal of the American Geriatrics Society, 42,* 545–552.

Schirm, V., Baumgardner, J., Dowd, T., Gregor, S., & Kolcaba, K. (2004). Development of a healthy bladder education program for older adults. *Geriatric Nursing, 25,* 301–306.

Van Dijk, M., de Boer, J. B., Koot, H. M., Tibboel, D., Passchier, J., & Duivenvoorden, H. J. (2000). The reliability and validity of the COMFORT scale as a postoperative pain instrument in 0 to 3-year old infants. *Pain (84),* 367–377.

Vendlinski, S., & Kolcaba, K. (1997). Comfort care: A framework for hospice nursing. *American Journal of Hospice and Palliative Care, 14,* 271–276.

Wagner, D., Bryne, M., & Kolcaba, K. (2006). Effects of comfort warming on preoperative patients. *AORN Journal, 84,* 427–430.

GLOSSARY*

Abstract concept. An image of something neither observable nor measurable.

Achievement subsystem. (Johnson) The behavioral subsystem relating to behaviors that attempt to control the environment and lead to personal accomplishment.

Adaptation. (Levine) Process of adjusting or modifying behavior or functioning to fit the situation and to achieve conservation; life process by which people maintain wholeness.

Adaptation. (Mishel) All of the person's behaviors (biological, psychological, social) as they occur within that person's usual range of behavior.

Adaptation. (Roy) Process and outcome of the use, by thinking and feeling people as individuals and groups, of conscious awareness and choice to create human and environmental integration.

Adaptation level. (Roy) Internal pooling of stimuli with three levels:

Integrated processes are working as a whole to meet human system needs.

Compensatory processes occur when response systems have been activated.

Compromised processes occur when the integrated and compensatory processes are not providing for adaptation.

Adaptive potential. (Erickson, Tomlin, and Swain) The person's ability to mobilize resources to cope with stressors.

Adaptive responses. (Roy) Behaviors that positively affect health through promotion of the integrity of the person in terms of survival, growth, reproduction, mastery, and transformation of the system and environment.

Affiliated-individuation. (Erickson, Tomlin, and Swain) The individual's simultaneous needs to be attached to others and separate from them.

Agency. (Benner) The ability to influence the situation.

Agent. (Wiedenbach) The practicing nurse, or the nurse's delegate, who serves as the propelling force in goal-directed behavior.

Aggressive subsystem. (Johnson) The behavioral subsystem that relates to behaviors concerned with protection and self-preservation.

Animate environment. (Barnard) Social aspects of the situation.

Arousal. (Erickson, Tomlin, and Swain) A stress state in which the person needs assistance to mobilize resources.

Assessment of behaviors. (Roy) Behavioral assessment; the gathering of output behaviors of the person in relation to the four adaptive modes.

Assessment of stimuli. (Roy) The collection of data about focal, contextual, and residual stimuli impinging on the person.

Assumption. Statement or view that is widely accepted as true.

Assumption. (Wiedenbach) The meaning a nurse attaches to an interpretation of a sensory impression.

Assumptions, expectations, and set. (Benner) Beliefs generated from past experiences that influence the nurse's view and understanding of the current situation.

Attachment or affiliative subsystem. (Johnson) The behavioral subsystem that is the first formed and provides for a strong social bond.

Authentic commitment. (Paterson and Zderad) The nurse is actively present with

---

*When a term relates specifically to a theorist, the name of the theorist appears in parentheses after the term.

the whole of the nurse's being, both personally and professionally.

Authority.   (King) An active, reciprocal relationship that involves values, experience, and perceptions in defining, validating, and accepting the right of an individual to act within an organization.

Automatic actions.   (Orlando) Nursing actions decided on for reasons other than the patient's immediate need.

Authentic commitment.   (Paterson and Zderad) The nurse being actively present with the whole of the nurse's being.

Background meaning.   (Benner) Culturally acquired meanings, accumulated from birth, that influence one's perceptions.

Basic conditioning factors.   (Orem) Aspects that influence the individual's self-care ability; include age, gender, stage of development, state of health, sociocultural orientation, health care system and family system factors, patterns of living, environment, and availability and adequacy of resources.

Being and doing.   (Paterson and Zderad) The interrelationship of existence and action.

Body image.   (King) Individuals' perceptions of their own bodies, influenced by the reactions of others.

Call and response.   (Paterson and Zderad) Simultaneous, sequential transactions, both verbal and nonverbal and possibly all-at-once.

Care.   (Hall) The exclusive aspect of nursing that provides the patient bodily comfort through "laying on of hands" and provides an opportunity for closeness.

Care.   (Leininger) (noun) Phenomena related to assistive, supportive, or enabling behavior toward or for another individual (or group) with evident or anticipated needs to ameliorate or improve a human condition or lifeway.

Care.   (Leininger) (gerund) Action directed toward assisting or helping another individual (or group) toward healing and wellbeing.

Caring.   (Benner) An essential skill of nurses; a basic way of being in the world.

Caring.   (Boykin and Schoenhofer) Intentional and authentic presence recognizing the other as living and growing in caring.

Caring occasion/moment.   (Watson) The coming together of a nurse and another in human-to-human transaction.

Central purpose.   (Wiedenbach) The commitment of the individual nurse, based on a personal philosophy, that defines the desired quality of health and specifies the nurse's special responsibility in providing care to assist others in achieving or sustaining that quality.

Choice point.   (Newman) Degree of disorganization indicating change is needed.

Chronic illness.   (Corbin and Strauss) Any condition (physical or mental) that requires monitoring or management for symptom control and to shape the course of the disease for longer than six months.

Clinical forethought.   (Benner) The ability to anticipate likely events and create a plan of action in order to prevent problems.

Clinical judgment.   (Benner) The ability to recognize important aspects of a situation and act appropriately.

Clinical knowledge.   (Benner) Practical knowledge that includes qualitative distinctions; common meanings; assumptions, expectations, and sets; paradigm cases and personal knowledge; maxims; and unplanned practices.

Clinical reasoning.   (Benner) The process of understanding a patient's condition at a particular time, based upon observed changes.

Clinical transitions.   (Benner) Detection of subtle or not-so-subtle changes that require reconsideration of patient needs.

Cocreating.   (Parse) Participation of humanuniverse in creating pattern.

Cognator mechanism. (Roy) Coping mechanism or control subsystem that relates to the higher brain functions of perception, information processing, learning, judgment, and emotion.

Cognitive schema. (Mishel) One's interpretation of illness-related events; by its nature, this interpretation is subjective.

Comfort. (Kolcaba) The immediate sense of being strengthened by feeling relief from having a specific need met, experiencing a state of calm or contentment (ease), and rising above problems or pain (transcendence) in the four contexts of physical, psychospiritual, environmental, and sociocultural human experience.

Communication. (King) A direct or indirect process in which one person gives information to another.

Community. (Paterson and Zderad) Two or more persons striving together, living–dying all-at-once.

Concept. An abstract notion; a vehicle of thought that involves images; words that describe objects, properties, or events.

Connecting–separating. (Parse) The rhythmical process of moving together and moving apart.

Consciousness. (Newman) The information of the system; the system's capacity to interact with the environment.

Conservation. (Levine) Defense of the wholeness of a living system through the most economical use of resources; ensures ability to confront change appropriately and retain unique identity.

Conservation of energy. (Levine) Balancing energy output with energy input to avoid excessive fatigue.

Conservation of personal integrity. (Levine) Maintaining or restoring the patient's sense of identity and self-worth.

Conservation of social integrity. (Levine) Acknowledging the patient as a social being.

Conservation of structural integrity. (Levine) Maintaining or restoring the structure of the body.

Contextual stimuli. (Roy) Stimuli of the human system's internal or external world, other than those immediately confronting the system, that influence the situation and are observable, measurable, or subjectively reported by the system as having a positive or negative effect.

Coping. (Barnard) The ability to respond to novel or stressful situations.

Core. (Hall) The aspect of client interaction shared with any health professional who therapeutically uses a freely offered closeness to help the patient discover who he or she is.

Core. (Neuman) The basic structure and energy resources of the system.

Covert problem. Hidden or concealed condition of concern.

Critical thinking. A disciplined intellectual process of applying knowledge, experience, abilities, and attitudes to guide actions and beliefs.

Cultural imposition. (Leininger) Efforts of an outsider, subtle and not so subtle, to impose his or her own cultural values, beliefs, or behaviors upon an individual, family, or group from another culture.

Culture. (Leininger) Learned, shared, and transmitted values, beliefs, norms, and lifeway practices of a particular group that guide thinking, decisions, and actions in patterned ways.

Culture values. (Leininger) Values that are derived from the culture, identify desirable ways of acting or knowing, guide decision making, are often held over long periods, and have a powerful influence on behavior.

Culture care. (Leininger) Assistive, supportive, or facilitative caring acts (toward self or others) that are culturally constituted and focus on needs, either evident or anticipated, for health and well-being or to face disabilities, death, or other human conditions.

Culture care accommodation/negotiation. (Leininger) Creative professional actions and decisions that assist, accommodate, facilitate, or enable clients of a particular culture to adapt to, or negotiate for, safe, effective, and culturally congruent care for health and well being or to deal with illness or dying.

Culture care diversity. (Leininger) The variability or differences of culture care meanings, patterns, values, lifeways, symbols, or other features of care that relate to the provision of beneficial care in a designated culture.

Culture care preservation/maintenance. (Leininger) Professional actions and decisions that assist, support, facilitate, or enable clients of a particular culture to keep, preserve, or maintain helpful care beliefs or to face handicaps and death.

Culture care repatterning/restructuring. (Leininger) Professional actions or decisions that assist, support, facilitate, or enable clients change, reorder, modify, or restructure their lifeways and institutions for new or different patterns that are culturally meaningful and satisfying, or that support beneficial and healthy life patterns, practices, or outcomes.

Culture care universality. (Leininger) Aspects or features of culture care that are commonly shared by human beings or a group; these features have recurrent meanings, patterns, values, lifeways, or symbols and serve as a guide for caregivers to assist, support, facilitate, or enable people toward healthy outcomes.

Culture shock. (Leininger) Experiencing feelings of discomfort, helplessness, disorientation while attempting to comprehend or adapt effectively to a different cultural group.

Cure. (Hall) An aspect of nursing shared with medical personnel in which the nurse helps the patient and family through medical, surgical, and rehabilitative care.

Decision making in organizations. (King) An active process in which choice, directed by goals, is made and acted upon.

Deliberative actions. (Orlando) Nursing actions that ascertain or meet the patient's immediate need.

Dependency subsystem. (Johnson) The behavioral subsystem in which behaviors evoke nurturing behaviors in others.

Disciplined intellectual approach. (Travelbee) Use of logic, reasoning, reflection, and deliberation to validate, analyze, and synthesize information.

Discrepancy. (Johnson) Action that does not achieve the intended goal.

Dominance. (Johnson) Primary use of one behavioral subsystem to the detriment of the other subsystems and regardless of the situation.

Drive. (Johnson) Stimulus to behavior.

Eliminative subsystem. (Johnson) The behavioral subsystem that relates to socially acceptable behaviors surrounding the excretion of waste products from the body.

Embodied knowledge. (Benner) Information "known" by the body that affects habits related to attentiveness, thinking, and acting; a method of reasoning and learning.

Emic. (Leininger) Personal knowledge or explanation of behavior; indigenous, not universal; the insider's view of a culture.

Empirical. Measured or observed through the senses.

Enabling–limiting. (Parse) Making choices results in helping an individual in some ways while restricting in others.

Energy field. (Rogers) The dynamic, infinite, fundamental unit of both the living and nonliving.

Environment. (Neuman) Those forces that surround humans at any given point in time; may be internal, external, or created.

Environment. (Nightingale) External conditions and influences that affect life and development.

Environment. (Rogers) Pan-dimensional, negentropic energy field identified by pattern and integral with the human energy field.

Environment. (Roy) All conditions, circumstances, and influences surrounding and affecting the development and behavior of human systems. Special attention is to be paid to person and earth resources.

Environmental context. (Leininger) The totality of an event, situation, or particular experience that gives meaning to human expressions, including physical, ecological, social interactions, emotional, and cultural dimensions.

Epistemology. The study of the history of knowledge, including the origin, nature, methods, and limitations of knowledge development.

Equilibrium. (Erickson, Tomlin, and Swain) A nonstress state. In adaptive equilibrium all subsystems are in harmony. In maladaptive equilibrium, one or more subsystems are placed in jeopardy to maintain the nonstress state.

Ethnonursing. (Leininger) The in-depth study of multiple cultures and care factors in a rigorous and systematic manner; such study occurs within people's familiar environments and focuses on the interrelationships of care and culture; the goal is identification and provision of culturally congruent care services.

Etic. (Leininger) Knowledge reflected in the professional perspective; may also be considered the stranger's or outsider's view of a culture.

Evidence-based practice. Practice supported by research pertinent to that clinical area.

Existential experience. (Paterson and Zderad). The experience that involves being at the same moment unique and like others (uniqueness-otherness), being in touch with one's self and open to others (authenticity-experiencing), increasing awareness of our own responses and the possibilities called forth by others (moreness-choice), and genuine presence occurring only when presence is valued (value-nonvalue).

Existential psychology. The study of human existence using phenomenological analysis.

Extrapersonal stressors. (Neuman) Forces occurring outside the system that generate a reaction or response from the system.

Flexible line of defense. (Neuman) Variable and constantly changing biological-psychological-sociocultural-developmental and spiritual ability to respond to stressors.

Focal stimulus. (Roy) Stimulus of the human system's internal or external world that immediately confronts the system.

Framework. (Wiedenbach) The human, environmental, professional, and organizational facilities that make up the context in which nursing is practiced and that constitute its currently existing limits.

General system theory. A general science of wholeness.

Generic care system. (Leininger) Traditional or local indigenous health care or cure practices that have special meanings and uses to heal or assist people and are generally offered in familiar home or community environmental contexts with their local practitioners.

Goal. (Wiedenbach) Outcome the nurse seeks to achieve.

Grand theory. Theory that covers broad areas of a discipline; may not be testable.

Growth and development. (King) The process in the lives of individuals that involves changes at the cellular, molecular, and behavioral levels and helps them move from potential to achievement.

Health promotion. (Pender) Behavior that arises from the desire to increase well-being and to achieve one's health potential.

Helicy. (Rogers) The nature and direction of human and environmental change; change that is continuously innovative, unpredictable, and characterized by increasing diversity of the human field and environmental field pattern emerging out of the continuous, mutual, simultaneous interaction between the human and environmental fields and manifesting nonrepeating rhythmicities.

Historicity. (Levine) Aspect of adaptation in which responses are based on past experiences.

Holism. A theory that the universe and especially living nature are correctly seen in terms of interacting wholes that are more than the mere sum of the individual parts.

Human potential. (Paterson and Zderad) All possible responses of a human being, both those that limit and those that help.

Illness. (Levine) State of altered health.

Illness. (Neuman) State of insufficiency in which needs are yet to be satisfied.

Imaging. (Parse) The picturing or making real of events, ideas, and people, explicitly or tacitly.

Impoverishment. (Erickson, Tomlin, and Swain) A stress state in which the person needs external resources, including affliation.

Inanimate environment. (Barnard) The non-social aspects of one's surroundings that can impact the senses, such as space, materials, toys, sounds, richness, or deprivation.

Incompatibility. (Johnson) Two behavioral subsystems in the same situation being in conflict with each other.

Ineffective responses. (Roy) Behaviors that do not promote the integrity of the human system in terms of survival, growth, reproduction, mastery, and transformation of the system and environment.

Ingestive subsystem. (Johnson) The behavioral subsystem that relates to the meanings and structures of social events surrounding the occasions when food is eaten.

Innovator system. (Roy) A group control mechanism that involves change and growth.

Insufficiency. (Johnson) A behavioral subsystem that is not functioning adequately.

Integrality. (Rogers) The continuous, mutual, simultaneous process of human and environmental fields.

Interactions. (King) The observable, goal-directed, behaviors of two or more persons in mutual presence.

Interdependence mode. (Roy) The social context in which relationships occur; involves nurturing, respect, values, context, infrastructure, and resources.

Interpersonal stressors. (Neuman) Forces that occur between two or more individuals and evoke a reaction or response.

Intersubjective transaction. (Paterson and Zderad) The shared situation in which nurturance occurs.

Intrapersonal stressors. (Neuman) Forces occurring within a person that result in a reaction or response.

Languaging. (Parse) Reflection of images and values through speaking and moving.

Lines of resistance. (Neuman) The internal set of factors (biological, psychological, sociocultural, developmental, and spiritual) that seek to stabilize the system when stressors break through the normal line of defense; the defense closest to the core.

Logical empiricism. Worldview in which truth must be confirmed by objective, sensory experiences that are to be relatively value free.

Mastery. (Meleis) The extent to which an individual can use the necessary skills and behaviors to deal with a new situation or environment.

Means. (Wiedenbach) The activities and devices that enable the nurse to attain the desired goal.

Meeting. (Paterson and Zderad) The coming together of human beings characterized by the expectation that there will be a nurse and a nursed and each have some control over what is disclosed.

Metaparadigm. Core context of a discipline, stated globally.

Metatheory. Theory about theory development.

Modeling. (Erickson, Tomlin, and Swain) Process used by the nurse to gain an understanding of the client's world as the client perceives it.

More-being. (Paterson and Zderad) The process of becoming all that is humanly possible within one's life circumstances.

Movement. (Newman) Change that occurs between two states of rest.

Need for help. (Orlando) A requirement for assistance in decreasing or eliminating immediate distress or in improving the sense of adequacy.

Normal line of defense. (Neuman) The biological-psychological-sociocultural-developmental-spiritual skills developed over a lifetime to achieve stability and deal with stressors.

Nurse–patient relationship. (Travelbee) The series of experiences between a nurse and a patient.

Nurse reaction. (Orlando). Portion of the nursing process discipline in which the nurse responds to the patient's behavior through expressing the nurse's perception, thought, or feeling and seeking congruence between these and the patient's immediate need.

Nursing problem. (Abdellah) A condition faced by the client or client's family with which the nurse can assist through the performance of professional functions.

Nursing process. A deliberate, intellectual activity by which the practice of nursing is approached in an orderly, systematic manner. It includes the following components:

Assessment. The process of data collection and analysis that results in a conclusion or nursing diagnosis.

Diagnosis. A behavioral statement that identifies the client's actual or potential health problem, deficit, or concern that can be affected by nursing actions.

Outcomes identification. Establishing the desired results in terms that are culturally appropriate and realistic.

Planning. The determination of what can be done to assist the client, including setting goals, judging priorities, and designing methods to resolve problems.

Implementation. Action initiated to accomplish defined goals.

Evaluation. The appraisal of the client's behavioral changes that result from the action of the nurse.

Nursing situation. (Boykin and Schoenhofer) Shared living experience in which personhood is enhanced through caring between nurse and nursed.

Nursing system. (Orem) Plan of care developed by the nurse to meet the person's self-care deficit:

Partly compensatory nursing system. A situation in which both nurse and patient perform care measures or other actions involving manipulative tasks or ambulation.

Supportive-educative nursing system. A situation in which the patient is able to, or can and should learn to, perform required therapeutic self-care measures but needs assistance to do so.

Wholly compensatory nursing system. A situation in which the patient has no active role in the performance of self-care.

Nurturer. (Hall) A fosterer of learning, growing, and healing.

Ontology. A branch of metaphysics that studies the nature of being and of reality.

Organization. (King) An entity made up of individuals who have prescribed roles and positions and who use resources to achieve goals.

Orientation phase. (Peplau) The first phase of Peplau's nurse–patient relationship. Through assessment, the patient's health needs, expectations, and goals are explored, and a care plan is devised. Concurrently, the roles of nurse and patient are being identified and clarified.

Originating. (Parse) A continuing process of creating personal uniqueness.

Overt problem. Apparent or obvious condition of concern.

Paradigm. (Rogers) A way of viewing the world; a particular perspective of reality.

Pattern. (Newman) Movement, diversity, and rhythm that depict the whole.

Pattern. (Rogers) The distinguishing or identifying characteristic of an energy field.

Perceived view. Worldview that focuses on the person as a whole and values the lived experience of the person.

Perception. (King) An individual's view of reality that gives meaning to personal experience and involves the organization, interpretation, and transformation of information from sensory data and memory.

Phenomenologic dialogue. (Paterson and Zderad) Description involving the what (the nurse's views and responses, the knowable responses of the nursed, and the reciprocal call and response in the nursing situation), the why (knowledge and understanding of the nursing situation), and the how (use of everyday language to describe the nursing situation in a deliberate, disciplined, and nonjudgmental way).

Phenomenologic nursology. (Paterson and Zderad) The five-phase research methodology proposed for humanistic nursing.

Phenomenology. The study of the meaning of phenomena to a particular individual; a way of understanding people from the way things appear to them.

Physiological-physical mode. (Roy) Involves the human system's physical response to and interaction with the environment.

Potential comforter. (Hall) The role of the nurse seen by the patient during the care aspect of nursing.

Potential painer. (Hall) The role of the nurse seen by the patient during the cure aspect of nursing.

Power. (King) A social force and ability to use resources to influence people to achieve goals.

Powering. (Parse) An energizing force the rhythm of which is the pushing–resisting interhuman encounters.

Praxis. Putting theoretical knowledge into practice; doing.

Prescription. (Wiedenbach) A directive for activity that specifies both the nature of the action and the necessary thought process.

Prescriptive theory. (Wiedenbach) A theory that conceptualizes both the desired situation and the activities to be used to bring about the desired situation.

Presence. (Paterson and Zderad) The quality of being open, receptive, ready, and available to another in a reciprocal manner.

Primary prevention. (Neuman) The application of general knowledge in a client situation to try to identify and protect against the potential effects of stressors before they occur.

Problem-solving process. Identifying the problem, selecting pertinent data, formulating hypotheses, testing hypotheses through the collection of data, and revising hypotheses.

Professional nursing action. (Orlando) What the nurse says or does for the benefit of the patient.

Professional nursing care. (Leininger) Professional care or cure services offered by nurses who have been prepared through formal professional programs of study in special educational institutions to provide care that seeks to improve a human health condition, disability, or lifeway, or to work with a dying client.

Proposition. A statement explaining relationships among concepts.

Qualitative research. Dynamic, organized investigations of the thoughts, feelings, and experiences of human beings.

Quantitative research. Systematic studies that involve empirical data analyzed through statistical methods.

Realities in the immediate situation. (Wiedenbach) At any given moment, all factors at play in the situation in which nursing actions occur; realities include the agent, the recipient, the goal, the means, and the framework.

Received view. *See* Logical empiricism.

Recipient. (Wiedenbach) The vulnerable and dependent patient who is characterized by personal attributes, problems, and capabilities, including the ability to cope.

Reconstitution. (Neuman) The increase in energy that occurs in relation to the degree of reaction to a stressor.

Redundancy. (Levine) Aspect of adaptation related to numerous levels of response available for a given challenge.

Reflective technique. (Hall) The process of helping the patient see who he or she is by mirroring what the person's behavior says, both verbally and nonverbally.

Regulation. (Barnard) Child's ability to be self-calming and to evoke desired responses from caregivers.

Regulator mechanism. (Roy) Coping mechanism subsystem that includes chemical, neural, and endocrine transmitters and autonomic and psychomotor responses.

Relating. (Paterson and Zderad) The process of nurse–nursed doing with each other, being with each other.

Residual stimuli. (Roy) Internal or external factors of the human system whose current effects are unclear.

Resonancy. (Rogers) The identification of the human field and the environmental field by wave pattern manifesting continuous change from lower-frequency longer waves to higher-frequency shorter waves.

Resources. (Barnard) What is available to support or hinder the parent–child relationship, including other people and finances.

Revealing–concealing. (Parse) Actions in interpersonal relationships that reveal one part of oneself and, as a result, conceal other parts.

Role. (King) The set of behaviors and rules that relate to an individual in a position in a social system.

Role function mode. (Roy) This mode involves knowing the relationship of the system to others so the system can behave appropriately.

Role-modeling. (Erickson, Tomlin, and Swain) Planning and implementing individualized care based on the client's model of the world to facilitate health.

School of thought. (Parse) A scholarly theoretical point of view.

Secondary prevention. (Neuman) Treatment of symptoms of stress reaction to lead to reconstitution.

Self-care. (Orem) Practice of activities that individuals personally initiate and perform on their own behalf to maintain life, health, and well-being.

Self-care action. (Erickson, Tomlin, and Swain) Use of self-care knowledge and self-care resources.

Self-care agency. (Orem) The human ability to engage in self-care.

Self-care deficit. (Orem) The inability of an individual to carry out all necessary self-care activities; self-care demand exceeds self-care agency.

Self-care knowledge. (Erickson, Tomlin, and Swain) Knowledge about what has made one sick, lessened one's effectiveness, or interfered with one's growth; also includes knowledge of what will make one well, fulfilled, or effective.

Self-care requisites. (Orem) The impetus for self-care activities. Three types follow:

Developmental self-care requisites. Maintaining conditions to support life and development or to provide preventive care for adverse conditions that affect development.

Health deviation self-care requisites. Care needed by individuals who are ill or injured; may result from medical measures required to correct illness or injury.

Universal self-care requisites. Those requisites, common to all human beings throughout life, associated with life processes and the integrity of human structure and function.

Self-care resources. (Erickson, Tomlin, and Swain) An individual's strengths and supports that will help gain, maintain, and promote optimal health.

Self-concept-group identity mode. (Roy) Behaviors related to integrity; involves self-concept, body sensation, body image, self-consistency, self-ideal, moral-ethical-spiritual self, interpersonal relationships, and social milieu.

Sensitivity to cues. (Barnard) The appropriateness of the caregiver's response to cues initiated by the child.

Set. (Johnson) An individual's predisposition to behave in a certain way.

Sexual subsystem. (Johnson) The behavioral subsystem that reflects socially acceptable behaviors related to procreation.

Simultaneity paradigm. (Parse) A view of humans as unitary beings who are in continuous interrelationship with the environment and whose health is a negentropic unfolding determined by the individual.

Space. (King) A universal area, known also as territory, that is defined in part by the behavior of those who occupy it.

Specificity. (Levine) Aspect of adaptation in which responses are task specific and particular challenges lead to particular responses.

Stabilizer subsystem. (Roy) A group control mechanism that involves the structures, values, and daily activities that accomplish the work of the group.

Status. (King) The relationship of an individual to a group or a group to other groups, including identified duties, obligations, and privileges.

Stress. (King) A positive or negative energy response to interactions with the environment in an effort to maintain balance in living.

Stressors. (Neuman) Stimuli that result in tensions and have the potential to create system instability.

Temperament. (Barnard) Child's level of maturity, neurological status, activity, responsiveness to external stimuli, alertness, habituation, and irritability.

Termination phase. (Peplau) The third and final phase of Peplau's nurse–patient relationship. This phase evolves from the successful completion of the previous phases. The patient and nurse terminate their therapeutic relationship as the patient's needs are met and movement is made toward new goals.

Tertiary prevention. (Neuman) Activities that seek to strengthen the lines of resistance after reconstitution has occurred.

Theory. Creative and systematic way of looking at the world or an aspect of it to describe, explain, predict, or control it.

Therapeutic interpersonal relationship. (Peplau) A relationship between patient and nurse in which their collaborative effort is directed toward identifying, exploring, and resolving the patient's need productively. The relationship progresses along a continuum as each experiences growth through an increasing understanding of one another's roles, attitudes, and perceptions.

Therapeutic self-care demand. (Orem) The sum or total of self-actions needed, during some period, to meet self-care requisites.

Therapeutic use of self. (Travelbee) Conscious use of one's personality to seek to establish a relationship and to structure nursing intervention.

Time. (King) The relation of one event to another, uniquely experienced by each individual.

Totality paradigm. (Parse) View of man as a summative being, a combination of bio-psycho-social-spiritual aspects, surrounded by an environment of external and internal stimuli. Man interacts with the environment to maintain equilibrium and achieve goals. Health is a state of well-being measured against norms.

Trajectory. (Corbin and Strauss) The course of an illness over time, including any actions taken by individuals, families, or health professionals to manage or shape that course.

Trajectory projection. (Corbin and Strauss) One's perception or vision of the course of an illness, including the meaning of the illness, what symptoms will be like, how it will affect one's life, and the time frame in which it occurs.

Trajectory scheme. (Corbin and Strauss) One's plan for shaping the course of an illness, controlling immediate symptoms, and handling any disability.

Transactions. (King) Observable behaviors between individuals and their environment that lead to the attainment of valued goals.

Transcultural nursing. (Leininger) The discipline of study and practice in nursing that focuses on culture care differences and similarities among and between cultures in order to help human beings attain and maintain meaningful and therapeutic culturally based health care practices.

Transformation. (Newman) Change occurring all-at-once.

Transforming. (Parse) The changing of change apparent in increasing diversity.

Transition. (Meleis) Moving from one state, condition, or place to another.

Transpersonal caring relationship. (Watson) A relationship that occurs with a caring consciousness in which the life space of another is entered, the other's state of being detected and experienced with a response that provides for the release of the other's feelings, thoughts, or tensions.

Uncertainty. (Mishel) A person's lack of ability to determine the meaning of illness-related events; occurs when the person cannot assign definite values to objects and events or cannot predict outcomes with any accuracy.

Unitary humans. (Rogers) Pandimensional, negentropic energy fields identified by pattern and manifesting characteristics and behaviors different from those of the parts and that cannot be predicted from knowledge of the parts.

Valuing. (Parse) The process of living cherished beliefs while adding to one's worldview.

Veritivity. (Roy) A philosophical assumption related to the richness of being rooted in an absolute truth leading to conviction, commitment, and caring.

Well-being. (Paterson and Zderad) Those aspects of nursing that deal with the quality of personal survival.

Working phase. (Peplau) The second phase of Peplau's nurse–patient relationship. The perceptions and expectations of the patient and nurse become more involved while building a working relationship of further identifying the problem and deciding on appropriate plans for improved health maintenance. The patient takes full advantage of all available services while feeling an integral part of the helping environment. Goals are met through a collaborative effort as the patient becomes independent during convalescence.

Worldview. (Leininger) The way in which people look at the world, or universe, and form a value stance about the world and their lives.

INDEX

('f' indicates a figure; 't' indicates a table)